SYNAPTIC FUNCTION

THE NEUROSCIENCES INSTITUTE
of the Neurosciences Research Program

The Neurosciences Institute was founded in 1981 by the Neurosciences Research Program to promote the study of scientific problems within the broad range of disciplines related to the neurosciences. It provides visiting scientists with facilities for planning and review of experimental and theoretical research with emphasis on understanding the biological basis for higher brain function.

As part of the Institute's active publishing program, this volume, the third in a continuing series of edited volumes, addresses the central issue of synaptic function and its modification. Combining experimental and theoretical approaches at levels of analysis ranging from molecular to network interactions, the book reviews the biological processes that underlie learning, memory, and behavior.

Support for the Neurosciences Research Foundation, Inc., which makes the Institute's programs possible, has come in part from generous gifts by The Vincent Astor Foundation, Lily Auchincloss, Francois de Menil, Sibil & William T. Golden Foundation, Doris & Ralph E. Hansmann Foundation, Lita Annenberg Hazen, Lita Annenberg Hazen Charitable Trust, Carl B. Hess, The IFF Foundation, Inc., Johnson & Johnson, Harvey L. Karp, John D. & Catherine T. MacArthur Foundation, Josiah Macy, Jr. Foundation, Pittway Corporation Charitable Foundation, Rockefeller Brothers Fund, Alfred P. Sloan Foundation, Timber Hill, Inc., van Ameringen Foundation, The G. Unger Vetlesen Foundation, and The Vollmer Foundation.

The Neurosciences Institute Publications Series

Neurophysiological Approaches to Higher Brain Functions
Edward V. Evarts, Yoshikazu Shinoda, and Steven P. Wise

Protein Phosphorylation in the Nervous System
Eric J. Nestler and Paul Greengard

Dynamic Aspects of Neocortical Function
Gerald M. Edelman, W. Einar Gall, and W. Maxwell Cowan, Editors

Molecular Bases of Neural Development
Gerald M. Edelman, W. Einar Gall, and W. Maxwell Cowan, Editors

The Cell in Contact: Adhesions and Junctions as Morphogenetic Determinants
Gerald M. Edelman and Jean-Paul Thiery, Editors

Synaptic Function
Gerald M. Edelman, W. Einar Gall, and W. Maxwell Cowan, Editors

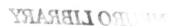

SYNAPTIC FUNCTION

Edited by

GERALD M. EDELMAN

W. EINAR GALL

W. MAXWELL COWAN

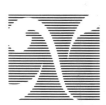

A Neurosciences Institute Publication

JOHN WILEY & SONS

New York • Chichester • Brisbane • Toronto • Singapore

Library of Congress Cataloging in Publication Data:

Synaptic function.

(The Neurosciences Institute publications series)
Based on the third annual symposium of the
Neurosciences Institute of the Neurosciences Research
Program held at the Salk Institute in 1984.
1. Synapses—Congresses.   2. Neuroplasticity—
Congresses.   3. Neurotransmitters—Congresses.
I. Edelman, Gerald M.   II. Gall, W. Einar.
III. Cowan, W. Maxwell.   IV. Neurosciences Institute
(New York, N.Y.)   V. Series. [DNLM: 1. Neuroregulators—
physiology—congresses.   2. Synapses—physiology—
congresses. WL 102.8 S9915 1984]

QP364.S969   1987   599'.01'88   86-24765
ISBN 0-471-85557-X
ISBN 0-471-63708-4 (PBK.)

Printed in the United States of America

10   9   8   7   6   5   4   3

Preface

This is the third in a continuing series of reports of the annual symposia of The Neurosciences Institute of the Neurosciences Research Program. The choice of subject matter was made by the Institute's Scientific Advisory Committee, whose members are Floyd E. Bloom, Research Institute of Scripps Clinic; W. Maxwell Cowan (Chairman), Washington University; Gerald M. Edelman, The Rockefeller University; John J. Hopfield, California Institute of Technology; Eric R. Kandel, Columbia University; Alvin M. Liberman, The Haskins Laboratories; and Vernon B. Mountcastle, The Johns Hopkins University.

The chosen topic of synaptic function underlies all of neurobiology and provides a link between the first symposium on dynamic aspects of neocortical function and the second on molecular approaches to neural development. It is a particularly apropriate topic at this time, when new insights into the molecular bases of learning and memory are beginning to emerge. The volume is organized into five sections: biochemical and biophysical mechanisms of changes in pre- and postsynaptic cells; the neurochemistry of transmitters and their release; the interactions of cells in small networks; synaptic plasticity related to long-term changes; and theoretical models of synaptic function. Its contents summarize current knowledge of synaptic function in these various contexts and herald the new views that are beginning to emerge as cellular and molecular approaches are combined.

We are grateful to Susan Hassler, Editor of The Neurosciences Institute, and to Jennifer Rish and Victoria Ball of the Institute's staff for their central roles in assembling this volume. We again recognize the generous hospitality of The Salk Institute, where the symposium was held, and thank the participants and contributors for their enthusiastic and scholarly exchanges in an exciting area of neuroscience.

G. M. E.
W. E. G.
W. M. C.

Contents

Introduction

PAUL GREENGARD

The concepts that were *au courant* twenty years ago concerning synaptic transmission appear relatively incomplete today. It is worth summarizing some of those ideas: A nerve impulse traveled along the presynaptic axon to the terminal, propagated by the sequential opening and closing of sodium and potassium ion "channels," according to the Hodgkin–Huxley equations. Upon reaching the nerve terminal, the wave of depolarization opened voltage-sensitive calcium channels. Calcium ions flowed into the nerve terminal, causing quantal release of neurotransmitter, as demonstrated by Katz and his colleagues, presumably by causing fusion of neurotransmitter-containing synaptic vesicles to the plasma membrane. The released neurotransmitter diffused to "receptors" in the postsynaptic membrane and, through the activation of these receptors, opened channels. Studies at one specific synapse, the neuromuscular junction, indicated that opening nonspecific channels caused an increased permeability to sodium and potassium, resulting in depolarization of the postsynaptic plasma membrane. When the depolarization reached threshold, a new Hodgkin–Huxley impulse was generated and propagated along the postsynaptic membrane. Based in large part on the work of Eccles and his colleagues, it was conceded that inhibitory synaptic transmission also took place; little was known about the ionic mechanisms underlying this inhibition, although it seemed likely that increases in chloride and/or potassium ion conductances were involved. Acetylcholine and norepinephrine were believed to be the only neurotransmitters involved in synaptic transmission in the peripheral nervous system and were suspected of being neurotransmitters in the central nervous system. The molecular mechanisms that coupled calcium ion influx and neurotransmitter release were not understood and were not even considered to be approachable experimentally. The nature of receptors was not understood, and even the existence of receptors was a matter of controversy.

Many insights into synaptic function have evolved in the intervening years. We now know of three distinct classes of neurotransmitters, namely, amino acids, biogenic amines, and peptides. It is estimated that the human brain contains 10^{10}–10^{12} neurons, each of which makes an average of 10^2–10^4 connections with other neurons. It is believed that approximately 90% of these synaptic connections are involved in fast excitatory or fast inhibitory synaptic transmission. Amino acids seem to *mediate* this fast synaptic transmission, the major excitatory neurotransmitters apparently being glutamate and possibly aspartate, and the major inhibitory neurotransmitters apparently being γ-aminobutyrate and glycine.

The biogenic amines and peptides are believed to *modulate* fast synaptic transmission. The known list of biogenic amines that appear to act as neuromodulators in the central nervous system (norepinephrine, epinephrine, dopamine, serotonin, histamine, and acetylcholine) has remained relatively constant during the past decade. In contrast, the list of peptides that appear to act as neuromodulators grows almost monthly and now includes several dozen. One remarkable advance in our knowledge of peptide neuromodulators is their colocalization, in nerve terminals, with other peptides as well as with classical neurotransmitters. Insights into the possible physiological significance of this colocalization have also been developed during the past few years.

Another advance in our understanding of synaptic transmission derives from the discovery of presynaptic receptors for neurotransmitters. There are autoreceptors on many types of nerve terminals, that is, receptors for the neurotransmitter released by those nerve terminals; in at least some instances, these autoreceptors serve a negative feedback role with respect to the release of neurotransmitter. There are also many types of heteroreceptors on axon terminals, that is, receptors for neurotransmitters released by other nerve terminals. Axoaxonal communication mediated by these presynaptic heteroreceptors can involve either immediately adjacent axonal elements or axonal elements separated by considerable distances.

It seems safe to predict that specific receptors will be found for each newly discovered neurotransmitter/neuromodulator. One would not necessarily have predicted that multiple receptors would be found for individual neurotransmitters, but such multiple receptors now appear to be commonplace. Similarly, multiple types of channels for individual ions have been found, the most noteworthy being the numerous types of calcium and potassium channels.

The molecular nature of the events by which the binding of the neurotransmitter to its receptor is coupled to the alteration of the ionic properties of the nerve cell membrane is beginning to be understood. There appear to be two general classes of mechanism by which this process can occur. In one class, the neurotransmitter receptor is thought to be coupled directly to an ionophore in such a manner that binding of the neurotransmitter to the receptor induces a conformational change in the ionophore, leading to a change in the permeability of the membrane to specific ions. One receptor that has been intensively studied, and which appears to work in this manner, is the nicotinic cholinergic receptor. A second general class of mechanisms by which a neurotransmitter affects the electrical properties of postsynaptic neurons is through a process in which the binding of the neurotransmitter to its receptor on the outer surface of the cell membrane leads to the production of another molecule, a second messenger, within the cell. This second messenger then initiates a sequence of biochemical reactions that ultimately result in a change in the electrophysiological properties of the neuronal membrane.

One might anticipate that the synaptic potentials caused by activation of the two different classes of receptors would have different characteristics. In the first case, in which the binding of the neurotransmitter to the receptor induces a conformational change in an ionophore, the synaptic potential resulting from this one-step, nonenzymatic process characteristically has a very short latency and duration, on the order of several milliseconds. In contrast, the effects of second messengers on the electrical properties of neuronal membranes appear to be mediated by means of a sequence of biochemical reactions, and the post-synaptic potential generated in this manner characteristically tends to have a much longer latency and duration, on the order of several hundred milliseconds to several seconds.

Our concepts concerning the chemical specificity of neurons have also changed considerably. Twenty years ago it was considered by most students of the nervous system that all neurons were identical, or nearly so, in their chemical composition. This has turned out to be an oversimplification. That there is an enormous amount of chemical heterogeneity within the mammalian brain is now clear from several distinct lines of investigation, which indicate specific distributions of a large number of: (1) neurotransmitters/neuromodulators as discussed above; (2) neuron-specific proteins (including phosphoproteins); and (3) brain-specific antigens (of unknown chemical nature and function, discovered by using monoclonal antibody techniques).

The multiple neurotransmitters/neuromodulators, the multiple receptors for these ligands, the multiple ion channels, and the multiple intracellular regulatory molecules that have been discovered provide some biochemical equipment for investigating the molecular basis of neuronal function, for example, the mechanisms by which different types of nerve cells respond to various extracellular signals with appropriate physiological responses. This investigation will undoubtedly be facilitated by the powerful new methodologies that have been developed in recent years: patch clamping, monoclonal antibodies, immunocytochemistry, radioactive ligands, and tissue culture techniques (e.g., *in vitro* reaggregation of dispersed brain cells into histiotypic patterns); intracranial transplantation techniques, techniques for the isolation of intraneuronal organelles (e.g., small synaptic vesicles and postsynaptic densities), and procedures for the purification of receptors, ion channels, and other integral membrane proteins; techniques for the functional reconstitution of receptors and ion channels into artificial membranes, the cloning of receptors and ion channels, site-directed mutagenesis of receptors and ion channels, and so forth.

Systems approaches to the study of higher brain function represent another very active area of neuroscience that is included in the last section of this volume, and that was in its infancy twenty years ago. Molecular approaches and systems approaches to the study of the nervous system, now almost completely separate disciplines, may ultimately merge to become a unitary approach to our understanding of the brain.

Section 1

Presynaptic and Postsynaptic Mechanisms

The recognition of the polar relationship between pre- and postsynaptic cells sets the stage for an analysis of the molecular machinery mediating transmitter release by the presynaptic cell and effector responses at the postsynaptic cell. Modern techniques now allow correlation of the electrophysiology and pharmacology with the chemical properties of supramolecular assemblies and the molecular structure of channels. In this first section, a reasonably comprehensive sample is given of approaches to defining synaptic function at the molecular level.

The first three chapters by Llinás, Magleby, and Korn and Faber concern presynaptic mechanisms of transmitter release. Llinás defines the nature of the interaction between the transmembrane electric field and intracellular chemistry in the classical system of the squid giant synapse. In particular, he details the role of local calcium and vesicle binding in transmitter release.

One of the most important characteristics of synaptic function is its historical property, as reflected by changes in synaptic efficacy. These changes are related to the fundamental system properties of plasticity, learning, and memory. In his chapter, Magleby points out that transmitter release involves at least four separate components of modification affecting overall function, each with characteristic buildup and decay.

Quantal transmitter release has a statistical, probabilistic property, which Korn and Faber take as their starting point. They make a strong case for statistical properties that underlie exocytosis not only in neuromuscular systems but also in the central nervous system. A binomial model is favored over competing models, and these authors find that the statistical measures correlate well with the number of anatomical release sites.

In addition to the now classical chemical and electrical synapses, electronic synaptic transmission can occur via gap junctions. Bennett and Spray provide a survey of the dynamics and molecular components involved in such junctions. They suggest that the evidence favors a fixed dipole moment between the open and closed states of these junctions, that the system appears best characterized as two gates in series, and that a variety of factors, including protein concentration, calcium concentration, local voltage, and second messengers affect junctional activity. This activity can also be modulated by other synapses, as shown in the case of horizontal cells in the retina.

One of the great advances in the understanding of postsynaptic mechanisms has come from the ability to study individual channels. Channels are the basic molecular units of postsynaptic response and comprise a highly diverse set of submembrane molecules. Catterall et al. provide specific details of the subunits of a sodium channel from rat brain and of a calcium channel from rabbit skeletal muscle. Both are multisubunit proteins, and both are protein kinase substrates, suggesting that the modulation of structure and response may occur by these enzymatic means. The sodium channel can be incorporated into phospholipid bilayers with subsequent restitution of properties; this result should provide enhanced opportunities to test modulation hypotheses.

One of the most remarkable properties of channels is their variety, as Hille points out in his scholarly review. With the evolution of excitable cells, one may see a reflection of the ubiquitousness of these structures and a two-stage evolutionary "transcendence": (1) the elaboration of voltage-sensitive sodium and calcium channels in the transition from prokaryotes to eukaryotes; and (2) the emergence of sodium channels along with synaptic transmission in the transition from protozoa to metazoa. This emergence freed the transmission chain from sole dependence on calcium ions and opened the possibility of efficient long-range transmission.

Characterization of the molecular hardware of synapses and its connection with electrophysiology and ultrastructural analysis opens up the possibility of a more refined analysis of the role of neurotransmitters. This is elaborated in the succeeding section.

Chapter 1

Functional Compartments in Synaptic Transmission

RODOLFO R. LLINÁS

ABSTRACT

Synaptic transmission has been studied in the squid giant synapse for three decades. These studies have yielded important insights into the relation between calcium and transmitter release. The role of calcium in the release process, the role of synaptic modulators, and some aspects of the molecular mechanisms of the release process itself have been central topics of investigation in more recent years. Present research suggests that synaptic transmission comprises a set of functional and anatomical compartments involving changes in the transmembrane electric field as well as in intracellular chemistry.

Historically, questions regarding the mechanisms of chemical synaptic transmission have been divided into those pertaining to either pre- or postsynaptic issues. Those that relate to the release process are often, but not exclusively, taken to be attributes of the presynaptic element, whereas those that address the response to a given transmitter substance are attributed mainly to the postsynaptic element. Issues concerning postsynaptic receptors have now been disembodied from the purely synaptic frame of reference and can be studied in lipid bilayers in a very propitious manner. In at least one case (the acetylcholine receptor), both the biochemical structure of the channel and much of its molecular organization are quite well known (cf. Numa et al., 1983).

The process of presynaptic release, however, continues to be a fair challenge, and important gaps in our understanding in the electrophysiological and morphological spheres are clearly evident. At this stage, the questions being asked refer to three main areas: (1) the role of calcium in the release process; (2) the role of modulators in the release process; and (3) the molecular mechanisms of the release process itself. These issues are, however, intertwined to such an extent that establishing clear separations between them may ultimately be quite difficult. It has become evident that transmitter release phenomena are dependent on a precisely timed entry of calcium ions prior to transmitter release, confirming the initial postulate of Katz (1969) that calcium should be the main trigger in this secretory process. More recent work has further supported the view that calcium is not only necessary but, in order to effect synaptic transmission with the observed speed, calcium entry must be coupled with a highly structured cellular machinery capable of rapidly transforming the calcium ion flow into transmitter release (Llinás, 1979). As a result, a rather important working relationship has developed between ultrastructural morphologists (using transmission and freeze-fracture electron microscopy techniques) and electrophysiologists.

REQUIREMENTS AND DEFINITION OF AN ACTIVE ZONE

The Preterminal Channel, Synaptic Vesicle, and Postsynaptic Channel Trilogy

From a morphological point of view, the idea of the existence of an active zone was first proposed by Couteaux and Pécot-Dechavassine (1970) at the neuromuscular junction (Figure 1). The concept related to the fact that synaptic transmitter was most probably released, not by the whole presynaptic terminal, but rather by a set of specialized sites. The active zone of the neuromuscular junction was

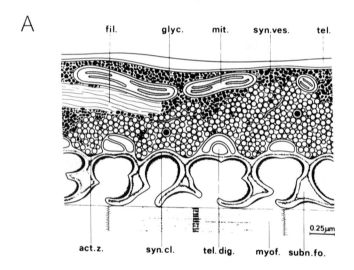

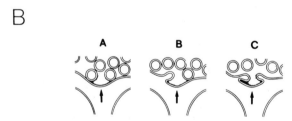

Figure 1.   *A: Schematic drawing of a neuromuscular junction (frog).* fil., neurofilaments; glyc., glycogen; mit., mitochondrion; syn. ves., synaptic vesicle; tel., teloglia; act. z., active zone; syn. cl., synaptic cleft; tel. dig., teloglial fingers; myof., myofibril; subn. fo., subneural fold. *B:* Diagrams of active zones (frog neuromuscular junctions). The active zones are seen in sections parallel to the axis of the nerve branch. (Modified from Couteaux and Pécot-Dechavassine, 1970.)

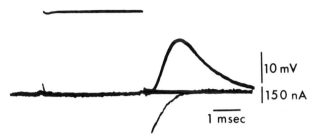

Figure 2. *Synaptic delay for the "off" excitatory postsynaptic potential.* Response seen following a depolarizing voltage clamp step to the "suppression potential" (140 mV). The latency between calcium entry (seen as a tail current) and the postsynaptic response is 200 μsec. (Modified from Llinás et al., 1981b.)

defined as that part of the presynaptic fiber situated immediately in front of the postsynaptic fold (Couteaux and Pécot-Dechavassine, 1970). This particular area of terminal is known to be the place where synaptic vesicles (De Robertis and Bennett, 1955; Palay, 1956) fuse onto the external membrane (Ceccarelli et al., 1972; Heuser et al., 1974), and is close to the point at which vesicular membrane is taken up for vesicular recycling (Ceccarelli et al., 1973; Heuser and Reese, 1973). It was also demonstrated to be in close spatial relation with the postsynaptic channels known to respond to iontophoresis of acetylcholine (Katz and Miledi, 1964, 1965; Kuffler and Yoshikami, 1975).

From a physiological point of view, experimental work initially performed in the squid giant synapse demonstrated that the latency between calcium entry and transmitter release could be as short as 200 μsec (Figure 2; Llinás, 1979; Llinás et al., 1976, 1981b, 1982). This immediately suggested that the release process had to be encompassed in an anatomically compact morphological unit, where not only were the release sites close to the sites of postsynaptic response, but where calcium entry would occur close to the release sites as well. It was proposed, for the squid giant synapse, that the calcium entry that triggers transmitter release should occur close to, if not precisely at, the active zone (Llinás et al., 1976). Freeze-fracture replicas of the active zone demonstrated that, in addition to its specialized location with respect to the postsynaptic target, it bore a very special relation to the presynaptic vesicles and a set of presynaptic membrane-bound particles (Pfenninger et al., 1971, 1972). These particles generally have a special order and, in the frog neuromuscular junction, are organized into a double row situated at right angles to the main axis of the terminal and immediately opposite the foldings of the postsynaptic membrane (cf. Heuser and Reese, 1977).

Based on these findings, it was then proposed (Pumplin et al., 1981) that the membrane-bound particles might be calcium channels. In this case, the precise morphological structure itself began to explain the rather short latency for release. Indeed, calcium channels identified by their diameter in freeze-fracture micrographs were situated in the immediate vicinity of the presynaptic vesicles, which upon exocytosis address the postsynaptic channels situated immediately across the synaptic cleft. Such a morphological unit was understood to be the subcellular basis for synaptic release.

A similar set of morphological studies in other synapses also provided grounds for the calcium channel, synaptic vesicle, and postsynaptic target channel trilogy (Figure 3). Physiological studies, employing voltage clamp techniques, of the presynaptic terminal of the squid giant synapse indicated that synaptic transmission is always accompanied by calcium entry. Furthermore, by using a presynaptic voltage clamp circuit as the source of a simulated action potential, calcium entry was elicited that was capable of generating synaptic transmission which precisely mimicked that produced by a presynaptic action potential (Llinás et al., 1982). This calcium entry occurred at the falling phase of the action potential, simulating more closely the "off" response than the "on" current observed during the presynaptic voltage clamp step depolarization. Because synaptic transmission could be mimicked in detail by an artificial action potential, it became apparent that the main role of the action potential was to allow a very well-timed entry of calcium into the presynaptic terminal at the active zone; this process would then trigger transmitter release. However, at this stage several other questions became of great interest: (1) Exactly how does calcium entry produce transmitter release? (2) How does the calcium current generated by the presynaptic action potential change the distribution of intracellular calcium concentration in the cytosol? (3) How does the calcium current relate to the ultimate cytosolic concentration of calcium at different points?

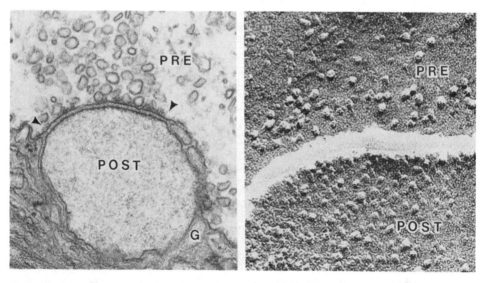

Figure 3. *Left: Thin section through an active zone from the giant synapse of* Loligo pealei. The presynaptic axon (Pre) contacts the postsynaptic axon spine (Post) without an intervening glial element (G). The active zone (*arrowheads*) is marked by parallel cell membranes separated by a cleft, an electron-dense fuzz associated with these membranes, and the presence of synaptic vesicles nearby. × 52,000. *Right*: Freeze-fracture micrograph through an active zone of a squid giant synapse. Large intramembrane particles occur in patches on the cytoplasmic leaflet of the presynaptic membrane and the external leaflet of the postsynaptic membrane. Densities of these particles were obtained from this and similar micrographs. × 200,000. (From Pumplin et al., 1981.)

Profile of the Intracellular Calcium Concentration

In a 1981 paper, Steinberg, Walton, and I came to the unexpected conclusion that, given the size of the calcium current per action potential, the calcium concentration against the membrane could reach rather high levels (Llinás et al., 1981b). In fact, as shown in Figure 4, the concentration was shown to be close to 400 μM during calcium flow. This model, however, assumed that calcium entry was not limited to any particular part of the membrane, but rather that such entry occurred throughout the presynaptic terminal in a nondiscriminative manner. The next obvious step was to combine our measurements of calcium current and calcium fluxes with the idea that calcium entry actually occurs at particular sites, and more particularly through channels having a particular spatial organization. With this in mind, Sanford Simon and I proceeded to tackle the problems at the single channel level. After a set of calculations and computer modeling (Simon and Llinás, 1984, 1985), we concluded that the calcium concentration immediately against the membrane and in the immediate cytosolic volume could not be easily determined from a study of the macroscopic voltage clamp currents actually measured during synaptic release. The reason for this is quite obvious in retrospect. If it is assumed that calcium enters through single channels, as it must, and that calcium moves away from the points of entry by diffusion, the calcium isoconcentration contour near each channel at the cytosolic level will resemble a hemisphere. At the time of maximum ion flow, the ions entering through a single channel will form a hemispherical isoconcentration profile with a minimum value of, let us say, 5 mM, 250 Å from the channel mouth (Simon and Llinás, 1984).

Furthermore, at a given level of depolarization, the maximum intracellular calcium concentration in front of a given channel is maximal at membrane potentials very close to the membrane resting level (-70 mV). At less negative values, the calcium concentration profile is smaller because the driving force for calcium rapidly decreases with membrane depolarization. Indeed, as illustrated in Figure 5, the flux per channel has an inverse relationship with respect to voltage. The process envisaged then suggests that as the membrane begins to be depolarized, few channels open but the flux per channel is maximal and so is the intracellular calcium concentration in the vicinity of the open calcium channels. With further depolarization, a larger total current flows through the membrane as more channels open, but the flux per channel decreases rather abruptly, reducing the maximal local calcium concentration immediately in front of each open channel. Two points become clear at this time: (1) With increased depolarization, the number and spatial distribution of open channels are quite different from that observed at smaller depolarizations, but (2) at increasing levels of membrane depolarization, the calcium concentration in front of a channel decreases.

Two parameters are of interest when considering intracellular calcium concentration: (1) the microscopic calcium concentration and (2) the spatial distribution of open channels over the preterminal membrane (Chad and Eckert, 1984; Simon and Llinás, 1984). The conclusion that as the membrane is further depolarized more calcium channels open but the concentration of calcium opposite each channel decreases made it evident that it is not possible to directly equate macroscopic calcium current with transmitter release. Moreover, an almost inverse

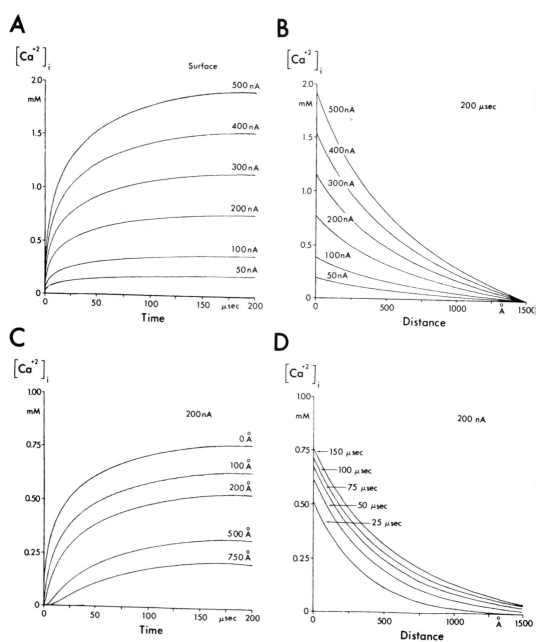

Figure 4. *Distribution of intracellular calcium concentration ([Ca²⁺]ᵢ).* A constant flux of calcium is assumed to flow radially into the cytoplasm through a hemisphere of 750 Å radius. *A:* $[Ca^{2+}]_i$ at the surface of the hemisphere as a function of time for various calcium currents. *B:* Distribution of $[Ca^{2+}]_i$ within the presynaptic terminal 200 μsec after the beginning of a constant flux of calcium of various amplitudes. *C:* Changes in $[Ca^{2+}]_i$ with time at various distances within the presynaptic terminal for a 200-nA current. *D:* Distribution of $[Ca^{2+}]_i$ within the presynaptic terminal at various times after the onset of a 200-nA calcium current. (From Llinás et al., 1981b.)

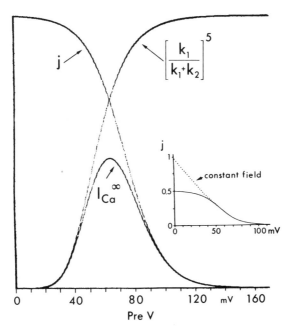

Figure 5. *Contribution of the current flow per open channel (j) and the number of open channels (given by [k₁/k₁ + k₂]⁵) to the determination of I*$\bar{C}_a$ *as a function of voltage (V). Inset:* Comparison of *j*, assuming a constant *(dots)* and a nonuniform *(solid line)* field across the length of the calcium channel. Extracellular calcium concentration ($[Ca^{2+}]_o$) is 10 mM. (From Llinás et al., 1981a.)

relation exists between the microscopic calcium concentration and the macroscopic calcium current. This inverse relation begins to explain some oddities of synaptic release (Simon et al., 1983). It was observed by several investigators (Llinás et al., 1981b; Charlton et al., 1982) that when the amounts of transmitter released for a given macroscopic calcium current at two levels of membrane potential are compared, synaptic release is larger at the more depolarized membrane potential. This experiment is easily performed, given the bell-shaped curve relating calcium current to prevoltage (Figure 6). Thus, the same amount of total calcium flows through the membrane at 45-mV depolarization from rest (−70 mV) as from a depolarization of 80 mV, yet at 80 mV there is more transmitter release than at 45 mV. This was initially taken to indicate that voltage dependence as well as calcium dependence was necessary for transmitter release (Llinás et al., 1980). Although the requirement of voltage dependence for release seems clear (Simon et al., 1983), a second variable to be considered is that while the total calcium current is clearly similar at the levels of depolarization described above, *the spatial distribution of the calcium concentration against the membrane is very different.* That is, since more channels are open at 80 mV than at 45 mV, the spatial distribution of calcium concentration is such as to trigger more transmitter release at 80 mV, because the probability of a given channel opening in association with a vesicle being ready to release is larger than at the lower membrane potential (Simon and Llinás, 1984).

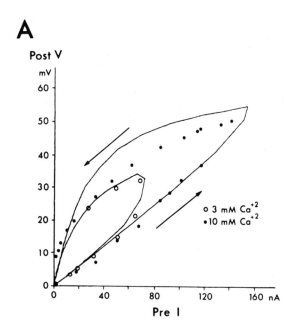

A

Post V

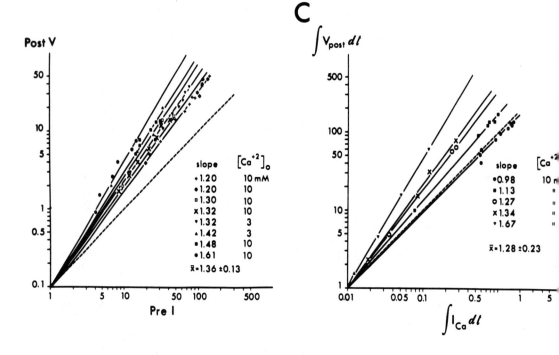

14

More than One Compartment in the Release Process?

The question at hand, then, concerns the compartmentalization of calcium concentration near the presynaptic membrane. At present, experimental and theoretical work is being performed in an attempt to define parameters that would be of importance in transforming cytosolic punctate calcium concentration into the release process. Specifically, the issue of the transmitter released by simultaneous channel opening in the vicinity of a vesicle (the so-called near-neighbor effect) (Simon and Llinás, 1984) and the question of the stoichiometric relationship between calcium and transmitter release are under scrutiny.

The question of the modulation of synaptic release is an issue quite close to the previous one. The relation between calcium and transmitter release is brought into this discussion by the observation that the amount of transmitter released by a given action potential can vary, depending on the immediate previous history of the release process. Thus, both facilitation (del Castillo and Katz, 1954; Dudel and Kuffler, 1961) and depression (Wachtel and Kandel, 1971) of transmission have been observed at chemical junctions. Because this modulation will probably be of great importance in the understanding of plasticity, these issues have been seriously considered for many decades (cf. Kandel, 1978). The mechanism by which intracellular calcium releases transmitter is most often considered as a single reaction in which a certain number of calcium ions interact with a vesicle to produce its exocytosis. The power relation between macroscopic calcium current and transmitter release has been determined as fluctuating between one and three in the squid giant synapse (Llinás et al., 1981b; Charlton et al., 1982; Augustine and Eckert, 1984). Little or nothing is known, however, about the exact mechanism by which increased intracellular calcium concentration produces the release of transmitter.

The assumptions are that calcium entry, by some intermediate step, produces the fusion of vesicles containing the synaptic transmitter substance in a concentration-dependent manner. Beyond this, however, there is the question of whether calcium itself can modify future release either by a maintained high intracellular concentration or by a calcium-dependent secondary mechanism. One possible mechanism much in favor today is the so-called "residual calcium hypothesis" (Katz and Miledi, 1968). This hypothesis proposes that after a given presynaptic action potential, calcium accumulates in the preterminal and adds

---

Figure 6. *Relationship between presynaptic calcium current and postsynaptic response.* A: Excitatory postsynaptic potential amplitude is plotted against presynaptic current for two $[Ca^{2+}]_o$. *Arrow* pointing to the *right* corresponds to voltage clamp pulses up to 60 mV; *arrow* pointing to the *left* corresponds to voltage clamp pulses above 60 mV. B: Excitatory postsynaptic potential amplitude (Post V) is plotted against presynaptic current (Pre I) for five synapses, using double logarithmic coordinates. For clarity, presynaptic current for 0.1 mV was set to 1 nA. C: Area under "on" excitatory postsynaptic potential ($V \cdot s$) is plotted as a function of total calcium entering the presynaptic terminal (nC). Presynaptic charge displacement for 1 $V \cdot s$ postsynaptic response was set to 0.001 nC. In B and C, only excitatory postsynaptic potentials after presynaptic depolarizations less than 60 mV were plotted. $[Ca^{2+}]_o$ is 10 mM unless indicated. *Dashed lines* in B and C are values given by the mathematical model. Note double logarithmic coordinates in B and C. (From Llinás et al., 1981b.)

to further calcium entry by subsequent spikes to increase the amount of transmitter released. A second possibility is that the modulation of the amount of transmitter to be released may be mediated by biochemical steps capable of regulating the number of immediately available synaptic vesicles after calcium entry (Llinás, 1977; Simon et al., 1984). This possibility was recently studied by Sugimori, Leonard, and myself in collaboration with Greengard and McGuinness from The Rockefeller University (McGuinness et al., 1984; Llinás et al., 1985). The experiments were carried out by using the squid giant synapse and involved the injection of a protein discovered and isolated by Greengard and his collaborators (see Nestler and Greengard, 1984). This protein, called synapsin I, is known to adhere to the surface of synaptic vesicles, but not to other secretory organelles, and can be phosphorylated at, among other places, a structural point of adherence between synapsin I and the synaptic vesicles (De Camilli et al., 1983). The phosphorylation, which is calcium-dependent, occurs via the activation of cal-modulin kinase II, a protein kinase that is both calcium- and calmodulin-dependent (Huttner et al., 1983). Kinase II phosphorylation of the tail of synapsin I results, we hypothesize, in the transformation of vesicles from a nonreleasable "caged" condition, to a free "decaged" releasable state by the partial denudation of the synaptic vesicles, as synapsin I is phosphorylated at site II. In this decaged condition, vesicles are then available for release. Direct physiological experiments that used both synapsin I (obtained from calf brain) and calmodulin kinase II demonstrated, respectively: (1) a reduction of synaptic release after synapsin I injection, to be expected if the binding of synapsin I to vesicles removes them from the immediately available pool; and (2) an increase in the amount of transmitter released by a voltage clamp depolarizing step after injection of calmodulin kinase II, without modifying the initial macroscopic calcium current. This would be expected if an increased phosphorylation of synapsin I were to increase the number of vesicles available for release (Llinás et al., 1985). Clearly, much needs to be done to understand the exact manner in which this particular biochemical machinery modulates synaptic release. However, the experiments do suggest a set of important biochemical steps that can modulate the release process.

The third query concerning depolarization–release coupling relates to the manner in which transmitter is released. Presently, the vesicular hypothesis seems to be the most consistent with the available facts. Freeze-fracture studies by Heuser et al. (1974) and by Ceccarelli and Hurlbut (1980) have demonstrated that transmitter release follows vesicle fusion and that the fusion occurs in the vicinity of the active zone. While the ultimate demonstration that this is a necessary and sufficient mechanism for synaptic release would require a direct observation of the release process, it is also clear that several other possibilities are being considered by different groups around the world. The experimental evidence in favor of nonvesicular transmitter release seems to be the presence of submini-ature postsynaptic potentials, as described by Kriebel and Gross (1974). These workers demonstrated that synaptic release at the neuromuscular junction can occur in quantities smaller than the miniature level initially described by Fatt and Katz (1952), that is, the level taken to be the product of the exocytosis of the content of a single vesicle. Because these subminiature potentials require that a preterminal contain a number of vesicles larger than those seen in anatomical studies, the findings have been considered a direct challenge to the vesicular hypothesis. This is not necessarily the case, however, as mechanisms such as the release of a partially filled vesicle (Bennett et al., 1976) are possible alternatives. Equally plausible is the possibility that transmitter may be released from vesicles by either complete or incomplete exocytosis. In the latter case, momentary fusion of a vesicle with the plasma membrane, not going to exocytotic completion, may then return to the cytosol having released only a small part of its contents.

This possibility is made more feasible by the finding that the fusion of secretory vesicles seems to consist of two components: (1) attachment of vesicles to the plasmalemma membrane and a partial fusion of those two elements; and (2) the actual exocytosis of the content of the vesicle with total emptying of vesicular content into the extracellular medium (Neher and Marty, 1982). Indeed then, the possibility exists that these two stages correspond, respectively, to the subminiature and the miniature potentials observed postsynaptically.

Nevertheless, the experimental fact of subminiature release seems to be with us. A second and more unconventional view is that presented by Israel et al. (1970) concerning the possible nonvesicular release of transmitter. Their point of view arises from a biochemical study in which they have demonstrated that acetylcholine release during synaptic transmission does not correspond to the vesicular fraction but to a nonvesicular cytosolic fraction that seems to have a higher turnover rate. The authors generated a set of cogent statements which propose that synaptic release may occur by a type of membrane gating of at least acetylcholine and that such gating, being calcium-dependent and having all the other requirements for chemical transmission, could in fact explain much of what is known about synaptic transmission. In their view, vesicles would serve as storage containers that keep the transmitter substance at the right sites, but are not susceptible to release by presynaptic action potential invasion.

Three objections can be brought against this hypothesis: (1) The volume of substance released. Synaptic transmission involves, at least in the squid giant synapse and the neuromuscular junction, a rather large release of intracellular substance. Assuming that the quantal content for the squid synapse is on the order of 1200 units, a sizeable reduction of cytosolic material would have to occur in order to release such a large amount of transmitter through channels. Such release, if generated by the opening of channels, should be observed as a large conductance change during the release process. This is, however, not the case. (2) Synaptic release, if occurring through the activation of special channels, should not involve any secondary membrane changes. However, in synaptic transmission (Gillespie, 1979) and during other secretory processes (Neher and Marty, 1982), an increased total capacitance during release has been measured, implying an increase of the surface membrane of the preterminal. This is only consistent with an exocytotic phenomenon accompanying the release process and thus with something very much akin to the vesicular release hypothesis. (3) Transmitter release via vesicular exocytosis is not inconsistent with nonvesicular release, so the two mechanisms do not have to challenge each other. Indeed, Katz and Miledi (1977) have demonstrated that the preterminal is constantly releasing acetylcholine in the absence of either calcium or changes in presynaptic membrane potential level. This indicates that the presynaptic membrane is somewhat permeable to acetylcholine and that a certain amount of acetylcholine turnover (not related to vesicles) is in fact quite possible. This is not necessarily a demonstration of the inadequacy of the vesicular hypothesis, however. Ultimately, in those cells in which the vesicles are large enough to be observed directly by microscopy, a direct correlation has been made between the secretory process and the exocytotic phenomenon (Douglas, 1975). Thus, at least by analogy, transmitter release seems to be very much associated with exocytosis.

From the above then, it is possible to conclude that while much has been gained in the understanding of the release process in synaptic transmission, much remains to be done. It is also true, however, that with further understanding of the release process we find ourselves closer to solving one of the truly challenging questions related to brain function—the molecular basis for synaptic transmission.

ACKNOWLEDGMENTS

This research was supported by U.S. Public Health Service grant NS-14014 from the National Institute of Neurological and Communicative Disorders and Stroke.

REFERENCES

Augustine, G. J., and R. Eckert (1984) Divalent cations differentially support transmitter release at the squid giant synapse. *J. Physiol. (Lond.)* **346**:257–271.

Bennett, M. V. L., P. G. Model, and S. M. Highstein (1976) Stimulation-induced depletion of vesicles, fatigue of transmission and recovery processes at a vertebrate central synapse. *Cold Spring Harbor Symp. Quant. Biol.* **40**:25–35.

Ceccarelli, B., and W. P. Hurlbut (1980) Vesicle hypothesis of the release of quanta of acetylcholine. *Physiol. Rev.* **60**:396–441.

Ceccarelli, B., W. P. Hurlbut, and A. Mauro (1972) Depletion of vesicles from frog neuromuscular junctions by prolonged tetanic stimulation. *J. Cell Biol.* **54**:30–38.

Ceccarelli, B., W. P. Hurlbut, and A. Mauro (1973) Turnover of transmitter and synaptic vesicles at the frog neuromuscular junction. *J. Cell Biol.* **57**:499–524.

Chad, J. E., and R. Eckert (1984) Calcium "domains" associated with individual channels may account for anomalous voltage relations of Ca-dependent responses. *Biophys. J.* **45**:993–999.

Charlton, M. P., S. J. Smith, and R. S. Zucker (1982) Role of presynaptic calcium ions and channels in synaptic facilitation and depression at the squid giant synapse. *J. Physiol. (Lond.)* **232**:173–193.

Couteaux, R., and M. Pécot-Dechavassine (1970) Vésicules synaptiques et poches au niveau des zones actives de la jonction neuromusculaire. *C. R. Soc. Biol. (Paris)* **271**:2346–2349.

De Camilli, P., R. Cameron, and P. Greengard (1983) Synapsin I (Protein I), a nerve terminal-specific phosphoprotein. I. Its general distribution in synapses of the central and peripheral nervous system demonstrated by immunofluorescence in frozen and plastic sections. *J. Cell Biol.* **96**:1337–1354.

del Castillo, J., and B. Katz (1954) Quantal components of the end-plate potential. *J. Physiol. (Lond.)* **124**:560–573.

De Robertis, E. D. P., and H. S. Bennett (1955) Some features of the submicroscopic morphology of synapses in frog and earthworm. *J. Biophys. Biochem. Cytol.* **1**:47–58.

Douglas, W. W. (1975) Secretomotor control of adrenal medullary secretion: Synaptic, membrane and ionic events in stimulus-secretion coupling. *Handb. Physiol., Endocrinology* **6**:367–388.

Dudel, J., and S. W. Kuffler (1961) Presynaptic inhibition at the crayfish neuromuscular junction. *J. Physiol. (Lond.)* **155**:543–562.

Fatt, P., and B. Katz (1952) Spontaneous subthreshold activity at motor nerve endings. *J. Physiol. (Lond.)* **117**:109–128.

Gillespie, J. I. (1979) The effect of repetitive stimulation on the passive electrical properties of the presynaptic terminal of the squid giant synapse. *Proc. R. Soc. Lond. (Biol.)* **206**:293–306.

Heuser, J. E., and T. S. Reese (1973) Evidence for recycling of synaptic vesicle membrane transmitter release at the frog neuromuscular junction. *J. Cell Biol.* **57**:315–344.

Heuser, J. E., and T. S. Reese (1977) Structure of the synapse. *Handb. Physiol., The Nervous System* **1**:261–294.

Heuser, J. E., T. S. Reese, and D. M. D. Landis (1974) Functional changes in frog neuromuscular junctions studied with freeze-fracture. *J. Neurocytol.* **3**:109–131.

Huttner, W. B., W. Schiebler, P. Greengard, and P. De Camilli (1983) Synapsin I (Protein I), a nerve terminal-specific phosphoprotein. III. Its association with synaptic vesicles studied in a high-purified synaptic vesicle preparation. *J. Cell Biol.* **96**:1374–1388.

Israel, M., J. Gautron, and B. Lesbats (1970) Fractionnement de l'organe électrique de la torpille: Localisation subcellulaire de l'acetylcholine. *J. Neurochem.* **17**:1441–1450.

Kandel, E. R. (1978) *A Cell-Biological Approach to Learning*, Grass Lecture Monograph 1, Society for Neuroscience, Bethesda, Maryland.

Katz, B. (1969) *The Release of Neural Transmitter Substance*, Sherrington Lecture X, Charles C Thomas, Springfield, Illinois.

Katz, B., and R. Miledi (1964) The development of acetylcholine sensitivity in nerve-free segments of skeletal muscle. *J. Physiol. (Lond.)* **170**:389–396.

Katz, B., and R. Miledi (1965) The measurement of synaptic delay, and the time course of acetylcholine release at the neuromuscular junction. *Proc. R. Soc. Lond. (Biol.)* **161**:483–495.

Katz, B., and R. Miledi (1968) The role of calcium in neuromuscular facilitation. *J. Physiol. (Lond.)* **19**:481–492.

Katz, B., and R. Miledi (1977) Transmitter leakage from motor nerve endings. *Proc. R. Soc. Lond. (Biol.)* **196**:59–72.

Kriebel, M. E., and C. E. Gross (1974) Multimodal distribution of frog miniature end-plate potentials in adult, denervated and tadpole leg muscle. *J. Gen. Physiol.* **64**:85–103.

Kuffler, S. W., and D. Yoshikami (1975) The distribution of acetylcholine sensitivity at the postsynaptic membrane of vertebrate skeletal twitch muscles: Iontophoretic mapping in the micron range. *J. Physiol. (Lond.)* **244**:703–730.

Llinás, R. (1977) Calcium and transmitter release in squid synapse. *Soc. Neurosci. Symp.* **2**:139–160.

Llinás, R. (1979) Calcium regulation of neuronal function. In *The Neurosciences: Fourth Study Program*, F. O. Schmitt and F. G. Worden, eds., pp. 555–571, MIT Press, Cambridge, Massachusetts.

Llinás, R., I. Z. Steinberg, and K. Walton (1976) Presynaptic calcium currents and their relation to synaptic transmission. Voltage clamp study in giant synapse and theoretical model for the calcium gate. *Proc. Natl. Acad. Sci. USA* **73**:2918–2922.

Llinás, R., I. Z. Steinberg, and K. Walton (1980) Transmission in the squid giant synapse: A model based on voltage clamp studies. *J. Physiol. (Paris)* **76**:413–418.

Llinás, R., I. Z. Steinberg, and K. Walton (1981a) Presynaptic calcium currents in squid giant synapse. *Biophys. J.* **33**:289–321.

Llinás, R., I. Z. Steinberg, and K. Walton (1981b) Relationship between presynaptic calcium current and postsynaptic potential in squid giant synapse. *Biophys. J.* **33**:323–351.

Llinás, R., M. Sugimori, and S. M. Simon (1982) Transmission by presynaptic spike-like depolarization in the squid giant synapse. *Proc. Natl. Acad. Sci. USA* **79**:2415–2419.

Llinás, R., T. L. McGuinness, C. S. Leonard, M. Sugimori, and P. Greengard (1985) Intraterminal injection of synapsin I or calcium/calmodulin-dependent protein kinase II alters neurotransmitter release at the squid giant synapse. *Proc. Natl. Acad. Sci. USA* **82**:3035–3039.

McGuinness, T. L., C. S. Leonard, M. Sugimori, R. Llinás, and P. Greengard (1984) Possible roles of synapsin I and Ca^{++}/calmodulin-dependent protein kinase II in synaptic transmission as studied in the squid giant synapse. *Biol. Bull. (Woods Hole)* **167**:530.

Neher, E., and A. Marty (1982) Discrete changes of cell membrane capacitance observed under conditions of enhanced secretion in bovine adrenal chromaffin cells. *Proc. Natl. Acad. Sci. USA* **79**:6712–6716.

Nestler, E. J., and P. Greengard (1984) *Protein Phosphorylation in the Nervous System*, Wiley, New York.

Numa, S., M. Noda, H. Takahashi, T. Tanabe, M. Toyosato, Y. Furutani, and S. Kikyotani (1983) Molecular structure of the nicotinic acetylcholine receptor. *Cold Spring Harbor Symp. Quant. Biol.* **48**:57–70.

Palay, S. L. (1956) Synapses in the central nervous system. *Biochim. Biophys. Acta* **2**:193–201.

Pfenninger, K., K. Akert, H. Moor, and C. Sandri (1971) Freeze-etching of presynaptic membranes in the central nervous system. *Philos. Trans. R. Soc. Lond. (Biol.)* **261**:387–389.

Pfenninger, K., K. Akert, H. Moor, and C. Sandri (1972) The fine structure of freeze-fractured presynaptic membranes. *J. Neurocytol.* **1**:129–149.

Pumplin, D. W., T. S. Reese, and R. Llinás (1981) Are the presynaptic membrane particles the calcium channels? *Proc. Natl. Acad. Sci. USA* **78**:7210–7213.

Simon, S. M., and R. Llinás (1984) Residual free calcium hypotheses may not account for facilitation of transmitter release in the squid giant synapse. *Soc. Neurosci. Abstr.* **10**:194.

Simon, S. M., and R. Llinás (1985) Compartmentalization of the submembrane calcium activity during calcium influx and its significance in transmitter release. *Biophys. J.* **48**:485–498.

Simon, S. M., M. Sugimori, and R. Llinás (1983) Resting potential affects transmitter release in the squid giant synapse. *Biophys. J.* **41**:136a.

Simon, S. M., M. Sugimori, and R. Llinás (1984) Modelling of submembranous calcium-concentration changes and their relation to rate of presynaptic transmitter release in the squid giant synapse. *Biophys. J.* **45**:264a.

Wachtel, H., and E. R. Kandel (1971) Conversion of synaptic excitation to inhibition at a dual chemical synapse. *J. Neurophysiol.* **34**:56–68.

Chapter 2

Short-Term Changes in Synaptic Efficacy

KARL L. MAGLEBY

ABSTRACT

The efficacy of chemical synapses changes as a function of the history of the synapses' activity. This chapter discusses some of the properties and possible mechanisms for short-term, stimulation-dependent changes in synaptic efficacy. Decreases in synaptic efficacy can arise from desensitization of postsynaptic receptors or decreased transmitter release from the presynaptic terminal (depression). Increases in synaptic efficacy can be accounted for by four kinetically and pharmacologically separable components of increased transmitter release: potentiation, augmentation, and the first and second components of facilitation. These components build up during repetitive stimulation and decay thereafter with characteristic time courses. The components may reflect the buildup and decay of calcium ions, calcium-activated factors, and other factors such as sodium in the nerve terminal. Some speculations on the possible functions of short-term changes in synaptic efficacy are presented.

Chemical synaptic transmission is the major means by which nerve cells communicate with each other and with their effector organs. The efficacy of chemical synapses is not static, but typically changes with activity and time, depending on the history of use of the synapse. Some changes in synaptic function have long-term time courses of hours to days. Examples of such plasticity include long-term depression (Ito, this volume), long-term potentiation (Andersen, and Siman et al., this volume), sensitization (Kandel et al., this volume), and classical conditioning (Kandel et al., and Tsukahara, this volume). While these long-term changes have been identified at a limited number of synapses, practically all synapses, including neuromuscular junctions, display stimulation-induced, short-term changes in synaptic efficacy that last from milliseconds to minutes. These short-term changes, which include facilitation, augmentation, potentiation, depression, and desensitization, are considered in this chapter.

Such changes in synaptic efficacy are interesting for at least two reasons. First, the nervous system typically operates through trains or bursts of impulses rather than through single isolated ones. Thus, in order to understand the operation of the nervous system, it will be necessary to determine for each synapse how its efficacy changes as a function of the stimulation pattern. Only then will it be possible to predict the synaptic output resulting from a given input of action potentials to a nerve terminal. Second, investigation of changes in synaptic efficacy is a way to explore the mechanisms of synaptic transmission and to gain insight into the inner workings of pre- and postsynaptic cells.

BACKGROUND

The basic steps involved in chemical synaptic transmission are now well established (for reviews, see Katz, 1969; Steinbach and Stevens, 1976; Ceccarelli and Hurlbut, 1980; and see Llinás, this volume). When the presynaptic nerve terminal is depolarized by the invading action potential, voltage-sensitive calcium channels open, allowing an influx of calcium into the nerve terminal. The entering calcium triggers the release of transmitter, which diffuses to the postsynaptic membrane and binds to receptors. Some of the bound receptors open their channels, allowing the passage of specific ions across the postsynaptic membrane, thus generating the postsynaptic potential. Transmitter is released from the nerve terminal in quantal packets of about 6000 molecules, and each quantal packet may represent the contents of a synaptic vesicle discharged by exocytosis into the synaptic cleft. Synaptic vesicles appear to be discharged at distinct release sites in the terminal. Quantal packets of transmitter are also occasionally released in the absence of or between impulses, giving rise to miniature end-plate potentials (MEPPs).

Transmitter release can be reduced by decreasing the calcium concentration or increasing the magnesium concentration of the bathing solution. Such changes decrease calcium entry, thus decreasing the number of packets of transmitter released.

The mechanism by which calcium acts to trigger transmitter release is not yet established, but the observation that the number of packets released by each nerve impulse is related to the fourth power of calcium in the bathing solution (for the neuromuscular junction) has led to the suggestion that four calcium ions may act together to cause the release of a quantum of transmitter (Dodge and Rahamimoff, 1967).

It is apparent from this brief description that changes in synaptic efficacy can result from changes in calcium entry or sequestration, changes in the number or positions of synaptic vesicles, changes in the number of active release sites or the factors that lead to the fusion of synaptic vesicles with the nerve terminal, and changes in the number of functional postsynaptic receptors. Other factors may also be involved.

MEASURING SHORT-TERM CHANGES IN SYNAPTIC EFFICACY

Much of the experimental data presented here is from the neuromuscular junction, as this preparation has served as a model synapse for the study of both synaptic transmission and short-term changes in synaptic efficacy. Most of the phenomena described have also been observed at central and peripheral synapses.

Under normal physiological conditions at the frog neuromuscular junction, a nerve impulse releases about 200 quantal packets of transmitter, generating an end-plate potential (EPP) that depolarizes the muscle cell to threshold, resulting in a muscle action potential and contraction. Synaptic function can be studied in the absence of contraction by measuring end-plate currents under voltage clamp conditions, by using curare to block some of the postsynaptic receptors to reduce EPPs below threshold, or by decreasing transmitter release by decreasing the calcium concentration or increasing the magnesium concentration of the bathing solution (for a review, see Barrett and Magleby, 1976).

Short-term changes in synaptic efficacy at the neuromuscular junction have traditionally been studied by conditioning the motor nerve with one or more impulses and then applying testing impulses at various intervals after the conditioning impulses to map out the time course of the resulting change in efficacy, measured as a change in EPP amplitude or end-plate current amplitude. Changes in amplitude can result from either pre- or postsynaptic factors.

OVERVIEW OF SHORT-TERM CHANGES IN SYNAPTIC EFFICACY

Table 1 presents a list of short-term changes in synaptic efficacy for the frog neuromuscular junction. Since different experimental conditions favor the expression of some components while masking others, this table should only be considered a list of *potential processes*. Each of the processes listed is considered below.

Components of Increased Transmitter Release

Facilitation, augmentation, and potentiation result from an increase in the number of quantal packets of transmitter released from the nerve terminal by each impulse (del Castillo and Katz, 1954b; Liley, 1956; Magleby and Zengel, 1976a). These components have traditionally been identified on the basis of their time constants of decay, measured as the time required for the increased transmitter release to decay to $1/e$ (37%) of its initial magnitude.

Facilitation (Feng, 1941), which decays in two components with time constants of about 50 msec and 300 msec (Mallart and Martin, 1967), can double transmitter release after a single impulse. Augmentation, which decays with a time constant of about 7 sec, increases release about 1% after a single impulse and can increase release severalfold during long conditioning trains (Magleby and Zengel, 1976a; Zengel and Magleby, 1982). Potentiation, also called posttetanic potentiation or PTP, decays with a time constant of 30 sec to minutes, increases release about 1% after a single impulse, and can increase release severalfold after hundreds of impulses (Liley, 1956; Hubbard, 1963; Rosenthal, 1969; Magleby, 1973b; Magleby and Zengel, 1975a,b).

The first and second components of faciliation (F_1 and F_2), augmentation (A), and potentiation (P) are all defined in a similar manner as the fractional increase in a test EPP amplitude over a control when the other components equal zero, such that

$$F_1 = EPP/EPP_0 - 1 \quad \begin{matrix} F_2 = 0 \\ A = 0 \\ P = 0 \, , \end{matrix} \quad (1)$$

$$F_2 = EPP/EPP_0 - 1 \quad \begin{matrix} F_1 = 0 \\ A = 0 \\ P = 0 \end{matrix} \tag{2}$$

$$A_1 = EPP/EPP_0 - 1 \quad \begin{matrix} F_1 = 0 \\ F_2 = 0 \\ P = 0 \end{matrix} \tag{3}$$

$$P = EPP/EPP_0 - 1 \quad \begin{matrix} F_1 = 0 \\ A = 0 \\ A = 0 \end{matrix} \tag{4}$$

where EPP is the testing EPP amplitude and EPP_0 is the control EPP amplitude in the absence of repetitive stimulation. The components of increased transmitter release, F_1, F_2, A, P, as well as EPP amplitude, are all functions of time and the stimulation pattern. Notice from these equations that a magnitude of one for any component doubles the EPP amplitude. A more detailed discussion of the components is presented later.

Depression of Transmitter Release

During repetitive stimulation under conditions of normal or increased levels of transmitter release, EPP amplitudes first typically increase as a result of facilitation, augmentation, and potentiation and then decrease below the control level. This decrease typically reflects depression and results from a decrease in the number of quantal packets of transmitter released from the nerve terminal by each impulse (del Castillo and Katz, 1954b; Otsuka et al., 1962). Both fast (Takeuchi, 1958; Mallart and Martin, 1968) and slow (Rosenthal, 1969; Lass et al., 1973) components of depression have been described. In characterizing fast-component depression, Takeuchi (1958) found that a testing EPP applied 100 msec after a single conditioning EPP decreased about 15% below the conditioning EPP amplitude under conditions of normal quantal content and decreased about 25% when the extracellular calcium concentration was five times normal. In both cases, this depression of transmitter release returned exponentially to the control level with a time constant

Table 1.   Short-Term Processes That Can Affect Synaptic Efficacy

Presynaptic Factors	Magnitude[a] After One Impulse	Time Constant[b]
Components of increased transmitter release		
Facilitation[1]		
First component	0.8	50 msec
Second component	0.12	300 msec
Augmentation[2]	0.01[c]	7 sec
Potentiation (PTP)[3]	0.01	20 sec to minutes[c]
Components of decreased transmitter release		
Depression		
Fast component[4]	0–0.15[d]	5 sec
Slow component[5]	0–0.001[d]	minutes[c]
Postsynaptic factors		
Desensitization of postsynaptic receptors[6]	0–0.001[e]	5–20 sec

Values for frog neuromuscular junction: [1]Mallert and Martin, 1967; Magleby, 1973a,b. [2]Magleby and Zengel, 1976a; Zengel and Magleby, 1982. [3]Rosenthal, 1969; Magleby and Zengel, 1975a,b. [4]Takeuchi, 1958; Mallart and Martin, 1968; Betz, 1970. [5]Rosenthal, 1969; Lass et al., 1973. [6]Katz and Thesleff, 1957; Magleby and Pallotta, 1981.

[a]Magnitude of the components of increased release is the fractional increase in release over the control level (Equation 1); a magnitude of 0.8 increases release by 80%. Magnitude for the components of decreased release is the fractional decrease in release below the control level; a magnitude of 0.15 decreases release by 15%. Magnitude for desensitization is the fractional decrease in end-plate potential amplitude resulting from a decreased number of functional postsynaptic receptors.

[b]Time constant is the time required to decay (or recover) to 37% of the initial magnitude of increased release (or decreased release or desensitization).

[c]Increases with the number of impulses.

[d]Depression is negligible under conditions of low quantal content and increases with increased extracellular calcium concentrations, which in turn increase quantal content.

[e]Not present under conditions of reduced transmitter release or normal physiological conditions. Can develop during extended high-frequency stimulation at increased levels of transmitter release.

of about 5 sec. This recovery from depression can be expressed as

$$EPP/EPP_0 = 1 - D_0 e^{-(t/\tau)} , \qquad (5)$$

where EPP is the EPP amplitude at time t, EPP_0 is the EPP amplitude in the absence of depression, D_0 is the depression immediately after the conditioning impulse, measured as the fractional decrease in EPP amplitude, and τ is the time constant for recovery from depression. In normal calcium, D_0 would be 0.15 and τ would be 5 sec.

In characterizing the slow-component depression, Lass et al. (1973) found that EPP amplitudes slowly decreased with an exponential time course to about 10% of the control level during 3 min of repetitive stimulation at 20 impulses/sec and then recovered exponentially with a time constant of about 4 min. Slow-component depression is minimal following short conditioning trains, and both its magnitude and its time constant for recovery increase with the number of conditioning impulses (Rosenthal, 1969; Magleby, 1973b). While depression is usually associated with normal levels of transmitter release, slow-component depression can also develop during extended periods of stimulation under conditions of greatly reduced transmitter release (Magleby and Zengel, 1976b).

That depression is correlated with the amount of transmitter released has led to the suggestion that depression may be due to a depletion of the quantal packets of transmitter immediately available for release (Takeuchi, 1958; Thies, 1965; Mallart and Martin, 1968; Glavinović, 1979; Charlton et al., 1982; and see Betz, 1970). Depression is not well characterized, and it is possible that other factors may also be involved, such as a reduction or depletion of the sites where exocytosis of the synaptic vesicles occurs, or decreased calcium entry because of the inactivation of calcium channels. Chad et al. (1984) have described calcium-dependent inactivation of calcium current in neuron somata.

Desensitization of Postsynaptic Receptors

Under some experimental conditions, postsynaptic receptors may desensitize by entering an inactivated state, giving rise to a decreased synaptic response. Densensitization can occur when receptors are exposed to an agonist for prolonged periods of time (Katz and Thesleff, 1957; Changeux and Heidmann, this volume) or when two pulses of agonist are applied within less than 30 msec of one another (Magleby and Pallotta, 1981). This postsynaptic effect can be distinguished from presynaptic depression by examining quantal content. Desensitization to nerve-released transmitter can occur at the frog neuromuscular junction during high-frequency, prolonged stimulation when the quantal content is elevated above normal physiological levels by increased extracellular calcium concentration or when acetylcholinesterase is inhibited (Magleby and Pallotta, 1981). While desensitization to nerve-released transmitter can occur, it is important to note that significant desensitization does not occur at the frog neuromuscular junction under normal physiological conditions or stimulation rates (Magleby and Pallotta, 1981), and that desensitization does not occur under the conditions of decreased transmitter release used in the experiments presented in later sections of this chapter (Magleby and Zengel, 1976a). The extent, if any, to which desensitization occurs at other synapses needs to be investigated.

EXPERIMENTAL DEMONSTRATION OF FACILITATION, AUGMENTATION, AND POTENTIATION

Facilitation has traditionally been studied by applying a single testing nerve impulse at various intervals after a conditioning impulse to track the resulting increase in transmitter release (Feng, 1941). Under these conditions, the testing EPP stimulated immediately after the conditioning EPP can be double in amplitude. As the interval between the two impulses exceeds several hundred milliseconds, the second EPP amplitude becomes similar to the first, indicating that facilitation has decayed. Mallart and Martin (1967) and Magleby (1973a) described this decay with a double exponential time course. As mentioned earlier, the faster decaying component, referred to as the first component of facilitation, had a time constant of about 50 msec, and the slower decaying component, referred to as the second component of facilitation, had a time constant of about 300 msec.

The facilitation of EPP amplitudes added by a single impulse is described by

$$EPP/EPP_0 = 0.8 \, e^{-(t/50)} + 0.12 \, e^{-(t/300)} + 1 , \qquad (6)$$

where EPP and EPP_0 are the testing and conditioning EPP amplitudes, separated by an interval of t milliseconds (Magleby, 1973a).

In contrast to facilitation, potentiation has traditionally been studied after conditioning trains of hundreds to thousands of impulses. This is because the potentiation added by each impulse is too small to study effectively after a few impulses, but builds up during a train. Under conditions of normal quantal content, potentiation typically develops with a delay of many seconds and then decays away with a time course of minutes (Feng, 1941). The delayed onset of potentiation is present only if depression developed during the conditioning train, suggesting that the delay is due to depression (Magleby, 1973b). Because depression masked any facilitation that might have been present, it was not known in these earlier experiments whether facilitation retained its properties during the train, or whether it changed its properties, becoming the slower time-course potentiation (Feng, 1941; Hubbard, 1963; Rosenthal, 1969). To examine this question, Dr. Zengel and I examined the decay of EPP amplitudes under conditions of decreased transmitter release when depression was no longer present.

Four-Component Decay of Increased Transmitter Release

Figure 1 shows the response of the neuromuscular junction to 5-sec trains of repetitive stimulation delivered at seven different stimulation rates under conditions of low quantal content. EPP amplitudes increased progressively during each conditioning train: The higher the stimulation rate, the greater the rate of increase, and there was no suggestion of depression.

Figure 2 examines the decay of EPP amplitudes after a 300-impulse train delivered at 20 impulses/sec. In contrast to Figure 1, which plots the actual EPPs, Figure 2 plots points for the EPP amplitudes. The nerve was first stimulated at a rate of once every 5 sec for six impulses to establish a control response. During the conditioning train, transmitter release increased about 14 times. Testing impulses applied after the train followed the time course of return of the nerve terminal to the control condition. This occurred with four exponential components. The slowest, with a time constant of 51 sec, represents the decay of potentiation (Figure 2B). Augmentation decayed with a time constant of 6.5 sec in this experiment (Figure 2C), and the first and second components of facilitation decayed with time constants of 60 msec (Figure 2E) and 500 msec (Figure 2D). This figure shows that the four components of transmitter release are clearly present after long conditioning trains. Thus, facilitation does not turn into the slower decaying potentiation or augmentation during repetitive stimulation. The magnitudes of

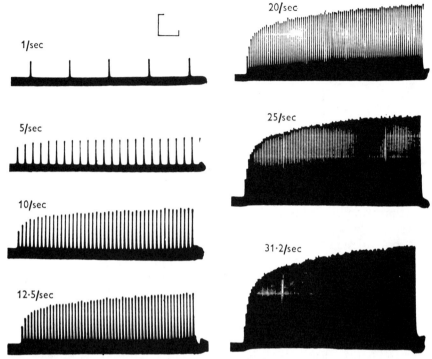

Figure 1. *Effect of stimulation rate on transmitter release.* End-plate potentials (EPPs) were recorded with a surface electrode from the frog neuromuscular junction at the indicated stimulation rates. Surface recording averages the responses from many end plates, reducing the expected quantal fluctuation. EPP amplitude gives a good measure of transmitter release under the low quantal content conditions of the experiments presented in this chapter. *Vertical bar* = 0.5 mV; *horizontal bar* = 0.5 sec. (From Magleby, 1973a.)

the various components depend on the assumed model for transmitter release. The time constants are relatively independent of the assumed model and can be used to identify the components.

Figure 3 shows that facilitation is also present and retains its characteristic properties during repetitive stimulation. In this experiment, impulses were deleted during a train to determine the facilitation that would have been added by the deleted impulses, and impulses were added to determine the facilitation added by the extra impulses. The rapid changes in EPP amplitudes resulting from the added or deleted facilitation are superimposed on the slower increases in EPP amplitude resulting from the buildup of augmentation and potentiation. Figure 3C, which plots the estimates of facilitation, shows that facilitation is present during the conditioning train, and that its magnitude increases while its time course of decay remains unchanged. Similar types of experiments have shown that the magnitude of augmentation also increases during conditioning trains, while its time constant remains unchanged (Magleby and Zengel, 1976a,b; Zengel and Magleby, 1982).

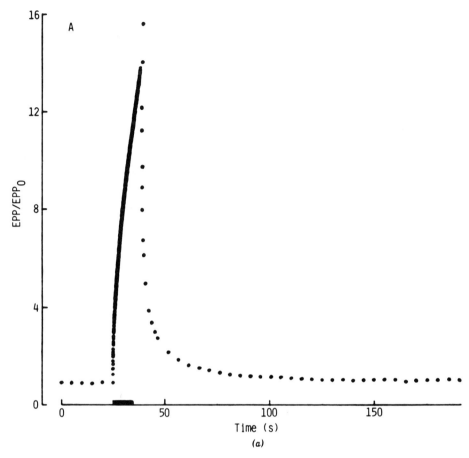

Figure 2. *Facilitation, augmentation, and potentiation of EPP amplitude after a 300-impulse conditioning train. A:* Plot of the average response of EPP amplitude for 71 conditioning–testing trials. Stimulation (20 impulses/sec) was applied during the period marked by the *horizontal bar*. During the train, the points start to overlap, forming a thick line. Other stimulation details in text. (*Figure continues on p. 30.*)

Barium and Strontium Can Separate the Components of Increased Transmitter Release

Figures 2 and 3 show a separation of the components of increased transmitter release, based on differences in the time constants of decay and the kinetic properties of these components. These components have also been separated on the basis of their differential sensitivities to the effects of barium and strontium in the bathing solution. Replacement of calcium with strontium leads to a selective increase in both the magnitude and time constant of decay of the second component of facilitation but has little effect on the other components of increased transmitter release. Addition of small amounts (0.1–0.2 mM) of barium to the calcium-containing medium results in a selective increase in the magnitude of augmentation,

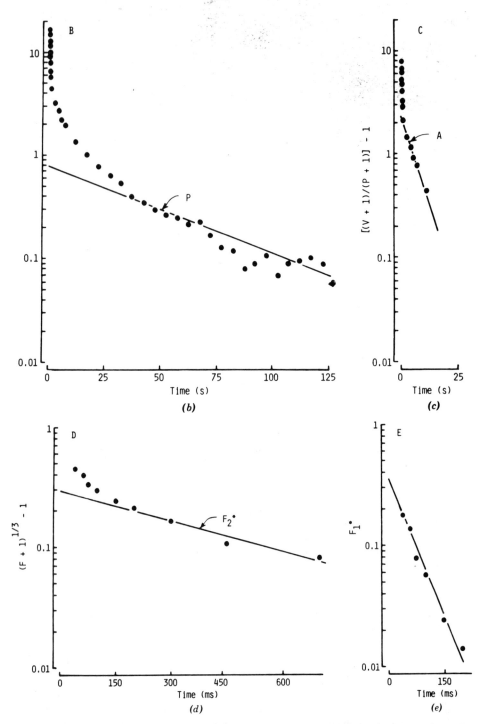

Figure 2. (*continued*) B: Decay of the fraction increase in EPP amplitudes, V, after the conditioning train in A, plotted semilogarithmically against time. The decay of potentiation is indicated by P. C: Decay of augmentation, A, after correcting the data in B for potentiation. D: Decay of the second component of facilitation, F_2^*, after correcting the data in C for augmentation. E: Decay of the first component of facilitation after correcting the data in D for the first component. The four components were separated on the assumption that they interact as described by Scheme II. (From Zengel and Magleby, 1982.)

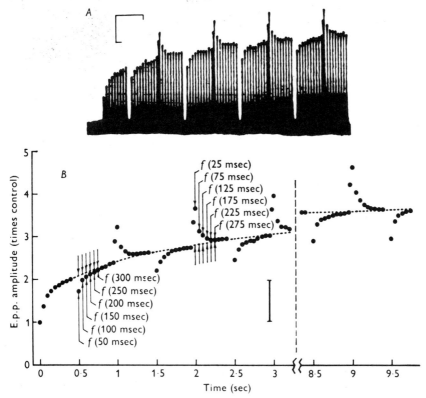

Figure 3. *Facilitation retains its properties during repetitive stimulation.* A: Surface-recorded EPPs under conditions of low quantal content. The basic stimulation rate was 20 impulses/sec. Each gap and subsequent decrease in EPP amplitude results from the deletion of an impulse. Each of the four step increases in EPP amplitude results from the addition of an impulse. *Horizontal bar*: 0.5 sec; *vertical bar*: 1 mV. B: EPP amplitudes plotted against time for the stimulation pattern in A (*filled circles*) and for continuous 20 impulses/sec stimulation (*dashed line*). Average of four trains for each pattern. The distance between the *vertical arrows* indicates the facilitation that would have been added by the deleted impulse (*left set*) or was added by the added impulse (*right set*). The *vertical bar* indicates a facilitation of one. (*Figure continues on p. 32.*)

while it has little effect on the time constant of augmentation or on the other components of increased transmitter release (Zengel and Magleby, 1980, 1981).

The mechanisms of action for the selective effects of strontium and barium are not known, but these ions do enter the nerve terminal, presumably by passing through calcium channels (Katz and Miledi, 1969; Silinsky, 1978; Mellow et al., 1982; Augustine and Eckert, 1984). Their effects may result from actions on calcium sequestration or removal systems, or perhaps from actions on other factors that may affect transmitter release. The observation of selective effects on some components and no effects on others places a number of restrictions on the mechanisms of action of the components. For example, whatever the underlying mechanism of potentiation, it will have to display similar kinetic properties in the presence of calcium, strontium, and small amounts of barium, as replacing calcium with strontium or adding a small amount of barium has

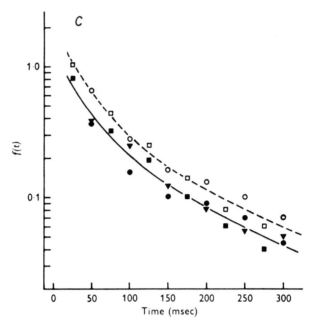

Figure 3. (*continued*) C: Semilogarithmic plot of facilitation contributed by a single impulse, $f(t)$, during a conditioning train, determined as in B. *Filled symbols* represent facilitation at the start of the train. *Open symbols* represent facilitation after 9 sec of stimulation. Estimates obtained by adding or deleting an impulse were the same. Note that the time course of the apparent two-component decay of facilitation remains constant during the train. The apparent increase in the magnitude of facilitation can be accounted for by the multiplicative effect of augmentation and potentiation on facilitation described by Scheme II. (From Magleby, 1973a.)

little effect on the magnitude or decay of potentiation (Zengel and Magleby, 1980, 1981).

It should be noted that the four components of increased transmitter release are also present and retain their kinetic properties under conditions of normal quantal content (Pallotta and Magleby, 1979). Thus, while conditions of low quantal content favor the study of these processes, such conditions are not a requirement for their expression.

FACILITATION, AUGMENTATION, AND POTENTIATION ARE ASSOCIATED WITH CALCIUM

Katz and Miledi (1968) suggested that a residue of calcium that enters the nerve terminal during the nerve impulse is responsible for facilitation. This residual calcium would combine with the calcium that enters at the time of a second nerve impulse, giving rise to an increased release of transmitter by that second impulse. In support of this hypothesis, they found that the facilitating effect of a nerve impulse depends, at least in part, on the presence of calcium in the external solution at the time of that impulse.

Rosenthal (1969) and Weinreich (1971) examined the calcium dependence of the potentiation of EPP amplitudes after long conditioning trains and found that the time course of potentiation increased with the concentration of external calcium during the conditioning train. Lev-Tov and Rahamimoff (1980) have found that external calcium ions are not an absolute requirement for the potentiation of MEPP frequency, but that they are responsible for a major part of the effect. Potentiation can be observed in the absence of external sodium (Weinreich, 1971; Lev-Tov and Rahamimoff, 1980), suggesting that the entry of sodium is not essential.

Augmentation also appears to be associated with calcium, as the augmentation component of MEPP frequency is missing under conditions of reversed calcium gradient across the nerve terminal. This suggests that augmentation may arise from an increased permeability of the membrane to calcium (Erulkar and Rahamimoff, 1978).

Sodium entry into the nerve terminal can increase transmitter release in the absence of external calcium, and this effect has been attributed to a sodium-induced increase in intracellular calcium because of the release of calcium from such intracellular stores as mitochondria or endoplasmic reticulum (for a review, see Rahamimoff et al., 1980). Magleby and Zengel (1976c) have characterized a stimulation-dependent factor (time-constant factor) that increases the time constant of decay of potentiation. This factor may reflect the kinetics of sodium in the nerve terminal.

The discussion above suggests that facilitation, augmentation, and potentiation are all associated with calcium in some manner. As pointed out by Katz and Miledi (1968), there are two ways that calcium may act to increase transmitter release: directly, as residual calcium that accumulates in the nerve terminal and combines with entering calcium to increase transmitter release; or indirectly, such that the role of calcium in increased release may reside in one of the steps between calcium entry and transmitter release. Thus, it is possible that one or more of the components of increased release may arise from a change in a calcium-activated factor, rather than from a direct effect of the residual calcium itself. Nevertheless, the idea that residual calcium directly increases transmitter release is attractive, since calcium does build up in nerve cells during repetitive stimulation, and the time course of the buildup and decay of residual calcium in the nerve terminal is similar to the time courses of some of the components of increased release (Baker et al., 1971; Ahmed and Connor, 1979; Charlton et al., 1982; Kretz et al., 1982).

While models for stimulation-induced changes in transmitter release can be developed based entirely on residual calcium, it also appears worthwhile to explore other types of models, since so little is known about the actual mechanism of transmitter release, and what factors in the nerve terminal modulate that release. To accomplish this goal, several different types of models were considered and tested.

WHAT DETERMINES THE DECAY OF FACILITATION, AUGMENTATION, AND POTENTIATION?

Under conditions of low quantal content at the frog neuromuscular junction, the time constants of decay of the first and second components of facilitation and augmentation are essentially independent of their magnitudes: The decay rates of these components remain unchanged during and after repetitive stimulation, when transmitter release can change as much as 20-fold (Figures 2, 3; Mallart and Martin, 1967, 1968; Magleby, 1973a,b; Magleby and Zengel, 1976a; Zengel and Magleby, 1982).

This observation—decay rates are independent of magnitude—excludes models which propose that the multiexponential decay that gives rise to the components of transmitter release is due to nonlinear, concentration-dependent uptake of calcium from its site of action (Linder, 1974). In such a model, calcium would be removed at a faster rate when its concentration was high, giving rise to the faster decaying components, and be removed at a slower rate when its concentration was low, giving rise to the slower decaying components. Thus, according to nonlinear models, decay rates should become faster with greater magnitudes, a prediction inconsistent with the experimental observations.

The experimental observation of decay rates independent of magnitude also excludes mechanisms for the decay of facilitation and augmentation of the type considered by Parnas and Segel (1980) that include saturation in the removal of calcium from its site of action.

Unlike facilitation and augmentation, the decay of potentiation is dependent on the stimulation parameters. A model in which the decay rate of potentiation is a function of the concentration of an additional factor (sodium?) with a time course longer than that of potentiation can account for the decay of potentiation (Magleby and Zengel, 1976c).

What, then, determines the decay of the four components? If all four components are due to residual calcium, diffusion and multicompartmental calcium buffering and removal may give rise to the four different decay rates (Blaustein et al., 1978; Zucker and Stockbridge, 1983). Potentiation, being the slowest component, may reflect the extrusion of calcium from the nerve terminal, and this may be sodium-dependent (Blaustein et al., 1978). Facilitation, because of its rapid time course, may reflect diffusion from the release sites and the rapid binding of calcium (Zucker and Stockbridge, 1983). If augmentation reflects the increased calcium permeability of the nerve terminal membrane (Erulkar and Rahamimoff, 1978), then whatever determines the decay of this increased permeability would determine the decay of augmentation.

If factors in addition to residual calcium are involved in the four components of increased transmitter release, the decay rates of the different components will depend on the decay of the different factors. In either case, barium and strontium may have selective effects on the factors in the nerve terminal that determine the kinetics of augmentation and the second component of facilitation.

Since so little is known about the mechanisms for the decays of the different components, it seems reasonable, for the purpose of testing general models for stimulation-induced changes in transmitter release, to use first-order kinetic descriptions for the decay of each component to match the experimental observations. This assumption allows different models to be tested independently of whether the decays arise from more complex mechanisms.

MODELS FOR STIMULATION-INDUCED INCREASES IN TRANSMITTER RELEASE

In developing models for release, it is necessary to know the relationship between calcium and transmitter release. Dodge and Rahamimoff (1967) observed a fourth-power relationship between extracellular calcium concentration and the number of quantal packets of transmitter released by a nerve impulse, and suggested that transmitter release might require the cooperative action of four calcium ions at some site. Such a fourth-power relationship holds to the very lowest levels of transmitter release (Andreu and Barrett, 1980). The major assumption in the interpretation of the results, that the entry of calcium through the calcium channels is proportional to the extracellular calcium concentration, seems reasonable under the conditions of the experiments. Llinás et al. (1981) have observed a linear relationship between calcium current and release at the squid giant synapse. However, as they point out, such a relationship does not exclude a power relationship between intracellular calcium concentration and transmitter release, as the sigmoidal (power) part of the relationship would only be apparent at low intracellular calcium concentrations, before possible saturation of the calcium binding sites involved in release becomes significant.

Fourth-Power Residual Calcium Model

If all transmitter release is proportional to the fourth power of calcium concentration at the release sites, then

$$\text{release} = k(Ca^*)^4 , \tag{7}$$

where K is a constant, and Ca^* represents calcium ions or a calcium complex at the release sites. Ca^* may be divided into three components such that

$$\text{release} = k(Ca_S + Ca_E + Ca_R)^4 , \tag{8}$$

where Ca_S is the steady-state level of Ca^* in the absence of action potentials in the nerve terminal, Ca_E is the phasic (evoked) increase in Ca^* at the time of the nerve impulse because of calcium entry through the voltage-dependent calcium channels, and Ca_R is the residual Ca^* that builds up during repetitive stimulation because of the incomplete removal of Ca_E after each impulse. It is the phasic pulse of Ca^*, Ca_E, that gives rise to the EPPs.

   If all four components of increased transmitter release are due to residual calcium, or directly to a calcium-activated factor, and if release is proportional to the fourth power of calcium, then transmitter release would be given by

$$EPP/EPP_0 = (F_1^* + F_2^* + A^* + P^* + 1)^4 , \tag{IV}$$

where EPP is EPP amplitude during or following repetitive stimulation, EPP_0 is the control EPP amplitude in the absence of repetitive stimulation, and F_1^*, F_2^*, A^*, and P^* represent the changes in residual calcium (expressed in units) that give rise to the four components of increased transmitter release. In this relationship (Scheme IV), Ca_E is expressed as one unit, and Ca_S is assumed to be negligible.

Joint Probability Model

If the four components of increased transmitter release reflect changes in four different underlying factors in the nerve terminal whose joint action determines the probability of transmitter release, then stimulation-induced changes in transmitter release would be determined by

$$EPP/EPP_0 = (F_1^* + 1)(F_2^* + 1)(A^* + 1)(P^* + 1) , \qquad \text{(I)}$$

where F_1^*, F_2^*, A^*, and P^* represent fractional changes in the different factors involved in release.

Scheme I is consistent with the selective effects of barium on augmentation and of strontium on the second component of facilitation (Zengel and Magleby, 1980, 1981), as the components in this scheme can act independently of one another. Scheme I is also consistent with the observed multiplicative relationship between facilitation, augmentation, and potentiation (Landau et al., 1973; Magleby, 1973b; Zengel and Magleby, 1982).

A model with multiplicative factors would also be consistent with some of the statistical properties of transmitter release. Del Castillo and Katz (1954a) found that quantal fluctuations in release could be accounted for by a model in which release, m, was assumed to arise from the product of two factors, n and p. If increases in n and p give rise to different components of increased transmitter release, then a multiplicative relationship between such components would be appropriate. The statistical factors n and p can change during repetitive stimulation (Wernig, 1972; Bennett and Fisher, 1977; Glavinović, 1979).

A model with some multiplicative factors might also be expected from the structural aspects of transmitter release. If a quantum of transmitter is released every time a synaptic vesicle successfully interacts with specific release sites on the inner side of the presynaptic nerve terminal (del Castillo and Katz, 1956; for a review, see Ceccarelli and Hurlbut, 1980), then release would be determined by the effective number of synaptic vesicles, times the number of active release sites, times the probability of successful interaction. If increases in these factors reflect some of the components of increased transmitter release, then a multiplicative relationship between such components would be appropriate. The population of synaptic vesicles at release sites does appear to change with repetitive stimulation (Quilliam and Tamarind, 1973).

Combined Models for Transmitter Release

Schemes I and IV represent extreme models for stimulation-induced increases in transmitter release (Magleby and Zengel, 1982). In Scheme I, the four exponential components of increased release arise from four independent factors, each with rather simple kinetics. In Scheme IV, they arise from a single factor (calcium), which decays with four exponentials. Two other schemes that combine properties of both of these models are

$$EPP/EPP_0 = (F_1{}^* + F_2{}^* + 1)^3(A^* + 1)(P^* + 1) \tag{II}$$

$$EPP/EPP_0 = (F_1{}^* + F_2{}^* + A^* + 1)^3(P^* + 1) . \tag{III}$$

Parallel (Linear) Model

One final model to be considered for the four components of stimulation-induced increases in transmitter release is one in which each component results from a separate factor, and each of these factors acts independently and in parallel with the others. For example, although it seems unlikely, there may be four classes of transmitter release sites within the nerve terminal. Each class would have different properties, so that the probability of release at each site would be elevated by a nerve impulse and then decay with, depending on the site, a time constant similar to that of one of the four components of increased transmitter release. Such a parallel model requires that the four components of transmitter release should sum, such that

$$EPP/EPP_0 = F_1{}^* + F_2{}^* + A^* + P^* + 1 . \tag{V}$$

Scheme V is also a linear version of Scheme IV, and therefore also represents a residual calcium model in which there is a linear relationship between Ca* and transmitter release. In this case, $F_1{}^*$, $F_2{}^*$, A^*, and P^* represent the components of the residual calcium in the nerve terminal.

DESCRIPTION OF FACILITATION, AUGMENTATION, AND POTENTIATION

One test of Schemes I–V is to determine whether they can account for stimulation-induced changes in transmitter release. In order to do this, it is necessary to incorporate kinetic descriptions of each of the four components of increased transmitter release into the models. Detailed kinetic descriptions of each of the components are presented in Zengel and Magleby (1982) and Magleby and Zengel (1982) and are summarized only briefly here. Each component is assumed to arise from the change in some factor in the nerve terminal. Each impulse adds an incremental increase to the factor, and the factor decays back to the unstimulated level with first-order kinetics. For example, the change in the underlying factor, $F_1{}^*$, which gives rise to the first component of facilitation, is described by $dF_1{}^*/dt = J(t)f_1{}^* - k_{F_1}{}^*F_1{}^*$, where $f_1{}^*$ is the incremental change in $F_1{}^*$ with each impulse; $k_{F_1}{}^*$ is the rate constant for removal of $F_1{}^*$ from its site of action; and $J(t)$ is one at the time of the nerve impulse and zero at all other times, representing a train of unit impulses (delta functions) occurring at an interval of 1/(stimulation rate).

Similar differential equations are assumed to describe the change in F_2^*, A^*, and P^* during and after repetitive stimulation. The different properties of the components arise from differences in the magnitudes of the increments added by each impulse (f_1^*, f_2^*, a^*, and p^*) and differences in the rate constants of decay ($k_{F_1}^*$, $k_{F_2}^*$, k_A^*, and k_P^*). For potentiation, the decay rate decreases as the number of conditioning impulses increases to account for the experimental observation that potentiation decays more slowly after longer trains (Rosenthal, 1969; Magleby and Zengel, 1975a). For augmentation and the two components of facilitation, the rate constants of decay are fixed and independent of the stimulation pattern or the magnitude of the components, which is consistent with the experimental findings (Mallart and Martin, 1967; Magleby and Zengel, 1975a; Zengel and Magleby, 1982). The increment of augmentation, a^*, added by each impulse during a train typically increases (Zengel and Magleby, 1982), while the increments added for the other components remain constant.

Linear or Power Models

Facilitation.   Mallart and Martin (1967) and Magleby (1973a) found that facilitation of EPP amplitudes during short trains of stimulation could be predicted by assuming that each nerve impulse adds an increment of facilitation similar to that described by Equation 6, and that these increments sum linearly. However, as the duration of stimulation was extended, the linear facilitation model underpredicted transmitter release (Magleby, 1973a). This underprediction occurred for two reasons. The models considered did not account for the increments of augmentation and potentiation added by each impulse (Magleby, 1973b), and the underlying factor or factors that give rise to facilitation appear to be expressed as a third or fourth power rather than linearly (Barrett and Stevens, 1972; Younkin, 1974; Zengel and Magleby, 1982; Zucker and Lara-Estrella, 1983). Models in which the two components of facilitation have a multiplicative relationship can also account for facilitation under some conditions (Zengel and Magleby, 1982). Interestingly, both linear and exponential facilitation models apply to different synapses at the crayfish neuromuscular junction (Linder, 1974), suggesting that all these models may be somewhat limited. The difference between various models for facilitation of EPP amplitudes becomes significant only for large values of facilitation. Linear, power, and multiplicative models for facilitation are described in Schemes I–V. In the absence of augmentation and potentiation ($A^* = 0$, $P^* = 0$), Scheme I becomes a multiplicative facilitation model, Schemes II–IV become power facilitation models, and Scheme V becomes a linear facilitation model. In calculating facilitation with these models, F_1^* is calculated as described in the previous two paragraphs, and F_2^* is calculated in a similar manner.

Augmentation.   Augmentation of EPP amplitudes can be described by either linear or power models, consistent with Schemes I–V if the other components are set equal to zero (Zengel and Magleby, 1982). A clear distinction cannot be made between linear or power models for augmentation because the increment of transmitter release added by each impulse increases during the train. The increase is different for linear models and power models, but both describe the data.

Potentiation.   Potentiation is described by a linear model, consistent with Schemes I–III and V when the other components are set equal to zero (Magleby and Zengel, 1975b; Zengel and Magleby, 1982).

QUANTITATIVE DESCRIPTION OF STIMULATION-INDUCED CHANGES IN TRANSMITTER RELEASE

Predicting the Increase in EPP Amplitudes During Repetitive Stimulation

Figure 4 shows that Scheme II, together with the kinetic properties of potentiation, augmentation, and the two components of facilitation, is sufficient to account for stimulation-induced changes in transmitter release under conditions of low quantal content. During the trains in Figure 4A, predicted EPP amplitudes are almost exactly superimposed on the observed EPP amplitudes so that the predicted points are not visible. For both stimulation rates, the predicted response was slightly higher than the observed amplitudes at the ends of the trains. Figure

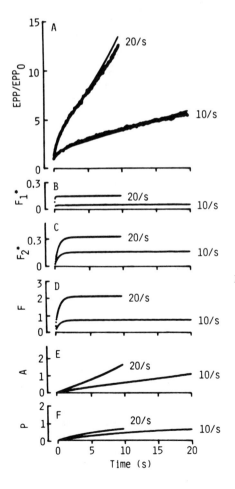

Figure 4. *Predicting the effect of stimulation rate on transmitter release during trains of repetitive stimulation. A: Plot of observed and predicted EPP amplitudes during 200-impulse conditioning trains delivered at 10 and 20 impulses/sec. The observed (large dots forming thick line) and predicted (smaller dots forming thinner line) EPP amplitudes superimpose except at the ends of the trains. The predicted response was calculated using Scheme II and the kinetic properties of potentiation, augmentation, and the first and second components of facilitation. B–F: Calculated increases in the components underlying stimulation-induced changes in transmitter release. (From Magleby and Zengel, 1982.)*

4D–F plots the calculated increase in potentiation (*P*), augmentation (*A*), and facilitation (*F*) underlying the stimulation-induced changes in transmitter release. The factors that give rise to the two components of facilitation, F_1^* and F_2^*, are also plotted separately in Figure 4B and C. These combine, as described by Scheme II, to give rise to *F*. Notice that the rapid increase in EPP amplitudes at the start of each train is mainly due to the increase in the two components of facilitation. Thereafter, facilitation is in a steady state and the increase in EPP amplitudes reflects the increase in augmentation and potentiation. Transmitter release is greater during the 20 impulses/sec stimulation than during the 10 impulses/sec stimulation, because facilitation increases more rapidly to a higher steady-state level, and because augmentation and potentiation also increase at a greater rate. The parameters used in the equations to predict transmitter release were obtained from conditioning–testing trials with 20 impulses/sec stimulation. The 10 impulses/sec train was then predicted without any free parameters.

Predicting the Decay of EPP Amplitudes After Repetitive Stimulation

Figure 5 shows that Scheme II can predict the decay of EPP amplitudes after a conditioning train. The calculated rise and decay of facilitation, augmentation, and potentiation underlying the predicted response are shown in Figure 5B–D. Facilitation decays to insignificant levels by the time of the first testing impulse, 2 sec after the train. Augmentation contributes to the decay for about 20 sec after the train, and potentiation decays slower still. Predicted EPP amplitudes were calculated without free parameters. As above, the values of the parameters used in the equations were obtained with 20 impulses/sec trains.

Predicting Step Changes in Transmitter Release

Step changes in stimulation rate during repetitive stimulation would lead to rapid changes in facilitation because of its short time course. These changes

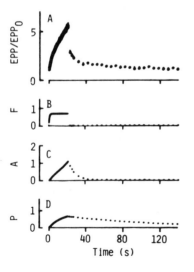

Figure 5. *Predicting the decay of transmitter release after a conditioning train. A:* Plot of observed and predicted EPP amplitudes during and after a 200-impulse conditioning train delivered at 10 impulses/sec. The observed response (*large dots*) and predicted response (*smaller dots*) are essentially superimposed and appear as single dots. Predicted response was calculated by using Scheme II. *B–D:* Calculated changes in the components underlying the predicted response. (From Magleby and Zengel, 1982.)

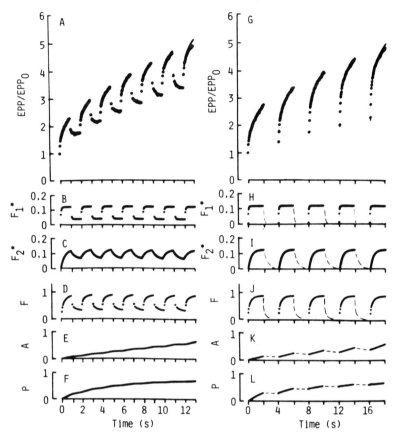

Figure 6. *Predicting transmitter release during step changes in the stimulation rate.* A and G: Observed and predicted EPP amplitudes during step changes in the stimulation rate. In *A*, the stimulation rate alternated between 20 impulses/sec for 1 sec and 10 impulses/sec for 1 sec. In *G*, the stimulation alternated between 20 impuludes/sec for 2 sec and 2-sec latency periods. The observed (*large dots* forming *thick lines*) and predicted (*smaller dots*) EPP amplitudes are essentially superimposed. Predicted responses were calculated by using Scheme II. *B–F* and *H–L*: Calculated changes in the components underlying the predicted responses. (From Magleby and Zengel, 1982.)

would be superimposed on the slower changing augmentation and potentiation. Examination of whether a transmitter release model can account for step changes in stimulation rate thus provides a means to examine whether the model can predict the interactions between the faster and slower decaying components.

Figure 6A and G plot EPP amplitudes during two different stimulation patterns. In Figure 6A, the nerve was stimulated in an alternating pattern of 20 impulses/sec for 1 sec, 10 impulses/sec for 1 sec. In Figure 6G, the nerve was stimulated in a repeating pattern of 20 impulses/sec for 2 sec, followed by a 2-sec latency period. The predicted EPP amplitudes were calculated as in Figures 4 and 5, and again the predicted amplitudes are essentially superimposed on the observed EPP amplitudes so that the predicted points are not visible. Notice that the model describes the step changes in EPP amplitude following the step changes in stimulation rate. The data were predicted without free parameters. As before, the values of the parameters used in the equations were obtained from trains with constant 20 impulses/sec stimulation.

Notice in Figure 6B–F and H–L that the rapid changes in predicted EPP amplitude with step changes in stimulation rate are mainly due to rapid changes in facilitation. The step changes in EPP amplitude become greater as augmentation and potentiation build up because of the multiplicative effect of these components on facilitation.

Which Model?

Although the data in experiments of the type shown in Figures 4–6 were typically best described by Scheme II, Schemes I and III could describe the data about as well. Thus, a multiplicative relationship between the components (Scheme I), or a combination of multiplicative and power models (Schemes II and III), could account for stimulation-induced changes in EPP amplitudes. Schemes II and III fit about equally well with either a third or fourth power. Scheme II is thus consistent with a fourth-power residual calcium model for the two components of facilitation, with additional factors required for augmentation and potentiation. Scheme III is consistent with a power residual calcium model for the two components of facilitation and augmentation, with an additional factor for potentiation.

Scheme IV, which is a fourth-power residual calcium model for all components of stimulation-induced changes in transmitter release, underpredicted the step changes in EPP amplitude that followed step changes in stimulation rate by about 20% at the end of the stimulation patterns. Increasing the power made the fit better; decreasing it made the fit worse. Thus while the fourth-power residual calcium model was generally consistent with the facilitation and augmentation of EPP ampltude, it did not describe the relationship between all the components of increased release as well as did Schemes I–III, and it will be shown in a later section that a simple fourth-power residual calcium model also does not account for stimulation-induced changes in MEPP frequency.

It is interesting, however, that power models like Scheme IV can approximate the apparent multiplicative relationships between facilitation, augmentation, and potentiation. This suggests that such models should not be rejected, but explored further in terms of different underlying assumptions for the models.

Scheme V, which is a linear model, underpredicted the step changes in transmitter release by about 50% and can be excluded. Such an underprediction is to be expected because of the apparent multiplicative or power type of relationship among the components (Magleby, 1973b; Zengel and Magleby, 1982).

Some readers may find it discouraging that such apparently different models as Schemes I–IV can describe, or at least approximate, stimulation-induced changes in EPP amplitude. Such a demonstration just reinforces the well-known fact that showing that a model can describe the data does not establish the model. It simply provides a working hypothesis for further investigations of mechanisms. In this case, there are four working hypotheses, some of which are more likely than others.

All four models have some features in common, and these features provide the significance of the quantitative description and our working hypothesis.

Stimulation-induced changes in EPP amplitude can be accounted for by the properties of four kinetically and pharmacologically distinguishable components of increased transmitter release: potentiation, augmentation, and the first and second components of facilitation. Additional components are not needed (or are not significant) under the conditions of low levels of transmitter release used in our experiments. This quantitative description extends by two orders of magnitude, over the pioneering experiments of Mallart and Martin (1967), the duration of stimulation that can be accounted for.

The Effects of Barium and Strontium Are Consistent with the Model

The model described by Scheme II can also account for the selective effects of barium and strontium on transmitter release during and after short trains of stimulation (Zengel and Magleby, 1977).

A further test of our working hypothesis would be to determine whether it can account for the selective effects of strontium and barium during patterned stimulation. If the predicted changes in the components underlying stimulation-induced changes in transmitter release shown in Figure 6H–L are correct, and if strontium selectively increases the magnitude and time constant of decay of the second component of facilitation (Zengel and Magleby, 1981), then strontium should lead to a greater rate of increase in EPP amplitude when the second component of facilitation is increasing, displace EPP amplitude upward when the second component is present but not increasing, and have no effect on EPP amplitude when the second component of facilitation is not present.

These are just the effects that were observed, as can be determined from Figures 6I and 7A. Strontium led to a greater increase in EPP amplitude during the first second of each stimulation period, when the second component of facilitation was calculated to be increasing most rapidly; strontium displaced EPP amplitude during the remainder of each 2-sec burst of stimulation, when the second component of facilitation was calculated to be in a steady state; and strontium had no effect on the first EPP amplitude of each block of stimulation, when facilitation was calculated to be absent.

Similarly, if barium selectively increases the magnitude of augmentation, then barium should increase EPP amplitude when augmentation is present. These expected effects of barium were also observed, as can be determined from Figures 6K and 7B. Barium led to a greater increase in EPP amplitude throughout each 2-sec block of stimulation, when augmentation was calculated to be increasing, and barium led to a progressive increase in the first EPP amplitude of each stimulation block, consistent with the calculated increase in augmentation.

The observations in Figures 6 and 7 lend further support to our working hypothesis, but the mechanisms underlying the selective effects of barium and strontium are not clear. They might arise from specific selective effects on factors that determine the kinetic properties of the individual components, as was assumed to account for the selective effects of these ions in Zengel and Magleby (1977), or they might arise from more complicated nonlinear models (Parnas and Segel, 1983).

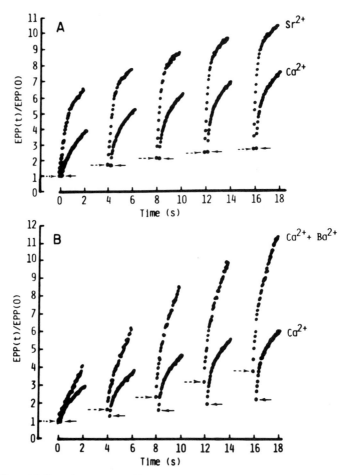

Figure 7. *Differential effects of strontium and barium on transmitter release.* Stimulation alternated between 20 impulses/sec for 2 sec and 2-sec latency periods. *A*: Superimposed plots of EPP amplitudes recorded during stimulation in a Ringer's solution with 0.7 mM calcium (*lower points*) and a Ringer's solution with 1.4 mM strontium replacing calcium (*upper points* displaced to the *left* for clarity). The *arrows* indicate the first EPP amplitude of each 2-sec train of impulses. *B*: Superimposed plots of EPP amplitudes recorded during stimulation in a Ringer's solution with 0.4 mM calcium (*lower points*) and a Ringer's solution with 0.4 mM calcium plus 0.3 mM barium (*upper points*). (From Zengel and Magleby, 1980.)

STIMULATION-INDUCED CHANGES IN MEPP FREQUENCY

Quantal transmitter release can be divided into two types: phasic release, which produces the EPP; and residual release, which gives rise to MEPPs (del Castillo and Katz, 1954a). Similar to stimulation-induced changes in EPP amplitude, MEPP frequency also increases during repetitive stimulation and decays thereafter (Hubbard, 1963; Hurlbut et al., 1971; Miledi and Thies, 1971; Erulkar and Ra-hamimoff, 1978). Figure 8, which presents an intracellular recording from a muscle fiber at an end-plate region during repetitive stimulation under conditions of low quantal content, shows this phenomenon. Notice that both EPP amplitude

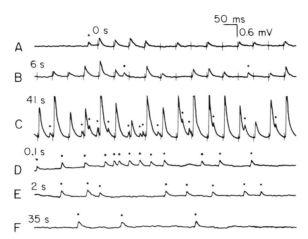

Figure 8. *Effect of repetitive stimulation on EPP amplitude and miniature end-plate potential (MEPP) frequency.* Records of intracellular recording are presented. The nerve was stimulated with 1000 impulses at a rate of 20 impulses/sec. The records were obtained at the indicated times during (A–C) and after (D–F) the conditioning train. The *thin vertical lines* in A–C (shock artifacts) indicate when the nerve was stimulated. The responses immediately after the stimulation indicate EPPs (phasic transmitter release). The quantal responses indicated by the *dots* are MEPPs (residual transmitter release). The EPPs in C are flat-topped because the penwriter reached its limit of travel. (From Zengel and Magleby, 1982.)

and MEPP frequency increase during the conditioning train. After the train, the MEPP frequency returns to the control level. The results shown in Figure 9 represent the average MEPP frequency obtained from 123 trials. MEPP frequency increased about 10 times during a 200-impulse conditioning train and then decayed away. The time course of decay was described by four exponential components with time constants of 69 sec (potentiation), 9.1 sec (augmentation), 560 msec (second component of facilitation), and 44 msec (first component of facilitation). These decay rates are similar to those in Figure 2 for the decay of EPP amplitude. In a series of experiments of this type, the time constants of decay of the four corresponding components of stimulation-induced changes in EPP amplitude and MEPP frequency were similar (Zengel and Magleby, 1981).

Strontium and barium had the same selective effects on the components of stimulation-induced changes in MEPP frequency as have been described for EPP amplitude (Zengel and Magleby, 1981). The observation that stimulation-induced changes in MEPP frequency and EPP amplitude have similar multiexponential decays and similar sensitivities to barium and strontium suggests that stimulation-induced changes in these two types of releases have similar underlying mechanisms.

The demonstration that residual changes in the nerve terminal that give rise to potentiation, augmentation, and the first and second components of facilitation are present and retain their kinetic properties between nerve impulses and after the conditioning train in the total absence of nerve impulses shows that these components are not due to changes in the size or shape of the presynaptic nerve impulses or to changes in the entry of calcium at the time of each nerve impulse.

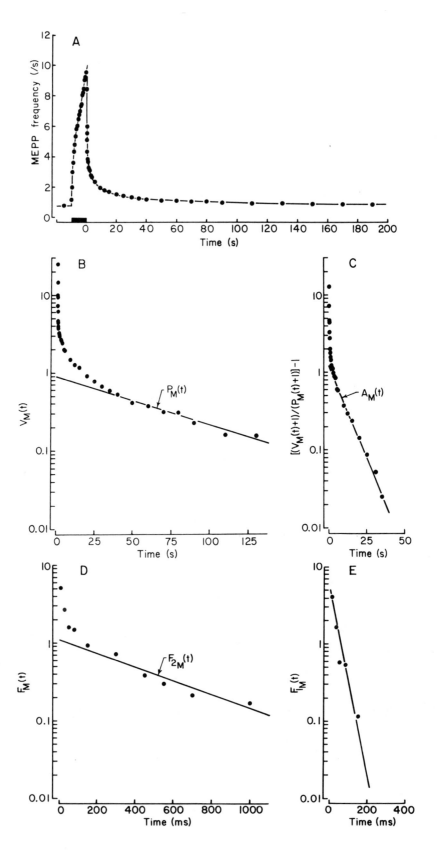

This conclusion is consistent with those reached in other studies (Martin and Pilar, 1964; Erulkar and Rahamimoff, 1978; Zucker and Lara-Estrella, 1979; Charlton et al., 1982).

Stimulation-induced changes in MEPP frequency thus reflect residual changes in the nerve terminal that give rise to stimulation-induced changes in EPP amplitude. They lend support for models such as Schemes I–V, which are based on such residual changes.

FURTHER TEST OF THE RESIDUAL CALCIUM MODEL

Scheme IV did not describe the data as well as did Schemes I–III. This poorer fit may indicate that the fourth-power residual calcium model is inadequate, or that some of the assumptions used to develop and test the model were incorrect.

A direct test of the residual calcium hypothesis would require simultaneous measurement of both transmitter release and intracellular calcium concentration at the release sites. This is not yet possible because the calcium-measuring systems currently available give the average intracellular concentration, which may differ from that at the release sites because of diffusion, the discrete entry of calcium at calcium channels, and differential uptake and buffering in various parts of the nerve terminal.

One method of circumventing these problems is to estimate residual calcium at the release sites from MEPP frequency. A comparison of MEPP frequency (residual release) and EPP amplitude (phasic release) then allows a test of the residual calcium hypothesis (Miledi and Thies, 1971). Such a test is made by: (1) Estimating Ca_R from the stimulation-induced increase in EPP amplitude; (2) using this value and Equation 8 to predict MEPP frequency; and (3) comparing the observed and predicted MEPP frequency.

Figure 10 shows that the simple fourth-power residual calcium model described by Equation 8 cannot account for stimulation-induced changes in MEPP frequency during a train of repetitive stimulation. The predicted MEPP frequency is typically an order of magnitude greater than the observed frequency, and the shape of the curve is incorrect. The fourth-power residual calcium model also predicts that the components of MEPP frequency should decay about four times faster than the corresponding components of EPP amplitude, a prediction inconsistent with the experimental data shown in Figures 2 and 9 (Zengel and Magleby, 1981).

Figure 9. *Stimulation-induced changes in MEPP frequency.* The data were averaged from 12 cells in six preparations (123 trials, 47,295 MEPPs). A: Rise and decay of MEPP frequency during (*horizontal bar*) and after repetitive stimulation of 200 impulses at 20 impulses/sec. B: Decay of the fraction increase in MEPP frequency, $V_M(t)$, after the conditioning train in A was plotted semilogarithmically against time after the train. The decay of potentiation of MEPP frequency is indicated by $P_M(t)$. C: Decay of augmentation of MEPP frequency, $A_M(t)$, after correcting the data in B for potentiation. D: Decay of the second component of facilitation of MEPP frequency, $F_{2M}(t)$, after correcting the data in C for augmentation. E: Decay of the first component of facilitation of MEPP frequency, $F_{1M}(t)$, after correcting the data in D for the second component. The four components were separated on the assumption that they interact as described by Scheme II. (From Zengel and Magleby, 1981.)

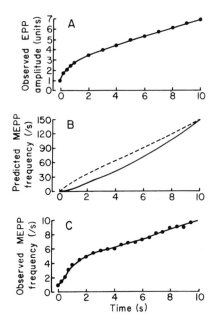

Figure 10. *Test of the fourth-power residual calcium model for stimulation-induced changes in transmitter release. A:* Increase in EPP amplitude during the conditioning train for the experiment in Figure 9. *B:* Predicted increase in MEPP frequency during the train in *A,* calculated with Equation 8, using values of Ca_R determined from the increase in EPP amplitude. *Continuous line:* $k = 1000$ quanta/sec; $Ca_E = 1$; and $Ca_S = 0.001$. *Dashed line:* $k = 100$ quanta/sec; $Ca_E = 1$; and $Ca_S = 0.3$. *C:* Observed increase in MEPP frequency during the conditioning train, which differs markedly from the predicted increase shown in *B.* (From Zengel and Magleby, 1981.)

A simple linear residual calcium model for stimulation-induced changes in transmitter release obtained by substituting one for the exponent of four in Equation 8 is even less satisfactory. For example, the assumption of a linear relationship predicts that MEPP frequency should be two to three orders of magnitude greater than is observed at the end of the conditioning train. The calculation is done as follows: Under the low quantal content conditions of the experiment shown in Figure 10, a typical nerve impulse at the start of the train released about one quanta of transmitter, and a typical nerve impulse at the end of the train after 10 sec of stimulation released about seven quanta of transmitter. Since the phasic transmitter release that gives rise to EPPs lasts about 1 msec (Katz and Miledi, 1965), the transmitter release rate during the phasic release period associated with each EPP was 1000 quanta/sec (1 quanta/msec) at the start of the train and 7000 quanta/sec at the end of 10 sec of stimulation. If the phasic calcium concentration at the release sites (Ca_E) that gives rise to the EPP is assumed to be one unit, then the residual calcium, Ca_R, would be six units at the end of the train for a linear model (calculated with Equation 8, assuming that $k = 1000$ quanta/sec and $Ca_S \ll 1$, because the resting MEPP frequency is less than 1 quanta/sec). From Equation 8, the predicted MEPP frequency at the end of the train for a linear model with $Ca_R = 6$ is 6000 impulses/sec, 600 times greater than the observed rate of 10 impulses/sec. This predicted frequency is so high that the EPP would not return to the baseline between nerve impulses. Thus the predictions of simple linear and power residual calcium models are clearly inconsistent with the experimental data shown in Figures 8–10.

These experiments do not exclude the possibility that residual calcium is responsible for stimulation-induced increases in transmitter release. But they do show that simple models which assume that transmitter release is simply determined by the concentration of calcium at the release sites, and that all stimulation-induced changes in transmitter release are due to changes in residual calcium at the release sites, are inadequate. It should be noted that this type of test of the residual calcium model is valid independently of whether the residual calcium enters from the extracellular solution or is released from internal stores.

Since the facilitation of MEPP frequency after one or a few impulses appears somewhat consistent with a simple fourth-power residual calcium model (Barrett and Stevens, 1972; Zucker and Lara-Estrella, 1983), the deviation with longer trains may be due to the buildup of augmentation and potentiation or factors other than residual calcium. Consistent with this possibility, Scheme II, which gave the best description of stimulation-induced changes in EPP amplitude, incorporates a residual calcium model for facilitation, and has additional factors for augmentation and potentiation.

The simple residual calcium model tested in Figure 10 greatly overpredicted MEPP frequency. If the residual calcium had been calculated from observed MEPP frequency instead of observed EPP amplitude, this model would have underpredicted the increase in EPP amplitude. If depolarization of the nerve terminal membrane both opens calcium channels and directly accelerates transmitter release, as suggested by Dudel (1983) and Parnas et al. (1984), then such a direct voltage-dependent effect might account for why a simple residual calcium model overpredicts MEPP frequency and/or underpredicts EPP amplitude.

USE OF QUANTITATIVE DESCRIPTION TO EVALUATE MODELS

One purpose of the kinetic studies presented here is to describe stimulation-induced changes in transmitter release in sufficient detail that proposed mechanisms for such changes can be evaluated critically. Certainly, any viable model for mechanism should be able to account for the detailed kinetics of the observed changes in transmitter release summarized by our quantitative description.

Although no models currently in the literature can account for these changes in terms of underlying mechanisms, progress is being made; investigators are now exploring mechanisms that could give rise to the components of increased transmitter release (see, e.g., Rahamimoff et al., 1980; Parnas and Segel, 1983; Zucker and Stockbridge, 1983). Most of these models focus on the kinetics of calcium and invoke various assumptions about its entry, its possible release from internal stores, its uptake, and its removal from the nerve terminal; such models do not directly address the question of how calcium may affect transmitter release.

These models will undoubtedly have to be expanded to include additional factors involved in transmitter release. Changes in these additional factors may result from either the direct or indirect effects of calcium and may include, for example, changes in the numbers of synaptic vesicles or active release sites. These additional factors may have time courses different from that of calcium.

COMPONENTS OF INCREASED TRANSMITTER RELEASE
AT OTHER SYNAPSES

Facilitation, augmentation, and potentiation are common features of synaptic transmission at both peripheral and central synapses (Kuno, 1964; Martin and

Pilar, 1964; Porter, 1970; McNaughton, 1980; Hirst et al., 1981; Ohmori et al., 1981). However, the kinetic properties of the components of increased transmitter release are often different for different synapses. For example, the increments of the first and second components of facilitation added by each impulse are about twice as large in the toad as in the frog (Zengel and Magleby, 1982), and the increments of augmentation and the second component of facilitation added by each impulse are about 6–10 times larger in the mammalian sympathetic ganglion than at the frog neuromuscular junction (Zengel el al., 1980). Interestingly, even though the time constants of decay of the four components of increased transmitter release are highly temperature-dependent, the decay rates in mammalian sympathetic ganglion at 34°C (Zengel et al., 1980) are about the same as those listed in Table 1 for the frog neuromuscular junction at 20°C, and the time constants of decay and general properties of augmentation and potentiation in the fascia dentata of rat hippocampus at 35°C (McNaughton, 1980, 1982) are similar to those at the frog neuromuscular junction at 20°C.

Because the components of transmitter release can have different properties at different synapses, it has been useful to distinguish among the components by examining the selective effects of barium and strontium. This technique has been used to identify augmentation and the second component of facilitation in the mammalian sympathetic ganglion (Zengel et al., 1980). It should also be kept in mind that, under conditions of normal quantal content, depression, which was not present in the experiments presented here, can be a dominant factor during synaptic transmission.

SPECULATIVE FUNCTIONS FOR SHORT-TERM CHANGES IN TRANSMITTER RELEASE

Short-Term Synaptic Memory

The physiological functions of the short-term, stimulation-induced changes in transmitter release summarized in Table 1 are not clear. They may simply reflect a by-product of synaptic activity; consequently, the nervous system may be designed to compensate for these changes so that it operates effectively in spite of the changes in transmitter release that can occur with repetitive stimulation. If this is the case, then some of the parallel pathways, circuitry, and properties of nervous system elements may be present to compensate for the variable information transfer across synapses.

An alternative possibility is that, at least at some synapses, the highly predictable behavior of variable synaptic efficacy may be used to store, integrate, and manipulate information on a short-term basis of milliseconds to minutes. Simply put, the synapse "remembers" its previous stimulation, and this memory is stored in terms of the magnitudes and interactions between depression, potentiation, augmentation, and the first and second components of facilitation. The memory is expressed as either an increase or a decrease (depending on the magnitude of depression) in the amount of transmitter released to the next nerve impulse. Thus each synapse keeps a running summary of its history of use and alters its output based on this history.

The next sections consider possible consequences or functions of short-term synaptic memory. These sections are *highly speculative* and are presented simply to provoke discussion or to initiate investigations of possible functions.

Integration of Information

It is well established (see Rall and Segev, this volume) that nerve cells act to integrate information in the nervous system. Potential changes resulting from synaptic input to the soma and dendrites of neurons are integrated, and when the cell is depolarized to threshold an action potential is generated. Synaptic information can be integrated over a period of time (10–20 msec) determined by the location and time course of synaptic inputs, the structure of the neuron, and the effective time constant of the motoneuron membrane.

Another means of integrating information might be through changes in synaptic efficacy. Each impulse to a synapse might produce increments in the components of increased transmitter release, and the synapse would reflect the record of previous activity by releasing different amounts of transmitter to subsequent impulses. The rules of integration would be complicated and, depending on the synapse, might be expressed by equations similar to Schemes I–III, with additional equations for depression, if present. Examples of integration of information are shown in Figures 1–9. Information about the frequency, duration, and pattern of previous stimulation, as well as the number of impulses, might be passed on in terms of changes in transmitter release. For example, Figures 3 and 6 show examples of a synapse passing on information about both the frequency and the duration of stimulation. Rapid changes in transmitter release result from step changes in the frequency of stimulation, and the magnitude of these changes increases with the duration of stimulation.

Because the four components of increased transmitter release have widely separated time constants that differ from one another by 1–3 orders of magnitude (Table 1), it would be possible to design synapses that are selectively responsive to a wide range of stimulation rates by changing the magnitude of the increments of each component added by each impulse. Consider two extreme examples. If each impulse added an increment only to the first component of facilitation, while having little effect on the other three components, then the synapse would have a short memory and integrate information over about a 100-msec time period, releasing greater amounts of transmitter for each impulse if the stimulation rate were greater than about 10 impulses/sec. Conversely, if each impulse only added an increment to potentiation, while having little effect on the other three components, the synapse would have a longer memory and integrate information over several minutes, keeping track of the average stimulation rate or number of impulses delivered over this period rather than the pattern of stimulation.

The nervous system might use synapses with these different properties to preprocess information selectively. For example, if neural function required that a postsynaptic cell respond to high-frequency bursts of action potentials in the synapse, the synapse might be designed with large amounts of facilitation, which would greatly increase transmitter release for high-frequency stimulation but have little effect on transmitter release for low-frequency stimulation. A synapse with the opposite properties might be made by implementing depression: The synapse would depress rapidly to high-frequency stimulation but not to lower-frequency stimulation.

Multiplication

The multiplicative relationship between the components of increased transmitter release (Magleby and Zengel, 1982) provides for a multiplicative relationship between the cumulative and short-term effects of repetitive stimulation. Rapid changes in the facilitation of transmitter release because of step changes in the stimulation rate would be multiplied by the slower cumulative effects of augmentation and potentiation. This multiplicative effect (apparent in Figures 3 and 6) might occur between inputs from two or more pathways by having each pathway drive the same neuron. The multiplicative interaction between inputs would then occur at synapses originating from the driven neuron.

Learning and Memory

Some forms of learning and memory may involve permanent or long-lasting changes in synaptic function (see the chapters by Siman et al., Kandel et al., Andersen, Edelman and Finkel, and Tsukahara in this volume). In addition to long-term changes in synaptic efficacy, which can be assessed with single testing impulses, there may be other, more dynamic, long-term changes that can only be detected with patterned stimulation. Since the nervous system typically operates through trains of impulses rather than single impulses, such changes would give the nervous system much more flexibility in storing various types of information.

Depression, potentiation, augmentation, and the two components of facilitation allow a synapse to remember for milliseconds to several minutes. Long-term changes in one or more of the properties of these components might lead to long-term changes in the response of a synapse to trains of impulses, without necessarily having any effect on the response to single testing impulses. For example, perhaps some form of synaptic modification involved in learning or memory leads to a doubling in the increments of the first and second components of facilitation added by each impulse. Such an increase might occur through a long-lasting change in the properties of calcium buffering in the nerve terminal (or whatever determines the magnitudes of the increments of facilitation). Such a long-term change in facilitation properties would not necessarily affect the amount of transmitter released by a single nerve impulse, but might double the amount of transmitter released during short trains of high-frequency stimulation and consequently have large long-term effects on the dynamic function of the synapse. Little is known about whether such long-term changes might occur in the properties of the components of increased transmitter release, but the possibility is worthy of investigation. Crick (1984) has proposed one way in which long-term structural changes in synapses might occur.

CONCLUSION

This chapter described some of the dynamic properties of synaptic transmission and speculated about possible functions of these dynamic properties. In order to understand the detailed operation of the nervous system, it may well be necessary to understand the input–output relationship of each synapse as a function of its history of activity. The equations developed to describe this relationship for the neuromuscular junction under conditions of low quantal content may serve as a starting point for the development of equations for other experimental conditions and synapses.

ACKNOWLEDGMENTS

The work described was supported by grant NS-10277 from the National Institutes of Health and a grant from the Muscular Dystrophy Association.

REFERENCES

Ahmed, Z., and J. A. Connor (1979) Measurement of calcium influx under voltage clamp in molluscan neurones using the metallochromic dye arsenazo III. *J. Physiol. (Lond.)* **286**:61–82.

Andreu, R., and E. F. Barrett (1980) Calcium dependence of evoked transmitter release at very low quantal contents at the frog neuromuscular junction. *J. Physiol. (Lond.)* **308**:79–97.

Augustine, G. J., and R. Eckert (1984) Divalent cations differentially support transmitter release at the squid giant synapse. *J. Physiol. (Lond.)* **346**:257–271.

Baker, P. F., A. L. Hodgkin, and E. B. Ridgway (1971) Depolarization and calcium entry in squid giant axons. *J. Physiol. (Lond.)* **218**:709–755.

Barrett, E. F., and K. L. Magleby (1976) Physiology of cholinergic transmission. In *Biology of Cholinergic Function*, A. M. Goldberg and I. Hanin, eds., pp. 29–100, Raven, New York.

Barrett, E. F., and C. F. Stevens (1972) The kinetics of transmitter release at the frog neuromuscular junction. *J. Physiol. (Lond.)* **227**:691–708.

Bennett, M. R., and C. Fisher (1977) The effect of calcium ions on the binomial parameters that control acetylcholine release during trains of nerve impulses at amphibian neuromuscular synapses. *J. Physiol. (Lond.)* **271**:673–698.

Betz, W. J. (1970) Depression of transmitter release at the neuromuscular junction of the frog. *J. Physiol. (Lond.)* **206**:629–644.

Blaustein, M. P., R. W. Ratzlaff, and E. S. Schweitzer (1978) Calcium buffering in presynaptic nerve terminals. II. Kinetic properties of the non-mitochondrial calcium sequestration mechanism. *J. Gen. Physiol.* **72**:43–66.

Ceccarelli, B., and W. P. Hurlbut (1980) Vesicle hypothesis of the release of quanta of acetylcholine. *Physiol. Rev.* **60**:396–441.

Chad, J., R. Eckert, and D. Ewald (1984) Kinetics of calcium-dependent inactivation of calcium current in voltage-clamped neurones of *Aplysia californica*. *J. Physiol. (Lond.)* **347**:279–300.

Charlton, M. P., S. J. Smith, and R. S. Zucker (1982) Role of presynaptic calcium ions and channels in synaptic facilitation and depression at the squid giant synapse. *J. Physiol. (Lond.)* **323**:173–193.

Crick, F. (1984) Memory and molecular turnover. *Nature* **312**:101.

del Castillo, J., and B. Katz (1954a) Quantal components of the end-plate potential. *J. Physiol. (Lond.)* **124**:560–573.

del Castillo, J., and B. Katz (1954b) Statistical factors involved in neuromuscular facilitation and depression. *J. Physiol. (Lond.)* **124**:574–585.

del Castillo, J., and B. Katz (1956) Biophysical aspects of neuro-muscular transmission. *Prog. Biophys.* **6**:241–266.

Dodge, F. A., and R. Rahamimoff (1967) Co-operative action of calcium ions in transmitter release at the neuromuscular junction. *J. Physiol. (Lond.)* **193**:419–432.

Dudel, J. (1983) Transmitter release triggered by a local depolarization in motor nerve terminals of the frog: Role of calcium entry and of depolarization. *Neurosci. Lett.* **41**:133–138.

Erulkar, S. D., and R. Rahamimoff (1978) The role of calcium ions in tetanic and post-tetanic increase of miniature end-plate potential frequency. *J. Physiol. (Lond.)* **278**:501–511.

Feng, T. P. (1941) Studies on the neuromuscular junction. XXVI. The changes of the end-plate potential during and after prolonged stimulation. *Chin. J. Physiol.* **16**:341–372.

Glavinović, M. I. (1979) Change of statistical parameters of transmitter release during various kinetic tests in unparalyzed voltage-clamped rat diaphragm. *J. Physiol. (Lond.)* **290**:481–497.

Hirst, G. D. S., S. J. Redman, and K. Wong (1981) Post-tetanic potentiation and facilitation of synaptic potentials evoked in cat spinal motoneurones. *J. Physiol. (Lond.)* **321**:97–100.

Hubbard, J. I. (1963) Repetitive stimulation at the mammalian neuromuscular junction, and the mobilization of transmitter. *J. Physiol. (Lond.)* **169**:641–662.

Hurlbut, W. P., H. B. Longenecker, Jr., and A. Mauro (1971) Effects of calcium and magnesium on the frequency of miniature end-plate potentials during prolonged tetanization. *J. Physiol. (Lond.)* **219**:17–38.

Katz, B. (1969) *The Release of Neural Transmitter Substances*, Charles C Thomas, Springfield, Illinois.

Katz, B., and R. Miledi (1965) The effect of temperature on the synaptic delay at the neuromuscular junction. *J. Physiol. (Lond.)* **181**:656–670.

Katz, B., and R. Miledi (1968) The role of calcium in neuromuscular facilitation. *J. Physiol. (Lond.)* **195**:481–492.

Katz, B., and R. Miledi (1969) Tetrotoxin-resistant electric activity in presynaptic terminals. *J. Physiol. (Lond.)* **203**:459–487.

Katz, B., and S. Thesleff (1957) A study of the "desensitization" produced by acetylcholine at the motor end-plate. *J. Physiol. (Lond.)* **138**:63–80.

Kretz, R., E. Shapiro, and E. R. Kandel (1982) Post-tetanic potentiation at an identified synapse in *Aplysia* is correlated with a Ca^{2+}-activated K^+ current in the presynaptic neuron: Evidence for Ca^{2+} accumulation. *Proc. Natl. Acad. Sci. USA* **79**:5430–5434.

Kuno, M. (1964) Mechanism of facilitation and depression of the excitatory synaptic potential in spinal motoneurones. *J. Physiol. (Lond.)* **175**:100–112.

Landau, E. M., A. Smolinsky, and Y. Lass (1973) Post-tetanic potentiation and facilitation do not share a common calcium-dependent mechanism. *Nature New Biol.* **244**:155–157.

Lass, Y., Y. Halevi, E. M. Landau, and S. Gitter (1973) A new model for transmitter mobilization in the frog neuromuscular junction. *Pfluegers Arch. Eur. J. Physiol.* **343**:157–163.

Lev-Tov, A., and R. Rahamimoff (1980) A study of tetanic and post-tetanic potentiation of miniature end-plate potentials at the frog neuromuscular junction. *J. Physiol. (Lond.)* **309**:247–273.

Liley, A. W. (1956) The quantal components of the mammalian end-plate potential. *J. Physiol. (Lond.)* **133**:571–587.

Linder, T. M. (1974) The accumulative properties of facilitation at crayfish neuromuscular synapses. *J. Physiol. (Lond.)* **238**:223–234.

Llinás, R., I. Z. Steinberg, and K. Walton (1981) Relationship between presynaptic calcium current and postsynaptic potential in squid giant synapse. *Biophys. J.* **33**:323–352.

McNaughton, B. L. (1980) Evidence for two physiologically distinct perforant pathways to the fascia dentata. *Brain Res.* **199**:1–19.

McNaughton, B. L. (1982) Long-term synaptic enhancement and short-term potentiation in rat fascia dentata act through different mechanisms. *J. Physiol. (Lond.)* **324**:249–262.

Magleby, K. L. (1973a) The effect of repetitive stimulation on facilitation of transmitter release at the frog neuromuscular junction. *J. Physiol. (Lond.)* **234**:327–352.

Magleby, K. L. (1973b) The effect of tetanic and post-tetanic potentiation on facilitation of transmitter release at the frog neuromuscular junction. *J. Physiol. (Lond.)* **234**:353–371.

Magleby, K. L., and B. S. Pallotta (1981) A study of desensitization of acetylcholine receptors using nerve-released transmitter in the frog. *J. Physiol. (Lond.)* **316**:225–250.

Magleby, K. L., and J. E. Zengel (1975a) A dual effect of repetitive stimulation on post-tetanic potentiation of transmitter release at the frog neuromuscular junction. *J. Physiol. (Lond.)* **245**: 163–182.

Magleby, K. L., and J. E. Zengel (1975b) A quantitative description of tetanic and post-tetanic potentiation of transmitter release at the frog neuromuscular junction. *J. Physiol. (Lond.)* **245**: 183–208.

Magleby, K. L., and J. E. Zengel (1976a) Augmentation: A process that acts to increase transmitter release at the frog neuromuscular junction. *J. Physiol. (Lond.)* **257**:449–470.

Magleby, K. L., and J. E. Zengel (1976b) Long-term changes in augmentation, potentiation, and depression of transmitter release as a function of repeated synaptic activity at the frog neuromuscular junction. *J. Physiol. (Lond.)* **257**:471–494.

Magleby, K. L., and J. E. Zengel (1976c) Stimulation-induced factors which affect augmentation and potentiation of transmitter release at the neuromuscular junction. *J. Physiol. (Lond.)* **260**:687–717.

Magleby, K. L., and J. E. Zengel (1982) Quantitative description of stimulation-induced changes in transmitter release at the frog neuromuscular junction. *J. Gen. Physiol.* **80**:613–638.

Mallart, A., and A. R. Martin (1967) An analysis of facilitation of transmitter release at the neuromuscular junction of the frog. *J. Physiol. (Lond.)* **193**:679–694.

Mallart, A., and A. R. Martin (1968) The relation between quantum content and facilitation at the neuromuscular junction of the frog. *J. Physiol. (Lond.)* **196**:593–604.

Martin, A. R., and G. Pilar (1964) Presynaptic and postsynaptic events during posttetanic potentiation and facilitation in the avian ciliary ganglion. *J. Physiol. (Lond.)* **175**:17–30.

Mellow, A. M., B. D. Perry, and E. M. Silinsky (1982) Effects of calcium and strontium in the process of acetylcholine release from motor nerve endings. *J. Physiol. (Lond.)* **328**:547–562.

Miledi, R., and R. Thies (1971) Tetanic and post-tetanic rise in frequency of miniature end-plate potentials in low-calcium solutions. *J. Physiol. (Lond.)* **212**:245–257.

Ohmori, H., S. G. Rayport, and E. R. Kandel (1981) Emergence of posttetanic potentiation as a distinct phase in the differentiation of an identified synapse in *Aplysia*. *Science* **213**:1016–1018.

Otsuka, M., M. Endo, and Y. Nonomura (1962) Presynaptic nature of neuromuscular depression. *Jpn. J. Physiol.* **12**:573–584.

Pallotta, B. S., and K. L. Magleby (1979) Effect of Ca^{++}, Ba^{++}, and Sr^{++} on the kinetics of transmitter release at the frog neuromuscular junction under conditions of normal quantal content. *Soc. Neurosci. Abstr.* **5**:487.

Parnas, H., and L. A. Segel (1980) A theoretical explanation for some of the effects of calcium on the facilitation of neurotransmitter release. *J. Theor. Biol.* **84**:3–29.

Parnas, H., and L. A. Segel (1983) A case study of linear versus non-linear modeling. *J. Theor. Biol.* **103**:549–580.

Parnas, I., J. Dudel, and H. Parnas (1984) Depolarization dependence of the kinetics of phasic transmitter release at the crayfish neuromuscular junction. *Neurosci. Lett.* **50**:157–162.

Porter, R. (1970) Early facilitation at corticomotoneuronal synapses. *J. Physiol. (Lond.)* **207**:733–745.

Quilliam, J. P., and D. L. Tamarind (1973) Some effects of preganglionic nerve stimulation on synaptic vesicle populations in the rat superior cervical ganglion. *J. Physiol. (Lond.)* **235**:317–331.

Rahamimoff, R., A. Lev-Tov, and H. Meiri (1980) Primary and secondary regulation of quantal transmitter release: Calcium and sodium. *J. Exp. Biol.* **89**:5–18.

Rosenthal, J. (1969) Post-tetanic potentiation at the neuromuscular junction of the frog. *J. Physiol. (Lond.)* **203**:121–133.

Silinsky, E. M. (1978) On the role of barium in supporting asynchronous release of acetylcholine quanta by motor nerve impulses. *J. Physiol. (Lond.)* **274**:157–171.

Steinbach, J. H., and C. F. Stevens (1976) Neuromuscular transmission. In *Frog Neurobiology,* R. Llinás and W. Precht, eds., pp. 33–92, Springer-Verlag, Berlin.

Takeuchi, A. (1958) The long-lasting depression in neuromuscular transmission of frog. *Jpn. J. Physiol.* **8**:102–113.

Thies, R. E. (1965) Neuromuscular depression and the apparent depletion of transmitter in mammalian muscle. *J. Neurophysiol.* **28**:427–442.

Weinreich, D. (1971) Ionic mechanism of post-tetanic potentiation at the neuromuscular junction of the frog. *J. Physiol. (Lond.)* **212**:431–446.

Wernig, A. (1972) Changes in statistical parameters during facilitation at the crayfish neuromuscular junction. *J. Physiol. (Lond.)* **226**:751–759.

Younkin, S. G. (1974) An analysis of the role of calcium in facilitation at the frog neuromuscular junction. *J. Physiol. (Lond.)* **237**:1–14.

Zengel, J. E., and K. L. Magleby (1977) Transmitter release during repetitive stimulation: Selective changes produced by Sr^{++} and Ba^{++}. *Science* **197**:67–69.

Zengel, J. E., and K. L. Magleby (1980) Differential effects of Ba^{2+}, Sr^{2+}, and Ca^{2+} on stimulation-induced changes in transmitter release at the frog neuromuscular junction. *J. Gen. Physiol.* **76**:175–211.

Zengel, J. E., and K. L. Magleby (1981) Changes in miniature end-plate potential frequency during repetitive nerve stimulation in the presence of Ca^{2+}, Ba^{2+}, and Sr^{2+} at the frog neuromuscular junction. *J. Gen. Physiol.* **77**:503–529.

Zengel, J. E., and K. L. Magleby (1982) Augmentation and facilitation of transmitter release: A quantitative description at the frog neuromuscular junction. *J. Gen. Physiol.* **80**:583–611.

Zengel, J. E., K. L. Magleby, J. P. Horn, D. A. McAfee, and P. J. Yarowsky (1980) Facilitation, augmentation, and potentiation of synaptic transmission at the superior cervical ganglion of the rabbit. *J. Gen. Physiol.* **76**:213–231.

Zucker, R. S., and L. O. Lara-Estrella (1983) Post-tetanic decay of evoked and spontaneous transmitter release and a residual-calcium model of synaptic facilitation at crayfish neuromuscular junctions. *J. Gen. Physiol.* **81**: 355–372.

Zucker, R. S., and N. Stockbridge (1983) Presynaptic calcium diffusion and the time courses of transmitter release and synaptic facilitation at the squid giant synapse. *J. Neurosci.* **3**:1263–1269.

Chapter 3

Regulation and Significance of Probabilistic Release Mechanisms at Central Synapses

HENRI KORN
DONALD S. FABER

ABSTRACT

Although the quantal aspect of transmitter release has been firmly established at the neuromuscular junction for a long time, the question of whether the same mechanism is also at work in the central nervous system has remained a matter of controversy. Evidence resolving this issue is given here: It is based primarily on the observation that postsynaptic responses produced by a single presynaptic neuron fluctuate in integer steps, the maximum possible number of which corresponds to the total number of release sites issued by a given cell. The probabilistic nature of release (defined by the statistical parameter p), which refers to the chance that each site undergoes exocytosis, constitutes the focus of this chapter. Of the different models that have been proposed, it appears that the binomial model, which assumes equal probability of release at each active zone, most appropriately accounts for the physiological and morphological observations. The slight discrepancies observed between theoretical binomial predictions and the experimental data do not negate this conclusion. Instead, they reflect a previously unreported transformation of the stochastic input by the activated postsynaptic membrane, which acts as a nonlinear processor favoring the occurrence of the "most likely" responses evoked by presynaptic impulses. This finding was obtained by comparing the experimental and theoretical entropies of the underlying variables. The applicability of the Shannon equation to such a problem favors the concept, also developed in this chapter, that quanta are more involved in information processing at central synapses than was previously suspected. It is suggested here that the probabilistic factor, p, is the primary element of the message coded and transmitted at this level. This proposition is founded on several arguments, the major one being that p is a critical presynaptic element that can account for the plasticity of release. A general scheme is advanced to incorporate variations of this parameter occurring in either direction.

The principal feature of evoked transmitter release is undoubtedly its probabilistic nature. Briefly stated, amplitude fluctuations of evoked, chemically mediated, postsynaptic potentials can be described by mathematical models that share one common assumption: Namely, that the response is made up of an integral number of equal basic units called quanta. This notion was derived from observations at the neuromuscular junction (for references, see Katz, 1969), which established that each junction contains n such units capable of being released in response to a nerve impulse with a probability p. Thus, variations of postsynaptic potentials (PSPs) occur in discrete steps, corresponding to quanta of the same size, q. Statistical analysis of such fluctuating responses was facilitated by the fact that spontaneously occurring, miniature end-plate potentials (MEPPs) turn out to be equivalent to single quanta. Poisson statistics adequately describe the composition of evoked potentials: that is, the probability p_x that a given response is made of 1, 2, 3, . . . , x miniature components is given by $p_x = e^{-m} \cdot m^x/x!$ (with m being the average number of packets released, or mean quantal content). This description implies a low probability of release and a large number of packets, and led to the hypothesis that each unit of transmitter represents a synaptic vesicle (del Castillo and Katz, 1954). This formulation has a potentially serious limitation in that it is impossible to give independent meaning to n and p. But in a number of preparations (for references, see McLachlan, 1978), it appears that binomial predictions of the form $p_x = \binom{n}{x} p^x (1 - p)^{n-x}$ fit the data more adequately. Indeed, the argument can be made that this model is more representative of normal physiological events because agreement with the more extreme Poisson predictions was the consequence of artificially lowering p pharmacologically.

The precise statistical properties of quantal release have an importance at central synapses beyond the question of whether a single event occurs. Specifically, although evoked release is probabilistic, some exocytosis from a pool of quantal units is essentially guaranteed, as the probability of getting a response is often close to one. The critical issue, then, seems to be that of the reliability of transmission. However, attempts to gain insight into these questions have been confronted by a great number of difficulties specific to central nervous system neurons and networks. Technical limitations usually preclude reliable simultaneous recordings from pre- and postsynaptic identified cells. Also, these neurons receive numerous distributed inputs. As a consequence, even if a single afferent can be selectively activated, there is no way to distinguish its corresponding MEPPs from background synaptic activity in the target cell. Finally, noise from various sources adds to the evoked PSPs in an unpredictable manner, and distorts their true amplitude. Therefore, it is not surprising that pioneer data about transmitter release in rat (Katz and Miledi, 1963), cat (Kuno, 1964a,b; Burke, 1967; Kuno and Miyahara, 1969; Mendell and Weiner, 1976), and amphibian (Shapovalov and Shiriaev, 1980) motoneurons have essentially been dependent on concepts established at the periphery.

In this chapter we first give some historical background showing that various arbitrarily chosen methods used to analyze the mechanisms of central chemical transmission led, at least initially, to rather conflicting conclusions that are only now being clarified.

Second, the accessibility of the teleost Mauthner cell (M-cell) (Furshpan and Furukawa, 1962) and its inhibitory afferents (Korn and Faber, 1975, 1976) for simultaneous pre- and postsynaptic intracellular recordings at a central synapse has made it a good experimental system in which to solve some of the difficulties mentioned above. More specifically, we found that the binomial representation best fit the probability density functions (or probability density "histograms") of the fluctuating responses, and that for each experiment the value of the binomial parameter n equaled the number of active sites established by the presynaptic cell. In turn, it appears that the action of a single releasing terminal is functionally similar to that of one synaptic vesicle's content. If this conclusion is correct, release at central synapses would have a binary character, with p defining the probability of signal transmission at each site.

Next, although mathematical models can give adequate descriptions of the release properties of central afferent synapses, slight differences between experimental and predicted probability density functions are often observed with an excess number of responses around the means. These (and other) discrepancies have often been taken as an argument to reject the simple binomial model. In reality, they can provide an additional perspective on synaptic function: We show that the discrepancies can be quantified by comparing experimental and theoretical entropies by applying Shannon's equation (1948a,b), which concerns information transfer, to central junctions. A model based on the experimentally derived assumption that the postsynaptic membrane "reorganizes" the binomial input can then be considered.

If q, the quantal size, and n, which is determined structurally, are invariable, it follows that they cannot account for the phenomena underlying synaptic plasticity. Short-term changes in synaptic efficacy are generally due to the regulation of transmitter release accomplished through a modification of p's value. This raises two different, although somewhat related, issues. The first issue is that of the factors which can alter the behavior of this critical parameter. The second issue is that if the quantal parameters of transmission can be used to quantify information transfer at a synapse, in the classic sense of the term, then the critical variables for encoding a message can only be n (although it is prewired) or p, which indeed varies as a function of presynaptic activity, or more likely their product, which is m.

HISTORICAL BACKGROUND

Evidence that Unitary PSPs Fluctuate in Amplitude

The type of paradigm available for the quantal analysis of fluctuating synaptic potentials is illustrated in Figure 1. This example is from an experiment performed in the teleost M-cell system. The technical requisites for recording synaptic potentials while activating an identified input are shown in Figure 1A. In this case, an inhibitory interneuron and its target cell were *simultaneously* impaled by intracellular microelectrodes. Direct stimulation of the interneuron produced inhibitory postsynaptic potentials (IPSPs), which appeared as depolarizing potentials as a result of the iontophoretic injection of chlorine ions into the M-cell. Samples of these potentials and a typical presynaptic impulse are shown in Figure 1B. It is obvious that the IPSP amplitudes vary over a wide range, but that their times to peak and half-decay times remain relatively constant. Qualitatively similar fluctuations have been observed at all central synapses studied in this manner. The difficulties encountered while measuring the size of individual response (obscured by spontaneous potentials or by background noise from different sources) have been discussed extensively elsewhere (Korn et al., 1982) and have been the same in all the experimental models used so far. For example, the noise that distorts the responses is apparent in the single sweep that occurred

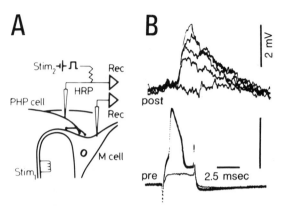

Figure 1. *Quantal fluctuations of unitary inhibitory postsynaptic potentials (IPSPs). A:* Experimental setup for simultaneous intracellular recording (Rec) from the M-cell and a presynaptic interneuron (passive hyperpolarizing potential or PHP cell), both identified by their responses to antidromic stimulation (Stim$_1$). The postsynaptic electrode was filled with potassium chloride so that the inhibitory potentials were depolarizing; the presynaptic electrode was used for intracellular stimulation (Stim$_2$) and for subsequent iontophoretic injections of horseradish peroxidase (HRP) for the histological reconstruction of the stained interneurons. *B:* Unitary IPSPs of variable amplitudes (*upper traces*) produced in the M-cell by single impulses directly evoked in the presynaptic neuron (*lower traces*). Stimulus current (not illustrated) straddled the threshold for spike initiation. (From Korn and Mallet, 1984.)

in the absence of a presynaptic impulse (Figure 1B). Because of these difficulties, and because of the complexity of the inputs impinging on individual neurons, it took years of investigation (and controversy) to ascertain that the primary process underlying the potential fluctuations is the algebraic summation of discrete basic units, or quanta.

A further problem, that of determining whether the potential fluctuations could be related to presynaptic morphology, was only solved even more recently, by staining the presynaptic cell with horseradish peroxidase (HRP) (Figure 1A).

First Hints of Quantal Release at Central Synapses

After the tremendous progress made at the level of the neuromuscular junction, the question naturally arose as to whether chemical transmission in central and autonomic ganglion cells results from the same quantal mechanisms. For example, evidence slowly accumulated that, in autonomic ganglion cells, the mean amplitude of spontaneous potentials approximates that of the smallest evoked synaptic response (unit potential) that constitutes the excitatory postsynaptic potential (EPSP) (Blackman et al., 1963; Martin and Pilar, 1964; Blackman and Purves, 1969; Dennis et al., 1971), and that there is a close resemblance in behavior between these potentials and the spontaneous MEPPs at the neuromuscular junction (Fatt and Katz, 1952). These observations supported the conclusion that such spontaneous potentials are the unit components of normal EPSPs (for further details, see Kuno, 1971), but at most only added to the suggestion that the same conclusion would pertain to central junctions.

Small depolarizing potentials, similar in size and time course to the minimal EPSP evoked by afferent nerve stimulation, were recognized from the very first intracellular recordings performed in cat spinal motoneurons (Brock et al., 1952). They were attributed to synaptic excitation triggered by afferent impulses and/ or by the background discharge of interneurons (see also Kolmodin and Skoglund, 1958; Eccles, 1961a). In the first systematic investigation of central "miniature potentials," which was achieved in the spinal motoneuron of the frog, Katz and Miledi (1963) confirmed that these small depolarizations arose locally from individual synaptic terminals through a mechanism similar to that of MEPPs. However, these authors failed to demonstrate that such units form the building blocks of normal synaptic responses: The amplitude distribution of EPSPs evoked in motoneurons by successive constant stimuli did not show satisfactory agreement with Poisson predictions.

This question was analyzed more successfully by Kuno and his collaborators. Although some of their conclusions were fragmentary, particularly because the binomial model had not yet been recognized as a more powerful analytical tool, their work represents the first important step toward understanding the nature of chemical transmission in central neurons. Monosynaptic activation of cat spinal motoneurons was studied (Kuno, 1964a) by stimulating a limited number of group IA afferent fibers. Fine dissections allowed successful activation of as few as a single filament in some cases. Yet the way in which the recorded EPSPs fluctuated in amplitude suggested "that the mechanism involved in the spinal monosynaptic transmission" might be similar to that at neuromuscular junctions. Two independent and indirect methods were used to calculate the quantal content (del Castillo and Katz, 1954). These relations are

$$ m = \frac{\text{mean amplitudes of EPSP responses } (\bar{v})}{\text{mean amplitudes of spontaneous potentials } (q)} \tag{1} $$

and

$$ m_f = \text{Log}_e \frac{\text{number of afferent impulses } (N)}{\text{number of failures of EPSP responses } (n_0)}, \tag{2} $$

the latter being known as the method of failures.

Although it was impossible to distinguish which spontaneous miniature potentials arose from the fibers under observation, m was calculated from Equation 1 and compared to that obtained with Equation 2. It ranged from 0.63 to 5.4 for both methods; occasionally, there was recruitment of miniature EPSPs following afferent stimulation. These responses were used to evaluate the mean size and variance of the postulated basic unit potential (Figure 2A$_2$), m was obtained from Equation 1, and the expected EPSP distribution was then calculated from the Poisson equation (Figure 2A$_1$). These predictions were generally in good agreement with the observed distributions, and as indicated in the figure, the number of observed failures was quite close to the value predicted by Equation 2. The method was only satisfactory with low m's, discrepancies being observed when the analysis was extended to larger EPSPs ($m > 3$). Attempts to relate m to

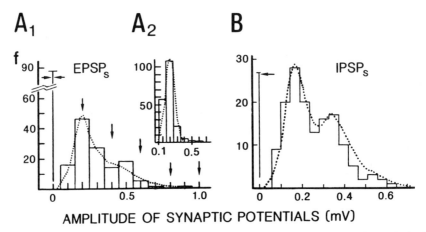

Figure 2. *Early presumptive evidence of the quantal nature of central synaptic transmission obtained with cat spinal motoneurons. A_1 and A_2: Applicability of Poisson's law. A_1: Histogram showing the amplitude distribution of monosynaptic excitatory postsynaptic potentials (EPSPs) evoked by stimulation of a single Ia afferent fiber (response failures are shown by the* vertical line *at 0). The theoretical distribution and number of failures are indicated by the* dotted curve *and the* horizontal arrows, *respectively; the peaks of the EPSP amplitudes corresponding to multiples of the putative unit size are indicated by* vertical arrows. *A_2: Amplitude distribution of miniature EPSPs recorded during the same experiment. (From Kuno, 1964a.) B: Demonstration that amplitude fluctutions of monosynaptic IPSPs produced by stimulation of local interneurons can be described by binomial estimations (dotted curve). The* arrow *points toward the number of predicted failures. (From Kuno and Weakly, 1972.)*

structure were unwarranted, since the assumption that the fibers usually have about three knobs on a motoneuron seems unrealistic on the basis of recent data obtained with HRP staining (Burke et al., 1979).

The first inference for quantal release of transmitter at vertebrate inhibitory synapses was based on the presence of spontaneous miniature IPSPs in spinal motoneurons of the frog (Katz and Miledi, 1963; Colomo and Erulkar, 1968) and of the cat (Blankenship and Kuno, 1968). But despite their small amplitude, and their persistence after application of tetrodotoxin in the cat, it was not clear whether the IPSPs were composed of all-or-none unit potentials until Kuno and Weakly (1972) investigated their fluctuations in cat motoneurons. Attempts were made to fit Poisson predictions with amplitude histograms of monosynaptic IPSPs evoked by intraspinal stimuli. Since some of these histograms showed several peaks (three of them can be distinguished in Figure 2B), it was assumed that the first peak represented the mean amplitude of the basic unit potential (called v_1), which would be distributed normally about the mean with a coefficient of variation (CV) of 30% (Martin, 1966). The mean quantal content, m, was estimated from the relation $m = v/v_1$, where v is the mean amplitude of observed IPSPs. However, the Poisson equations did not adequately predict the number of failures or the distribution of recorded IPSPs.

Two alternative explanations were considered: nonlinear summation of unit potentials (del Castillo and Katz, 1954; Martin, 1955) or a high probability of release (see also Johnson and Wernig, 1971). These two possibilities were tested by comparing the m values obtained with the method of failures, f, and with the CV technique, where

$$m_{cv} = \frac{1}{(\text{CV})^2} \cdot \tag{3}$$

For a Poisson distribution, the calculated m's should be equal, but m_{cv} was always greater than m_f, ruling out that model, as well as a nonlinear summation of unit potentials.

On the other hand, the fit of the curve obtained with binomial predictions for the same observed distribution was remarkably good, as shown in Figure 2B. The parameters of this second description were again derived in a somewhat indirect manner, starting with the notion that, for a binomial prediction, there should be a linear relationship between m_{cv} and m_f if p is constant. This relation is given (Kuno, 1964a; Johnson and Wernig, 1971) by

$$m_{cv} = \frac{-p}{(1 - p) \cdot \ln(1 - p)} m_f \cdot \tag{4}$$

Once the value of p is known (here approximately 0.5 from the slope of the relation between m_{cv} and m_f), the number of failures can be predicted from

$$m = \frac{-p}{\ln(1 - p)} \ln \frac{N}{n_0}, \tag{5}$$

and the number of responses with x quanta by

$$n_x = n_{x-1} \frac{m - p(x - 1)}{x(1 - p)}, \tag{6}$$

where $x = 1, 2, 3, \ldots, n$ quanta, from which the curve of Figure 2B was computed.

In retrospect, one can say that these data laid the groundwork for further analysis of the nature of release in the central nervous system. To our surprise, we even noted that the conductance increase resulting from a unit IPSP was calculated as $5\text{–}8 \times 10^{-9}$ S, which is about two to three times greater than that for a unit EPSP in motoneurons (Kuno, 1964a; Kuno and Miyahara, 1969) and is comparable to our own results with the M-cell (Korn et al., 1982; see also below). However, rather fortunate conditions were probably encountered at that time from which generalizations could not yet be made. For instance, from the relation $n = m/p$, n was estimated to be very low, which is unrealistic, as was already indicated by Kuno and Weakly themselves. It is also surprising that, although the contribution of noise was not considered (synapses being treated as similar to neuromuscular junctions), the binomial fit of the data was so good.

Clearly, no conclusion could be reached about the preferred model for central transmission. Along this line, in a subsequent quantal analysis of Ia-EPSPs in single motoneurons, Mendell and Weiner (1976) used the method of failures in 33 cases: Twenty-two satisfied the Poisson Law and six satisfied the bino-mial predictions, while the remaining ones satisfied neither. These discrepancies were not explained by the authors, although the contributions of synaptic ac-tivity noise to shunting EPSPs and of nonlinear summation of PSPs were dis-cussed briefly.

SEARCH FOR NEW PARADIGMS

Because the Poisson and the classic binomial models of quantal release failed to match all experimental data in the central nervous system, alternative analytical procedures were adopted. Despite major conceptual progress resulting in part from their mathematical sophistication, these analyses did not initially lead to a clarification of the specific mechanisms of transmission at central neurons, nor to a better characterization of their morphological bases (in this section we adhere to the symbols and terminology adopted in the various studies).

Removing the Masking Effects of Noise

Focusing their work on the distortion of synaptic potentials by noise, Redman and his collaborators analyzed the fluctuations of EPSPs evoked in cat spinal motoneurons by impulses in single Ia afferent fibers. Basically, three major assumptions were made. The first was that "true" uncontaminated synaptic potentials took a finite number of values, but that their distribution and probabilities of occurrence could not be postulated *a priori*. In other words, and in contrast to preceding investigations, no initial hypothesis was made about the type of distribution that best described the fluctuations. The second was that background activity contaminated the records; its statistical nature (i.e., its amplitude fluc-tuations) was found to be a Gaussian function, the mean and variance of which were assessed from recordings of the membrane potential at a particular time following the stimulus. Third, it was postulated that the noise fluctuations were independent from those of synaptic potentials, and that the two added linearly (the probability density of noisy peak voltage being a convolution of the probability density function of noise voltage with that of the noise-free synaptic potential). The integral resulting from this process was solved for the noise-free synaptic-potential probability density function through a process called deconvolution.

Principles of the Deconvolution Method.   The techniques, which have been described elsewhere (Edwards et al., 1976a,b; Wong and Redman, 1980), can be summarized by considering the probability density function Y of the noisy synaptic potentials as the convolution product of the noise-free probability density function S with that of noise N. Whether the measured parameter of the synaptic potential is the charge transfer (Edwards et al., 1976a) or its peak voltage (Jack et al., 1981a), S can be considered as representing a set of impulse functions

$$S(V) = S_1\delta(V - V_1) + S_2\delta(V - V_2) + \cdots + S_n\delta(V - V_n) ,$$

where $V_{k+1} - V_k = \Delta V$ (ΔV is also the bin width of the histogram classes into which potential values are allocated). The movements between successive amplitudes of the components is constrained by the intervals selected for the histogram. For the kth class, the probability that the noisy synaptic potential lies between V_{k+1} and V_k is

$$Y_k = \sum_{i=1}^{k} S_i N_{k+1-i} , \qquad (7)$$

where

$$N_k = \int_{(k-1)\Delta v + v^1}^{k\Delta v + v^1} N(v)dv .$$

In fact, Equation 7 results from discretization of the convolution formula

$$Y(v) = \int_{v_1}^{v_u} N(v - x) S(x)dx ,$$

where v_u and v_l are bounds selected according to practical considerations.

Figure 3 is a schematic illustration of the method: A deconvolved histogram with two separate peaks is shown in Figure 3A$_1$; the uncontaminated synaptic potentials have two possible values, v_1 and v_2. The solid curves represent the two convolution products ($NS_1\delta(v - v_1)$ and $NS_2\delta(v_1 - v_2)$, where N is the probability density function of the Gaussian noise. The sum of these two products is indicated by the dashed line; it is the convolution product and therefore would be the "histogram of the recorded potentials" (Edwards et al., 1976b). The probabilities S_1 and S_2 of the values v_1 and v_2 are indicated by the vertical bars in Figure 3A$_2$.

More practically, the problem was to recover S, the noise-free random variable, from sample estimates of Y and N; since the true values of those two functions were not known, conventional recursive methods would have been misleading. The Redman group made a compromise between the "classical recursive methods of deconvolution" and the more traditional approach of quantal analysis (which used *a priori* assumptions about the form of the noise-free EPSP fluctuations). Intuitively, they guessed the size and the probability of occurrence of components making up the uncontaminated Ia-EPSP, computed the convolution of this distribution and the Gaussian noise for each k, $W_k = \Sigma_{v=1} SN$, and evaluated the fit with the experimental histogram by using a square difference criterion: $\Sigma_{k=1}^{n}(Y_k - W_k)^2$. They implemented a nonlinear optimization algorithm to find the distribution of the probabilities that gave the best fit of the selected histogram (according to the defined criterion) with the experimental data.

An example of the results obtained with this procedure is presented in Figure 3B$_1$–B$_2$. The rectangles in Figure 3B$_3$ stand for the probabilities of the components identified from the experimental histogram (EPSP + noise) shown in Figure 3B$_2$. The components are actually located at the lower bound of each rectangle. The reliability of the uncontaminated EPSP fluctuation pattern was checked by convolving the estimated probability density function with that of the noise; the resulting probability density function was then compared with the experimental one by computing a chi-square test.

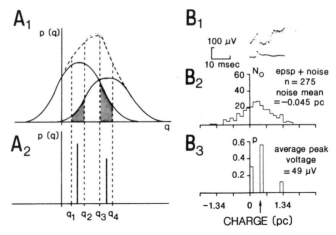

Figure 3.   *Removal of the masking effects of noise to reveal the underlying distribution of fluctuating synaptic potentials. A_1 and A_2:* Illustration of the convolution method showing two probability densities for amplitude indices. A_2 consists of two entries representing discrete EPSPs. When Gaussian noise is superimposed on these two peaks, overlapping probability densities (A_1, *solid curves*) are obtained; their addition gives the measured probability density function (A_1, *dashed curve*), which is the probability density function of the EPSPs + noise. The boundaries (q_1 and q_2; q_3 and q_4) that are selected for each peak determine the range (*shaded areas* in A_1) of the responses used to estimate the corresponding average time courses. (From Edwards et al., 1976b.) B_1– B_3: Results obtained with the procedure described above during the analysis of statistical fluctuations in charge transfer at Ia synapses. B_1: Standard deviation of the mean (*upper trace*) and mean time course (*lower trace*) of 275 EPSPs evoked by the stimulation of a single Ia fiber. B_2: Distribution of EPSP charges, with the indicated mean and standard deviation of the noise histogram. B_3: Computed result for charge variations resulting from the EPSP alone (mean indicated by *arrow*) showing two different charge contents and failures. (From Edwards et al., 1976a.)

Some of the constraints imposed by the deconvolution method were pointed out (Wong and Redman, 1980); they are the consequence of finite sampling and noise amplitude. These two limiting factors determine the bin width of the histograms and the resolution of the adjacent components. For the sample sizes used by the authors, that is, between 400 (Edwards et al., 1976a,b) and 1600 (Jack et al., 1981a), the number of classes should be no more than 25. Furthermore, the deconvolution of a simulated Poisson process and noise showed other limits of the technique (Wong and Redman, 1980): When the standard deviation of the noise was half the quantal size, the discrimination of discrete components could be carried out with accuracy, but for larger values equal to the quantum size, some components disappeared after the deconvolution, and the location of the remaining ones was sometimes unreliable.

In a further control, Wong and Redman tested the ability of their algorithm to resolve adjacent components. They showed that, if only two amplitudes occurred, the resolution limit: (1) depends on the respective probabilities of each component, being best when they are equal; and (2) is never less than the noise standard deviation (in extreme cases it was twice this value). Furthermore, discrete components with probability values of less than 0.05 were not considered (because they were taken to be statistically unreliable). *In our own experience, this requirement probably represents the weak point of the method in that it generates a serious contradiction.* That is, rare events are dropped, although in a probabilistic system they are a critical aspect of the expected data pool. Indeed, they provide hints about even rarer occurrences that are statistically unlikely to appear, even with a large number of counts.

Fluctuating Results of a Sophisticated Method

The "Nonquantal" Statement. To improve the rather poor signal-to-noise ratio, Edwards et al. (1976a) computed the total charge transfer to the Ia-evoked EPSPs (which is the integral of the EPSP over its complete time course divided by the input resistance at the soma) rather than its peak amplitude. Figure $3B_2$ illustrates a histogram of such charge transfers. With this procedure, the deconvolved histograms showed only a few components. Increments between them differed from one neuron to the other, and those extracted from a single neuronal pattern of fluctuations did not look like multiples of a basic unit. For example, in Figure $3B_3$, the magnitudes of the first and second entries are about 0.50 and 1.30 pC, respectively. It was thus suggested that the basic mode of transmission at a single terminal is all or none (rather than graded in quantal steps), and that the fluctuations resulted from the combined effect of failures at several terminals arising from a single afferent fiber. Yet the authors mentioned that their results were not unique, and they recognized that at least some of the histograms could be fit by either the Poisson or the binomial predictions. However, it must be pointed out that the way in which the quantal parameters were determined was not detailed by the authors. In fact, the classic models were not fully tested and thus were not given a real chance: They were rejected after simple comparisons between the standard deviation and the mean time course of the whole EPSP. Furthermore, it was necessary to postulate that the probability of release differed from one terminal to another.

Edwards et al. (1976a) also developed a method to determine the shape parameters of the components that build up single EPSPs.

Once deconvolution had been carried out, intervals were selected around each discrete component (Figure $3A_1$–A_2). The average contribution of each discrete component to the noisy EPSPs whose values fall within those limits can be computed. In Figure $3A_1$, the contribution of the larger component to the small EPSPs lying within q_1 and q_2 corresponds to the smallest shadowed area, and so on. If $v(t)$ is the mean value at time t of the EPSPs lying within those bounds, $v_1(t)$ is the value of the smaller component at time t, $v_2(t)$ is the value of the larger component at time t, and p and $1 - p$ are the respective contributions of those components, then $v(t) = p \cdot v_1(t) + (1 - p) \cdot v_2(t) + K_1$, where K_1 is an additive constant because of the noise, which can easily be removed.

Similar assumptions can be made about the EPSPs around the larger component. Thus, for any time t, a set of two linear equations with two unknowns $v_1(t)$ and $v_2(t)$ is available, and these variables can be extracted. The component shape indices were analyzed and, on the basis of their differences, distinct synaptic locations were deduced from a cable model.

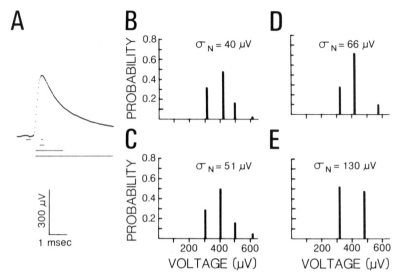

Figure 4. *Sensitivity of the deconvolution method to the signal-to-noise ratio.* A: Average of the Ia EPSP further analyzed in Figure 5. A region for baseline calculation is shown below the record, as well as four regions of integration, all of which enclose the peak of the synaptic potential. The average peak voltage over this period was 397 μV, and this scaling applied to all the components of the EPSP. The different scaled values of σ_N (noise variance) are indicated in B, C, D, and E, where the deconvolved peak voltages are also illustrated (B shows the shortest period). Note that there is little difference between B and C, but that as the period of integration is increased (and therefore so is σ_N), the results become unreliable, with adjacent components of the distribution amalgamating because of a reduced resolution of fluctuations. (From Jack et al., 1981a.)

Thus, the heterogeneity of the synaptic locations of the components of a unitary EPSP could already be demonstrated, although the noisy appearance of the records prevented a more detailed study of their time course.

Better Resolution of EPSP Components. A critical step forward was made when it became obvious (Jack et al., 1981a) that using charge transfer as an EPSP amplitude index was misleading: Instead, integration of noise throughout a length of time equivalent to the whole duration of the EPSP reduced the signal-to-noise level and, accordingly, the resolution of fluctuations, as illustrated in Figure 4. The different integration periods are shown in Figure 4A, and the corresponding *deconvolved* histograms in Figure 4B–E; they are arranged in order of increasing duration. There is little difference between Figure 4B and C, where four distinct peaks with a mean increment of about 100 μV are visible (see also Figure 5). The increase of N for the two longest periods of Figure 4D and E makes the results quite different, since adjacent components amalgamate under these conditions.

The discrepancies between the four distributions of the experiments described above led Jack et al. (1981a) to reevaluate the earlier hypothesis of nonquantal release. For the experiment illustrated in Figures 4 and 5, the apparent unit size was determined after measuring EPSP peak amplitudes, for a noise standard deviation of less than 50 μV. The question was critical, because the histogram shown in Figure 5A could be fit by either a Poisson distribution (assuming $q = 14$ μV and $m = 28$) or a binomial distribution (assuming $q = 50$ μV, $n = 11$, and $p = 0.75$). To rule out these alternative fits to the one illustrated in Figure 5B, which indicates only four distinct peaks, Jack et al. (1981a) extracted the shape indices of each of these four components. The smallest one is presented in Figure 5C. For each amplitude range delineated in Figure 5A$_1$, the variance of the associated EPSP sample was computed. Then the variance of the biased noise involved in the generation of the noisy EPSP was subtracted, and by so doing the variance of the supposed pattern of fluctuations of the noise-free EPSP was obtained. The conclusion was that each component identified by the deconvolution algorithm could not be the envelope of several other components because there

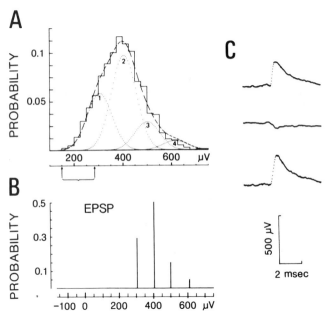

Figure 5. *Evidence that Ia EPSPs fluctuate between different components that are integer multiples of a unit synaptic potential.* For this study, peak voltage, instead of total charge, was measured for each individual EPSP. *A*: Histogram of the peak voltage of 800 EPSPs evoked in a spinal motoneuron following stimulation of a small branch of the nerve to the medial gastrocnemius. *B*: Deconvolved probabilities, calculated by using a Gaussian curve for noise (not shown), demonstrating that four components underlie the measured histogram in *A*. Their peak voltages are 302, 406, 505, and 607 μV, and their respective probabilities are 0.29, 0.50, 0.16, and 0.05. The *four curves* in *A*, labeled 1–4, are Gaussian distributions that have means equal to the corresponding peak amplitudes, and standard deviations equal to that of the noise (51.4 μV). They were scaled in area according to the associated probabilities of occurrence. The sum of these four distributions, indicated by the *dashed line*, matched the experimental histogram; the basic unit synaptic potential was about 100 μV. *C*: Extraction of an EPSP component following deconvolution. The *upper trace* shows an average EPSP obtained by selecting response ($n = 66$) with peak voltages in the range of 150–270 μV (indicated by the *vertical arrows* in the *lower left corner* of *A*). The *middle trace* shows average corresponding noise records ($n = 213$) for which the voltage was in the range of −152 to −32 μV. The *lower trace* is a record of the difference between the *upper* and *middle traces*. (From Jack et al., 1981a.)

was no significant variance remaining after the subtraction. Three other EPSPs with two, three, and five discrete entries, respectively, were analyzed with binomial and Poisson statistics. For this purpose, the quantum size, q, was defined as the mean increment found by the deconvolution method; for binomial parameters, n was the number of "quanta" in the largest identified component. This might have been a dangerous way of estimating such parameters; some loss of information might have occurred when histograms of the data were created. Furthermore, evaluation of the results was difficult: Since the models were not embedded, there was no theoretical way of testing these hypotheses against one another.

Nevertheless, this work showed that, in contrast to previous findings, Ia-evoked EPSPs fluctuated between different components of a particular discrete amplitude, which averaged about 90 μV for those generated at or near the soma. Yet the authors still argued against the notion that each component represented the addition of a further quantum of transmitter. Two sets of arguments were used. In the first, the lack of variability in amplitude of the increment of a single component (Edwards et al., 1976a; Jack et al., 1981a), which had a CV of less than 5%, led the authors to postulate that a saturation of the postsynaptic receptors accounted for the constancy of the postsynaptic response. Two points should be kept in mind here: The saturation of the postsynaptic receptors, with less than 5% response variability, was highly unlikely, at least in the context of present notions about transmitter–receptor interactions. More specifically, it is now well established that not all bound receptor–channel complexes are activated, particularly since rapid multiple binding is required for each (unless the Hill coefficient is 1!), which necessarily leaves a significant fraction available for an additional amount of transmitter. Such a constancy of unit amplitudes might actually indicate that the individual components are due to synchronous release from some or all terminal boutons disposed in separate clusters. Smaller potentials and/or smaller quanta would simply be buried in noise, or discarded during the analysis because of their rare occurrence (see above). In the second set of arguments, an analysis of the shape indices of the components showed that each was generated at a different synaptic location (Edwards et al., 1976a; Jack et al., 1981a). But although the electrotonic distance to the soma can reach one membrane space constant, and although linear cable theory would predict a 10-fold attenuation of the signal in such a situation, there was a constant increment of somatic responses. However, the number of receptors involved in response generation at remote synapses was assumed to be larger (as many as 10 times) than that involved at somatic junctions. Again, different groupings of some presynaptic terminals could account for these results as well.

The Ineffective Synapses Hypothesis.   New problems were raised when the results of the deconvolution method were confronted with histological data obtained by filling the Ia afferent fibers under study with HRP (Redman and Walmsley, 1983a,b). The deconvolutions were carried out on large sample sizes (1600 counts) and the EPSP shape indices were also determined: It then turned out that the number of connections established by the stimulated fiber on the target motoneuron was greater than or equal to the number of increments that must be added to produce the largest EPSP (Redmand and Walmsley, 1983b). This result was certainly consistent with the notion of an all-or-none release at terminals, but one had to postulate further that, at most cells, a fraction of the terminal boutons are silent at low rates of stimulation, while others release with a high p.

Data from two of the four pairs used for this study are shown in Figure 6. In the first case (Figure $6A_1$–A_2), three terminal boutons were identified, and the EPSP fluctuated between three discrete amplitudes in approximately 90-μV steps. Assuming that each bouton generated an identical EPSP at the soma, the computed p indicated that no transmission failure ($p = 1$) occurred at one of them, while the two others released independently, with p equaling 0.81 and 0.38, respectively. This result also seems to rule out the Poisson and binomial models, although the tests that were applied in Jack et al. (1981a) to search for additional (unresolved) amplitudes could not be used because of the considerable overlap of the distributions associated with each component.

The second reconstruction (Figure $6B_1$–B_2) illustrates another termination pattern with eight terminals and a single discrete component. As this single entry was located at about 200 μV, it was concluded that two of the boutons

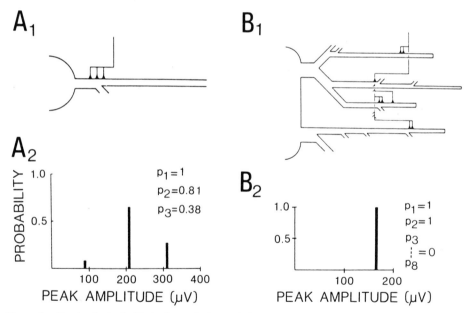

Figure 6. *Results obtained with the deconvolution method requiring the notion of silent synapses for conciliation with the morphological data. A_1 and A_2: Comparison of histological and fluctuation analysis events. A_1: Schematic diagram of an Ia terminal that was stimulated at a low rate and was subsequently filled with HRP for histological reconstruction. Three boutons are visible on a proximal dendrite of the postsynaptic cell. A_2: Fluctuation pattern of the EPSPs evoked in the motoneuron by the presynaptic connection. Three peaks are visible; they were interpreted as indicating that transmission always occurred at one bouton ($p_1 = 1$) and was intermittent at the others ($p_2 = 0.81$ and $p_3 = 0.38$). B_1 and B_2: Data from another experiment. B_1: Eight boutons were in contact with the motoneuron on four different dendrites. B_2: Deconvolved probability density function of the EPSP peak amplitude suggesting that the synaptic potential did not fluctuate in amplitude. These results were thought to indicate constant synaptic transmission at two boutons only (p_1 and $p_2 = 1$), the six others remaining inactive at this frequency of stimulation. (From Redman and Walmsley, 1983b.)*

were always active ($p = 1$), with discrete increments of about 100 μV, while the remaining six were always silent. But again, it seems to us that subcomponents with amplitudes of less than 200 μV could hardly have been separated, since the standard deviation of the noise in this case was 167 μV. Besides, there is no compelling reason to believe that every increment or quantum must be equal in all cells. It would, in fact, be surprising if this were the case.

Compound Binomial Models

The conclusion of Redman's group that p is not the same at all terminals leads to the more general question of the possible effects of spatial variations in p (nonuniformity) and of temporal variations in p or n (nonstationarity) on binomial estimations. In describing the quantal hypothesis, del Castillo and Katz (1954) had already stated that "different members of the population may not have the same chance of success, and that for large values of m, some units may have a high probability, while others have a low probability. . . ." Also, it was concluded that during depression at the Mauthner–giant fiber synapse of the hatchetfish, evoked release probability must approach unity at some release sites and zero at others (Highstein and Bennett, 1975). Detailed mathematical analyses and computer simulations have shown (Brown et al., 1976) that such variations can drastically bias the estimates, whereas the experimental histograms remain indistinguishable from those predicted by binomial law (at least with regard to minimal statistical tests; for a discussion of equivalence between different binomial fits, see Korn et al., 1982). Brown et al. used a hypothetical synapse that had 50 sites (n), each with a probability that a quantum was released ($p = 0.2$), leading to an expected m of 10. The computer was then "stimulated" 1000 times. Because we found (see above) that n is constant, we consider here only the possible effects of variations in p.

Nonuniformity of **p.** With a simple binomial model, the sample m and its variance S^2 can be used (see Ginsborg and Jenkinson, 1976) to derive

$$\tilde{p} = 1 - (S^2/m) , \tag{8}$$

with $\tilde{p}$ being the estimated p.

With n constant and p varying randomly among release sites (and remaining constant over time at each site), it can be shown (Brown et al., 1976) that Equation 8 overestimates the mean probability of p_1 (see also Zucker, 1973; Bennett et al., 1976) and leads to an underestimation of n (since $n = m/p$). An example of a distribution produced by modeling such conditions is shown in Figure 7A, where nonuniformity gave $\tilde{p} = 0.72$ and $\tilde{n} = 14$ (for the real values of 0.2 and 50, respectively). This indicates that considerable errors can result from the use of Equation 8 if variance of p exists.

As discussed by McLachlan (1978), the distribution of p (with $p = 0.103$ in his example) may contain a high proportion of $p \approx 0$. This raises the question, also considered by others (Barton and Cohen, 1977), of whether a unit with a very low probability really contributes to the value of n in a finite series of

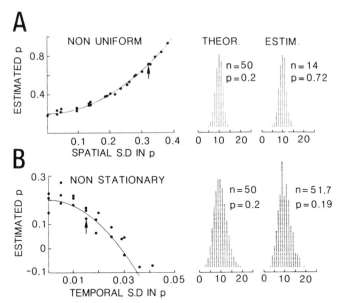

Figure 7. *Bias of binomial parameter* n *and* p *estimates when fitting data with a compound binomial model. A and B: Results of computer simulations of the distribution of quanta (n = 10,000) released at a hypothetical synapse at which n = 50 and p = 0.2. Left: Estimated p as a function of the spatial (A) or temporal (B) standard deviation; curves are theoretically derived, points are from computer experiments. Middle: Corresponding simple binomial histograms based on selected n and p. Right: Observed repartitions of quanta released with the indicated estimates of n and p, for the cases indicated by the arrows in the graphs at the left. Note that despite an incorrect estimation of the binomial parameters, the two histograms are nearly identical in A, whereas in B, reasonable estimates still result in a poor fit around the mean of the distribution: Spatial variation causes p to be overestimated; temporal variation has an opposite effect and leads quickly to negative values of p. (From Brown et al., 1976.)*

observations. If not, a model that gives n as the number of sites at which release can occur is inappropriate. This problem is in reality quite abstract, at least with regard to our experiments, as additional structure–function correlations have indeed shown the validity of the simple binomial model (see above).

Nonstationarity of **p**. If p varies temporally, its estimate, as obtained with Equation 8, will then be less than the actual mean probability (Brown et al., 1976), the discrepancy being slight, as in Figure 7B, or appreciably larger. A clear lack of fit of the observed distribution with that predicted from these estimates occurs around the mean, possibly reflecting some aspect of the program used in this study (see Barton and Cohen, 1977; McLachlan, 1978). Furthermore, unless n is very small, a large variance of p will give an estimated $\tilde{p}$ of negative value, suggesting that the simple model does not apply, because significant variation of this type is hardly conceivable.

There seems to be no need, in fact, to search for a perfect fit of biological data that are generally subjected to at least some measurement errors. It makes more sense to confront the "imperfect" fits with other known biological properties of the system being studied.

Does Presynaptic Release Combine Poisson and Binomial Statistics?

In an original work (Shapovalov and Shiriaev, 1980), the isolated frog spinal cord was used for quantal analysis of monosynaptic EPSPs evoked by activation of single dorsal root fibers. These EPSPs had two components: an early component resulting from electrical transmission and a later chemical component. Taking the electrotonic component as an index of the invasion of the presynaptic fiber, it was shown that replacement of external calcium by manganese could reversibly abolish chemical transmission or reduce m (which varied from 1 to 10) until the response fluctuated according to a Poisson distribution, with the unit EPSP equivalent to the (presumed) single quantum of transmitter. It was found that of 23 experiments, 7 were fit by a Poisson distribution (when m was less than 3) and 9 by a binomial distribution (p varied from 0.2 to 0.7). Neither set of predictions fit the histograms at the 7 remaining connections, but interestingly, the deviation from a stochastic distribution could be attributed to variable invasion of the terminal region by the nerve impulse, as determined from the behavior of the electrical component.

In further investigations with frog spinal cord (Grantyn et al., 1982, 1984a,b), attempts were made to correlate release parameters with structure after staining the primary afferent fibers with HRP (Figure 8A–B). The reconstruction of the labeled elements showed that some of the presynaptic boutons tended to be grouped into clusters termed synaptic contacts. The amplitude fluctuation of the EPSPs could be fit this time by both Poisson and binomial distributions. Since the unit potential, or quantal size estimated from Poisson equations, was two or three times smaller than that derived from binomial statistics, and since a similar quantitative relationship was found between the total number of contacting boutons and that of contact zones, it was concluded that, at single active sites, transmission results in the release of a single quantum of transmitter, whereas the binomial quantum reflects the multiquantal release occurring simultaneously at the boutons constituting a contact region. Data used to substantiate this conclusion are shown in Figure 8.

To obtain this result, the authors assumed that V_{max} (the largest recorded response) was brought about by the activation of the total number of active sites; they derived v, the Poisson quantal size, from $m = 1/CV^2$ and $v = \overline{V}/m$. Similarly, the binomial parameters were obtained from $p = V/V_{max}$ (V is the mean EPSP amplitude), $m = 1 - p/CV^2$, and $v = \overline{V}/m$; the number of units was then $n = m/p$. For the example shown in Figure 8, the derived Poisson m and n were 10.6 and 25, respectively ($v = 30$ μV and $p = 0.11$), and the binomial p and v were 0.20 and 69 μV, respectively ($n = 8$). It is surprising that the authors did not try to test their initial assumption that V_{max} was due to the activation of all the available release sites by calculating the chance that it would be observed, for instance, in a series of 400 EPSPs (their maximum number of trials). For the Poisson results, this expectation is given by e^{-m} $(m^n/n!) \cdot 400$, which here is no more than 2.7×10^{-2} (i.e., the largest possible response should occur once every 15,000 trials). For the binomial data, the expectation is given by $(p^n) \cdot 400$, which yields 1×10^{-3} (i.e., 400,000 responses are required to expect one in which all terminals are activated). Otherwise stated, it is clear that the basic assumption upon which this work was based is not experimentally supported.

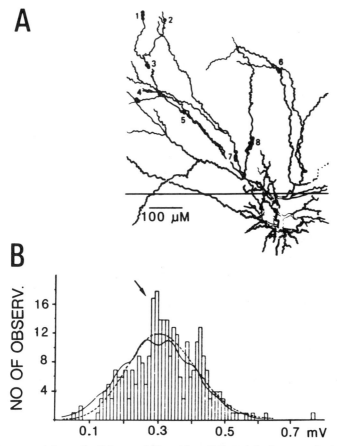

Figure 8. *Discrepancy between the Poisson and binomial predictions at the frog sensorimotor synapse, and its postulated interpretation. A*: Location of contacting boutons established on a motoneuron by a single HRP-filled presynaptic fiber (their total number was 26; each one is indicated by a *filled circle*). The numbers 1–8 refer to individual "contact regions," that correspond to a tight cluster of boutons. *B*: Histogram of amplitude distributions of EPSPs evoked by stimulation of this presynaptic afferent. The *dashed* and *continuous curves* were drawn according to the Poisson and binomial predictions, respectively. Assuming that the maximal EPSP amplitude was due to the activation of all release sites, and using the coefficient of variation technique, the number of release sites estimated from the Poisson model was 25, whereas the predicted binomial number of quanta was 9. These results were taken to mean (see text) that the difference between Poisson and binomial unit potentials reflects the difference between the quantum potentials produced by a single bouton and those produced by a tight cluster of terminals forming a contact zone. (From Grantyn et al., 1984b.)

BINOMIAL DESCRIPTION OF RELEASE AT A CENTRAL INHIBITORY SYNAPSE AND ITS MORPHOFUNCTIONAL IMPLICATIONS

The M-cell of teleosts triggers an escape reaction by means of a contralateral tail flip and is subjected to a powerful inhibitory control (reviewed in Faber and Korn, 1978). In this task, the M-cell displays all the major synaptic mechanisms identified to date in vertebrates and thus was rightly named a "miniature brain"

(Kuffler and Nicholls, 1976). It is ideally suited for quantal analysis of its IPSPs because both the M-cell and its individual presynaptic interneurons can be identified (Faber and Korn, 1973; Korn and Faber, 1975), and simultaneous intracellular recordings can be obtained from them (Korn and Faber, 1976). This alone would permit a mathematical treatment of evoked unitary IPSPs. In the M-cell, the voltage recorded during the IPSP is a fairly direct measure of the underlying conductance change; however, critical progress was also made by staining individual cells with HRP, which allowed some parameters to be related to physical entities.

A computer program enabled us to determine whether the Poisson or the binomial representation, combined with noise, gave the best fit with the histogram of the evoked responses. This part of our work was possible because the M-cell system satisfies the requirements for a reliable extraction of binomial parameters, including steady-state conditions (McLachlan, 1978) that can be maintained during the sampling period. To our surprise, we found that in each experiment the values of the binomial parameter n and the number of presynaptic knobs established on the M-cell were equal: Thus, each individual terminal bouton functions as an independent all-or-none unit. These results led to other investigations suggesting that the action of a single releasing terminal is functionally similar to that of a single synaptic vesicle's contents.

Methods

Because the techniques and theoretical considerations necessary for this work have been described extensively elsewhere, they are summarized only briefly here.

Electrophysiological Techniques and Data Analysis.   The experiments were performed on goldfish (*Carassius auratus*; see Furshpan and Furukawa, 1962; Korn and Faber, 1975). Because the IPSP in the M-cell is hard to detect as a potential change, chlorine ions were iontophoretically injected through the recording microelectrode; thus, unitary IPSPs appeared as depolarizing potentials (Figure 9A). Responses were evoked at the rate of one or two per second (unless otherwise stated) and stored on tape for measurement and statistical analysis. Values of peak amplitudes (sample size generally equaled 100–300) and estimated noise variances (Figure 9B) were fed to a computer, which was programmed (1) to calculate *with a free search* the probability density function of each series of counts and the optimal corresponding parameters that fit the histogram, assuming either a Poisson or binomial distribution; and (2) to estimate whether either model satisfied an independent test, the Kolmogorov. If necessary, the measured responses were corrected for any nonlinearity between postsynaptic voltage and conductance change (Martin, 1955).

The statistical analyses were based on a model in which fluctuations in both evoked IPSPs and background noise summate algebraically according to the equation $\mu = qX + B$, where μ is the observed random variable, q is the elementary or quantum size, X is either the Poisson or binomial variable, and B is the noise process. The latter was approximated as white (uncorrelated) and Gaussian (Jazwinski, 1970) with a constant variance, σ^2, which was assessed from direct

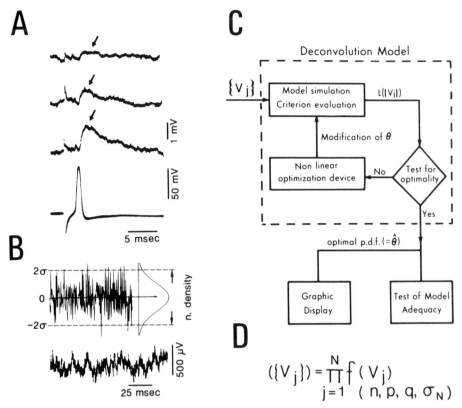

Figure 9. *Computer program used for quantal analysis of fluctuating postsynaptic potentials. A and B:* Samples of potentials *(V$_j$)* whose amplitudes were processed for computation. *A:* Fluctuating monosynaptic depolarizing IPSPs (indicated by *arrows* in the *three upper traces*) directly following evoked presynaptic spikes *(lower trace). B:* Characterization of noise amplitude. *Upper trace* is the record of a simulated random sample produced by a digital Gaussian uncorrelated sequence generator. The *solid horizontal line* represents the zero amplitude level, and regions where the absolute value of the noise amplitude is less than twice its standard deviation (2σ) are delineated by *dashed lines.* The *curve* to the *right* encompasses the theoretical distribution of this simulated background activity. *Lower trace* shows a sample of intracellularly recorded noise. *C:* Block diagram of main steps of the program. The sample of potentials {V$_j$} was used to calculate a likelihood criterion L({V$_j$}) based on either the Poisson or the binomial model; this criterion was maximized with θ, the estimated values of the model, until an optimal solution $\hat{\theta}$ was obtained. This whole sequence, enclosed in *dashed lines,* is equivalent to a constraint deconvolution process. *D:* Simplified equation indicating that, for the binomial model, the likelihood criterion *L* was determined by *N,* the sample size; *n* and *p* are the binomial parameters; *q* is the quantal size; and σ_N is the level of background activity. (From Korn et al., 1982.)

measurements of spontaneous activity. Estimation of the parameters defining the Poisson or binomial fits (Korn et al., 1981, 1982), on the basis of a sample of *N* responses, was treated as a problem of "constraint deconvolution," requiring definition of a goodness of fit criterion, which was chosen as the likelihood criterion, *L* (Kendall and Stuart, 1977). Its definition depended on the statistical characteristics of the background noise; if the observed individual responses had values of μ_i, with $i = 1, \ldots , N$, *L* could be expressed by

$$L(\{\mu_i\}, n, p, q) = \prod_{i=1}^{N} \sum_{x=0}^{n} \left[\begin{array}{ccc} \text{binomial} \\ \text{or} & \text{equation} \\ \text{Poisson} \end{array} \right] \cdot \frac{1}{\sqrt{2\pi}\sigma} \exp - \frac{(\mu_i - qx)^2}{2\sigma^2} .$$

$$(9)$$

These criteria were maximized by using a nonlinear optimization technique (Nelder and Mead, 1965) that yielded the optimal values of the binomial and Poisson parameters and indicated which model provided a better fit (Figure 9C, D).

It is important to point out that our approach is largely indebted to that described by Edwards et al. (1976a,b) for the concept of deconvolution, but differs significantly from it in its basic approach because we have fitted the observed fluctuations in response amplitude with models incorporating not only additive contributions of the noise but also different quantal processes.

Histological Techniques. After each experiment, HRP was iontophoretically injected into cells exhibiting a passive hyperpolarizing potential (PHP; one per fish) (Korn et al., 1978; Triller and Korn, 1981). The dye was revealed according to standard procedures (Triller and Korn, 1982), and terminal boutons were clearly distinguished in most cases; some of them were in contact with the M-cell soma and main dendrites, and others were situated within the axon cap. Both classic rounded boutons and occasional abrupt endings without swelling were taken as indicating synaptic sites. The validity of this procedure was demonstrated by electron microscope evidence that: (1) All such terminals exhibit a well-differentiated synaptic apparatus characteristic of the chemical type (Korn et al., 1981; Triller and Korn, 1981, 1982); and (2) *en passant* boutons were never apparent. There was little opportunity to overestimate the number of terminals because those within the axon cap necessarily innervated the M-cell soma or thin cap dendrites, which are their only possible targets in this area (Nakajima, 1974).

Quantal Nature of M-Cell IPSPs

PHP-exhibiting neurons belong to two classes; one group contains cells that are part of the M-cell's collateral network (Korn and Faber, 1975; Korn et al., 1978), and those of the second category are second-order commissural interneurons (Triller and Korn, 1978). Results obtained from these two different anatomical structures were essentially the same. When the HRP-filled inhibitory interneurons were reconstructed histologically from serial sections that included their target M-cell, the total number of terminal boutons that defined the histological n ranged from 3 to 93 (Triller and Korn, 1981, 1982). However, if n exceeded approximately 30, the binomial analysis of fluctuating responses sometimes led to indistinguishable solutions with several equivalent parametric values, as a result of the mathematical phenomenon called "degenerescence" (Kendall and Stuart, 1977). As a consequence, only cases with a binomial product less than or equal to 6.6 are considered here.

Physical Correlate of the Binomial Parameter **n.**   The data shown in Figures 10 and 11 illustrate two of our most striking initial results: (1) The binomial prediction provided a statistically more adequate definition of IPSP amplitude fluctuations than did the Poisson one; and (2) the value of the optimal binomial parameter n was the same as the number of stained presynaptic boutons.

The data shown in Figure 10 indicate that the background activity of the M-cells was moderate; the standard deviation of the noise was approximately 60 μV, and the unitary IPSPs evoked by presynaptic impulses varied from extremes of 0.26 to 2.05 mV, with a mean of 0.88 mV for 182 trials. The average records in Figure 10A$_1$–A$_2$ reflect the mean amplitude and time course. A visual evaluation of the computer-determined best fits, shown in Figure 10B, obviously suggests that the Poisson prediction was less acceptable than the binomial one. In confirmation, only the latter model passed the Kolmogorov test. This result was further borne out by statistical tests based on the comparison of the optimal likelihood criteria for the two models, the latter being, as in other experiments (for details, see Korn et al., 1982), more satisfactory than the former. The second conclusion was obtained from comparisons between the binomial parameters and the geometrical features of the presynaptic neurons: The camera lucida reconstruction of this cell, which was a commissural neuron, is illustrated in Figure 11A and B and shows that the number of synaptic boutons was six and equaled the binomial parameter n extracted by computer analysis.

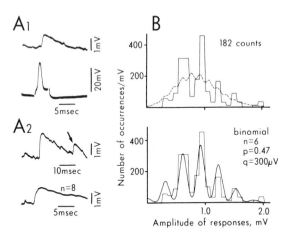

Figure 10.   *Probability density functions of IPSP fluctuations and computer-modeled fits with Poisson and binomial predictions. A$_1$:* Sample unitary IPSP (*upper trace*) evoked by a presynaptic impulse (*lower trace*). *A$_2$:* Evoked IPSP of larger amplitude recorded at a slower sweep, with a late-occurring spontaneous PSP (*arrow, upper trace*) and the on-line computed average (n = 8) of several responses (*lower trace*). *B:* Comparisons of the observed IPSP amplitude variations (stepwise distributions for 182 counts) with the best fits obtained by assuming a Poisson (*top*) or binomial (*bottom*) relationship. *Abscissae*, amplitude of the evoked responses; *ordinates*, density of observations expressed as the number of occurrences per millivolt. The likelihood criterion was better for the binomial prediction, which yielded a value of six for parameter n, while p and q were 0.47 μV and 300 μV, respectively. The binomial prediction satisfied the Kolmogorov test ($P > 0.05$) but the Poisson prediction did not ($P < 0.01$), and the test for possible equivalence between the models indicated that the binomial one was more satisfactory. (From Korn et al., 1982.)

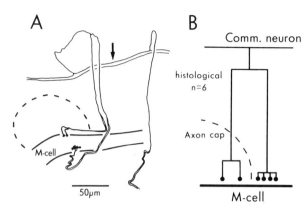

Figure 11. *Camera lucida reconstruction (A) and corresponding diagram (B) of the HRP-filled commissural interneuron that evoked the responses illustrated in Figure 10.* Six boutons that impinged on the M-cell's soma were visualized; two of them were in the axon cap (delineated by *dashed lines*), while the other four remained outside this region. The *arrow* indicates the recording and injection site, as determined by the track of the presynaptic microelectrode. For this neuron, the binomial parameter *n* and the number of synaptic knobs were the same. (From Korn et al., 1982.)

As demonstrated by the two examples in Figure 12, the total number of releasable quanta n ascertained by the computer treatment of unitary response fluctuations was also in agreement with the histological n in interneurons with a larger number of terminals, which were often clustered within tightly packed boutons. In these commissural cells, the binomial parameter n, which was 14 in Figure $12A_1-A_2$ and 17 in Figure $12B_1-B_2$, again corresponded to the number of histologically determined synaptic boutons. Thus, despite some close grouping, all endings functioned as distinct release units.

The data from 30 experiments involving 24 commissural and 6 collateral interneurons are summarized by the plot in Figure 13, which demonstrates that the equivalence between the n's derived by the statistical and the histological approaches was valid for values ranging from 3 to 28. Slight differences were noticeable for some of the cells, with binomial n sometimes being one or two units larger than histological n. This difference was always slight and suggests that either some terminals were lost during neuronal reconstruction, or some of them can bear more than one release site or presynaptic grid (see below). In any case, with this model, each synaptic knob can be equated to a quantal unit that releases in an all-or-none manner, and the quantum, defined by binomial terms, corresponds to the basic unit processed by the postsynaptic neuron.

Estimates of binomial parameters were resolved from these experiments. The probability of release, p, was consistently high, ranging from 0.17 to 0.75, with a mean of 0.42 (SDM = 0.16; $n = 30$). On the other hand, quantal sizes were expressed by normalizing these parameters with respect to the full-sized IPSP evoked by spinal stimulation and appeared to be constant in most experiments, except for two extreme cases. Normalized q ranged from 0.6 to 1.9% of that of the collateral IPSP, with a mean of 1.24 (SDM = 0.40; $n = 30$). This finding implies that transmitter action is relatively stable at each subsynaptic site.

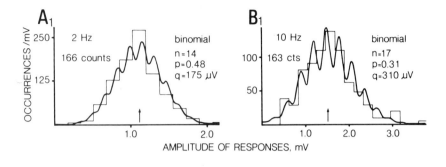

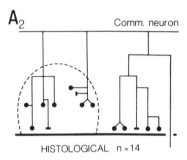

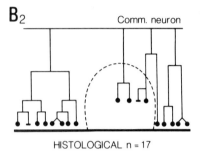

Figure 12. *More evidence that the binomial parameter* n *is equivalent to the number of presynaptic endings.* A_1: Probability density histogram for 166 trials, computer-determined optimal curve, and parameters assuming a binomial curve (Kolmogorov test satisfied with $P > 0.65$). A_2: Schematic representation of the reconstructed terminals issued by the HRP-filled interneuron that were in contact with the M-cell. This commissural (Comm.) neuron established 14 synaptic boutons (*filled circles*) in relation to the M-cell soma (*thick line*); nine of them were located within the axon cap (*dashed circle*), and five were situated outside this region. B_1 and B_2: Comparison of the quantal parameters provided by the probability density functions (163 counts) and best fits (B_1), using a binomial model (Kolmogorov test satisfied with $P > 0.75$), and of the histological features of another stimulated commissural neuron (B_2). Note that in each experiment, the number of presynaptic terminals (14 and 17, respectively) strictly equaled that of the binomial term *n*. (From Korn, 1984.)

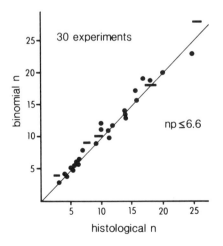

Figure 13. *One-to-one correspondence between the binomial parameter* n *and the number of synaptic boutons.* Plot of the correlation between the binomial (*ordinate*) and histological (*abscissa*) *n*'s, as determined in 30 experiments for which the product *np* was ≤ 6.6. The *horizontal bars* encompass the range of possible histological values in several cases of uncertainties, and the *solid line* is the identity relationship. The correlation suggests that, for each of the investigated neurons, the quantal unit corresponds to the transmitter released by one synaptic bouton. (From Korn, 1984.)

Comparison of Constraint and Sequential Deconvolution Models. Since our quantal analysis gave very different results from those of Redman's group, we decided to confront both methods with the same set of data, as illustrated in Figure 14. In this experiment (which was used for the plot in Figure 13), the binomial n was 10 and was strictly equivalent to the number of stained presynaptic terminals, as shown in Figure 14A$_1$ and A$_2$. Five distinct peaks can be distinguished on the probability density function of the recorded unitary IPSPs, which fluctuated between 0.40 and 4.5 mV (for a full-sized collateral IPSP of about 40 mV), with a mean of 1.66 mV.

Owing to the courtesy of S. Redman, who kindly analyzed our data, we first obtained the apparent fluctuation pattern of the same series of IPSPs, as determined by the deconvolution procedure (using the same value of 130 μV for σ_N). That histogram, shown in Figure 14B$_1$, is slightly different from those in Figure 14A$_1$ because the data were binned for the former (with a bin width of 125 μV), but

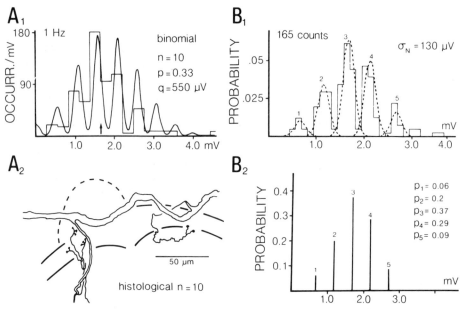

Figure 14. *Analysis of an M-cell's fluctuating IPSPs: Comparison of results obtained with the binomial model, and those obtained with the deconvolution method. A_1 and A_2: Correlation of the statistical properties of an M-cell's responses with the morphological features of a presynaptic neuron. A_1: Probability density histogram for 165 unitary IPSPs evoked by stimulations of a presynaptic neuron at a low rate (1 Hz) and a superimposed computer-modeled curve generated with binomial equations. A_2: Camera lucida reconstruction of the HRP-filled presynaptic cell. For this neuron, the binomial term n and the number of active sites (histological n) were strictly the same. B_1 and B_2: Fluctuating pattern determined by the deconvolution procedure. B_1: Histogram of the evoked IPSP amplitudes and its underlying components (dotted curves) obtained as for Figure 4A; the peaks are labeled 1–5. B_2: Deconvolved probabilities calculated by using the histogram shown in B_1 and the indicated value (σ_N) for noise variance, the IPSP seems to fluctuate between five discrete peaks, with the indicated probabilities. Because five other terminals of the presynaptic neuron were undetected, one would have to postulate that they establish "ineffective synapses." (B_1 and B_2 are from a collaboration with S. Redman.)*

again five peaks were identified. The deconvolved peak voltage distribution calculated from this histogram shows five entries separated by steps of about 550 μV, as in Figure 14A$_1$; their respective probabilities are indicated in Figure 14B$_2$. However, the recorded unitary responses with amplitudes above 3 mV were discarded by the program (presumably because of their infrequent occurrence). Therefore, the deconvolution of noise alone suggests that only 5 synapses of 10 were active, with the remaining 5 being ineffective at this rate of stimulation (1 Hz). This conclusion is in sharp contrast to the results from the constraint deconvolution with a simple binomial model, which accurately identified all presynaptic terminals.

Five other cells were analyzed in this manner; the full complement of boutons was recognized by both methods for two of them, which had histological n's of 4 and 6. The remaining three had 5, 11, and 14 terminals, and the two-step method showed 4, 10, and 8 entries, respectively, the quantal size of the last two appearing to be half that of the binomial one. Perhaps these differences would have been minimized by larger sample sizes or by a better evaluation of the noise, but in general, these and all the data presented above do not support the notion of ineffective synapses and rather confirm the validity of the simple binomial model for quantal analysis in the central nervous system.

Physical Correlate of the Binomial q.   The identity of a terminal as a quantal unit means that its postsynaptic effect is relatively constant. Therefore, in the context of the vesicular theory of transmitter release (e.g., Katz, 1971), each fundamental unit represents either the effect of a relatively high and fixed number of released vesicles or the effect of only one. These alternative possibilities were evaluated by estimating the size of the population of channels opened by the transmitter released at each synaptic bouton. The problem was formalized in a simple analogue circuit of the M-cell, illustrated in Figure 15A; a detailed justification of this model has been given elsewhere (Faber and Korn, 1982a; Korn, 1984). One should, however, indicate here that: (1) The M-cell's membrane capacitance and distributed dendritic cable properties could be neglected because the neuron's time constant is extremely short with respect to IPSP kinetics (Faber and Korn, 1980), and because the synapses are electrotonically close to the recording site (Korn et al., 1981); and (2) all potentials were measured with respect to the resting level.

With this circuit, some equations were derived (Faber and Korn, 1982a,b). The PSP amplitude is $V = E \cdot g_{psp}/(g_{psp} + G_m)$, where E is the driving force, G_m is the input conductance, and g_{psp} is the synaptic one. Solving for the latter yields $g_{psp} = V \cdot G_m/(E - V)$, which for small responses, such as quantal ones, becomes

$$g_q = (q/E)\, G_m \; , \tag{10}$$

where g_q and q are the quantal conductance and voltage, respectively. Since q was known from the binomial analysis, and G_m had been determined by standard techniques, the critical parameter to estimate was E, which varied greatly from one experiment to the next. However, the use of double intracellular impalements

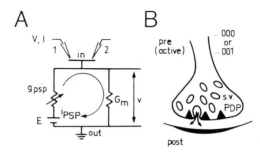

Figure 15. *Electrical analogue of the postsynaptic cell and an illustration of the proposition that a quantal unit equals the action of a single vesicle's transmitter content.* A: Circuit diagram of the synaptic membrane under conditions for generating a depolarizing IPSP. E and g_{psp} stand for the driving force and for the increment of conductance contributed by a single unitary IPSP, respectively; G_m is the resting conductance of the unactivated part of the postsynaptic membrane; V is the transmembrane potential change during the response recorded by an intracellular (in) micro-electrode, with reference to the external potential (out). It follows that if G_m and E are known, g_{psp}, the quantal conductance, can be assessed to determine the number of channels opened across the membrane. These two variations were indeed measured by placing two microelectrodes in the M-cell, one for current and one for voltage. (Modified from Faber and Korn, 1982a.) B: At high magnification, a terminal bouton (pre) appears to contain many synaptic vesicles (s.v.) and regularly spaced presynaptic dense projections (PDP). When the terminal bouton is sufficiently depolarized (active), exocytosis of one vesicle may occur and the transmitter diffuses toward the postsynaptic (post) side. The binary notation (. . . 000 or . . . 001) emphasizes that, although there is a large number of apparently available vesicles, a maximum of one can be singled out after an impulse. (Modified from Faber and Korn, 1982b.)

led to the important finding that the peak amplitude of the full-sized collateral IPSP, which is easily obtained by antidromic activation of the M-cell, is about one half of E. Thus, Equation 10 can be rewritten as

$$g_q = (0.5_q / V_{coll})\, G_m ,\tag{11}$$

where V_{coll} is the amplitude of the collateral IPSP. G_m was shown to be 6.08×10^{-6} S (Faber and Korn, 1982a) and, as indicated above, the mean value of the normalized quantum size is 1.15%. Then the conductance increase associated with the action of a single binomial quantum would be in the range of 3.5×10^{-8} S. By assuming that a single channel conductance is about 25 pS (see Neher and Stevens, 1977; Dudel et al., 1980), we concluded that approximately 1400 channels are opened by each releasing synaptic bouton, with extreme ranges of 400–2800. This estimate leads to the tentative postulate (Korn et al., 1981, 1982; Faber and Korn, 1982a), illustrated in Figure 15B, that at each individual release site (or bouton) apparently no more than one vesicle can normally undergo exocytosis after one presynaptic impulse.

Our calculations are consistent with those obtained at other inhibitory junctions (Dudel et al., 1977; Barker and McBurney, 1979; Gold and Martin, 1983). In fact, Eccles (1961a,b) originally proposed that a single Ia terminal knob may release no more than one quantum, or at most two or three. The same conclusion was reached after the analysis of Ia-EPSPs fluctuations (Kuno, 1964a) and at the crayfish neuromuscular junction (Zucker, 1973; Wernig, 1975, 1976). These important suggestions were later overshadowed by the use of toxins and drugs to provoke massive but nonphysiological transmitter output (see Heuser et al., 1979). But strong arguments substantiated by structural data and morphofunctional correlations suggest that the "one vesicle hypothesis" may be valid not only in the central nervous system but also in the periphery (see discussion in Korn et al., 1982; Korn, 1984).

NONLINEAR PROCESSING OF THE STOCHASTIC MESSAGE BY THE POSTSYNAPTIC MEMBRANE

Although the binomial model gives an adequate description of the release properties of central afferent synapses, the best binomial predictions do not always fit exactly the histograms of evoked responses, most often because of an excess number of responses observed around the means. These differences, which can be of statistical significance, was taken as a justification to search for other models that might provide better fits. However, in view of the striking morphofunctional correlation given by the simple binomial, it becomes counterproductive to struggle for a perfect fit in the sole context of mathematical considerations. Thus, we have asked (Korn and Mallet, 1984) if the discrepancy mentioned above actually has significance.

The fundamental concept of quantal analysis is based on two principles: (1) That release at a given active zone is a random process, independent of exocytosis at other release sites; and (2) that the PSPs or currents classically used to estimate n and p directly reflect the release phenomena. We have obtained evidence suggesting that the latter need not be the case at central synapses, where information carried by the input can be reorganized by the postsynaptic side of the junction. By using experimental and theoretical entropies as a means of quantification, we put forward an experimentally supported model according to which the postsynaptic membrane functions as a nonlinear processor of multiple adjacent events. The nonlinearity is most likely a result of a localized interaction between the effects of simultaneously activated neighboring synapses.

Entropies: A Quantitative Measure of Deviations from the Model

The diagrams of Figure 16A are similar to the earlier ones that showed that binomial predictions provide a satisfactory definition of IPSP amplitude fluctuations. The optimal values of binomial p and n were 0.45 and 13, respectively, and the total number of HRP-stained synaptic boutons established on the M-cell by this presynaptic neuron was also 13 (for the morphology of this cell, see Figure 19A). However, a close inspection of the probability density functions showed that they were systematically biased, with fewer unitary IPSPs in the extreme values than expected from the binomial predictions and with an excess of responses around the means (see also Figures 10B, 12A$_1$, and 14A$_1$). These differences are also apparent in the cumulative distributions of Figure 16B.

Discrepancies between the recorded and predicted probability density functions were quantified by using as an index the entropies of their underlying random variables. Specifically, if Y is a discrete random variable with a set of t-possible

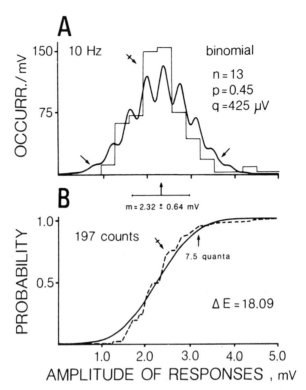

Figure 16. *Enhancement of postsynaptic response frequencies within the range of their predicted mean amplitude. A: Probability density histogram (stepwise distribution for 197 counts) of unitary IPSP fluctuations and computer-modeled binomial best fit. The stimulus was 10 Hz. Abscissa, amplitude of evoked responses; ordinate, density of observations expressed as the number of occurrences per millivolt. The Kolmogorov test was poorly satisfied (P > 0.040) and the number of recorded PSPs was less than that predicted at the extremes of the spectrum (arrows). By contrast, the number of recorded PSPs was in excess around the mean (crossed arrow). Vertical arrow and horizontal bar indicate the mean (m) ± one standard deviation. B: Cumulative probability functions of the predicted IPSP amplitudes (solid curve) and of the potentials recorded in the M-cell (dashed curve). E_{exp} was less than E_{th}, with ΔE = 18.09. Mean of the computed result for variations resulting from the IPSPs alone is indicated by the arrow; crossed arrow as in A. (From Korn and Mallet, 1984.)*

values associated with the probabilities p_x, $x = 1, \ldots, t$, the entropy of Y, which is a measure of the uncertainty of the estimate of Y resulting from random sampling experiments (Shannon, 1948; see also Kullback, 1959), can be defined by

$$E_Y = -\sum_{x=1}^{t} p_x \operatorname{Log} p_x \,. \tag{12}$$

This relation was used to determine the entropies of the experimental results, E_{exp}, and of the binomial predictions, E_{th}, through an adapted discretization scheme (for the mathematical details, see Korn and Mallet, 1984), and a parameter

$\Delta E = 100 \cdot (E_{th} - E_{exp})/E_{th}$ was defined. At low stimulation frequencies (up to 10 Hz), ΔE ranged from 0.4 to 21.76, with a mean of 11.27 (SD = 4.74; $n = 35$), E_{exp} thus being consistently smaller than E_{th}. For instance, in Figure 16, ΔE was as large as 18.09. Otherwise stated, the postsynaptic responses were grouped around the means and were less variable than predicted by the binomial relation.

Nevertheless, as indicated above, a simple binomial description of release remains appropriate, as it has generated a powerful structure–function correlation; tests with a nonuniform (compound) binomial model with various values of p at each terminal compromised this correlation (e.g., Figure 14). Also, presynaptic structural and quantal parameters did not affect ΔE. For instance, in cells with terminals restricted within the axon cap, ΔE was in the same range and was not modified when cells were grouped according to different classes of p and n (details in Korn and Mallet, 1984).

Data indicating that the grouping of responses was of postsynaptic origin were obtained by using strychnine, which is a competitive blocker of glycine, the putative transmitter at these junctions (Roper et al., 1969; Diamond et al., 1973; see also Faber et al., 1983). Two experimental approaches were employed, both involving pre- and postsynaptic intracellular recordings, with stimulating rates of ~2 Hz and a binomial analysis of the response fluctuations. In a first series, control and experimental data were obtained prior to and after iontophoretic application of strychnine through a third microelectrode placed extracellularly near the M-cell soma. As expected, unitary IPSPs were then either abolished or reduced. In five cases in which individual responses were still large enough for reliable measurements, binomial statistics showed that the major effect was indeed on q, with n and p remaining unaffected. This result is illustrated in Figure 17, where q dropped substantially after injection of the drug although n and p were quite stable. In this and the other experiments, ΔE also decreased by an average of 9.77 (SDM = 6.87; $P < 0.025$; paired t test, $n = 5$). In the second set of experiments ($n = 8$), strychnine was administered intramuscularly and each interneuron was injected with HRP to determine if, as predicted, the binomial n still equaled the number of presynaptic boutons (Figure 18A$_1$–A$_2$). Such was the case for a range of 4–31 stained terminals (bin n/hist $n = 1.04 \pm 0.14$). Values of p and q were consistent with those above. In this series, ΔE was also unusually low, with a mean of 1.65 ± 0.40, the value of 1.22 computed in Figure 18A$_3$ being quite typical of these results.

Evidence for Synaptic Interactions

These data raised questions about the notion that postsynaptic conductance changes at adjacent synaptic loci are independent. A postsynaptic transfer function (Figures 18A$_4$, 19B) was derived by relating the amount of transmitter released to the resultant conductance change, such that the theoretical probability density function was transformed to the experimental one (Korn and Mallet, 1984). This function was computed on the basis of f, the estimated (binomial) probability density function of the release process, and ψ, that of the recorded potentials. ψ represents the output variable, that is, the conductance increments resulting

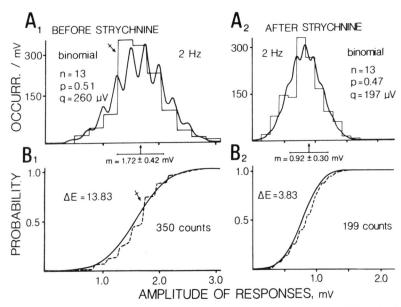

Figure 17. *Evidence that the lack of fit of the observed distribution of fluctuating M-cell IPSPs by the optimal binomial predictions has a postsynaptic origin. A_1 and B_1:* Control probability density function with computer-modeled best fit (A_1), and control cumulative probability function (B_1) of predicted and recorded IPSPs (same disposition as for Figure 16A,B). The Kolmogorov test was not satisfied. Note that the recorded IPSPs were in excess around the mean *(crossed arrow)*. A_2 and B_2: After iontophoretic application of strychnine close to the M-cell's soma, which lowered the amplitude of the collateral IPSP from 41 to 35 mV (not shown), the binomial parameters n and p remained unaffected, but the quantum size and the mean unitary IPSP were reduced by the effect of this competitive blocker. The lack of fit between experimental and estimated curves was abolished, as ΔE dropped from 13.83 to 3.83.

from transmitter action; f corresponds to the input variable, namely the amount of transmitter released after each impulse, and is expressed in quantal units. *We found that this transform is unique and is defined by* $r = \phi^{-1} \circ F$, *where F and ϕ are the cumulative functions associated with f and ψ, respectively, and o stands for the composition of functions.*

Figures 18A_4 and 19B are typical of the transforms so obtained. In Figure 19B, the amplitude of the response to several quanta is less than that predicted by the proportionality assumption, suggesting that the postsynaptic membrane adds quantal conductances nonlinearly. The magnitude of this nonlinearity was largely dependent on the grouping of the presynaptic terminals in distinct clusters. For instance, the five cells that had the lowest ΔE's, ranging from 0.4 to 5.31 ($m = 3.04$; SDM = 2.42), were morphologically exceptional because their terminals were separated considerably (no less than 30 μm). Thus, r presumably reflects the degree of a postsynaptic interaction that has not been described previously, and that is characterized by a progressive decrease in the mean response per bouton when several nearby terminals are activated simultaneously.

This postulate (Figure 19C) was computer modeled. The program, based on the geometrical characteristics of the reconstructed presynaptic neurons, distinguished two classes: (1) terminals clustered within a radius of up to 20 μm that released independently but had intersecting zones of influence, such that response increment per activated knob was less than the quantal size (for a first approximation, the magnitude of interaction was constant throughout the cluster regardless of the specific locations of the release sites, varying only with the number of activated terminals); and (2) isolated boutons. The simulation procedure computed the expected distribution of responses generated according to the derived binomial parameter p and the modeled interaction within the cluster. Finally, a theoretical transfer function was derived for comparison with r. For instance, the histological reconstruction of the neuron of Figure 19A showed two widely disposed clusters of eight and five terminal boutons, respectively. The program used the transmitter/response relationship illustrated in Figure 19D for both clusters. In this and other experiments, the theoretial r function quite satisfactorily fit its experimental counterpart, as shown in Figure 19B.

Thus, the transfer function that eliminates the discrepancies between experimental and theoretical probability density functions can be simulated by modeling nonlinear increments in quantal conductances, restricted to the effects of simultaneously activated, closely located terminals. The basis for such a postsynaptic interaction is unclear; the properties of M-cell responses suggest that voltage

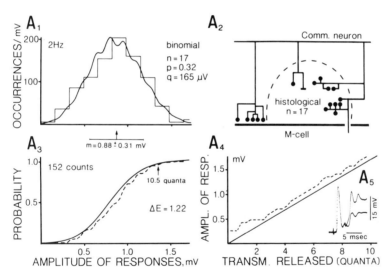

Figure 18. *Persistence of the equivalence between binomial and histological* n *after strychnine. A_1*: Probability density histogram for 152 trials, computer-determined optimal curve, and corresponding binomial parameters; Kolmogorov test ($P > 0.60$) was satisfied. A_2: Schematic representation of the reconstructed terminals issued by the HRP-filled presynaptic interneuron. Despite an intraperitoneal injection of strychnine, the binomial term ($n = 17$) strictly equaled the number of presynaptic sites. A_3: Cumulative probability functions of the predicted IPSP amplitudes (*solid curve*) and of the potentials recorded in the M-cell (*dashed curve*). A_4: Corresponding computed r function. Note that the predicted and experimental curves did not differ substantially and that, accordingly, ΔE was low (1.22). A_5: Superimposed traces of the M-cell collateral IPSP recorded before and after strychnine, showing that the antidromic spike was not affected by the blocker, whereas the IPSP amplitude fell from 23 to 15 mV.

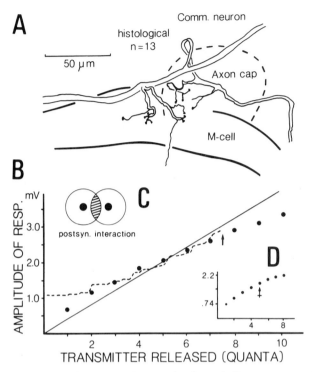

Figure 19. *Evidence for localized interaction between the effects of adjacent synapses. A: Camera lucida reconstruction of the HRP-filled commissural (Comm.) neuron that evoked the responses shown in Figures 1 and 16. B: Plot of the relationship between the amount of transmitter released (abscissa) and the amplitudes of the postsynaptic responses (ordinate). Solid line represents the linear relationship that would pertain if the responses were directly proportional to transmitter output. Dashed curve is the plot of the calculated r function that, if applied to the theoretical probability density function, would produce conductance changes similar to those accompanying the IPSPs over the range of reliability, that is, to 7.5 quanta (arrow). The marked deviation of this curve from the solid line suggests a localized interaction between synaptic effects when several terminals are simultaneously active. Filled dots represent the computer-modeled r function (see text). C: Schematic representation of the postulated locus of interactions occurring when two synapses (filled circles) of a cluster are simultaneously active and their zones of influence (intersecting open circles) overlap (hatched area). D: Plot of the modeled relationship between response amplitudes (ordinate) and the number of activated synaptic knobs (abscissa). These amplitudes, normalized to equate the mean binomial response with that obtained after transform, were 0.74, 1.03, 1.29, 1.55, 1.77, 1.96, 2.11, and 2.22 mV, respectively, as one to eight synapses were active. The crossed arrow indicates the maximum response produced by the second cluster of five terminals. (From Korn and Mallet, 1984.)*

dependence of quantal PSPs or transient, increased local conductances (Koch et al., 1983) are unlikely (Furshpan and Furukawa, 1962; Fukami et al., 1965; see Faber and Korn, 1978). The effects produced by release at each synaptic bouton may be due to a diffuse action of the transmitter over domains larger than those restricted under a given release site. The cooperation between adjacent synapses described previously (McNaughton et al., 1978) could also be accounted for by such a mechanism (Korn and Faber, 1983). Alternatively, the synaptic current produced at clustered junctions may be saturated, for example, by local ionic movements and shifts in the IPSP driving force. In the latter case, the reduction in quantal size after strychnine administration would then minimize the non-linearities.

RELATION OF p TO SYNAPTIC PLASTICITY

The experimental paradigms that have been favored for studies of short-term, activity-dependent changes in synaptic efficacy have involved the use of paired presynaptic stimuli and repetitive stimulation. It is well accepted that a conditioning stimulus induces at least two separate processes, depression and facilitation, which are of presynaptic origin (Hubbard, 1963; Kuno, 1971; McLachlan, 1978). These two processes are often superimposed in time, and one or the other may dominate in a given system. Because attempts to correlate facilitation and depression with changes in quantal parameters have been limited in the case of central synapses and have frequently depended on the use of pharmacologically manipulated preparations from peripheral nervous systems, data from both sets of preparations are reviewed here, in order to evaluate the idea that p is the critical presynaptic modifiable variable.

Quantal Correlates of Synaptic Depression

Synaptic depression can be subdivided into the short-term reduction in synaptic responses produced either by a single conditioning stimulus or by a brief period of high-frequency stimulation, and the long-term fatigue associated with prolonged repetitive activity. The latter has been primarily studied at peripheral junctions and is commonly attributed to a depletion of transmitter or quanta. The reduction in quantal content is associated with a decrease in binomial n, either alone (e.g., Bennett and Florin, 1974; Bennett et al., 1976) or in conjunction with a decrease in p (McLachlan, 1975; Hatt and Smith, 1976).

Short-term depression has been studied at a number of central synapses. Typically, it has been the predominant effect observed with low-frequency stimulation of most junctions in the vertebrate central nervous system, such as those between Ia afferents and spinal motoneurons (Curtis and Eccles, 1960; Kuno, 1964b; Honig et al., 1983), Ia and Ib connections with neurons of the dorsal and ventral spinocerebellar tracts (Eccles et al., 1961a,b), corticorubral connections (Tsukahara and Kosaka, 1968), and those at the longer intervals used (≥ 200 msec) during paired pulse activation of the perforant input to dentate granule cells (Lømo, 1971). However, there has been a limited number of quantal analyses of this phenomenon, in part because it is often complicated by a superimposed facilitatory process. Kuno (1964b) used a Poisson model to analyze the depression observed at Ia synapses on motoneurons with stimulus frequencies of 1–4 Hz and concluded that, since m decreased, the effect was presynaptic, as is the case for other junctions (Otsuka et al., 1962; Elmqvist and Quastel, 1965; Thies, 1965).

The inhibitory synapses on the M-cell provided an opportunity to study, for the first time, possible changes in n, p, and q during depression (Korn et al., 1982, 1984), because complications posed by a superimposed facilitatory process are not present there (Faber and Korn, 1982a). The presynaptic cell was stimulated at frequencies ranging from 2 to 33 Hz, and the binomial parameters were derived separately for each frequency (Korn et al., 1984). As before, the findings could be correlated with the morphology of the reconstructed interneurons. Results from a typical experiment are illustrated in Figure 20. When stimulus frequency was increased from the control level of 2 Hz, the average unitary IPSP amplitude decreased steadily, from a maximum of about 1.01 mV to 0.28 mV at 33 Hz (Figure 20A). In this case, the presynaptic neuron was a commissural cell that established 14 terminal boutons on the M-cell (Figure 20B). The binomial statistics indicated that q and n, the latter of which equaled the number of terminals, changed minimally over this range, whereas p dropped steadily from 0.44 at 2 Hz to 0.25 at 33 Hz (Figure 20C). Data from the 12 experiments, in which the number of stained terminals ranged from 3 to 18, are summarized in Figure 21. Normalized quantal size and binomial n were remarkably constant, with the former being essentially equal to histological n for all frequencies of stimulation. In contrast, p decreased exponentially as a function of frequency, and appeared to have a minimum of about 0.15. *Thus, all of the synaptic boutons remained functional under conditions of high-frequency stimulation, and the decreased amplitude of the post-synaptic responses could be attributed solely to a lowered probability of release.* The mechanism underlying this reduction has not been established, but in view of the hypothesis that at these junctions an active zone releases, at most, one synaptic vesicle after each presynaptic impulse, we have proposed that it reflects incomplete recovery of the release mechanism from a block triggered by the preceding exocytotic event (Korn et al., 1984; for the concept that there is a transient refractoriness of release sites that have undergone exocytosis at the neuromuscular junction, see Betz, 1970).

It is possible that, in addition to the effect of prior activity on p, n may be depressed in systems in which there is either a rapid depletion of transmitter vesicles available for release, as suggested for the output synapses of the hatchetfish M-cell (Highstein and Bennett, 1975; Model et al., 1975), and junctions between hair cells and eighth-nerve fibers in the goldfish (Furukawa and Matsuura, 1978; Furukawa et al., 1978, 1982). In the latter, fluctuations in sound-evoked EPSPs have been fitted with a binomial model and quantal analysis has established that in conditions characterized by decrementing responses, p remains constant and n drops. Furukawa and colleagues have advanced an explanation, based on structural evidence, suggesting that the vesicles gain access to the presynaptic grid from its edges. They propose that there are n release sites within an active zone, with different thresholds for release, and that p is fixed once the threshold is exceeded. The preferred release sites are in the center of the grid and their vesicles will be rapidly depleted during repetitive activity, leading to an apparent drop in n. This elegant model may be appropriate for these specialized junctions, where a large dense body in the presynaptic ending does seem to protect the center of the active zone, but it may be less relevant to synapses with more conventional structural restraints.

Quantal Correlates of Facilitation

An initial facilitation following a conditioning stimulus has been observed at most other central and peripheral junctions studied thus far (reviewed in Eccles,

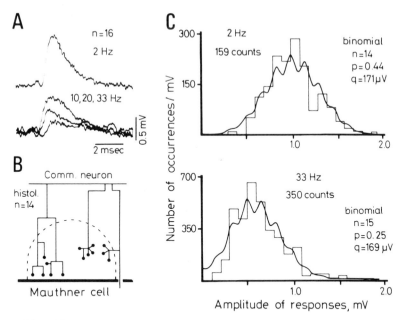

Figure 20. *Binomial parameters* n, p, *and* q *during synaptic depression. A:* Computer-averaged IPSPs (*n* = 16) recorded in the M-cell as the presynaptic inhibitory neuron was stimulated at different frequencies. Calculated for more than 150 counts, the mean amplitude of the evoked responses, which was about 1.01 ± 0.27 mV at a frequency of 2 Hz (*upper trace*), fell progressively as the stimulus rate was increased to the indicated values (*lower trace*). *B:* Schematic representation of the reconstructed presynaptic cell's terminals. This commissural (Comm.) neuron established 14 synaptic boutons (*filled circles*) in relation with the M-cell soma (*thick line*). *C:* Comparison of the probability density functions and best fits obtained with a binomial model, using 159 counts at 2 Hz (*top*) and 350 counts at 33 Hz (*bottom*). Note that the synaptic depression was essentially associated with a lower *p*, whereas *n* and *q* remained almost constant. The Kolmogorov test was satisfied with *P* > 0.09 (*top*) and *P* > 0.05 (*bottom*). (From Korn et al., 1984.)

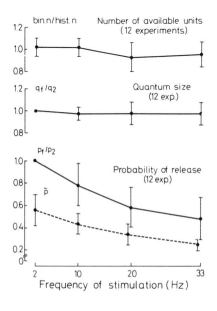

Figure 21. *Relative changes in the statistics of transmitter release during depression, as observed in 12 experiments. Top:* Plot of the mean normalized number of units available for release, represented by the expression bin.*n*/hist.*n*, which is the ratio between the computer-estimated *n* at each of the indicated frequencies and the histologically determined number of synaptic boutons. *Middle:* Plot of the mean normalized quantum size, represented by q_f/q_2, that is, by the ratio between the size of the quanta at each frequency and its control value at 2 Hz. *Bottom:* Mean probability of release, normalized with reference to its control value (p_f/p_2) or represented in absolute value ($\bar{p}$). *Vertical bars* throughout indicate standard deviations of the means. (From Korn et al., 1984.)

1964; McLachlan, 1978; Mendell, 1984), but there have only been a limited number of studies of its quantal aspect. In fact, the assumption that the underlying mechanism is situated presynaptically is substantiated in only a few instances (e.g., Dudel and Kuffler, 1961; Kuno and Weakly, 1972; Wernig, 1972a; Zucker, 1973; McLachlan, 1975), at most, an increase in m was reported.

Two apparently more detailed studies in cat spinal motoneurons did not provide more insights. In the case of IPSPs (Kuno and Weakly, 1972), facilitation appeared to parallel an increase in n, while p, which was already 0.5 in the controls, seemed unchanged; the limitations of the techniques used then have already been emphasized. In the case of EPSPs, Redman and his colleagues applied their method to study facilitation by using single and tetanic conditioning stimuli (Edwards et al., 1976b; Hirst et al., 1981) and 4-aminopryridine (4-AP; Jack et al., 1981b). In general, they found that the probability of failures had decreased, and that in the case of 4-AP, previously ineffective synapses may have been recruited. Unfortunately, these descriptions do not provide specific information regarding the quantal parameters.

> Changes in synaptic transmission during depression and/or facilitation are some-times considered to reflect frequency-dependent effects on impulse propagation within preterminal arborizations (Edwards et al., 1976b; Luscher et al., 1979, 1983). Certainly, axonal branch points can be regions of low safety factor for impulse propagation, and branch point failure has been documented (reviewed in Waxman, 1975). However, our analysis of normal and depressed transmitter release in the M-cell system argues against this hypothesis: Action potentials do not actively propagate in the presynaptic processes penetrating this neuron's axon cap (Furukawa and Furshpan, 1963; Faber and Korn, 1978), yet the depolarization passively conducted to the terminals is above threshold for transmitter release. Similarly, Jack et al. (1981a) argued that branch point failure cannot account for the fluctuations in Ia-EPSPs in cat spinal motoneurons, since the time course of averaged EPSPs and of their standard deviations are the same. This correspondence would not be expected if time course and latency varied as a result of fluctuations in the timing of transmitter release.

DISCUSSION

Our current perspective on transmitter release in the central nervous system is based on the primary finding that the binomial parameter n is the same as the number of release sites established by a given presynaptic cell on its target. This relation laid the grounds for a better definition of q and p; the main purpose of this chapter was to focus attention on the probabilistic aspects of transmission. Despite the fact that little is known about the physical determinants of p, various aspects of its behavior and its crucial role in higher functions, such as information processing, can be synthesized.

Relation of n to Release Sites

Chemical synapses are morphologically characterized by active zones (Couteaux and Pécot-Dechavassine, 1970a,b) with a specific arrangement of membrane densities around which synaptic vesicles are clustered and undergo exocytosis; these densities exhibit various geometrical forms, such as dense bands at neuromuscular junctions (or bars; they were first termed release sites in crustacea; see Atwood, 1976) or hexagonal lattices in central synapses (for references, see Llinás and Heuser, 1977). Electron-dense specializations with vesicles clustered around them were first noticed in motor nerve terminals by Birks et al. (1960), and the opening of vesicles was demonstrated to occur at their borders (Couteaux and Pécot-Dechavassine, 1970a,b). In that system, the terminal axon contains numerous active zones, aligned as 100-nm-wide parallel bars, and disposed, with their tight row of associated vesicles, perpendicular to the long axis of the axon (Dreyer et al., 1973; Heuser et al., 1974; Heuser and Reese, 1977).

Interneurons inhibitory to the M-cell provide favorable conditions for a careful analysis of presynaptic ultrastructure, as almost all boutons contain only one active zone. The HRP-stained terminals are segregated inside and outside the axon cap of the M-cell, and they exhibit the distinct characteristics of unmyelinated club endings and small vesicle boutons (Nakajima, 1974), both of which display the characteristics typical of Gray type II synapses. Electron microscope analysis of the HRP-stained endings confirmed that the synaptic complexes are comparable to those seen at other central junctions (Triller and Korn, 1981, 1982). All the boutons examined are filled by numerous pleiomorphic vesicles; the mean diameter, elongation coefficient, and surface area of these vesicles are the same as those of adjacent unstained terminals from the same classes. The presynaptic specializations can also be compared to those of other investigated central synapses: In the latter, they are formed (Gray, 1959, 1963) by electron-opaque patches called presynaptic dense projections, which are disposed in triagonal arrays and are linked at their bases (Bloom and Aghajanian, 1966, 1968; Pfenninger et al., 1969). Thus, they are referred to as part of a "presynaptic grid" (Akert et al., 1972), which guides the vesicles toward the plasma membrane, as suggested by freeze-fracture studies (Pfenninger et al., 1972). Transverse sections of our material demonstrated a similar organization. Finally, E-PTA staining (Triller and Korn, 1982) provided a definition of the boundaries of single terminals and their synaptic grids, showing in *en face* views that at least 95% of the terminals, if not more, contain only one presynaptic grid. *Thus, the striking equivalence found during the quantal analysis of fluctuating unitary IPSPs between the binomial term* n *and the number of stained presynaptic boutons can also be expressed as indicating a one-to-one correspondence with the number of presynaptic grids present in terminals of investigated inhibitory interneurons.*

That "release sites" represent a correlate for n at the neuromuscular junction was hinted at on the basis of indirect arguments. For instance, binomial n's calculated at crayfish motor nerve terminals (Johnson and Wernig, 1971; Wernig, 1972a, 1975; Zucker, 1973) most likely correspond to the number of release sites presumably detected by the postsynaptic microelectrode (Atwood and Johnston, 1968; Jahromi and Atwood, 1974). At the neuromuscular junction of the frog, there also seems to be (Zucker, 1973) a positive correlation between calculated n's (Katz and Miledi, 1965) and the number of sites present along the length of a presynaptic fiber that contribute to the recordings (Birks et al., 1960). More recently, m was correlated with the number and size of presynaptic dense bars in single lobster muscle fibers (Meiss and Govind, 1980) during the formation of neuromuscular junctions (Bennett et al., 1973; Bennett and Florin, 1974; Bennett and Pettigrew, 1974; Bennett and Raftos, 1977). To some extent, n was associated with the number of terminals in cultured spinal neurons (Neale et al., 1983). Finally, since some central terminals may contain more than one active site (Rethelyi, 1970), the binomial term n is certainly not always related to the number of presynaptic boutons. Caution is thus necessary before making morphofunctional correlates on the basis of light microscope observations.

How Do Variations in p Account for Synaptic Plasticity?

Because knowledge of p in the central nervous system is fragmentary, perspectives on its regulation are derived mainly from the periphery. At the crayfish neuromuscular junction, p is quite small following a single presynaptic impulse, but it is raised by conditioning (Zucker, 1973; see also Wernig, 1972a,b). In that system, it was not possible to determine clearly whether facilitation was also associated with any changes in n. However, studies at sympathetic ganglia (McLachlan, 1975; Bennett et al., 1976) and treated mammalian neuromuscular junctions (Bennett et al., 1975) suggested that either n changed alone, or n and p both increased. These apparently conflicting observations can be reconciled if we assume that there is a major effect on p, unless this parameter is already maximal in the unconditioned state (Wernig, 1972a,b; Zucker, 1973; see discussion in McLachlan, 1978).

Zucker (1973, 1977) split p into two multiplicative factors (Vere-Jones, 1966), one representing the probability that a release site is occupied by a quantum, and the other that a presynaptic impulse is effective in evoking release. The notion that p can be broken down into at least two independent variables reconciles some apparently conflicting data, and allows us to put into one scheme the apparently separate mechanisms underlying depression. As summarized in Figure 22, we propose that p be treated as the product of two probability factors, p_1 and p_2, where p_1 undergoes immediate facilitation following a conditioning stimulus, and p_2 is rather decreased at the same time. The variable p_1 would then represent the step or steps in release that are enhanced by the residual intracellular calcium concentration (see below), and p_2 the component of the release mechanism that becomes refractory. In the model curves illustrated, we have assumed that recovery from both processes is exponential, with facilitation decaying more rapidly as depression seems to be longer lasting. This certainly appears to be the case at those central junctions where a single conditioning stimulus triggers both (e.g., Lømo, 1971). Such a simple model reproduces conditions in which initial facilitation is followed by a late depression (Figure 22A), or in which depression dominates at all interstimulus intervals (Figure 22B) by regulating the unconditioned value of the facilitating parameter p_1, which is referred to as p_1^∞. In the first case, which is similar to the perforant pathway synapses on dentate granule cells (Lømo, 1971), p_1 is about 0.2 in the absence of a prior stimulus. Its fivefold increase after a stimulus is sufficient to overcome the effect of a simultaneous decrease in p_2. In the second case, which is comparable to the inhibitory synapses on the M-cell (Faber and Korn, 1982a), the unconditioned value of p_1 is closer to 0.5, and its facilitation is too weak to overcome the depression; thus release is not enhanced. This model, therefore, provides a

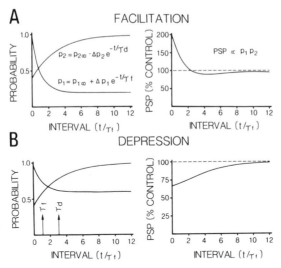

Figure 22. *Synaptic facilitation and depression modeled by the interaction of two independent processes regulating* p. *A and B: Examples corresponding to facilitation and depression, respectively. In each case, the time courses of the two probability factors, p_1 and p_2, are plotted to the left; the curves on the* right *were constructed under the assumption that transmitter release, and thus the amplitudes of the resulting PSP, are directly proportional to the product of p_1 and p_2. Immediately following a conditioning stimulus, p_1 increases to its maximum, while p_2 drops to its minimal value. Both parameters recover exponentially to their unconditioned levels (p_1^∞ and p_2^∞) according to the equations indicated in A. The time constant of recovery of p_1 from its maximal value is τ_f; the corresponding parameter for the recovery of p_2 from its minimal value is τ_d, with $\tau_d = 3 \times \tau_f$ (vertical arrows in B). In A, facilitation dominates during the short intervals because the unconditioned level of p_1 is low, but at longer times a slight depression is apparent. In B, the control level of p_1 is greater than in A; consequently, depression is dominant at all stimulus intervals. Abscissae, the interval between a conditioning and a test stimulus, normalized with respect to the time constant of recovery from facilitation (t/τ_f); ordinates, probabilities p_1 and p_2 (left) and PSP amplitude (right, expressed as a percentage of the control response).*

general framework that encompasses synapses exhibiting differing degrees and forms of activity-dependent plasticity.

Even though p is the product of at least two opposing processes, its calcium dependency has been well documented since Fatt and Katz (1952) first noted that a reduction in this ion's concentration reduced the amplitude of end-plate potentials in a stepwise fashion (see Katz, 1969). With respect to quantal aspects, Miyamoto (1975) observed that when the effective extracellular calcium concentration was raised or lowered at the frog neuromuscular junction, p (and occasionally n) changed in the same direction. At the crayfish neuromuscular junction (Wernig, 1972b), p and m increased in parallel with elevated calcium, while n remained constant. Thus, p is regulated by calcium. Indeed, the hypothesis that facilitation is due to a residual increase in the free intracellular calcium concentration after the initial influx triggered by the presynaptic impulse (Katz and Miledi, 1968) is now generally accepted, and detailed models that predict the time course of residual calcium disposition also accurately describe the process of facilitation (Zucker and Stockbridge, 1983; Stockbridge and Moore, 1984). On the other hand, there is no related explanation for the reduction in p during depression, unless one postulates that calcium channels are blocked or calcium binding sites are inactivated following exocytosis.

Boundaries of Quantal Analysis as a Function of n

It may seem that the proposal that each active zone releases transmitter in an all-or-none manner is incompatible with evidence that release is graded as a function of external calcium or presynaptic depolarization (e.g., Llinás et al., 1981, 1982). However, the evidence for graded release has been obtained from junctions that have a high quantal content and a correspondingly large number of presynaptic active zones, such as 200–300 at the frog neuromuscular junction and about 10,000 at the squid giant synapse (reviewed in McLachlan, 1978). Figure 23, in which the CV of the expected postsynaptic responses is plotted against n, provides an explanation of this apparent paradox. This measure of variability is defined as

$$CV = \frac{1}{\sqrt{n}} \cdot \sqrt{\frac{1 - p}{p}}, \tag{13}$$

for the binomial, and thus decreases in proportion to the square root of n. Consequently, under normal physiological conditions, synapses characterized by low values of n exhibit significant fluctuations, and the magnitude and stability

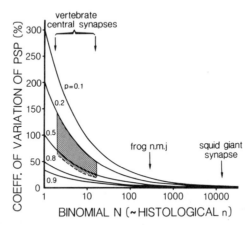

Figure 23. *Influence of quantal release parameters on the variability of synaptic responses.* The coefficient of variation of postsynaptic responses is plotted in percentages as a function of the number of available quantal units, or binomial n, for release probabilities of 0.1, 0.2, 0.5, 0.8, and 0.9. Values typical of binomial n for many vertebrate central synapses, for the frog neuromuscular junction, and for the squid giant synapse are indicated. In each, binomial n has been assumed to be comparable to the number of presynaptic active zones, that is, to histological n. Synapses with large n's have high safety factors for transmission, do not exhibit significant fluctuations, and are relatively insensitive to modifications in p. Synaptic units with lower values of n are associated with large response fluctuations; under such conditions, modifications of p can have significant effects on response variability.

of their output are sensitive to changes in p. Most input connections within the central nervous system fall within this category, and since their target cells process convergent information from a number of sources, modulation of p, for example, can alter transmission appreciably as a consequence of prior activity. Hence, when these synaptic connections are accessible for detailed quantal analyses, such as in the case of the M-cell input synapses, an appreciation of the release mechanisms can be achieved at a level different from that afforded by the larger, more accessible, models. In the latter models, typified by the frog neuromuscular junction and the squid giant synapse, quantal analysis is either precluded or can be achieved only after the bathing solution or temperature has been altered. These preparations provide important macroscopic information about mechanisms regulating release, but do not provide insights concerning its quantal or microscopic properties. Specifically, release may appear graded within the limits of resolution, but nevertheless the postsynaptic responses do vary by quantal increments under the influence of p.

Physiological Meaning of Nonlinear Interaction and Information Processing

The individual active zone (or release site) remains the quantal or functional unit, but the postsynaptic membrane seems to favor the occurrence of responses close to the mean; that is, it seems to reduce response variability by modifying those extreme potentials that have a small probability of appearance. This peculiar filtering mechanism may be significant in terms of stabilizing the sensory input to a highly integrative command neuron and is quite different in nature to other postulated coding strategies in which: (1) The redundancy of sensory messages would be discarded by eliminating the expected messages from the incoming data and by enhancing the more unusual ones (Barlow, 1961a,b, 1981); or (2) a neuron's capacity is maximized by ensuring that all response levels are used with equal frequency (Laughlin, 1981, 1983). Because nonlinear summation of the effects of clustered terminals could also account for the lack of fits observed in different preparations, including those at the Ia–motoneuron synapses, it is tempting to extend this concept to other central nervous system structures.

The fact that equations belonging to communication theory are useful for clarifying the apparent discrepancies between theoretical concepts and experimental data suggests that the quantal nature of chemical transmission is more critically involved in the process of information transfer than was previously suspected. Along this line, it can be pointed out that in reports by electrophysiologists, quanta (unlike nerve impulses, trains in single or several channels) are not considered candidate neural codes (e.g., Perkel and Bullock, 1968; Moore, 1980). But without being exceedingly metaphorical, one can certainly view the input–output relation at single synapses as one of several processes embedded in Shannon's encoding and decoding schemes that may operate in the central nervous system.

At this level, the symbolic communication system (Shannon and Weaver, 1949) may be viewed as consisting of five elements: (1) *The information source*, that is, the presynaptic axon and its branches, which select the desired message; in the context of the events described here, the latter are most likely represented by p, which is the only "plastic" element of chemical transmission. That is, given that a presynaptic impulse triggers the system, the physical representation of the message is np, but as noted before, n is fixed for each cell. (2) *The "transmitter" or encoding process*, which transforms this message into an output signal, is the release site at which the two-choice binary mode of a quantum is well suited to define the amount of information with the classical unity of a bit. If n is the number of release sites issued by one presynaptic cell, with a binomial sampling of vesicular release H, the amount of information at the source is given by $-\Sigma_{x=0}^{n} Px \, \mathrm{Log_2} p_x$, where $x = 0, \ldots, n$, and p_x is given by the binomial equation; hence $H = -\Sigma_{k=0}^{n} C_k^n p^k (1 - p)^{n-k} \log_2[C_k^n p^k (1 - p)^{n-k}]$. For instance, for a neuron with 16 terminals (which is about the average for M-cell inhibitory interneurons) and with p values of 0.5, 0.4, and 0.15 (the last two approximating the mean values for stimulating rates of 2 Hz and 33 Hz, respectively; see Korn et al., 1984), H, the entropy at the information source, is 3.05, 3.02, and 2.51 bits, respectively. In the case of $p = 0.4$ and 0.15, these quantities become 2.51 and 1.97 bits for $n = 8$, 3.51 and 3.04 bits for $n = 32$, and 4.01 and 3.52 bits for $n = 64$. Thus, the amount of information defined by the logarithm to the base two of the number of available choices is determined by both n and p. However, as a consequence of binomial sampling, dispersion expected from an increase of n is minimized: H increases by 0.5 instead of 1.0 when np is doubled. Finally, in a system with one channel, the maximum value of H for two equal possibilities (i.e., if $p = 0.5$) would be one bit. The values in excess are due to the stochastic nature of the release process (or model) and to the multiple release sites and are somewhat redundant. Presumably, this redundancy is useful in a discrete channel with noise for reducing the equivocation (or uncertainty of the message relative to the signal) that is therefore probably large in this system. (3) The physical substrate of the *channel of transmission* is the rather uniform amount of neurotransmitter issued by the synaptic vesicles, which is the carrier of information, but spatial and temporal variables introduce noise acting on the transmitted signal. Of interest here is that the principles underlying the fundamental theorem for a discrete channel with noise, which takes into account the capacity C [given by $C = \mathrm{Lim}_{T\to\infty} (\mathrm{Log} \, N(T)/T)$, where $N(T)$ is the number of allowed signals of duration T], and a discrete source of entropy H, may still be valid. However, the parameter C, which is thus the maximum rate (in bits per second) at which useful information (i.e., total uncertainty minus noise uncertainty) can be transmitted over the channel, has to be redefined, as the information transfer considered here is a nonsequential process: Following each impulse, the active zones release transmitter quasi-simultaneously. (4) *The receiver* and (5) *the destination of the message* may be viewed, in the most general terms, as the postsynaptic membrane and the spike-generating site, respectively.

Information is decoded postsynaptically, and the "reading" procedure is certainly part of the integrative function of the neuron. The precise role of noise is unclear because the characteristics of its physiological components (i.e., noninstrumental) are not determined yet. The assumption that it is uncorrelated is probably valid for thermal noise, but its synaptic part may be due less to chance than is commonly accepted. At this point, it is at least obvious that equivocation (i.e., the increase of average uncertainty of the received message over the emitted signal) introduced by noise is reduced by the interaction between quanta, which maximizes the responses around their mean, and increases the signal-to-noise ratio. In this manner, the receiver is reliably "informed" about the mean quantal content np of the activated presynaptic cell; as shown here, p is the parameter that varies. The "excess" of the total number n of presynaptic release sites over those that are activated by each impulse is clearly advantageous, since it guarantees that a stable fraction of the former will always be available for the coding process.

The question thus becomes whether any analogy can be drawn between the coding used at the synaptic level, and that used to reduce equivocation in a noisy channel. Our computations led to apparently paradoxical results: The entropy increases (and hence the equivocation) with the number of synaptic boutons. But a normalization should be undertaken here; since q is the physical unit that carries the information, entropy should be calculated per quantal site. Then, p being equal, the entropy per quantum decreases as n grows.

A similar phenomenon is observed when an efficient coding is implemented to transmit a message through a noisy channel. The theorem for noisy channels (Shannon and Weaver, 1949) predicts that, if the capacity of the channel is greater than the entropy of the original message, such a code exists. It will lead to the construction of a redundant message in which less information is carried by each symbol. Again, the redundancy is hard to define for a nonsequential process, but the decrease of the number of bits associated with a quantal channel (or symbol) is comparable to redundancy, and it presumably reduces equivocation introduced by the stochastic character of quantal release and by noise.

The increased reliability of neurons with larger n's, which is already suggested by the fact that, for an equal value of p, the number of bits per quantum is decreased (e.g., if $p = 0.4$, the normalized value of H is 0.31, 0.19, 0.11, and 0.06 for n's of 8, 16, 32, and 64, respectively), is further confirmed by the examination of the CV. As given in Equation 13, this normalized index of variability decreases with the square root of n, indicating the greater stability of responses to neurons with more terminals (p being equal). Similarly, as p decreases and n increases while m remains constant, calculations indicate that the entropy per available quantum decreases.

It would be interesting to demonstrate a possible analogy or formal equivalence between putative neuronal coding at the synaptic level and theoretically analyzed methods of coding. The most relevant possibility here may be one that best allows the correction of errors; it was described by Shannon and Weaver (1949) and was named the (n,k) code (see Atlan, 1972). In this code, the symbols of the original message are grouped by series of k symbols and replaced by clusters of n symbols ($n > k$) carrying the same quantity of information. The redundancy is raised, but proper decoding reduces equivocation to an arbitrarily low level. However, since these symbols and messages are still waiting for a precise physical definition as well as an adequate operational definition, the eventual meaning and values of n and k remain only tentative.

ACKNOWLEDGMENTS

We wish to thank S. Boucheron (E.N.S.) for his help with some of the theoretical formulations presented in this chapter.

REFERENCES

Akert, K., K. Pfenninger, C. Sandri, and H. Moor (1972) Freeze etching and cytochemistry of vesicles and membrane complexes in synapses of the central nervous system. In *Structure and Function of Synapses*, G. D. Pappas and D. P. Purpura, eds., pp. 67–86, Raven, New York.

Atlan, H. (1972) *L'Organisation Biologique et la Théorie de l'Information*, Hermann, Paris.

Atwood, H. L. (1976) Organization and synaptic physiology of crustacean neuromuscular systems. *Prog. Neurobiol.* 7:291–391.

Atwood, H. L., and H. S. Johnston (1968) Neuromuscular synapses of a crab motor axon. *J. Exp. Zool.* 167:457–470.

Barker, J. L., and R. N. McBurney (1979) Phenobarbitone modulation of postsynaptic GABA receptor function on cultured mammalian neurons. *Proc. R. Soc. Lond. (Biol.)* 206:319–327.

Barlow, H. B. (1961a) Possible principles underlying the transformations of sensory messages. In *Sensory Communication*, W. A. Rosenblith, ed., pp. 217–234, MIT Press, Cambridge, Massachusetts.

Barlow, H. B. (1961b) Three points about lateral inhibition. In *Sensory Communication*, W. A. Rosenblith, ed., pp. 782–786, MIT Press, Cambridge, Massachusetts.

Barlow, H. B. (1981) Critical limiting factors in the design of the eye and visual cortex. *Proc. R. Soc. Lond. (Biol.)* 212:1–34.

Barton, S. B., and I. S. Cohen (1977) Are transmitter release statistics meaningful? *Nature* 268:267–268.

Bennett, M. R., and T. Florin (1974) A statistical analysis of the release of acetylcholine at newly formed synapses in striated muscle. *J. Physiol. (Lond.)* 238:93–107.

Bennett, M. R., and A. G. Pettigrew (1974) The formation of synapses in striated muscle during development. *J. Physiol. (Lond.)* 241:515–545.

Bennett, M. R., and J. Raftos (1977) The formation and regression of synapses during the re-innervation of axolotl striated muscle. *J. Physiol. (Lond.)* 265:261–295.

Bennett, M. R., E. M. McLachlan, and R. S. Taylor (1973) The formation of synapses in reinnervated mammalian muscle. *J. Physiol. (Lond.)* 233:481–500.

Bennett, M. R., T. Florin, and R. Hall (1975) The effect of calcium ions on the binomial statistic parameters which control acetylcholine release at synapses in striated muscle. *J. Physiol. (Lond)* 247:429–446.

Bennett, M. R., T. Florin, and A. G. Pettigrew (1976) The effect of calcium ions on the binomial statistic parameters that control acetylcholine release at preganglionic nerve terminals. *J. Physiol. (Lond.)* 257:597–620.

Betz, W. J. (1970) Depression of transmitter release at the neuromuscular junction. *J. Physiol. (Lond.)* 206:629–644.

Birks, R., H. E. Huxley, and B. Katz (1960) Differentiation of nerve terminals in the crayfish opener muscle and its functional significance. *J. Physiol. (Lond.)* 150:134–144.

Blackman, J. G., and R. D. Purves (1969) Intracellular recordings from ganglia of the thoracic sympathetic chain of the guinea pig. *J. Physiol. (Lond.)* 203:173–198.

Blackman, J. G., B. L. Ginsborg, and C. Ray (1963) On the quantal release of the transmitter at a sympathetic synapse. *J. Physiol. (Lond.)* 167:402–415.

Blankenship, J. E., and M. Kuno (1968) Analysis of subthreshold activity in spinal motoneurons of the cat. *J. Neurophysiol.* 31:186–194.

Bloom, F. E., and G. K. Aghajanian (1966) Cytochemistry of synapses: Selective staining for electron microscopy. *Science* 154:1575–1577.

Bloom, F. E., and G. K. Aghajanian (1968) Fine structural and cytochemical analysis of the staining of synaptic junctions with phosphotungstic acid. *J. Ultrastruct. Res.* 22:361–375.

Brock, L. G., J. S. Coombs, and J. C. Eccles (1952) The recording of potentials from motoneurons with an intracellular electrode. *J. Physiol. (Lond.)* 117:431–460.

Brown, T. H., D. H. Perkel, and M. W. Feldman (1976) Evoked neurotransmitter release: Statistical effect of nonuniformity and nonstationarity. *Proc. Natl. Acad. Sci. USA* 73:2913–2917.

Burke, R. E. (1967) Composite nature of the monosynaptic excitatory postsynaptic potential. *J. Neurophysiol.* **30**:1114–1137.

Burke, R. E., B. Walmsley, and J. A. Hodgson (1979) HRP anatomy of group Ia afferent contacts on alpha motoneurons. *Brain Res.* **160**:347–352.

Colomo, F., and S. D. Erulkar (1968) Miniature synaptic potentials at frog spinal neurones in the presence of tetrodotoxin. *J. Physiol. (Lond.)* **199**:205–221.

Couteaux, R., and M. Pécot-Dechavassine (1970a) Vésicules synaptiques et poches au niveau des zones actives de la jonction neuro-musculaire. *C. R. Seances Acad. Sci. (Series D)* **271**:2346–2349.

Couteaux, R., and M. Pécot-Dechavassine (1970b) L'ouverture des vésicules synaptiques au niveau des zones actives. In *Microscopie Electronique*, Vol. III, P. Favard, ed., pp. 709–710, Seventh International Congress of Electron Microscopy, Grenoble, France.

Curtis, D. R., and J. C. Eccles (1960) Synaptic action during and after repetitive stimulation. *J. Physiol. (Lond.)* **150**:374–398.

del Castillo, J., and B. Katz (1954) Quantal components of the end-plate potential. *J. Physiol. (Lond.)* **124**:560–573.

Dennis, M. J., A. J. Harris, and S. W. Kuffler (1971) Synaptic transmission and its duplication by focally applied acetylcholine in parasympathetic neurons in the heart of the frog. *Proc. R. Soc. Lond. (Biol.)* **177**:509–539.

Diamond, J., S. Roper, and G. M. Yasargil (1973) The membrane effects and sensitivity of strychnine, of neural inhibition of the Mauthner cell, and its inhibition by glycine and GABA. *J. Physiol. (Lond.)* **232**:87–111.

Dreyer, F. K., K. Peper, K. Akert, C. Sandri, and H. Moor (1973) Ultrastructure of the active zone in the frog neuro-muscular junction. *Brain Res.* **62**:373–380.

Dudel, J., and S. W. Kuffler (1961) The quantal nature of transmission and spontaneous miniature potentials at the crayfish neuromuscular junction. *J. Physiol. (Lond.)* **155**:514–529.

Dudel, J., W. Finger, and H. Stettmeier (1977) GABA-induced membrane current noise and the time course of the inhibitory synaptic current in crayfish muscle. *Neurosci. Lett.* **6**:203–208.

Dudel, J., W. Finger, and H. Stettmeier (1980) Inhibitory synaptic channels activated by γ-aminobutyric acid (GABA) in crayfish muscle. *Pfluegers Arch. Eur. J. Physiol.* **387**:143–151.

Eccles, J. C. (1961a) The effect of frequency of activation on transmission across synapses. In *Proceedings of the Symposium on Bioelectrogenesis*, C. Chagas and M. C. de Carvalho, eds., pp. 297–309, Elsevier, Amsterdam.

Eccles, J. C. (1961b) The mechanism of synaptic transmission. *Ergebn. Physiol.* **51**:299–430.

Eccles, J. C. (1964) *The Physiology of Synapses*, Springer-Verlag, Berlin.

Eccles, J. C., J. I. Hubbard, and O. Oscarsson (1961a) Intracellular recording from cells of the ventral spino-cerebellar tract. *J. Physiol. (Lond.)* **158**:486–516.

Eccles, J. C., O. Oscarsson, and W. D. Willis (1961b) Synaptic action of group I and II afferent fibres of muscle on the cells of the dorsal cerebellar tract. *J. Physiol. (Lond.)* **158**:517–543.

Edwards, F. R., S. J. Redman, and B. Walmsley (1976a) Statistical fluctuations in charge transfer at Ia synapses on spinal motoneurones. *J. Physiol. (Lond.)* **259**:655–688.

Edwards, F. R., S. J. Redman, and B. Walmsley (1976b) Non-quantal fluctuations and transmission failures in charge transfer at Ia synapses on spinal motoneurones. *J. Physiol. (Lond.)* **259**:689–704.

Elmqvist, D., and D. M. J. Quastel (1965) Presynaptic action of hemicholinium at the neuromuscular junction. *J. Physiol. (Lond.)* **177**:463–482.

Faber, D. S., and H. Korn (1973) A neuronal inhibition mediated electrically. *Science* **179**:577–578.

Faber, D. S., and H. Korn (1978) Electrophysiology of the Mauthner cell: Basic properties, synaptic mechanisms, and associated networks. In *Neurobiology of the Mauthner Cell*, D. S. Faber and H. Korn, eds., pp. 47–131, Raven, New York.

Faber, D. S., and H. Korn (1980) Single-shot channel activation accounts for duration of inhibitory postsynaptic potentials in a central neuron. *Science* **208**:612–615.

Faber, D. S., and H. Korn (1982a) Transmission at a central inhibitory synapse. I. Magnitude of the unitary postsynaptic conductance change and kinetics of channel activation. *J. Neurophysiol.* 48:654–678.

Faber, D. S., and H. Korn (1982b) Binary mode of transmitter release at central synapses. *Trends Neurosci.* 5:157–159.

Faber, D. S., H. Korn, and A. Triller (1983) Quantal analysis of strychnine action at a presumed glycinergic central synapse. *Soc. Neurosci. Abstr.* 9:456.

Fatt, P., and B. Katz (1952) Spontaneous subthreshold activity at motor nerve endings. *J. Physiol. (Lond.)* 117:109–128.

Fukami, Y., T. Furukawa, and Y. Asada (1965) Excitability changes of the Mauthner cell during collateral inhibition. *J. Gen. Physiol.* 48:581–600.

Furshpan, E. J., and T. Furukawa (1962) Intracellular and extracellular responses of several regions of the Mauthner cell of the goldfish. *J. Neurophysiol.* 25:732–771.

Furukawa, T., and E. J. Furshpan (1963) Two inhibitory mechanisms in the Mauthner neurons of goldfish. *J. Neurophysiol.* 26:140–176.

Furukawa, T., and S. Matsuura (1978) Adaptive rundown of excitatory postsynaptic potentials at synapses between hair cells and eighth nerve fibers in the goldfish. *J. Physiol. (Lond.)* 276:193–209.

Furukawa, T., Y. Hayashida, and S. Matsuura (1978) Quantal analysis of the size of excitatory postsynaptic potentials at synapses between hair cells and afferent nerve fibers in goldfish. *J. Physiol. (Lond.)* 276:211–226.

Furukawa, T., M. Kuno, and S. Matsuura (1982) Quantal analysis of a decremental response at hair cell–afferent fibre synapses in the goldfish sacculus. *J. Physiol. (Lond.)* 322:181–195.

Ginsborg, B. L., and D. H. Jenkinson (1976) Transmission of impulses from nerve to muscle. *Handb. Exp. Pharmacol.* 42:229–364.

Gold, M., and A. R. Martin (1983) Inhibitory conductance changes at synapses in the lamprey brainstem. *Science* 221:85–87.

Grantyn, R., A. I. Shapovalov, and B. I. Shiriaev (1982) Combined morphological and electrophysiological description of connexions between single primary afferent fibres and individual motoneurones in the frog spinal cord. *Exp. Brain Res.* 48:459–462.

Grantyn, R., A. I. Shapovalov, and B. I. Shiriaev (1984a) Tracing of frog sensory-motor synapse by intracellular injection of horseradish peroxidase. *J. Physiol. (Lond.)* 349:441–458.

Grantyn, R., A. I. Shapovalov, and B. I. Shiriaev (1984b) Relation between structural and release parameters at the frog sensory-motor synapse. *J. Physiol. (Lond.)* 349:459–474.

Gray, E. G. (1959) Axo-somatic and axo-dendritic synapses on the cerebral cortex: An electron microscope study. *J. Anat.* 93:420–433.

Gray, E. G. (1963) Electron microscopy of presynaptic organelles of the spinal cord. *J. Anat.* 97:101–106.

Hatt, H., and D. O. Smith (1976) Non-uniform probabilities of quantal release at the crayfish neuromuscular junction. *J. Physiol. (Lond.)* 259:395–404.

Heuser, J. E., and T. S. Reese (1977) Structure of the synapse. *Handb. Physiol., The Nervous System,* 1:261–294.

Heuser, J. E., T. S. Reese, and D. M. D. Landis (1974) Functional changes in frog neuro-muscular junctions studied with freeze fracture. *J. Neurocytol.* 3:109–131.

Heuser, J. E., T. S. Reese, M. J. Dennis, Y. Yan, L. Yan, and L. Evans (1979) Synaptic vesicle exocytosis captured by quick freezing and correlated with quantal transmitter release. *J. Cell Biol.* 81:275–300.

Highstein, S. M., and M. V. L. Bennett (1975) Fatigue and recovery of transmission at the Mauthner fibre–giant synapse of the hatchetfish. *Brain Res.* 98:229–242.

Hirst, G. D. S., S. J. Redman, and K. Wong (1981) Post-tetanic potentiation and facilitation of synaptic potentials evoked in cat spinal motoneurones. *J. Physiol. (Lond.)* 321:97–109.

Honig, M. G., W. F. Collins, III, and L. M. Mendell (1983) α-motoneuron EPSPs exhibit different frequency sensitivities to single Ia-afferent fiber stimulation. *J. Neurophysiol.* 49:886–901.

Hubbard, J. I. (1963) Prolonged effects of stimulation at the mammalian neuromuscular junction. *J. Physiol. (Lond.)* **169**:641–662.

Jack, J. J. B., S. J. Redman, and K. Wong (1981a) The components of synaptic potentials evoked in cat spinal motoneurones by impulses in single group Ia afferents. *J. Physiol. (Lond.)* **321**:65–96.

Jack, J. J. B., S. J. Redman, and K. Wong (1981b) Modifications to synaptic transmission at group Ia synapses on cat spinal motoneurones by 4-aminopyridine. *J. Physiol. (Lond.)* **321**:111–126.

Jahromi, S. S., and H. L. Atwood (1974) Three-dimensional ultrastructure of the crayfish neuromuscular apparatus. *J. Cell Biol.* **63**:599–613.

Jazwinski, A. H. (1970) *Stochastic Processes and Filtering Theory*, Academic, New York, pp. 81–85.

Johnson, E. W., and A. Wernig (1971) The binomial nature of transmitter release at the crayfish neuromuscular junction. *J. Physiol. (Lond.)* **218**:757–767.

Katz, B. (1969) *The Release of Neural Transmitter Substances*, Charles C Thomas, Springfield, Illinois.

Katz, B. (1971) Quantal mechanism of neural transmitter release. *Science* **173**:123–126.

Katz, B., and R. Miledi (1963) A study of spontaneous miniature potentials in spinal motoneurones. *J. Physiol. (Lond.)* **168**:389–422.

Katz, B., and R. Miledi (1965) The effect of temperature on the synaptic delay at the neuromuscular junction. *J. Physiol. (Lond.)* **181**:656–670.

Katz, B., and R. Miledi (1968) The role of calcium in neurotransmitter facilitation. *J. Physiol. (Lond.)* **195**:481–492.

Kendall, M. and A. Stuart (1977) *The Advanced Theory of Statistics*, Vol. 1, C. Griffin and Co., London, pp. 109–110.

Koch, C., T. Poggio, and V. Torre (1983) Nonlinear interactions in a dendritic tree: Localization, timing and role in information processing. *Proc. Natl. Acad. Sci. USA* **80**:2799–2802.

Kolmodin, G. M., and C. R. Skoglund (1958) Slow membrane potential changes accompanying excitation and inhibition in spinal moto- and interneurons in the cat during natural activation. *Acta Physiol. Scand.* **44**:11–54.

Korn, H. (1984) What central inhibitory pathways tell us about mechanisms of transmitter release. *Exp. Brain Res. (Suppl. 9)*:201–224.

Korn, H., and D. S. Faber (1975) An electrically mediated inhibition in goldfish medulla. *J. Neurophysiol.* **38**:452–471.

Korn, H., and D. S. Faber (1976) Vertebrate central nervous system: Same neurons mediate both electrical and chemical inhibitions. *Science* **194**:1166–1169.

Korn, H., and D. S. Faber (1983) A possible cooperativity between synapses sharing a common postsynaptic locus. *Soc. Neurosci. Abstr.* **9**:456.

Korn, H., and A. Mallet (1984) Transformation of binomial input by the postsynaptic membrane at a central synapse. *Science* **225**:1157–1159.

Korn, H., A. Triller, and D. S. Faber (1978) Structural correlates of recurrent collateral interneurons producing both electrical and chemical inhibitions of the Mauthner cell. *Proc. R. Soc. Lond. (Biol.)* **202**:533–538.

Korn, H., A. Triller, A. Mallet, and D. S. Faber (1981) Fluctuating responses at a central synapse: *n* of binomial fit predicts number of stained presynaptic boutons. *Science* **213**:898–901.

Korn, H., A. Mallet, A. Triller, and D. S. Faber (1982) Transmission at a central synapse. II. Quantal description of release with a physical correlate for binomial *n*. *J. Neurophysiol.* **48**:679–707.

Korn, H., D. S. Faber, Y. Burnod, and A. Triller (1984) Regulation of efficacy at central synapses. *J. Neurosci.* **4**:125–130.

Kuffler, S. W., and J. G. Nicholls (1976) *From Neuron to Brain*, Sinauer Associates, Sunderland, Massachusetts.

Kullback, S. (1959) *Information Theory and Statistics*, Wiley, New York.

Kuno, M. (1963) The quantal nature of monosynaptic transmission in spinal motoneurons of the cat. *Physiologist* **6**:219.

Kuno, M. (1964a) Quantal components of excitatory synaptic potentials in spinal motoneurones. *J. Physiol. (Lond.)* **175**:81–99.

Kuno, M. (1964b) Mechanisms of facilitation and depression of the excitatory synaptic potential in spinal motoneurones. *J. Physiol. (Lond.)* **175**:100–112.

Kuno, M. (1971) Quantum aspects of central and ganglionic synaptic transmission in vertebrates. *Physiol. Rev.* **51**:647–678.

Kuno, M., and J. T. Miyahara (1969) Non-linear summation of unit synaptic potentials in spinal motoneurones of the cat. *J. Physiol. (Lond.)* **201**:465–477.

Kuno, M., and J. N. Weakly (1972) Quantal components of the inhibitory synaptic potential in spinal motoneurones of the cat. *J. Physiol. (Lond.)* **224**:287–303.

Laughlin, S. (1981) A simple coding procedure enhances a neuron's information capacity. *Z. Naturforsch.* **36c**:910–912.

Laughlin, S. (1983) Matching coding to scenes to enhance efficiency. In *Physical and Biological Processing of Images*, O. J. Braddick and A. Sleish, eds., pp. 42–52, Springer-Verlag, Berlin.

Llinás, R., and J. E. Heuser (1977) Depolarization release coupling systems in neurons. *Neurosci. Res. Program. Bull.* **15**:557–687.

Llinás, R., I. Z. Steinberg, and K. Walton (1981) Relationship between presynaptic calcium current and postsynaptic potential in squid giant synapse. *Biophys. J.* **33**:323–352.

Llinás, R., M. Sugimori, and S. M. Simon (1982) Transmission by presynaptic spike-like depolarization in the squid giant synapse. *Proc. Natl. Acad. Sci. USA* **79**:2415–2419.

Lømo, T. (1971) Potentiation of monosynaptic EPSPs in the perforant path–dentate granule cell synapse. *Exp. Brain Res.* **12**:46–63.

Luscher, H. R., P. Ruenzel, and E. Henneman (1979) How the size of motoneurons determines their susceptibility to discharge. *Nature* **282**:859–861.

Luscher, H. R., P. Ruenzel, and E. Henneman (1983) Composite EPSPs in motoneurons of different sizes before and during PTP: Implications for transmission failure and its relief in Ia projections. *J. Neurophysiol.* **49**:269–289.

McLachlan, E. M. (1975) Changes in statistical release parameters during prolonged stimulation of preganglionic nerve terminals. *J. Physiol. (Lond.)* **253**:477–491.

McLachlan, E. M. (1978) The statistics of transmitter release at chemical synapses. *Int. Rev. Physiol. Neurophysiol.* **17**:49–117.

McNaughton, B. L., R. M. Douglas, and G. V. Goddard (1978) Synaptic enhancement in fascia dentata: Cooperativity among coactive afferents. *Brain Res.* **157**:277–293.

Martin, A. R. (1955) A further study of the statistical composition of the end-plate potential. *J. Physiol. (Lond.)* **130**:114–122.

Martin, A. R. (1966) Quantal nature of synaptic transmission. *Physiol. Rev.* **46**:51–66.

Martin, A. R., and G. Pilar (1964) Quantal components of the synaptic potential in the ciliary ganglion of the chick. *J. Physiol. (Lond.)* **175**:1–16.

Meiss, D. E., and C. K. Govind (1980) Heterogeneity of excitatory synapses at the ends of single muscle fibers in lobster *Homarus americanus*. *J. Neurobiol.* **11**:381–395.

Mendell, L. M. (1984) Modifiability of spinal synapses. *Physiol. Rev.* **64**:260–324.

Mendell, L. M., and R. Weiner (1976) Analysis of pairs of individual Ia-EPSPs in single motoneurones. *J. Physiol. (Lond.)* **255**:81–104.

Miyamoto, M. D. (1975) Binomial analysis of quantal transmitter release at glycerol-treated frog neuromuscular junctions. *J. Physiol. (Lond.)* **250**:121–142.

Model, P. G., S. M. Highstein, and M. V. L. Bennett (1975) Depletion of vesicles and fatigue of transmission at a vertebrate central synapse. *Brain Res.* **98**:209–228.

Moore, G. P. (1980) Mathematical techniques for studying information processing by the nervous system. In *Information Processing in the Nervous System*, H. M. Pinker and J. D. Willis, eds., pp. 17–30, Raven, New York.

Nakajima, Y. (1974) Fine structure of the synaptic endings on the Mauthner cell of the goldfish. *J. Comp. Neurol.* **156**:375–402.

Neale, E. A., P. G. Nelson, R. L. Macdonald, C. N. Christian, and L. M. Bowers (1983) Synaptic interactions between mammalian central neurons in cell culture. III. Morphological correlates of quantal synaptic transmission. *J. Neurophysiol.* **49**:1459–1468.

Neher, E., and C. F. Stevens (1977) Conductance fluctuations and ionic pores in membranes. *Annu. Rev. Biophys. Biol.* **6**:345–381.

Nelder, J. A., and R. Mead (1965) A simple method for function minimization. *Computer J.* **7**:308–313.

Otsuka, M., M. Endo, and Y. Nonomura (1962) Presynaptic nature of neuromuscular depression. *Jpn. J. Physiol.* **12**:573–583.

Perkel, D. H., and T. H. Bullock (1968) Neural coding. *Neurosci. Res. Program Bull.* **6**:221–348.

Pfenninger, K., C. Sandri, K. Akert, and C. H. Eugster (1969) Contribution to the problem of structural organization of the presynaptic area. *Brain Res.* **12**:10–18.

Pfenninger, K., K. Akert, H. Moor, and C. Sandri (1972) The fine structure of freeze-fractured presynaptic membranes. *J. Neurocytol.* **1**:129–149.

Redman, S., and B. Walmsley (1983a) The time course of synaptic potentials evoked in cat motoneurones at identified group Ia synapses. *J. Physiol. (Lond.)* **343**:117–133.

Redman, S., and B. Walmsley (1983b) Amplitude fluctuations in synaptic potentials evoked in cat spinal motoneurones at identified group Ia synapses. *J. Physiol. (Lond.)* **343**:135–145.

Réthelyi, M. (1970) Ultrastructural synaptology of Clarke's column. *Exp. Brain Res.* **11**:159–174.

Roper, S., J. Diamond, and G. M. Yasargil (1969) Does strychnine block inhibition postsynaptically? *Nature* **223**:1168–1169.

Shannon, C. E. (1948a) A mathematical theory of communication. *Bell Syst. Tech. J.* **27**:379–423.

Shannon, C. E. (1948b) A mathematical theory of communciation. *Bell Syst. Tech. J.* **27**:623–656.

Shannon, C. E., and W. Weaver (1949) *The Mathematical Theory of Communication*, University of Illinois Press, Urbana.

Shapovalov, A. I., and B. I. Shiriaev (1980) Dual mode of junctional transmission at synapses between single primary afferent fibres and motoneurones in the amphibian. *J. Physiol. (Lond.)* **306**:1–15.

Stockbridge, N., and J. W. Moore (1984) Dynamics of intracellular calcium and its possible relationship to phasic transmitter release and facilitation at the frog neuromuscular junction. *J. Neurosci.* **4**:803–811.

Thies, R. E. (1965) Neuromuscular depression and the apparent depletion of transmitter in mammalian muscle. *J. Neurophysiol.* **28**:427–442.

Triller, A., and H. Korn (1978) Mise en évidence électrophysiologique et anatomique de neurones vestibulaires inhibiteurs commissuraux chez la tanche (*Tinca tinca*). *C. R. Seances Acad. Sci. (Series D)* **286**:89–92.

Triller, A., and H. Korn (1981) Morphologically distinct classes of inhibitory synapses arise from the same neurons: Ultrastructural identification from crossed vestibular interneurons intracellularly stained with HRP. *J. Comp. Neurol.* **203**:131–155.

Triller, A., and H. Korn (1982) Transmission at a central inhibitory synapse. III. Ultrastructure of physiologically identified terminals. *J. Neurophysiol.* **48**:708–736.

Tsukahara, N., and K. Kosaka (1968) The mode of cerebral excitation of red nucleus neurons. *Exp. Brain Res.* **5**:102–117.

Vere-Jones, D. (1966) Simple stochastic models for the release of quanta of transmitter from a nerve terminal. *Aust. J. Statist.* **8**:53–63.

Waxman, S. G. (1975) Integrative properties and design principles of axons. *Int. Rev. Neurobiol.* **18**:1–40.

Wernig, A. (1972a) Changes in statistical parameters during facilitation at the crayfish neuromuscular junction. *J. Physiol. (Lond.)* **226**:751–760.

Wernig, A. (1972b) The effects of calcium and magnesium on statistical release parameters at the crayfish neuromuscular junction. *J. Physiol. (Lond.)* **226**:761–768.

Wernig, A. (1975) Estimates of statistical release parameters from crayfish and frog neuromuscular junctions. *J. Physiol. (Lond.)* **244**:207–221.

Wernig, A. (1976) Localization of active sites in the neuromuscular junction. *Brain Res.* **118**:63–72.

Wong, K., and S. Redman (1980) The recovery of a random variable from a noisy record with application to the study of fluctuations in synaptic potentials. *J. Neurosci. Methods* **2**:389–409.

Zucker, R. S. (1973) Changes in the statistics of transmitter release during facilitation. *J. Physiol. (Lond.)* **229**:787–810.

Zucker, R. S. (1977) Synaptic plasticity at crayfish neuromuscular junctions. In *Identified Neurons and Behavior of Arthropods*, G. Hoyne, ed., pp. 49–65, Plenum, New York.

Zucker, R. S., and N. Stockbridge (1983) Presynaptic calcium diffusion and the time course of transmitter release and synaptic facilitation at the squid giant synapse. *J. Neurosci.* **3**:1263–1269.

Chapter 4

Intercellular Communication Mediated by Gap Junctions Can Be Controlled in Many Ways

MICHAEL V. L. BENNETT
DAVID C. SPRAY

ABSTRACT

Gap junctions are the usual morphological substrate of electrotonic synaptic transmission and of the passage of small molecules between cells, as exemplified by dye coupling. A number of treatments are now known that decrease junctional conductance, g_j. Treatments acidifying the coupled cells' cytoplasms decreases g_j, and in some cases good reversible titration curves can be obtained. Sensitivity to hydrogen ions varies in different tissues, presumably reflecting differences in the amino acid composition of the junctional protein. Block by cytoplasmic calcium can also be obtained, although much higher concentrations are required than for hydrogen. The same active sites may be involved. Decrease in g_j caused by acidification may be one effect of ischemia. Calcium sensitivity may act in the uncoupling produced by cell injury that disrupts the surface permeability barrier and lets in extracellular calcium. Junctions in amphibian embryos are quite sensitive to transjunctional voltage, V_j; g_j is decreased symmetrically by V_j of either sign. Steady-state conductances are well fit by a Boltzmann relation, implying a fixed dipole moment change between the open and closed states. Apparently there are two gates in series, one in each membrane. Because closing one gate should affect the potential seen by the other gate, an applied field may cause individual channels to cycle around a circular reaction scheme. Other junctions exhibit dependence on the voltage between the cytoplasm and the bath, inside–outside voltage or V_{i-o}. Presumably, V_{i-o} dependence is also simply a consequence of a dipole moment change but in the direction between the cytoplasm or channel and the extracellular space of the junctional gap. Dependence on V_j varies; in amphibians, it is comparable to although slower than that of sodium channels. Other tissues are less sensitive or insensitive. Sensitive junctions allow cells to exist in two stable states of coupling and may play a role in establishing borders in embryonic development. In a coupled neuronal system, the horizontal cells of the retina, g_j can be controlled by other synaptic inputs, apparently acting through cAMP. The degree of electrotonic spread between cells can also be modulated by inhibitory synapses. An anti-junction antibody is now available that blocks junctional communication when injected intracellularly. This antibody provides a highly specific tool for investigating the functional role of gap junctions. Junctional formation between sympathetic neurons can be induced by appropriate pharmacological treatments. The diverse biophysics of channel gating and the cellular controls of synthesis and turnover provide the gap junction with a wide range of functional capabilities. They also provide the experimenter with many methodologies and problems for investigation.

Gap junctions are a morphologically defined class of structures that join cells of the same or different types (cf. Bennett and Goodenough, 1978; Bennett and Spray, 1985). A single junctional unit apparently comprises two hemichannels (or connexons), one in each membrane, that form a channel connecting the interiors of the coupled cells. The apposed membranes are separated by a narrow gap that is bridged by the channel structure. The channel interiors are isolated from the extracellular space in the gap that is continuous with the surrounding medium; thus the junctions form a private pathway between cells. This pathway passes ions and small molecules up to a diameter of about 1.2 nm or a molecular weight of 1 kD. Proteins and polynucleotides are excluded.

A gap junction is characterized in thin sections perpendicular to the membranes as a reduction of extracellular space to about 2 nm (Figure 1). The channels bridging the gap are not well defined, and the channels' walls apparently do not stain well within the gap. Periodic substructure representing junctional units is sometimes seen and clearly distinguishes gap junctions from tight junctions (zonulae occludentes) and the artifactual close appositions that occur in a number of tissues (cf. Bennett, 1977). Negative staining also reveals the channel arrays, particularly in *en face* views.

In freeze-fracture micrographs, gap junctions are recognizable as aggregates of intramembrane particles associated with a narrowing of the intercellular cleft (Figure 2). In vertebrates, particles are generally found on the P face with corresponding pits on the E face. Single particles associated with narrowing of the cleft may represent junctions of the minimum size (Ginzberg et al., 1985).

Early electrophysiological studies mainly dealt with junctions that were electrically linear and quite fixed in their properties (Bennett, 1977). In the past few years, a number of methods have been found to alter junctional conductance, g_j, methods that have more or less widespread applicability to gap junctions in different tissues and different species (Bennett et al., 1984; Spray et al., 1984b; Spray and Bennett, 1985). These methods of altering, or gating, g_j are the subject of this chapter. The main message is that communication via gap junctions can be rapidly controlled by cellular mechanisms. Slower changes can also be produced by the formation of new junctions or the removal of existing ones, a subject only briefly mentioned here. In general, we have worked with pairs of cells that allow unambiguous measurement of junctional and nonjunctional resistances (cf. Bennett, 1966).

EFFECTS OF CYTOPLASMIC IONS

A dramatic way of changing g_j is by bathing coupled cells in CO_2-equilibrated saline (or other weak acids). CO_2 (or the undissociated acid) rapidly crosses the plasma membrane and acidifies the cell interior; upon rinsing in normal saline, the effect is rapidly reversed (Figure 3; Spray et al., 1979, 1981a). Experiments with strong acids and impermeant buffers show that external hydrogen ions have no effect on g_j. If one monitors intracellular pH (pH_i) with an ion-selective electrode and correlates g_j with pH_i, one obtains in many cell types a simple titration curve for which the points during recovery fall on the same line as

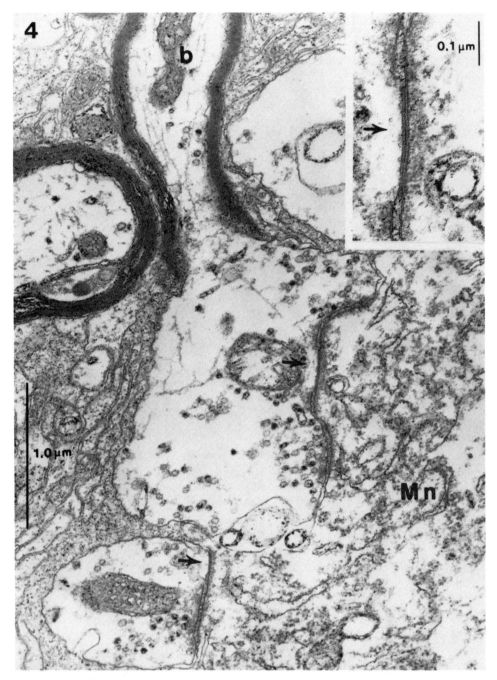

Figure 1. *Gap junctions at synaptic terminals on motoneurons in the hatchetfish.* An axon (b) looses its myelin sheath and forms a morphologically mixed synapse on a motoneuron (Mn) that has both a gap junction (*arrow*, enlarged in *inset*) and apparent chemically transmitting active zones. The active zones are characterized by synaptic vesicles, many with an electron-dense granule, and fuzz in the pre- and postsynaptic cytoplasm. At the gap junctions, there is a thick layer of increased density in the postsynaptic cytoplasm. Physiological data indicate that postsynaptic potentials at some or all of these synapses are purely rectifying, without a chemically mediated component (Auerbach and Bennett, 1969). (From Hall et al., 1985.)

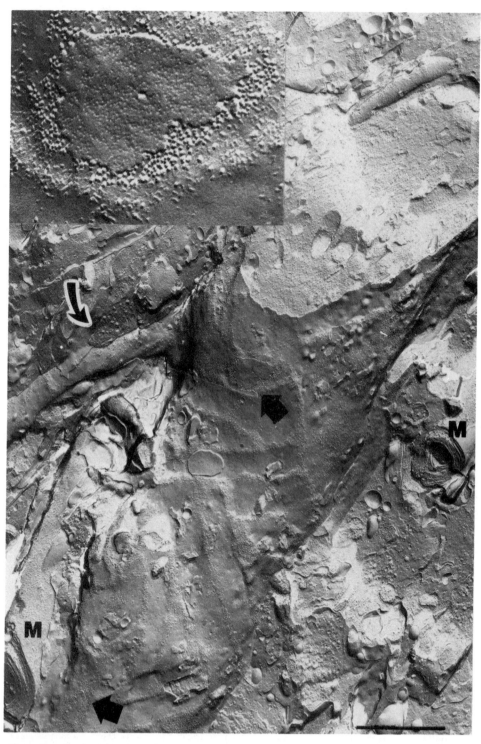

Figure 2. *Gap junctions* (straight arrows) *on the dendrite of a CA3 pyramidal cell from the hippocampus of a guinea pig.* The junction near the *center* of the figure is enlarged four times in the *inset* and shows a narrowed intercellular cleft and both *P*-face particles and *E*-face pits. The *curved arrow* indicates a synaptic bouton on a small dendritic branch. Two myelinated fibers (M) are cross-fractured. *Calibration bar* = 1 μm. (From Schmalbruch and Jahnsen, 1981.)

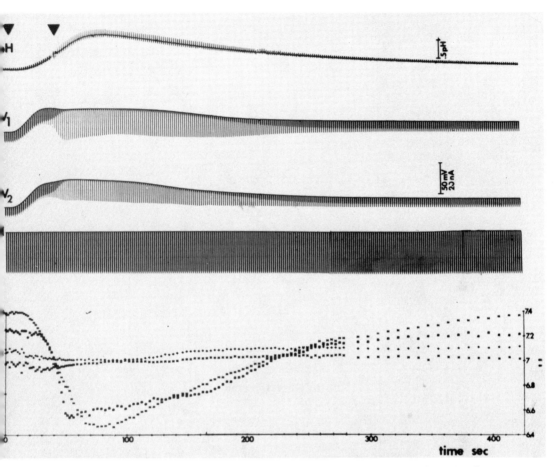

Figure 3. *The effect of* CO_2 *on electrotonic coupling between a pair of axolotl blastomeres.* Current pulses
(I) were alternately passed through cell 1 and cell 2 (V_1 and V_2), producing approximately equal
voltage deflections in the polarized cell and somewhat smaller potentials in the other cell.
Application of saline equilibrated with 100% CO_2 (between *arrowheads* at the *top* of the figure)
decreased cytoplasmic pH (*uppermost trace*; increased hydrogen activity shown by *rising trace*),
increased the input resistance of each cell, and decreased the spread of current from cell to cell
(seen as a decrease in the potential produced in each cell by current injected into the other).
Washing the cells with CO_2-free saline at normal pH restored pH_i and electrotonic coupling
over a similar but slower time course. Junctional and nonjunctional conductances calculated
from these data (second, third, and fourth plots, respectively, *ordinate* at *left*) and pH (first plot,
ordinate at *right*) are plotted on a log scale along the same time scale in the *bottom portion* of the
figure. Response time for the pH electrode to measure a change of 1 pH unit was < 10 sec;
measurements were made at intervals of 2 sec. Junctional conductance (g_j) decreased more than
two orders of magnitude and recovered gradually as pH_i returned. The nonjunctional conductances,
(g_{njs}) of the two cells decreased only slightly during the acidification. (From Spray et al., 1981a.)

during the initial decrease. The speed of response and lack of hysteresis suggest
a direct action on the channel macromolecules. In fish and amphibian blastomeres, the titration curve is well fit by a Hill plot with a pK_H of 7.3 and a Hill
coefficient of four or five (Figure 4A). The value of the coefficient suggests that
four or five highly cooperative sites are involved, or that there are more sites
with less cooperativity.

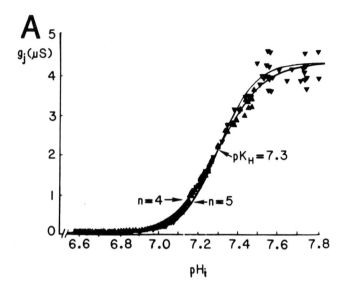

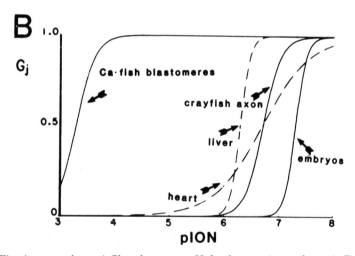

Figure 4. *Titration curves for* g$_j$. *A:* Plot of g_j versus pH$_i$ for the experiment shown in Figure 3. The *triangles (apexes down)* represent before and during acidification. The *triangles (apexes up)* represent recovery in normal saline. The points fell along the same curve, which was well fit by a Hill plot with $n = 4$ or 5 and pK$_H$ = 7.3. *B:* pH titration curves from other tissues show differences in slope and pK$_H$. The *leftmost curve* is for calcium in fish blastomeres (Spray et al., 1982) and illustrates a four-decade reduction in sensitivity to calcium as compared to hydrogen.

The effect on g_j of cytoplasmic acidification has been observed in most cells tested (Spray and Bennett, 1985), possible exceptions being adult lens fibers (Scheutze and Goodenough, 1982) and retinal rods in toad (E. R. Griff and L. H. Pinto, personal communication). In neither case have pH$_i$ and g_j been directly measured, and intracellular buffering or the presence of such large values of g_j that coupling coefficients are not greatly changed remain possible, if unlikely, explanations. As pH sensitivity can be reduced or blocked by certain pharmacological treatments (Spray et al., 1984b, 1986a), it is not unreasonable that some junctions are by their nature (or protein composition) very much less sensitive without experimental treatment. Differences in the titration curves for different tissues are now known and both pKs and Hill coefficients vary (Figure 4B). The differences could result from modest differences in the amino acid compositions of the different junctional proteins (cf. Nicholson et al., 1983; Revel and Yancey, 1985).

A physiological role for pH sensitivity has not been established. However, in amphibian and teleost blastomeres, normal pH_i is just above where g_j changes steeply, and small degrees of acidification produce significant uncoupling. In cardiac muscle, g_j may be reduced at normal pH, and pH changes may alter g_j in either direction. pH changes large enough to alter g_j in the more sensitive tissues certainly occur during ischemia and conceivably contribute to cardiac arrhythmias.

Although we have emphasized the titratability of the channels, reversibility is not always complete, depending on the tissue and the length of exposure (e.g., Campos de Carvalho et al., 1984). There may be secondary changes that occur, as the degree of recovery sometimes depends on the brevity of exposure. g_j may depend on phosphorylation (see below) or on other covalent modification, as well as on simple pH_i.

Another factor affecting g_j is an increase in free cytoplasmic calcium (Ca_i), although g_j in systems so far measured is relatively insensitive to Ca_i, compared to free cytoplasmic hydrogen (H_i). Using a preparation of fish blastomeres in which the junctions were perfused on one cytoplasmic aspect, we showed that Ca_i levels in excess of 0.1 mM were required to reduce g_j (Figure 4B; Spray et al., 1982). This level is not far above that given by Oliveira-Castro and Loewenstein (1971), who found that junctions in an arthropod preparation began to close between 40 and 80 μM. Dahl and Isenberg (1980) reported that cardiac junctions were blocked at about 5 μM, but under their conditions of dinitrophenol poisoning, pH_i (which they did not measure) may have been significantly lowered. In our hands, injured pairs of cardiac myocytes remain coupled even after they have let in enough calcium to cause irreversible contracture, presumably a level of at least 10 μM (White et al., 1985).

The concentrations of calcium required to decrease g_j are high compared to those involved in muscle contraction, secretion, or bioluminescence. Thus, it is unlikely that calcium would be a physiological mechanism for controlling g_j. However, if one of a pair of coupled cells is broken open in normal saline, there is a rapid decrease in g_j, presumably as external calcium reaches the now unprotected junctions (cf. Asada and Bennett, 1971). Injury uncoupling is very likely an important protective mechanism and in coupled tissues keeps intact cells from losing their contents through their junctions with injured cells.

It is plausible (but unproven) that hydrogen and calcium act at the same site on the channel molecules. Interaction between hydrogen and calcium has not been evaluated; however, the steepness of the g_j–Ca_i relation is about half that for H_i (in fish blastomeres), which supports a common site of action for the two ions. In *Chironomus* salivary gland, treatments raising H_i or Ca_i affect the voltage dependence of g_j similarly (Obaid et al., 1983; see below), again consistent with a common site of action.

VOLTAGE DEPENDENCE

Although most junctions originally characterized behaved liked fixed resistances, a few junctions between neurons were known to rectify as diodes do, and this property contributed to or accounted for unidirectional action at these electrical synapses (Furshpan and Potter, 1959; Auerbach and Bennett, 1969). Two other classes of voltage dependence are now known; g_j can depend symmetrically on transjunctional voltage, V_j, and it can depend on the potential between the inside and outside of the cell, V_{i-o} (Spray et al., 1984b). Gap junctions, unlike the channels of excitable membranes, form a three-terminal network, the cytoplasm at either end of the channel and the extracellular medium in the gap. The gap is accessible to markers of extracellular space, and without encircling tight junctions there is likely to be little resistive barrier between the gap and the distant medium. At least when cells are closely coupled, there is very little leakage out of the channels themselves, and thus V_{i-o} develops across the channel walls. It is not surprising, therefore, that some sensitivity to V_{i-o} exists.

Symmetrical dependence on V_j has been well characterized in amphibian blastomeres (Harris et al., 1981; Spray et al., 1981b). Under current clamp conditions, sufficiently small pulses do not change g_j and cells are stably coupled in the familiar way (Figure 5A). Somewhat larger currents produce a dramatically different result. After the potential in both cells rises and appears to be reaching a plateau, the voltage in the cell in which the current is applied accelerates upward to reach a new plateau while voltage in the second cell decreases markedly. At the beginning of the pulses the cells are well coupled; at the end they are poorly coupled. Clearly this change could be due to a decrease in junctional conductance, causing a decrease in the postcell voltage and an increase in the precell voltage. Because of the relatively slow time course of the voltage changes, it seemed probable that voltage clamp would be helpful. A method was devised in which each cell is independently clamped. If cell 1 is held clamped at its resting potential and cell 2 is stepped, current will flow through the junctions into cell 1 and also through the nonjunctional membrane of cell 2. The clamp on cell 1 will apply a current equal in magnitude to that flowing through g_j to keep V_1 constant. Thus $-I_1 = I_j$ and $g_j = I_j/V_2$, since V_1 is unchanged. A direct measure of g_j can be seen during the experiment, and any changes in g_j as a function of potential are immediately apparent.

As it turns out, g_j is quite simply dependent on potential. After a step change in voltage is made (on one side of $V_j = 0$), g_j relaxes exponentially to a new steady-state value (Figure 5B). The steady-state conductance is symmetrically dependent on voltage, decreasing for V_js of either sign in a manner well fit by the Boltzmann relation (Figure 5C). Exponential change suggests a first-order reaction in which each open channel has a constant probability over time of closing rapidly in an all-or-none fashion, and each closed channel has a fixed probability of opening, all the channels behaving independently of each other. Steady state is reached when the mean numbers for opening and closing are equal. The Boltzmann relation arises when the energy difference between open and closed states is a linear function of potential, a reasonable situation for an intrinsic membrane protein (Neher and Stevens, 1977). A diagram of a change in dipole moment that could lead to voltage dependence is shown in Figure 6A.

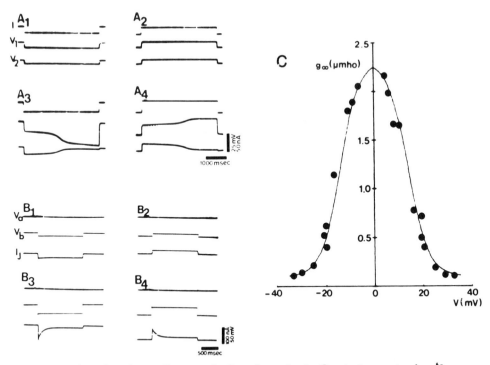

Figure 5. *Voltage-dependent* g_j: *Current and voltage clamp.* A_1–A_4: Constant current pulses {I, *upper traces*) were applied to cell 1 of a coupled pair. For the smaller currents (A_1 and A_2), the potentials in cell 1 (V_1) and cell 2 (V_2) remained nearly constant. During the larger currents (A_3 and A_4), V_1 increased and V_2 decreased; the cells went from well to poorly coupled. B_1–B_4: Voltage clamp records of junctional current. Cell 1 was clamped at its resting potential (V_a) and cell 2 was stepped to various values (V_b). The clamp current to cell 1 required to hold its potential constant gave junctional current (I_j). For small steps of either sign (B_1 and B_2), current remained constant during the pulse. For larger steps (B_3 and B_4), the current decayed exponentially to a lower steady-state value. C: Steady-state values of g_j obtained in a voltage clamp experiment are plotted as a function of transjunctional voltage, V_j. Steady-state g_j decreased steeply for increasing V_j of either sign, the half-maximum values occurring at about 15 mV. The points for each polarity of V_j are well fit by a Boltzmann relation (*smooth curve*). (From Spray et al., 1981b.)

Work would be done by the applied field in moving from the open to the closed configuration. The diagram shows two gates in series, one at either end of the channel. This arrangement is plausible because of the overall symmetry of the junctions, which are formed by presumably identical cells. It should be admitted that the polarity of sensitivity is unknown; there is no evidence showing on which side the gate is located that is closed by a given polarity V_j. Effects of suddenly reversing V_j confirm the presence of series gates (Harris et al., 1981). These data also suggest that the entire voltage drop occurs across a single closed gate, and that this gate must open before the gate in series with it sees the voltage and has an increased probability of closing.

An entertaining consequence of the series gates is that applied voltages should cause a small fraction of the channels to cycle around a circular reaction scheme (Figure 6B; Bennett and Spray, 1984). Consider a voltage closing the gate on side one so that the channel is in state C_1O_2. Since there is no current going

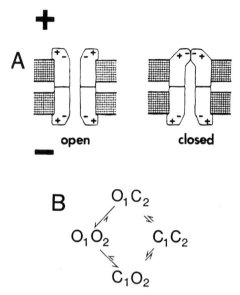

Figure 6. *Channel models with series gates. A: A distribution of charges that would produce a dipole moment shift in the transjunctional direction when one gate on the channel opened and closed. B: Cycling around this reaction scheme would occur when a voltage was applied that tended to drive the channels from the state of both gates open to the conformation gate 1 closed, gate 2 open (C_1O_2). (From Bennett et al., 1984.)*

through the channel, there will be no voltage drop across gate 2, and this gate will occasionally close spontaneously (a small percentage of the gates are closed at $V_j = 0$). When it closes, the voltage across gate 1 will be reduced, and there will be an increased probability of gate 1 opening, moving the channel to state O_1C_2. Now all the voltage will be across gate 2, and there will be a very strong tendency for the channel to move to state O_1O_2 with equal voltages across the two gates, whereupon most of the channels will move back to state C_1O_2. Calculations indicate that the rate of cycling will be small, but it might be detectable in recordings of single channel open and closed times. The cycling does not violate microscopic reversibility because energy is provided by the applied field. An analogous cycling has been hypothesized for voltage-sensitive channels of ordinary membrane (Finkelstein and Peskin, 1984).

In amphibian cells, g_j is independent of V_{i-o} over a range of ± 30 mV from the resting level. Furthermore, voltage and pH gates appear separate. A different situation is found in *Chironomus* salivary gland and squid blastomeres (Obaid et al., 1983; Spray et al., 1984b). In *Chironomus*, the cells are quite sensitive to V_{i-o}, and when $V_j = 0$, steady-state g_j can be accounted for in terms of two gates in series, each with the same V_{i-o} dependence. However, if V_js are present, the model no longer predicts g_j, and there appears to be a component of V_j sensitivity as well. Sensitivity to both V_j and V_{i-o} would occur if dipole moment changes associated with gating were significant in both the transjunctional direction and between the channel and the extracellular gap.

In *Chironomus*, the dependence on V_{i-o} is shifted in the depolarizing direction by increasing cytoplasmic hydrogen or calcium levels. Evidently, the same gating mechanism is affected by voltage and by cytoplasmic ions in this tissue.

A possibly homologous mechanism exists in squid blastulae (Spray et al., 1984b). At normal pH, the junctions appear to show little dependence on voltage, although not very large V_js have been applied, because the normal conductance is so high. The cells have very little resting potential, and a large inside negative value is clearly not necessary for coupling. Dependence on V_j appears when g_j is reduced following cytoplasmic acidification by bathing in weak acids; subsequent hyperpolarization of either cell increases g_j rather than decreases it (Figure 7A, C). The junctions also exhibit some degree of V_{i-o} sensitivity under these conditions.

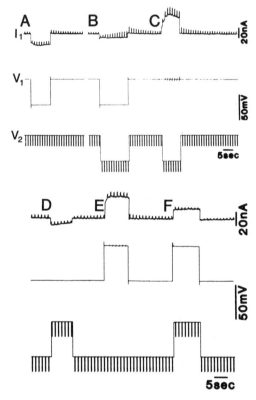

Figure 7. *In squid blastomeres, g_j depends on both V_j and V_{i-o}.* Pairs of blastomeres were independently voltage-clamped. Brief test pulses in cell 2 produced clamp currents in cell 1 (I_1) that reflected changes in g_j. Junctional conductance was decreased by bathing in CO_2 solution. A: Hyperpolarization of cell 1 increased g_j (the increase required about 5 sec; then there was a small decrease). The clamp current associated with the pulse in cell 1 is junctional plus nonjunctional current, but the slow increase and small decrease in current reflect changes in g_j, as shown by the changes in the test pulses. After the hyperpolarization, g_j decayed back to its initial level C in about 10 sec. B: Hyperpolarization of both cells also increased g_j. The steady component in I is entirely nonjunctional current, since the cells are hyperpolarized equally. (The same nonjunctional current would have flowed in A, allowing I_j to be determined by subtraction.) C: Hyperpolarization of cell 2 produced a larger increase in g_j and also a slight decrease toward the end of the pulse. D: Depolarization of cell 2 decreased g_j. E: Equal depolarization of cell 1 increased g_j. F: Depolarization of both cells decreases g_j. The effects of equal V_js for the depolarization and hyperpolarization of the two cells differ because of the additive effect of V_{i-o}. The effects of equal but opposite V_js also differ, presumably because of the additional factor of different pHs in the two cells.

Equal hyperpolarization of both cells increases g_j (Figure 7B), and equal depolarization of both cells decreases it (Figure 7F). Under these circumstances, V_j is zero, so only V_{i-o} can be acting.

When acid is injected into one cell of a coupled pair, the sensitivity to V_j is asymmetrical, and some degree of asymmetry is often seen when the cells are bathed in weak acids, presumably because of unequal cytoplasmic acidification (Figure 7). The polarity is such that depolarization on the injected side increases g_j and depolarization on the opposite side decreases g_j (Figure 7D,E). The production of a consistent asymmetry by unilateral acidification indicates that there are two gates in series. Since hydrogen ions should have a greater effect on the injected cell, it appears that V_j opens the gate on the positive side, and unlike the case in amphibians, one can assign a polarity of sensitivity to the gate in each membrane.

Several details of Figure 7 can be explained as arising from a combination of asymmetrical V_j sensitivity and V_{i-o} sensitivity. g_j is increased more for the same V_j with V_2 negative than with V_1 positive, because the effect of V_{i-o} is additive in one case and subtractive in the other (Figure 7C,E). Similarly, during equal and opposite V_j, g_j is decreased with V_2 positive while it is increased with V_1 negative (Figure 7A,D).

Granted that there are two gates in series, one can ask how V_j acts to open channels when it should act oppositely on the series gates. It is likely that V_j can only open singly closed channels, those that are closed only by the gate on the side of relatively greater positivity. The increases in g_j are always rather small, consistent with only a subpopulation being affected. Once the closed gate opens, the previously open series gate would tend to be closed by the same V_j, also reducing the increase in g_j. (This effect may be responsible for the late decreases in g_j in Figure 7A,C.) More extensive acidification causes the V_j sensitivity to disappear, perhaps because the channels become closed on both sides. During recovery from acidification, voltage dependence reappears, also consistent with double closure of gates at low pH_i, rendering the channels V_j-insensitive.

The gating in amphibians, and in squid and *Chironomus*, is interestingly different. In the former, V_j and pH mechanisms are independent. In the latter, there is interaction. All are reasonably explained in terms of a dipole moment shift associated with a conformational change of channel opening and closing. In amphibians, the dipole change is significant only in the V_j direction and is small or absent in the V_{i-o} direction. In *Chironomus*, the change has a large component in the V_{i-o} direction, but also some sensitivity to V_j. In squid, V_j sensitivity is apparently greater than in *Chironomus*, and sensitivity to V_{i-o} less. Different systems provide different degrees of voltage sensitivity (Figure 8). Rectification at the crayfish giant synapse implies unidirectional V_j dependence, and there may be only one gate in the channel. The voltage sensitivity is less than in the amphibian blastomeres (Margiotta and Walcott, 1983), but the conductance changes are at least 100 times faster. Responses to current pulses very similar to those in amphibia are seen in the *Limulus* lateral eye, but quantitative data are lacking (Smith and Baumann, 1969). Some teleost blastomeres show sensitivity but to a lesser degree than in amphibia. Several junctions in adult vertebrate tissues show no V_j sensitivity over ± 50 mV or more (liver, heart, and sympathetic

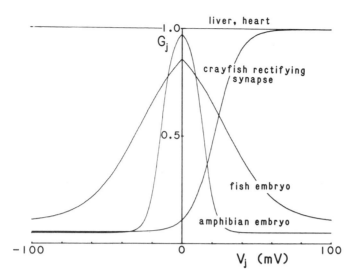

Figure 8. *Voltage sensitivity of different gap junctions.* Normalized conductance, G_j, is shown as a function of V_js of either sign. For the symmetrical cases of fish and amphibian blastomeres, the curves are Boltzmann relations for a single gate of either polarity; the effects of two gates in series are neglected. For amphibian blastomeres, the slope is greater and the voltage at which G_j is decreased by half is smaller. For the crayfish rectifying synapse, a single Boltzmann relation is assumed such that the gate is opened for positive V_j, that is, depolarization on the presynaptic side. Gap junctions in rat hepatocytes and ventricular myocytes are voltage-insensitive over a range of at least $\pm$ 60 mV. (From Spray and Bennett, 1985.)

ganglion neurons in culture). In leech ganglia, neurons may transmit depolarization in either direction but fail to pass hyperpolarization (Nicholls and Purves, 1972). These effects could arise from sensitivity to V_{i-o} but may also be a result of rectification in nonjunctional membranes (Zipser, 1979).

The role of voltage sensitivity of these several kinds remains to be determined (except for ordinary rectifying synapses, where a functional role is obvious). The exquisite sensitivity of junctions between amphibian blastomeres allows there to be bistability of coupling (Figures 9, 10; Harris et al., 1983). Thus, differences in nonjunctional membranes with respect to resting potential or electrogenic pumping can lead to a loss of coupling between cells, and in an epithelium, a transition between a smooth gradient and a sharp boundary could be triggered by a brief event. In *Xenopus*, action potentials may trigger uncoupling of Rohon-Beard cells (Spitzer, 1982). In *Fundulus* embryos, where voltage dependence is like that in amphibia but much less sensitive, a physiological role, if any, is obscure. In squid, voltage sensitivity is very low and is only expressed at low pH. This voltage dependence may merely reflect the dipole moment shift associated with the conformational change of the pH gating mechanism. In *Chironomus*, voltage sensitivity is reasonably high. It may be that changes in resting potential modulate the coupling, which could be important during the different stages of larval development. However, the same mechanism is quite pH-sensitive, and changes in this parameter could also provide a physiological control of coupling. Until we know what normally operates these gates, it will be unclear as to whether they are best termed pH or voltage gates (or both).

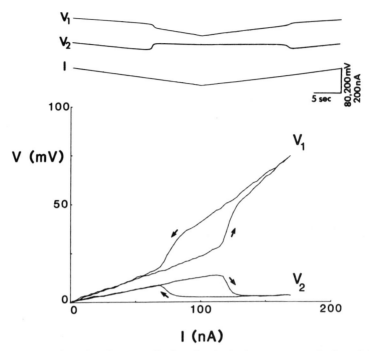

Figure 9. *Bistability of coupling during application of maintained current to a pair of coupled amphibian blastomeres.* A slowly rising and falling current (about 30 sec in each direction) was applied to cell 1 in order to obtain a quasi-steady voltage to current relation. The applied current (I) and the resulting voltages in the two cells (V_1 and V_2) are shown in the *upper portion* of the figure. In the *lower portion* of the figure, V_1 and V_2 are plotted as a function of I. As the current increased from zero (*arrows* indicate direction), the cells were well coupled, but then rapidly uncoupled at a current level of about 120 nA and remained uncoupled as the ramp of current continued upward. As the ramp decreased from its peak, the cells remained uncoupled until the current reached a level of about 80 nA, then rapidly recoupled. The observed hysteresis and the bistability of the voltage to current relation between currents of 80 and 120 nA follow from the voltage dependence of the junctional conductance and reflect the regenerative nature of the uncoupling and recoupling events. (From Harris et al., 1983.)

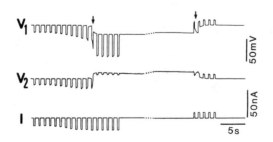

OTHER PHARMACOLOGY

A number of different kinds of agents affect g_j, and it is now possible to speak of a pharmacology of electrical transmission. Some years ago gap junctions were shown to be sensitive to aldehyde fixatives, which rapidly and irreversibly block g_j (cf. Bennett, 1977). Fixative concentrations were used because the goal was to determine the electrical state of the junctions after fixation. As aldehydes react with proteins, one would expect other group-specific protein reagents to be active, but not much has been done along these lines. Glutaraldehyde, EEDQ (Campos de Carvalho et al., 1986), and retinoic acid all act on gap junctions to reduce their pH sensitivity but, in amphibia, do not affect voltage sensitivity (Spray et al., 1986a). A different mode of action would appear to be required in each case.

Another class of agents is the permeant esters. Orthonitrobenzyl acetate is a neutral ester that can be photolyzed to give acetic acid as one product (Spray et al., 1984a). We had planned to use this compound to produce flash-induced jumps in hydrogen ion concentration, but discovered that the ester reduces pH_i and causes uncoupling without light flashes. Evidently, intracellular esterases hydrolyze the ester to generate acetic acid. The substituted benzyl acetates may well turn out to be useful uncoupling agents, as they can be used in millimolar quantities instead of one-tenth molar quantities, and a number of cell types tolerate the ester better than the high concentrations of weak acids required for uncoupling. At neutral pH, the permeant undissociated acid in acetate saline is about 1% of the total acetate, a concentration comparable to that at which benzyl acetates are effective. An important, if in retrospect obvious, aspect of this study is that one should be careful when loading cells with polar dyes, buffers, or other compounds (e.g., 6-carboxyfluorescein, BAPTA, and cAMP) by means of their neutral esters. A permeant ester that is hydrolyzed intracellularly to trap the active moiety will also acidify the cytoplasm.

A completely different class of agent that reduces g_j consists of higher alcohols, particularly heptanol and octanol. These alcohols act rapidly and reversibly on what is now a wide spectrum of junctions (crayfish septate axon; squid, fish, and amphibian blastomeres; rat cardiac myocytes and rat hepatocytes; Johnston

---

Figure 10. *Bistability of coupling of amphibian blastomeres in the absence of applied current.* Small hyperpolarizing current pulses (I) of increasing amplitude were delivered to cell 1 (V_1) and showed that it was well coupled to cell 2 (V_2). Partial uncoupling occurred during the pulses as they increased in amplitude. At the termination of the pulse at the *first arrow*, there was a sudden transition at which the cells assumed new steady-state potentials—cell 1 hyperpolarized and cell 2 depolarized from its previous potential. At this point, the cells had shifted to a poorly coupled state, as indicated by the stable difference in the resting potentials and by the decreased coupling during the current pulses following the *first arrow*. The steady potential required to maintain the cells uncoupled was presumably supplied by a difference in the nonjunctional membrane potentials. At the *second arrow*, depolarizing current pulses were applied to cell 1. The first pulse increased g_j to some extent, but the cells largely uncoupled following the pulse. The second pulse initiated recoupling that persisted, as indicated by the effects of brief pulses and by the restoration of the original membrane potentials. The *dotted line* indicates a gap of 100 sec. (From Harris et al., 1983.)

et al., 1980; Deleze and Herve, 1983; Spray et al., 1984b; White et al., 1985, and unpublished observations). It seems likely that these alcohols act by altering the lipid environment of the channels.

SYNAPTIC CONTROL OF JUNCTIONAL CONDUCTANCE AND OF COUPLING

A new mechanism of control of gap junctional communication between retinal horizontal cells has been found in both fish and turtles (Teranishi et al., 1984; Piccolino et al., 1984). Electrical coupling between horizontal cells is widespread and is responsible for the large receptive fields of these cells. Treatment of the retina with dopamine reduces the spread from the surround region into the center of the receptive field and also reduces the spread of dye between cells (Figure 11A,C). While the electrical measurements in intact retina could result from changes in nonjunctional membranes, the effects on dye coupling require a change in the junctions themselves. Furthermore, in isolated coupled pairs of horizontal cells, g_j is reversibly decreased by dopamine with little effect on non-junctional membrane (Lasater and Dowling, 1985).

The reduction in g_j caused by dopamine is mediated by intracellular cAMP, as indicated by the action of permeant cAMP derivatives and forskolin, an

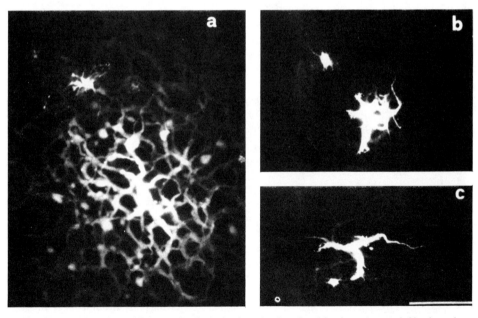

Figure 11. *Dye coupling of horizontal cells in turtle retina is reduced by dopamine, probably through an increase in cAMP. a:* A control injection. The dye has spread from the brighter axonal arbor near the center of the field to many surrounding axons. The soma of the injected cell (*upper left*) shows a number of small dendrites. Other somata are less fluorescent. *b:* An injection after bathing in 10 μM forskolin. Little dye has left the injected cell. *c:* An injection after bathing in 10 μM dopamine. Again, the dye is largely restricted to the injected axon and its cell body. Calibration bar = 10 μm. (From Piccolino et al., 1984.)

activator of adenylate cyclase (Figure 11B). From anatomical considerations, modulation by a chemical synapse of gap junctional conductance would almost have to be mediated by a second messenger. It is possible that junctional proteins are directly phosphorylated. We have recently shown that isolated gap junctions from liver are phosphorylated by the catalytic subunit of cAMP-dependent kinase (Saez et al., 1985). As discussed below, coupling in some systems is increased rather than decreased by cAMP.

Synaptic modulation of junctional conductance may occur at other central nervous system sites. Hormone treatment may modify junctional conductance in either direction (Caveney et al., 1980; Cole and Garfield, 1985). As these changes may involve no change in the number of junctions defined morphologically, a gating mechanism is presumably responsible.

As a coda to this section on the synaptic control of g_j, we add the changes in coupling mediated by changes in nonjunctional conductance, g_{nj}. Since the coupling coefficient ($k_{12} = V_2/V_1$ when current is applied in cell 1 of a coupled pair) is given by $k_{12} = g_j/(g_j + g_{nj})$, coupling can be increased or decreased by changes in g_{nj} without changes in g_j. An example occurs in the mollusk *Navanax*, where pharyngeal expansion motoneurons are coupled and also receive inhibitory inputs with a reversal potential near the resting potential (Spira et al., 1980). When the inhibitory synapses are active, g_{nj} is greater and the coupling coefficient from another cell coupled to it is reduced (Figure 12). The coupling pathway between the two cells has significant axial resistance, and the coupling coefficient

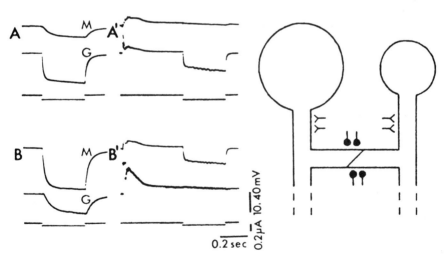

Figure 12. *Control of electrotonic coupling by inhibitory synapses. A and B:* Electrotonic coupling from G (giant)- to M (medium)- cells and from M- to G-cells, expansion motor neurons in the buccal ganglion of *Navanax inermis*. Current is shown in the *lower traces. A'* and *B':* Following a brief train of stimuli to the pharyngeal nerve, the neurons were no longer coupled. Their input conductances were increased, and there was a small depolarization owing to the activation of inhibitory synapses with a reversal potential just positive to the resting potential. The loss of coupling is explicable as short-circuiting by inhibitory synapses along the axonal pathway connecting the cells (*diagram at right*). The cells remained excitable to other synaptic inputs. Higher gain recording in G-cell in *B* and *B'*. (From Bennett et al., 1984.)

can be decreased virtually to zero without completely inhibiting the cells, thus allowing them to be excited independently by other inputs. The uncoupling may allow cells to fire asynchronously to participate in peristalsis. Coupling of the cells would help them to fire synchronously to mediate the rapid movement of pharyngeal expansion.

Suitable circuitry for synaptic control of coupling has been described in the mammalian inferior olive and probably occurs in the sensory cortex as well (Sotelo et al., 1972; Sloper and Powell, 1978). An instance in which postsynaptic potentials that decrease conductance increase coupling has also been described (Carew and Kandel, 1976).

A SPECIFIC BLOCKER

To study the function of gap junctional communication, particularly between inexcitable cells, it would be valuable to have a specific blocking agent (as, for example, curariform agents aided in the analysis of chemical transmission). Agents changing intracellular pH and the long-chain alcohols certainly have other effects, but the recently available antibodies appear to provide the required specificity. Polyclonal antibodies raised against isolated rat liver junctions react with a 27-kD protein in a variety of rat tissues and label localized regions that are consistent with the known distribution of junctions (Hertzberg and Skibbens, 1984). Cross-reactivity also occurs in vertebrates as distant as fishes, suggesting homology with conservation of functional groups between tissues and throughout the vertebrates (also implied by the formation of cross-coupling between disparate cells). The protein apparently differs in the few vertebrate tissues examined to date (Nicholson et al., 1983; Revel and Yancey, 1985). Comparison among proteins should give insight into the mechanisms of junctional formation.

Injection of the antibodies into coupled liver, heart, or cultured neurons blocks electrical and dye coupling (Figure 13; Hertzberg et al., 1985). Preimmune serum has no effect. External application of antibody is also without effect. Here then is a reagent that appears to have the desired specificity, although it is inconvenient in that it must be applied intracellularly. Certainly, intracellular application gives a high degree of localization, much better than bath application. Since the immunogen was isolated intact junctions, it is not surprising that the cytoplasmic face of the junctions is the site of reactivity. Moreover, intact antibodies are too large to get into the intercellular gap. If junctions form through the joining of hemichannels already present in apposed cell membranes, an antibody might be raised that prevents junctional formation. Also, antibodies that prevent cell adhesion by combining with cell adhesion molecules (Edelman, 1983) might block junctional formation.

Anti-junction antibodies have been used to indicate a role of gap junctions in the intercellular communication of developmental information (Warner et al., 1984). Injection of a particular blastomere of the Xenopus blastula with antibody reduces coupling to its neighbors and blocks differentiation of its progeny, although cell division continues apparently normally. Unfortunately, antibody binding to protein of the molecular weight of junctional protein in other species has not yet been demonstrated. Nevertheless, the experiments provide a paradigm for

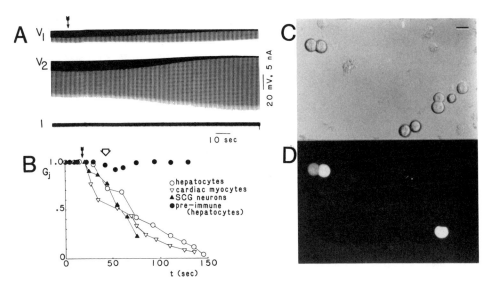

Figure 13. *Effects of an anti-junction antibody on* g_j. *A:* Injection of the antibody into one of a pair of coupled hepatocytes uncoupled the cells. (Display as in Figure 3.) *B:* A graph of the decrease in normalized conductance, G_j, after intracellular injection of the antibody into one cell of a coupled pair of rat hepatocytes, cardiac myocytes, and cultured sympathetic ganglion cells. A control injection of preimmune serum had little effect on g_j in another cell pair. *C* and *D:* Bright-field and fluorescence micrographs of rat hepatocyte pairs. After injection of one of a cell pair with Lucifer yellow and preimmune serum, the dye spread to the second cell (*upper left*, photographed 1 min after injection). The dye did not spread from a cell injected with antibody plus dye 5 min previously (*lower right*). *Calibration bar* = 20 μm. (From Hertzberg et al., 1985.)

future investigations that should validate the long presumed role of gap junctions in embryonic development (Potter et al., 1966; cf. Bennett et al., 1981). The problem of identifying the signaling molecule that passes through gap junctions will remain.

FORMATION AND REMOVAL

The gating processes described above do not, at least initially, involve the removal (or formation) of junctions. There is a modest literature of changes in junctional structure, particularly increases in the density and regularity of particle arrangement that are supposed to cause or at least be associated with decreases in junctional conductance (cf. Peracchia, 1980). However, the techniques with greatest resolution fail to reveal any obvious differences between junctions in high- and low-conductance states in intact tissues (Hanna et al., 1985). In some cases, regularization can apparently be a slow step that follows the rapid gating processes. Moreover, junctions are highly regular in the normal, presumably high-conductance, state in some tissues (Page et al., 1983). Conformational changes must surely underlie gating, and some hints are available from isolated junctions studied by low-dose electron microscopy or X-ray diffraction (Makowski et al., 1984; Unwin and

Ennis, 1984). Correspondence of the different structures observed to actual gating processes is uncertain.

Many different kinds of cells will form junctions when simply placed together or cocultured, and protein synthesis may not be necessary, as indicated by the short latency of development of coupling and the failure of protein synthesis inhibitors to block it (cf. Bennett and Goodenough, 1978). The general picture is one of promiscuity; cells from many different tissues and from amphibians to mammals will couple indiscriminately. The cross-coupling, like the antibody studies, suggests homology between interacting hemichannels based on the reasonable assumption that each cell contributes its own hemichannel. The problem is how specificity arises among communication-competent cells, as in the central nervous system, where glia couple only to glia and neurons interact highly specifically—for example, there may be axodendritic but no axoaxonal or dendrodendritic gap junctions in a particular nucleus. Cell adhesion molecules may be responsible, as gap junction formation requires that cells approach each other very closely.

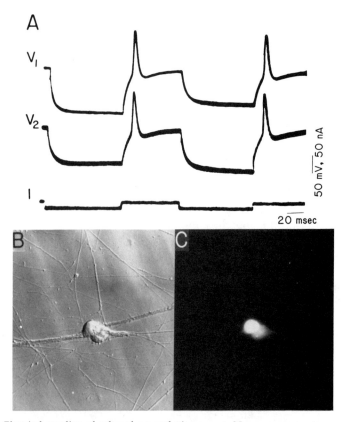

Figure 14. *Electrical coupling of cultured sympathetic neurons.* Neurons grown in serum-containing medium with 5 μg/ml added insulin became coupled, hyperpolarization spreading in either direction between cells. *A:* First pulse applied in the *upper trace* cell, second pulse in the *lower trace* cell. The hyperpolarizing pulses were followed by anode break responses. *B* and *C:* Bright-field and fluorescence micrographs of two closely apposed neurons (about 20 μm in diameter). Dye injected into the *left* cell spread to the *right* cell. (From Kessler et al., 1984.)

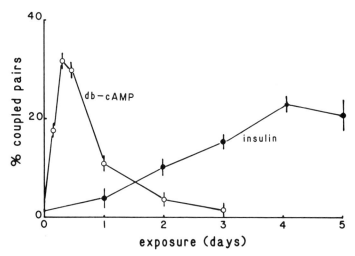

Figure 15.   *Promotion of coupling of cultured sympathetic ganglion cells by insulin and by cAMP.* Cells were cultured in serum-containing medium to which insulin (5 μg/ml) or dibutyryl cAMP (1 mM) had been added. The percentage of coupled cells was determined by sampling 30–50 pairs of cells in two or more culture dishes. (From Kessler et al., 1984.)

Numerous examples of factors inducing formation between cells already in contact have been described (cf. Spray and Bennett, 1985). Again, protein synthesis may or may not be required. The availability of antibodies should lead reasonably soon to a description of where the junctional protein comes from. An example is provided by dissociated neurons from neonatal superior cervical ganglion (Figure 14; Kessler et al., 1984). These cells do not become coupled in serum-containing medium, but do become coupled in a defined medium containing salts plus insulin, progesterone, putrescine, transferrin, and selenium (Figure 14; Higgins and Burton, 1982). We further examined this phenomenon in order to analyze the factors involved. When added separately to serum-containing medium, both insulin (Figure 15) and selenium induce the appearance of coupling. Dibutyryl cAMP also increases coupling (Figure 15); its effect is prolonged by caffeine, presumably because of the latter's phosphodiesterase activity. Serum decreases cAMP levels and probably inhibits the development of coupling through this mechanism. Insulin and selenium do not increase cAMP and so must increase coupling by a different mechanism. Thus, coupling in the defined medium results from both the removal of inhibitory factors and the addition of promoting factors. The appearance of coupling is reduced by protein synthesis inhibitors and is likely to involve the synthesis of junctional protein (a possibility that can now be tested with the antibody).

Removal of gap junctions (defined morphologically) occurs in at least two ways. Intact junctions may be torn out of one of the coupled cells, a common event in a number of tissues as well as in cell dissociation, and then be internalized by the cell on which they remain (Mazet et al., 1985). The internalized junctions eventually are degraded. Alternately, junctional membranes may separate, and the hemichannels may disperse over the cell surface (e.g., Lee et al., 1982; Hanna et al., 1984). Re-use of junctional material is an attractive possibility in the latter case, but might also occur with internalized junctions.

The signals for junction removal are unknown. One possibility is that the treatments that close the channels put them into a state in which the cell removes them by internalization or by splitting and dispersal. Dispersed hemichannels presumably have negligible conductance, based on teleological grounds and on the crayfish septate axon, in which loss of junctions, probably by splitting, is not associated with any change in nonjunctional conductance (Asada and Bennett, 1971; Hanna et al., 1984). When junctions are pulled out of one or the other cell, sealing of the holes must in general occur very rapidly. Closing of ruptured membranes over the intact junctions also occurs, as demonstrated morphologically. It is uncertain whether the junctions by which the small vesicles remain attached are of low or high conductance, and what triggers internalization is also unknown.

SUMMARY AND PROSPECTS

Gap junctions now prove to have properties corresponding to those of the channels of conventional excitable membrane. They can be gated chemically by an increase in cytoplasmic hydrogen or calcium. They can be gated by voltage, and because they involve three rather than two compartments, they can be sensitive to both V_j and V_{i-o}. Voltage sensitivity presumably arises from dipole moment changes associated with the conformational changes of channel gating. Chemical gating may or may not exhibit voltage sensitivity, which again can be accounted for in terms of the presence or absence of dipole moment changes. The chemical and voltage sensitivity of an apparently single mechanism may make describing the gate as either chemical or electrical misleading. Similar kinds of sensitivity of excitable channels in ordinary membranes to both chemical and electrical stimuli are now well established (Tsien and Siegelbaum, 1983).

Gap junctions have other pharmacological properties, the significance of which may be as obscure as it is for ordinary channels. Protein reagents should lead to information regarding the critical components and active sites involved in junctional responsiveness. Available antibodies block only at the cytoplasmic face.

There is now evidence that junctions can be covalently modified. Phosphorylation can be produced in vivo (Willecke et al., 1985) and in vitro. An increase in cAMP following hormone treatment or an increase in the action of synaptic transmitters can decrease junctional conductance. It is plausible that junctional macromolecules in formed junctions are phosphorylated and dephosphorylated to cause closing and opening, respectively. Conversely, channel formation is promoted in some systems by cAMP.

Junctional formation can be elicited between many cell types, indicating the conservation of interacting parts of the junctions in many tissues and vertebrate species. Such conservation is also found at the cytoplasmic face, as indicated by antibody cross-reactivity. The sites of protein synthesis and the mechanisms of junctional formation should become clearer as immunohistochemistry is extended to the ultrastructural level. The specificity observed in vivo may result from cell adhesion molecules rather than from the junctions themselves.

It should not be long before gap junction genes are cloned and sequenced. Then the interesting task will be to determine how the proteins are arranged in the membrane, and what is responsible for channel gating. Factors affecting the expression of gap junction genes are known. The detailed mechanisms of intracellular signaling remain, as do many other aspects of gene expression in excitable as well as inexcitable cells, subjects of speculation and investigation.

POSTSCSRIPT

While this manuscript was in the publication process, significant advances were made on several fronts. The cDNAs for gap junction protein mRNAs of rat and human liver were cloned and sequenced (Kumar and Gilula, 1986; Paul, 1986). Parallel measurements of levels of gap junction mRNA, protein, and conductance are now feasible; such measurements should shed light on the roles of transcriptional, translational, and posttranslational processing in the regulation of junctional communication by hormones and other factors. Quantitative measurements of transjunctional fluxes between embryonic cells were made for several larger ions by using ion-sensitive electrodes (Verselis et al., 1986). The permeability is proportional to junctional conductance as it is altered by transjunctional voltage, which implies that channel gating is all or none. Comparison of permeabilities to different ions by means of normalization with respect to conductance should provide information on the interactions of ions with the channel wall. These data must ultimately relate to the tertiary structure of the junctional protein.

Gap junctions of rat liver were shown to consist of a phosphoprotein (Saez et al., 1986), and phosphorylation by different kinases appears to be a mechanism of modulation of junctional conductance. Isolated liver gap junctions were incorporated into lipid membranes, and the open time of single channels (Spray et al., 1986c) was shown to be regulated by treatments that affect macroscopic conductance between cell pairs (Spray et al., 1986b). Consequently, the effects of modulatory treatments such as phosphorylation are now analyzable in terms of the gating properties of single channels.

ACKNOWLEDGMENTS

This work was supported in part by National Institutes of Health grants NS-19830 and NS-16524 to D.C.S. and grants NS-07512 and HD-04248 to M.V.L.B.; D.C.S. also received a grant-in-aid from the American Heart Association and a McKnight Foundation Development Award.

REFERENCES

Asada, Y., and M. V. L. Bennett (1971) Experimental alteration of coupling resistance at an electrotonic synapse. *J. Cell Biol.* **49**:159–172.

Auerbach, A. A., and M. V. L. Bennett (1969) A rectifying synapse in the central nervous system of a vertebrate. *J. Gen. Physiol.* **53**:211–237.

Bennett, M. V. L. (1966) Physiology of electrotonic junctions. *Ann. N.Y. Acad. Sci.* **37**:509–539.

Bennett, M. V. L. (1977) Electrical transmission: A functional analysis and comparison to chemical transmission. *Handb. Physiol., Cellular Biology of Neurons* **1**:357–416.

Bennett, M. V. L., and D. M. Goodenough (1978) Gap junctions, electrotonic coupling and intercellular communication. *Neurosci. Res. Program Bull.* **16**:373–486.

Bennett, M. V. L., and D. C. Spray (1984) Gap junctions: Two voltage-dependent gates in series allow voltage-induced steady-state cycling around a circular reaction scheme. *Biophys. J.* **45**:60a.

Bennett, M. V. L., and D. C. Spray, eds. (1985) *Gap Junctions*, Cold Spring Harbor Laboratory, Cold Spring Harbor, New York.

Bennett, M. V. L., D. C. Spray, and A. L. Harris (1981) Electrical coupling in development. *Am. Zool.* **21**:413–427.

Bennett, M. V. L., D. C. Spray, A. L. Harris, R. D. Ginzberg, A. C. Campos de Carvalho, and R. L. White (1984) Control of intercellular communication by way of gap junctions. *Harvey Lecture Series* **78**:23–57.

Campos de Carvalho, A. C., D. C. Spray, and M. V. L. Bennett (1984) pH dependence of transmission at electrotonic synapses of the crayfish septate axon. *Brain Res.* **321**:279–286.

Campos de Carvalho, A. C., F. Ramon, and D. C. Spray (1986) Effect of group-specific protein reagents on electrotonic coupling in crayfish septate axon. *Am. J. Physiol. (Cell Physiol. 20)* **251**:C99–C103.

Carew, T. J., and E. R. Kandel (1976) Two functional effects of decreased conductance EPSPs: Synaptic augmentation and increased electrotonic coupling. *Science* **192**:150–153.

Caveney, S., R. C. Berdan, and S. McLean (1980) Cell-to-cell ionic communication stimulated by 20-hydroxyecdysone occurs in the absence of protein synthesis and gap junction growth. *J. Insect Physiol.* **26**:557–567.

Cole, W. C., and R. E. Garfield (1985) Alterations in coupling in uterine smooth muscle. In *Gap Junctions*, M. V. L. Bennett and D. C. Spray, eds., pp. 215–230, Cold Spring Harbor Laboratory, Cold Spring Harbor, New York.

Dahl, G., and G. Isenberg (1980) Decoupling of heart muscle cells: Correlation with increased cytoplasmic calcium activity and with changes of nexus ultrastructure. *J. Membr. Biol.* **53**:63–75.

Deleze, J., and J. C. Herve (1983) Effect of several uncouplers of cell-to-cell communication on gap junction morphology in mammalian heart. *J. Membr. Biol.* **74**:203–215.

Edelman, G. M. (1983) Cell adhesion molecules. *Science* **219**:450–457.

Finkelstein, A., and C. S. Peskin (1984) Some unexpected consequences of a simple physical mechanism for voltage-dependent gating in biological membranes. *Biophys. J.* **46**:549–558.

Furshpan, E. J., and D. D. Potter (1959) Transmission at the giant motor synapses of the crayfish. *J. Physiol. (Lond.)* **145**:289–325.

Ginzberg, R. D., E. A. Morales, D. C. Spray, and M. V. L. Bennett (1985) Cell junctions in early embryos of squid (*Loligo pealei*). *Cell Tissue Res.* **239**:477–484.

Hall, D. H., E. Gilat, and M. V. L. Bennett (1985) Ultrastructure of rectifying electrical synapses between giant fibers and pectoral fin adductor motoneurons in the hatchetfish. *J. Neurocytol.* **14**:825–834.

Hanna, R. B., G. D. Pappas, and M. V. L. Bennett (1984) The fine structure of identified electrotonic synapses following increased coupling resistance. *Cell Tissue Res.* **235**:243–249.

Hanna, R. B., R. L. Ornberg, and T. S. Reese (1985) Structural details of rapidly frozen gap junctions. In *Gap Junctions*, M. V. L. Bennett and D. C. Spray, eds., pp. 23–32, Cold Spring Harbor Laboratory, Cold Spring Harbor, New York.

Harris, A. L., D. C. Spray, and M. V. L. Bennett (1981) Kinetic properties of a voltage-dependent junctional conductance. *J. Gen. Physiol.* **77**:95–117.

Harris, A. L., D. C. Spray, and M. V. L. Bennett (1983) Control of intercellular communication by a voltage-dependent junctional conductance. *J. Neurosci.* **3**:79–100.

Hertzberg, E. L., and R. V. Skibbens (1984) A protein homologous to the 27,000 Dalton liver gap junction protein is present in a wide variety of species and tissues. *Cell* **39**:61–69.

Hertzberg, E. L., D. C. Spray, and M. V. L. Bennett (1985) Reduction of gap junctional conductance by microinjection of antibodies against the 27,000 Dalton liver gap junction polypeptide. *Proc. Natl. Acad. Sci. USA* **83**:2412–2416.

Higgins, D., and H. Burton (1982) Electrotonic synapses are formed by fetal rat sympathetic neurons maintained in a chemically defined culture medium. *J. Neurosci.* **7**:2241–2253.

Johnston, M. F., S. A. Simon, and F. Ramon (1980) Interaction of anesthetics with electrical synapses. *Nature* **286**:498–500.

Kessler, J. A., D. C. Spray, J. C. Saez, and M. V. L. Bennett (1984) Determination of synaptic phenotype: Insulin and cAMP independently initiate development of electrotonic coupling between cultured sympathetic neurons. *Proc. Natl. Acad. Sci. USA* **81**:6235–6239.

Kumar, N. M., and N. B. Gilula (1986) Cloning and characterization of human and rat liver cDNAs coding for a gap junction protein. *J. Cell Biol.* **103**:767–776.

Lasater, E. R., and J. E. Dowling (1985) Electrical coupling between pairs of isolated fish horizontal cells is modulated by dopamine and cyclic AMP. In *Gap Junctions*, M. V. L. Bennett and D. C. Spray, eds., pp. 393–404, Cold Spring Harbor Laboratory, Cold Spring Harbor, New York.

Lee, W. M., D. G. Cran, and N. J. Lane (1982) Carbon dioxide-induced disassembly of gap junctional plaques. *J. Cell Sci.* **57**:215–228.

Makowski, L., D. L. D. Caspar, W. C. Phillips, and D. A. Goodenough (1984) Gap junction structures. V. Structural chemistry inferred from X-ray diffraction measurements on sucrose accessibility and trypsin susceptibility. *J. Mol. Biol.* **174**:449–481.

Margiotta, J. F., and B. Walcott (1983) Conductance and dye-permeability of a rectifying synapse. *Nature* **305**:52–56.

Mazet, F., B. A. Wittenberg, and D. C. Spray (1985) Fate of intercellular junctions in isolated adult rat cardiac cells. *Circ. Res.* **56**:195–204.

Neher, E., and C. F. Stevens (1977) Conductance fluctuations and ionic pores in membranes. *Annu. Rev. Biophys. Bioeng.* **6**:345–372.

Nicholls, J. G., and D. Purves (1972) A comparison of chemical and electrical synaptic transmission between single sensory cells and a motoneurone in the central nervous system of the leech. *J. Physiol. (Lond.)* **225**:637–656.

Nicholson, B. J., L. J. Takemoto, M. W. Hunkapiller, L. E. Hood, and J.-P. Revel (1983) Differences between the liver gap junction protein and lens MIP-26 from rat: Implications for tissue specificity of gap junctions. *Cell* **32**:967–978.

Obaid, A. L., S. J. Socolar, and B. Rose (1983) Cell-to-cell channels with two independently regulated gates in series: Analysis of junctional channel modulation by membrane potential, calcium and pH. *J. Membr. Biol.* **73**:69–89.

Oliveira-Castro, G. M., and W. R. Loewenstein (1971) Junctional membrane permeability: Effects of divalent cations. *J. Membr. Biol.* **5**:51–77.

Page, E., T. Harrison, and J. Upshaw-Early (1983) Freeze-fractured cardiac gap junctions: Structural analysis by three methods. *Am. J. Physiol.* **224**:H525–H539.

Paul, D. L. (1986) Molecular cloning of cDNA for rat liver gap junction protein. *J. Cell Biol.* **103**:123–134.

Peracchia, C. (1980) Structural correlates of gap junction permeation. *Int. Rev. Cytol.* **66**:81–104.

Piccolino, M., J. Neyton, and H. M. Gerschenfeld (1984) Decrease of gap junction permeability induced by dopamine and cyclic AMP in horizontal cells of turtle retina. *J. Neurosci.* **4**:2477–2488.

Potter, D. D., E. J. Furshpan, and E. S. Lennox (1966) Connections between cells of the developing squid as revealed by electrophysiological methods. *Proc. Natl. Acad. Sci. USA* **55**:328–336.

Revel, J.-P., and S. B. Yancey (1985) Molecular conformation of the major intrinsic protein of lens fiber membranes: Is it a junction protein? In *Gap Junctions*, M. V. L. Bennett and D. C. Spray, eds., pp. 33–48, Cold Spring Harbor Laboratory, Cold Spring Harbor, New York.

Saez, J. C., D. C. Spray, A. Nairn, E. L. Hertzberg, P. Greengard, and M. V. L. Bennett (1986) cAMP increases junctional conductance and stimulates phosphorylation of the 27-kDa principal gap junction polypeptide. *Proc. Natl. Acad. Sci. USA* **83**:2473–2477.

Scheutze, S. M., and D. A. Goodenough (1982) Dye transfer between cells of the embryonic chick lens becomes less sensitive to CO_2 treatment during development. *J. Cell Biol.* **92**:694–705.

Schmalbruch, H., and H. Jahnsen (1981) Gap junctions on CA3 pyramidal cells of guinea pig hippocampus shown by freeze fracture. *Brain Res.* **217**:175–178.

Sloper, J. J., and T. P. S. Powell (1978) Gap junctions between dendrites and somata of neurons in the primate sensori-motor cortex. *Proc. R. Soc. Lond. (Biol. Sci.)* **203**:39–47.

Smith, T. G., and F. Baumann (1969) The functional organization within the ommatidium of the lateral eye of the *Limulus. Prog. Brain Res.* **31**:313–349.

Sotelo, C., R. Llinás, and R. Baker (1972) Structural study of inferior olivary nucleus of the cat: Morphological correlates of electrotonic coupling between neurons. *Brain Res.* **37**:294–300.

Spira, M. E., D. C. Spray, and M. V. L. Bennett (1980) Synaptic organization of expansion motoneurons of *Navanax inermis. Brain Res.* **195**:241–269.

Spitzer, N. (1982) Voltage- and stage-dependent uncoupling of Rohon-Beard neurones during embryonic development of *Xenopus* tadpoles. *J. Physiol. (Lond.)* **330**:145–162.

Spray, D. C., and M. V. L. Bennett (1985) Physiology and pharmacology of gap junctions. *Annu. Rev. Physiol.* **47**:281–303.

Spray, D. C., A. L. Harris, and M. V. L. Bennett (1979) Voltage dependence of junctional conductance in early amphibian embryos. *Science* **204**:432–434.

Spray, D. C., A. L. Harris, and M. V. L. Bennett (1981a) Gap junctional conductance is a simple and sensitive function of intracellular pH. *Science* **211**:712–715.

Spray, D. C., A. L. Harris, and M. V. L. Bennett (1981b) Equilibrium properties of a voltage-dependent junctional conductance. *J. Gen. Physiol.* **77**:75–94.

Spray, D. C., J. H. Stern, A. L. Harris, and M. V. L. Bennett (1982) Comparison of sensitivities of gap junctional conductance to H and Ca ions. *Proc. Natl. Acad. Sci. USA* **79**:441–445.

Spray, D. C., J. Nerbonne, A. C. Campos de Carvalho, A. L. Harris, and M. V. L. Bennett (1984a) Substituted benzyl acetates: A new class of compounds that reduce gap junctional conductance by cytoplasmic acidification. *J. Cell Biol.* **99**:174–179.

Spray, D. C., R. L. White, A. C. Campos de Carvalho, A. L. Harris, and M. V. L. Bennett (1984b) Gating of gap junction channels. *Biophys. J.* **45**:219–230.

Spray, D. C., A. C. Campos de Carvalho, and M. V. L. Bennett (1986a) Sensitivity of gap junctional conductance to H ions is independent of voltage sensitivity. *Proc. Natl. Acad. Sci. USA* **83**: 3533–3536.

Spray, D. C., R. D. Ginsberg, E. A. Morales, Z. Gatmaitin, and I. N. Arias (1986b) Electrophysiological properties of gap junctions between dissociated pairs of rat hepatocytes. *J. Cell Biol.* **103**:135–194.

Spray, D. C., J. C. Saez, D. Brosius, M. V. L. Bennett, and E. L. Hertzberg (1986c) Isolated liver gap junctions: Gating of transjunctional current is similar to that in intact pairs of rat hepatocytes. *Proc. Natl. Acad. Sci. USA* **83**:5494–5497.

Teranishi, T., K. Negishi, and S. Kato (1984) Regulatory effect of dopamine on spatial properties of horizontal cells in carp retina. *J. Neurosci.* **4**:1271–1280.

Tsien, R. W., and S. A. Siegelbaum (1983) Modulation of gated ion channels as a mode of transmitter action. *Trends Neurosci.* **6**:307–310.

Unwin, N. T., and P. D. Ennis (1984) Two configurations of a channel forming protein. *Nature* **307**:609–613.

Verselis, V., R. L. White, D. C. Spray, and M. V. L. Bennett (1986) Gap junctional conductance and permeability are linearly related. *Science* **234**:461–464.

Warner, A. E., S. C. Guthrie, and N. B. Gilula (1984) Antibodies to gap junctional protein selectively disrupt junctional communication in the early amphibian embryo. *Nature* **311**:127–131.

White, R. L., D. C. Spray, A. C. Campos de Carvalho, B. A. Wittenberg, and M. V. L. Bennett (1985) Some electrical and pharmacological properties of gap junctions between adult ventricular myocytes. *Am. J. Physiol.* **249**:447.

Willecke, K., O. Traub, U. Janssen-Timmen, U. Frixen, R. Dermietzel, A. Leibstein, O. Paul, and
    H. Rabes (1985) Immunochemical investigations of gap junction protein in different mammalian
    tissues. In *Gap Junctions*, M. V. L. Bennett and D. C. Spray, eds., pp. 67–76, Cold Spring Harbor
    Laboratory, Cold Spring Harbor, New York.

Zipser, B. (1979) Voltage-modulated membrane resistance in coupled leech neurons. *J. Neurophysiol.*
    42:465–475.

Chapter 5

Molecular Properties of Voltage-Sensitive Sodium and Calcium Channels

WILLIAM A. CATTERALL
BENSON M. CURTIS
DANIEL J. FELLER

ABSTRACT

Conventional biochemical methods have been used to identify, solubilize, and purify protein components of the voltage-sensitive sodium and calcium channels. Sodium channels from rat brain consist of a complex of three subunits: α, with a molecular weight of 260 kD; β1, with a molecular weight of 36 kD; and β2, with a molecular weight of 33 kD. The β2-subunit is associated with the α-subunit by disulfide bonds, while the β1-subunit is noncovalently attached. Incorporation of this defined complex into phospholipid bilayers of appropriate composition restores the functional properties of sodium channels, as measured by neurotoxin binding, ion flux, and single channel recording. Calcium channels from rabbit skeletal muscle transverse tubules consist in part of a calcium antagonist receptor, which is a complex of three subunits: α, with a molecular weight of 135 kD; β, with a molecular weight of 50 kD; and γ, with a molecular weight of 33 kD. Both sodium and calcium channels are substrates for phosphorylation by protein kinases, suggesting that their physiological properties may be subject to long-term modulation by direct covalent modification of their subunits.

Nerve cells are electrically excitable because of the presence in their surface membranes of voltage-sensitive ion channels that are selective for sodium, potassium, or calcium. One class of sodium channels and multiple classes of calcium and potassium channels have been described in neurons. These channels open and close as a function of membrane voltage, allowing rapid movement of the appropriate ions down their concentration gradient carrying ionic current into or out of the cell, and thereby depolarizing or hyperpolarizing the membrane potential. The electrical excitability of neurons is influenced by the nature and functional properties of their ion channels, the density of ion channels in their surface membrane, and the location of ion channels in the different functional elements of the nerve cell. Neurons can be divided into four morphological elements that play different roles in signal transmission. Dendrites receive synaptic input from numerous presynaptic elements and respond with graded or, in some cases, propagated changes in membrane potential that are mediated by

137

potassium, calcium, and perhaps sodium channels. The cell body or soma also receives synaptic inputs. It acts as a summing point for membrane potential changes occurring in various dendrites and on the soma itself. Depolarization of the cell membrane beyond a threshold value elicits one or a series of conducted action potentials that are initiated by sodium channels in the cell soma or in the initial segment of the axon and are conducted down the axon to the nerve terminal. The sodium-dependent action potential invades the nerve terminal, causing depolarization, activation of calcium channels, release of neurotransmitter into the synaptic cleft, and excitation of succeeding neurons in the pathway or of effector cells such as skeletal muscle. Voltage-sensitive sodium, potassium, and calcium channels each contribute in a specific way to signal processing and transmission in neurons. Knowledge of the molecular properties of these critical components of the nervous system will allow new approaches to studies of neuronal function. In this chapter, we review the strategy that has been developed to identify the protein components of voltage-sensitive sodium and calcium channels, purify them, and analyze their functional properties and physiological regulation.

VOLTAGE-SENSITIVE SODIUM CHANNELS

Electrophysiological experiments using the voltage clamp technique have shown that the initial rapid depolarization during an action potential in nerve, skeletal muscle, and heart muscle results from rapid voltage-dependent increases in membrane permeability to sodium ions. Many different lines of evidence indicate that a selective transmembrane sodium channel is responsible for the rapid sodium permeability increase during the action potential. Selective ion permeation is mediated by a hydrophilic pore containing a sodium-selective ion coordination site, designated the ion selectivity filter (Hille, 1971, 1972). Ion conductance through the sodium channel is regulated or "gated" by two separate processes: activation, which controls the rate and voltage dependence of the sodium permeability increase following depolarization; and inactivation, which controls the rate and voltage dependence of the subsequent return of sodium permeability to the resting level during a maintained depolarization (Hodgkin and Huxley, 1952). Membrane-charge movements associated with voltage-dependent activation of sodium channels have been detected as gating currents and are thought to represent the movement of charged components of the sodium channel protein during the conformational changes leading to channel activation (Armstrong and Bezanilla, 1974). Sodium channel inactivation is thought to be a sequential, relatively voltage-insensitive process that is initiated by the voltage-dependent conformational changes that lead to channel activation (Armstrong and Bezanilla, 1977; Aldrich et al., 1983).

Analysis of sodium channel properties by voltage clamp methods has provided a detailed description of the three essential functional properties of sodium channels: voltage-dependent activation, voltage-dependent inactivation, and selective ion transport. However, an understanding of the molecular basis of electrical excitability requires the identification of the membrane macromolecules that make up the ionic channels, solubilization and purification of these channel components, and correlation of their structural features with the known functional properties of sodium channels. This task has required the development of new approaches.

Neurotoxins as Molecular Probes of Sodium Channels

Neurotoxins that bind with high affinity and specificity to voltage-sensitive sodium channels and modify their properties have provided the essential tools for identifying and purifying sodium channels. Four different groups of neurotoxins that act at four different neurotoxin receptor sites on the sodium channel have been useful in these studies (Table I). Neurotoxin receptor site 1 binds the water-soluble, heterocyclic guanidines, tetrodotoxin, and saxitoxin. These toxins inhibit sodium channel ion transport by binding to a common receptor site that is thought to be located near the extracellular opening of the ion-conducting pore of the sodium channel (for a review, see Narahashi, 1974; Ritchie and Rogart, 1977; Catterall, 1980).

Neurotoxin receptor site 2 binds several lipid-soluble toxins, including grayanotoxin and the alkaloids veratridine, aconitine, and batrachotoxin (for reviews, see Albuquerque and Daly, 1976; Catterall, 1980). The competitive interactions among these four toxins at neurotoxin receptor site 2 have been confirmed by direct measurements of the specific binding of [^{3}H]batrachotoxinin A 20-α-benzoate to sodium channels (Catterall et al., 1981). These toxins cause persistent activation of sodium channels at the resting membrane potential by blocking sodium channel inactivation and by shifting the voltage dependence of sodium channel activation to more negative membrane potentials (for a review, see Catterall, 1980). Therefore, neurotoxin receptor site 2 is likely to be localized on a region of the sodium channel involved in voltage-dependent activation and inactivation.

Neurotoxin receptor site 3 binds polypeptide toxins purified from North African scorpion venoms or sea anemone nematocysts. These toxins slow or block sodium channel inactivation. They also markedly enhance persistent activation of sodium channels by the lipid-soluble toxins acting at neurotoxin receptor site 2 (for a review, see Catterall, 1980). The affinity for the binding of ^{125}I-labeled derivatives of the polypeptide toxins to neurotoxin receptor site 3 is reduced by depolarization. The voltage dependence of scorpion toxin binding is closely correlated with the voltage dependence of sodium channel activation. These experiments indicate

Table 1. Neurotoxin Receptor Sites on the Sodium Channel

Site	Neurotoxins	Physiological Effect
1	Tetrodotoxin	Inhibit ion transport
2	Veratridine Batrachotoxin Grayanotoxin Aconitine	Cause persistent activation
3	North African α-scorpion toxins Sea anemone toxins	Slow inactivation
4	American β-scorpion toxins	Enhance activation

that neurotoxin receptor site 3 is located on a region of the sodium channel that undergoes a conformational change during voltage-dependent channel activation, leading to a markedly reduced affinity for scorpion toxin. Therefore, scorpion toxin and sea anemone toxin bind to the voltage-sensing or voltage-gating structures of sodium channels.

Neurotoxin receptor site 4 binds a new class of scorpion toxins that has also proved valuable in studies of sodium channels. Cahalan (1975) showed that the venom of the American scorpion *Centruroides sculpturatus* modifies sodium channel activation rather than inactivation. Pure toxins from several American scorpions have a similar action (Couraud et al., 1982; Meves et al., 1982; Wang and Strichartz, 1982). These toxins bind to a new receptor site on the sodium channel (Jover et al., 1980; Barhanin et al., 1982) and have therefore been designated β-scorpion toxins.

These several neurotoxins provide specific high-affinity probes for distinct regions of the sodium channel structure. They have been used to detect and localize sodium channels in neuronal cells, as well as to identify and purify the protein components of sodium channels that bind these toxins and to analyze their structural and functional properties.

Identification of Protein Components of Sodium Channels in Neurons

Measurements of the distribution and density of sodium channels indicate that, with the exception of the very small amount of specialized membrane at the node of Ranvier, sodium channels are a minor component of excitable membranes. These results emphasize the need for highly specific probes to identify the macromolecules that make up the sodium channel. The neurotoxins that bind to sodium channels with high affinity and specificity have provided the tools needed in such experiments. Direct chemical identification of sodium channel components *in situ* was first achieved by specific covalent labeling of neurotoxin receptor site 3 with a photoreactive azidonitrobenzoyl derivative of the α-scorpion toxin from *Leiurus quinquestriatus* (Beneski and Catterall, 1980). The photoreactive toxin derivative is allowed to bind specifically to sodium channels in the dark. Irradiation with ultraviolet light then chemically activates the arylazide group, which covalently reacts with the scorpion toxin receptor site on the sodium channel. Analysis of covalently labeled synaptosomes by polyacrylamide gel electrophoresis under denaturing conditions in sodium dodecyl sulfate (SDS) to separate synaptosomal proteins by size reveals the specific covalent labeling of two polypeptides that have subsequently been designated the α- and β1-subunits of the sodium channel. These proteins, as assessed by polyacrylamide gel electrophoresis in SDS, have molecular weights of 270 kD and 36 kD, respectively. The covalent labeling of these two polypeptides in synaptosomes was shown to be specific through inhibition of labeling by competition with excess unlabeled scorpion toxin or by block of the voltage-dependent binding of scorpion toxin by membrane depolarization.

The β-scorpion toxins derived from American scorpion venoms have also been used to label neurotoxin receptor site 4 on the sodium channel (Barhanin et al., 1983; Darbon et al., 1983). Toxin γ from *Tityus serrulatus* was covalently attached to its receptor site by cross-linking with disuccinimidyl suberate. A single polypeptide of 270 kD was labeled in rat brain synaptosomes. Photoreactive derivatives of toxin II from *Centruroides suffusus suffusus* covalently label polypeptides of 255 kD and 35 kD in rat brain synaptosomes that are likely to be the α- and β1-subunits of the sodium channel. Taken together, these covalent labeling results indicate that neurotoxin receptor sites 3 and 4 are both located near the contact regions of the α- and β1-subunits of the sodium channel.

Molecular Size of the Sodium Channel

The first indications of the molecular size of the neuronal sodium channel *in situ* were derived from radiation inactivation studies (Levinson and Ellory, 1973). In these experiments, membrane preparations from pig brain were irradiated with X-rays and the decrease in the number of functional tetrodotoxin binding sites was measured as a function of radiation dose. From these data, the size of the membrane target can be determined, since larger targets are more likely to be hit and are therefore inactivated at a lower radiation dose. Applying target theory, Levinson and Ellory concluded that a structure of 230 kD was required for toxin binding. These experiments have recently been repeated by Barhanin et al. (1983), who compared the target size of the sodium channel assessed by either tetrodotoxin binding or *Tityus serrulatus* toxin γ binding. In each case, the target size was approximately 270 kD, in reasonable agreement with the earlier work. This size estimate might correspond to the molecular weight of the 'entire sodium channel, or to the molecular weight of a protein subunit that is essential for binding these neurotoxins.

The molecular size of the intact sodium channel protein has been measured by hydrodynamic studies of the detergent-solubilized channel. The saxitoxin and tetrodotoxin binding component of sodium channels was first solubilized, with retention of the high affinity and specificity of toxin binding, from garfish olfactory nerve membrane by using nonionic detergents (Henderson and Wang, 1972; Benzer and Raftery, 1973). Similar techniques have now been applied to sodium channels in mammalian brain and skeletal muscle (Catterall et al., 1979; Krueger et al., 1979; Barchi et al., 1980). In contrast to the ease of solubilization of the sodium channel with retention of saxitoxin and tetrodotoxin binding activity at neurotoxin receptor site 1, both neurotoxin receptor site 2 and neurotoxin receptor site 3 lose high-affinity neurotoxin binding activity on solubilization. The molecular weight of the solubilized sodium channel from rat brain and skeletal muscle has been estimated by hydrodynamic studies to be 601 kD (Hartshorne et al., 1980; Barchi, 1983). Since the detergent–channel complex contains 0.9 gm Triton X-100 and phosphatidylcholine per gram of protein, the molecular weight of the sodium channel protein solubilized from rat brain is 316 kD. This represents the size of the entire sodium channel, as solubilized in detergents, and corresponds to a complex of three nonidentical protein subunits, as described below. If the channel protein is spherical in shape, the diameter indicated by these results is 118 Å. Thus, the channel protein is much larger than the postulated transmembrane pore through which sodium moves, the ion selectivity filter, which is proposed to be 3 Å × 5 Å at its narrowest point.

Purification of the Solubilized Saxitoxin–Tetrodotoxin Receptor of the Sodium Channel

Although the saxitoxin receptor of the sodium channel had been successfully solubilized several years earlier, the marked instability of the toxin binding activity prevented progress on the purification of the sodium channel until the discovery by Agnew et al. (1978) that the addition of phospholipid markedly stabilized the saxitoxin receptor from eel electroplax. These investigators were able to achieve substantial purification of the saxitoxin receptor by ion exchange chromatography and gel filtration, culminating in a preparation that was approximately 50% pure (Agnew et al., 1980). The only protein component of this partially purified preparation that was clearly correlated with toxin binding activity was a 260-kD polypeptide. This protein is likely to be analogous to the α-subunit of the sodium channel from mammalian brain that was identified in intact membranes by covalent labeling with a photoreactive scorpion toxin derivative (Beneski and Catterall, 1980).

Application of similar procedures to sodium channels solubilized from mammalian skeletal muscle and brain also gives substantial purification (Barchi et al., 1980; Hartshorne and Catterall, 1981). In addition, affinity chromatography on wheat germ lectin–Sepharose columns provides a further enrichment of the saxitoxin binding activity from these tissues. The specific adsorbtion and elution of the saxitoxin receptor from this lectin affinity column indicates that it is a glycoprotein containing N-acetylglucosamine and/or sialic acid residues. Saxitoxin receptor preparations that are highly purified can now be obtained from either rat skeletal muscle or rat brain by using a combination of these procedures, as assessed by the specific activity for the binding of saxitoxin and by the number of protein bands identified on polyacrylamide gels of the purified protein.

Subunit Composition of the Purified Mammalian Sodium Channel

The subunit compositions of these highly purified sodium channel preparations from eel electroplax, rat brain, and rat skeletal muscle differ somewhat, and therefore each is considered individually. Analysis of highly purified preparations of sodium channels from rat brain by polyacrylamide gel electrophoresis in the presence of SDS without the reduction of protein disulfide bonds reveals two protein components with molecular weights of approximately 300 kD and 36 kD, which are associated with saxitoxin binding activity (Hartshorne and Catterall, 1981, 1984; Hartshorne et al., 1982). These two polypeptide bands account for 90% of the protein stain intensity in silver-stained gels. Reduction of protein disulfide bonds by treatment with β-mercaptoethanol cleaves the 300-kD protein into two polypeptides with molecular weights of approximately 260 kD and 33 kD (Hartshorne et al., 1982). In previous experiments, the gel electrophoresis conditions used did not allow clear resolution of the approximately 36-kD and 33-kD polypeptides. Therefore, it was first necessary to separate the disulfide-linked complex of 260-kD and 33-kD polypeptides from the 36-kD polypeptide by gel filtration in SDS without reduction and then to demonstrate the presence of the 33-kD polypeptide by reduction of the complex followed by gel electrophoresis. We have now devised new conditions of gel electrophoresis that allow consistent resolution of these two polypeptides (Messner and Catterall, 1985). Electrophoresis in polyacrylamide gels with reduced cross-linking [(acrylamide)/ (methylene bisacrylamide) = 30/0.20] resolves three polypeptides of 260 kD, 36 kD, and 33 kD (Figure 1). They are designated the α-, β1-, and β2-subunits of the sodium channel (Hartshorne et al., 1982; Hartshorne and Catterall, 1984).

As illustrated in Figure 1, the α- and β2-subunits are covalently linked by one or more disulfide bonds, whereas the β1-subunit is associated with the complex by noncovalent forces. The total molecular weight of the subunits is 329 kD, in close agreement with the estimated molecular weight of the entire sodium channel complex of 316 kD. The ratio of stain intensities of the individual subunits is also in agreement with a molar ratio of subunits of 1:1:1. Thus, the data available at present are in best agreement with a subunit stoichiometry of α_1, $(\beta 1)_1$, and $(\beta 2)_1$ for the sodium channel from rat brain.

Photoaffinity labeling of neurotoxin receptor site 3 on the sodium channel with an azidonitrobenzoyl derivative of the α-scorpion toxin from *Leiurus quin-questriatus* results in reaction with the α- and β1-subunits, as described above (Beneski and Catterall, 1980; Hartshorne et al., 1982). Similarly, photoreactive derivatives of α-scorpion toxins that bind at neurotoxin receptor site 4 on the sodium channel also specifically label the α- and β1-subunits of the sodium channel (Barhanin et al., 1983; Darbon et al., 1983). Evidently, neurotoxin receptor

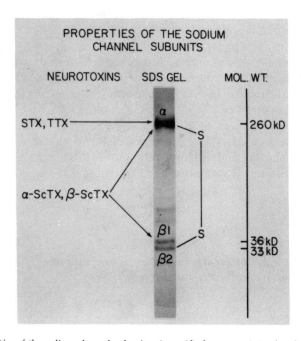

Figure 1. *Properties of the sodium channel subunits.* A purified preparation of sodium channels was dissociated by incubation at 100°C in sodium dodecyl sulfate (SDS) and β-mercaptoethanol and analyzed by electrophoresis in polyacrylamide gels with a low ratio of cross-linking [(acrylamide)/ (methylene bisacrylamide) = 30/0.2], as described by Messner and Catterall (1985). The α-, β1-, and β2-subunits, as visualized by silver staining, are indicated, along with the sites of covalent attachment of photoreactive neurotoxin derivatives, the intersubunit disulfide bonds, and the subunit molecular weights.

sites 3 and 4 are located near the regions of contact of the α- and β1-subunits, so that neurotoxins bound there can label either subunit. In contrast, covalent attachment of a specifically bound tetrodotoxin derivative through the use of bifunctional cross-linking reagents labels only a 260-kD protein, suggesting that neurotoxin receptor site 1 is located on the α-subunit. These neurotoxin labeling reactions are summarized in Figure 1. The results provide positive identification of the α-, β1-, and β2-subunits in intact synaptosomal membranes and verify that these components of the purified sodium channel also exist in intact membranes. Further support for this conclusion has been derived from experiments in which sodium channels were covalently labeled in membranes of a freshly prepared homogenate of rat brain in the presence of a cocktail of 11 protease inhibitors immediately after decapitation (Sharkey et al., 1984). The α-, β1-, and β2-subunits are all detected, indicating that they are likely to be the components of the sodium channel in the intact brain.

The initial analyses of the sodium channel purified from mammalian skeletal muscle (Barchi et al., 1980) revealed polypeptides with molecular weights of 64 kD, 60 kD, and 53 kD, but more recent work has shown that these were not components of the sodium channel. Barchi (1983) subsequently reported that the purified saxitoxin receptor from skeletal muscle contains three major polypeptide components with molecular weights of 125–250 kD, 48 kD, and a doublet at 38 kD. However, it now appears that only polypeptides with molecular weights of 260 kD and 38 kD are components of the sodium channel (Kraner et al., 1985). Thus it appears that the sodium channels from both rat brain and skeletal muscle have one large and one or two small subunits.

In contrast to these results with sodium channels from mammalian nerve and muscle, highly purified preparations of the tetrodotoxin binding component of the sodium channel from eel electroplax appear to consist of a single polypeptide with a molecular weight of 260 kD (Agnew et al., 1980; Nakayama et al., 1982; Miller et al., 1983; Norman et al., 1983b). Apparently, the β-subunits of the mammalian sodium channel are not present in the eel electroplax or not required for tetrodotoxin binding and are lost in the purification procedures. The subunit composition of sodium channels purified from these three sources is summarized in Table 2.

Table 2. Molecular Properties of the Sodium Channel Purified from Different Tissues

Tissue	Molecular Weight (kD)	Subunits (kD)
Electroplax	—	260
Brain	316	α: 260
		β1: 36
		β2: 33
Skeletal Muscle	314	260
		38

Reconstitution of Sodium Channel Function from Purified Components

The purified sodium channel binds [³H]saxitoxin and tetrodotoxin with the same affinity as the native sodium channel and therefore contains neurotoxin receptor site 1 of the sodium channel in an active form. The purified channel also contains the α- and β1-subunits that were identified as components of neurotoxin receptor site 3 by photoaffinity labeling with scorpion toxin, although after solubilization the binding activity for scorpion toxin is lost. However, the purified channel does not have binding activity for neurotoxins at receptor site 2 and cannot transport sodium in the detergent-solubilized state. Reconstitution of these sodium channel functions from purified components is the only rigorous proof that the proteins identified and purified on the basis of their neurotoxin binding activity are indeed sufficient to form a functional voltage-sensitive ion channel. In addition, successful reconstitution will provide a valuable experimental preparation for biochemical analysis of the structure and function of sodium channels.

Several groups have successfully restored aspects of sodium channel function from detergent-solubilized brain membranes, showing that detergent solubilization does not irreversibly destroy channel function. More recently, sodium channel ion transport has been successfully reconstituted from sodium channels substantially purified from eel electroplax, rat brain, and skeletal muscle (Talvenheimo et al., 1982; Weigele and Barchi, 1982; Tanaka et al., 1983; Rosenberg et al., 1984). We have applied these methods to essentially homogeneous preparations of sodium channels from rat brain (Tamkun et al., 1984). Purified sodium channels in Triton X-100 solution are supplemented with phosphatidylcholine dispersed in Triton X-100, and the detergent is removed by adsorbtion to polystyrene beads. As the detergent is removed, phosphatidylcholine vesicles with a mean diameter of 1800 Å are formed, containing an average of 0.75–2 sodium channels per vesicle. The functional activities of the sodium channel can then be assessed in neurotoxin binding and ion flux experiments.

Figure 2 illustrates the time course of sodium-22 influx into phosphatidylcholine vesicles containing purified sodium channels. In these experiments, the vesicle

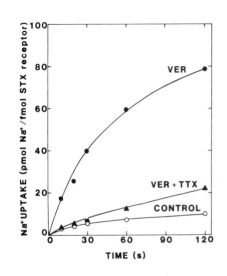

Figure 2. *Neurotoxin-activated sodium-22 influx mediated by purified and reconstituted sodium channels.* Sodium channels were purified, as described by Hartshorne and Catterall (1984), and incorporated into phosphatidylcholine vesicles, as described by Tamkun et al. (1984). The rate of sodium-22 influx was measured for the indicated times in the presence of no additions (*open circles*), 100 μM veratridine (*filled circles*), or 100 μM veratridine plus 1 μM tetrodotoxin (*filled triangles*) added to both sides of the membrane.

preparation was incubated for 2 min with veratridine to activate sodium channels and then diluted into medium containing sodium-22 to initiate influx into the vesicles. Influx into the vesicles under control conditions is slow. Incubation with veratridine increases the initial rate of influx 10- to 15-fold. When tetrodotoxin is present in both the intravesicular and extravesicular phases, the veratridine-dependent increase in the initial rate of sodium-22 influx is nearly completely blocked. Half-maximal activation is observed with 29 μM veratridine and half-maximal inhibition with 14 nM tetrodotoxin, in close agreement with the corresponding values for the action of these toxins on native sodium channels. These results show that the purified sodium channel regains the ability to mediate neurotoxin-stimulated ion flux after incorporation into phosphatidylcholine vesicles. Evidently, the purified channel retains neurotoxin receptor site 2 and the ion-conducting pore of the sodium channel.

Ion transport by neurotoxin-activated sodium channels in neural membranes is selective, although the rate of transport of large cations such as rubidium and cesium relative to the rate of transport of sodium is significantly greater than when channels are activated by membrane depolarization. The ion selectivity of the purified and reconstituted sodium channels has been determined by measuring the initial rate of influx of various radiolabeled cations through channels activated by veratridine or batrachotoxin (Tanaka et al., 1983; Tamkun et al., 1984). The purified and reconstituted sodium channels from mammalian brain and skeletal muscle retain ion selectivity with permeability ratios relative to sodium that compare favorably to those of native sodium channels activated by neurotoxins, as summarized in Table 3.

The results of Figure 2 show that at least a fraction of the sodium channels in the most highly purified preparations from rat brain can mediate selective neurotoxin-activated ion transport after incorporation into phospholipid vesicles. We have taken two approaches to estimate how many of the reconstituted sodium channels contribute to our ion flux measurements. First, we have compared the ion transport rates measured in purified and reconstituted sodium channel preparations to those measured for veratridine-activated sodium channels in neuroblastoma cells and synaptosomes. This comparison shows that the transport rate, measured in ions/min/saxitoxin receptor site, is 33–70% of that in native membranes, suggesting that at least 33–70% of the reconstituted sodium channels are active. In a second approach, we have compared the fraction of vesicles that

Table 3. Ion Selectivity of Native or Purified and Reconstituted Sodium Channels Activated by Neurotoxins

| | Permeability Ratios | | | |
| | Native Sodium Channels | | Purified Sodium Channels | |
Ion	Neuroblastoma	Node of Ranvier	Brain	Skeletal Muscle
Sodium	1.0	1.0	1.0	1.0
Potassium	0.17	0.45	—	0.15
Rubidium	0.08	0.27	0.25	0.02
Cesium	0.04	0.15	0.12	0.01

contain sodium channels to the fraction of vesicles whose internal volume is accessible to veratridine-activated sodium channels. Assuming that sodium channels are distributed among vesicles according to a Poisson distribution, this comparison leads to a range of 30–70% for the fraction of active channels, depending upon whether active vesicles containing more than one channel are assumed to have one active channel or all active channels. Both of these estimates indicate that a minimum of 30% of the reconstituted sodium channels are active. Since the sodium channel preparation from rat brain is 90% pure, and no single contaminant makes up as much as 2% of the protein, we conclude that the purified complex of the α-, β1-, and β2-subunits is sufficient to mediate selective neurotoxin-activated ion flux.

While sodium channels reconstituted into phosphatidylcholine vesicles can transport sodium, these channels do not bind α-scorpion toxin at neurotoxin receptor site 3. In contrast, if purified sodium channels from rat brain are incorporated into vesicles composed of a mixture of phosphatidylcholine and brain lipids, scorpion toxin binding is recovered. The toxin binding reaction is of high affinity (K_D = 43 nM), and a mean of 0.76 ± 0.08 mol of scorpion toxin is bound per mole of purified sodium channel (Tamkun et al., 1984). The brain lipid fraction was prepared through the use of $CHCl_3/CH_3OH$ extraction followed by silicic acid chromatography and was found to be protein-free by gel electrophoresis and sensitive silver staining. Therefore, we conclude that brain lipids are essential to restore the scorpion toxin receptor site to the same functional state as in native membranes. Since the affinity for scorpion toxin binding to synaptosomal sodium channels is dependent upon the functional state of the sodium channel, as reflected in the voltage dependence of toxin binding and its allosteric modulation by alkaloid toxins such as veratridine (Catterall, 1980), components of the brain lipid mixture may also be required for other functional activities of the channel.

The phospholipid components of the brain lipid mixture that are required for efficient restoration of scorpion toxin binding have been determined by the reconstitution of sodium channels in defined lipid mixtures. Addition of either phosphatidylethanolamine or phosphatidylserine from brain to the reconstitution mixture as 35–60% of the lipid mass restores high-affinity scorpion toxin binding as efficiently as the rat brain lipid mixture (Table 4). Other brain lipid components do not have a marked effect. Evidently, an appropriate mixture of brain phospholipids is necessary to restore the normal function of neurotoxin receptor site 3 on the sodium channel.

The results of these reconstitution experiments show that the purified sodium channel preparation from rat brain consisting of a stoichiometric complex of α-, β1-, and β2-subunits is sufficient to mediate most of the functions of the sodium channel that can be measured via biochemical methods. These include neurotoxin binding and action at neurotoxin receptor sites 1 through 3 and selective neurotoxin-activated ion flux. However, in excitable membranes, sodium channels are normally activated and inactivated by changes in membrane potential. In order to examine this aspect of the function of purified and reconstituted sodium channels, it is necessary to record their activity electrically on the millisecond time scale. As a first step in that direction, we have employed the methods of Montal (1974) and Krueger et al. (1983) to fuse reconstituted phospholipid vesicles to preformed planar phospholipid bilayers in a bath equipped for voltage clamp recording.

**Table 4.   Effect of Vesicle Phospholipid Composition
on Recovery of Scorpion Toxin Binding**

Phospholipid[a]	Ratio (%)	Scorpion Toxin Binding (fmol)
PC/BL	40/60	1.10
PC	100	0.24
PC/PE	65/35	1.25
PC/PS	65/35	0.71
PC/PE/PS	50/35/15	1.20

[a] PC, phosphatidylcholine; BL, brain lipid; PE, phosphatidylethanolamine; PS, phosphatidylserine.

Treatment of the bilayers with batrachotoxin causes the appearance of single
channel events of the type illustrated in Figure 3. These channels are characterized
by a single channel conductance of 23 pS at 20°C in 0.5 M sodium chloride
(Hartshorne et al., 1985), in close agreement with values for native sodium
channels activated by batrachotoxin (Krueger et al., 1983). The channels are
reproducibly blocked by tetrodotoxin, with a K_I of 10 nM at -60 mV. The fraction
of time an individual channel spends in the open state is strongly voltage-
dependent, between -130 mV and -60 mV, with a 50% open probability at
-98 mV (Hartshorne et al., 1985). These values are also in close agreement with
those for batrachotoxin-activated native sodium channels (Krueger et al., 1983).
Evidently, the purified and reconstituted sodium channel retains the high ionic

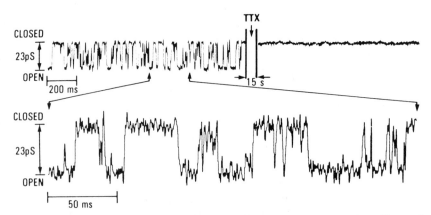

Figure 3. *Conductance mediated by single batrachotoxin-activated sodium channels in planar bilayers.* Sodium
channels were purified, as described by Hartshorne and Catterall (1984), and incorporated into
phospholipid vesicles composed of 65% phosphatidylethanolamine and 35% phosphatidylcholine,
as described by Feller et al. (1985). The reconstituted vesicles were placed in the *cis* compartment
of the planar bilayer chamber (Montal, 1974) and were allowed to fuse to the planar bilayer at
22°C (Krueger et al., 1983; Hartshorne et al., 1984). Batrachotoxin was added to the *trans* chamber
to activate the sodium channels. No activity was observed without toxin treatment, as is expected
for native sodium channels. Addition of tetrodotoxin (final concentration, 3 μM) to the *cis*
chamber rapidly blocked the observed single channel currents.

conductance and voltage sensitivity of native sodium channels. Recording of voltage-activated sodium currents requires more rapid time response than is possible with the present recording apparatus. Experiments are in progress to assess this final aspect of sodium channel function.

VOLTAGE-SENSITIVE CALCIUM CHANNELS

Voltage-sensitive calcium channels in brain produce action potentials in dendrites (Schwartzkroin and Slawsky, 1977; Llinás et al., 1981) and couple changes in membrane potential at the nerve terminals to the release of neurotransmitter (Katz and Miledi, 1969; Blaustein, 1975). In muscle tissue, they mediate calcium influx during cellular depolarization and play an important role in excitation–contraction coupling (for reviews, see Reuter, 1979; Hagiwara and Byerly, 1981) Calcium channels are nonconducting at the resting membrane potential. They are activated by membrane depolarization, with a half-maximal probability of activation at -20 to $+10$ mV in various tissues (for a review, see Tsien, 1983). Calcium channels in some tissues are slowly inactivated upon prolonged membrane depolarization, whereas in others inactivation is partial or absent. Inactivation results from a decrease in the probability of channel activation. Two different mechanisms have been described: inactivation produced by membrane depolarization per se, and inactivation because of increased intracellular calcium concentration (for a review, see Tsien, 1983). Calcium channels in secretory cells and skeletal muscle seem not to inactivate significantly, while those in cardiac muscle exhibit both voltage- and calcium-dependent inactivation mechanisms.

Under physiological conditions, calcium channels are highly selective, yet transport up to 3×10^6 ions/sec (Tsien, 1983). Calcium and barium are efficiently transported, while other divalent cations are poor permeants and block calcium and barium conductance (Hagiwara and Byerly, 1981). Surprisingly, in the absence of calcium ions, calcium channels are much less selective and will transport a variety of monovalent cations effectively (Almers and McCleskey, 1984; Almers et al., 1984; Hess and Tsien, 1984). Thus, calcium regulates channel selectivity. A model involving two high-affinity calcium binding sites within the ion-conducting pore, located close enough for strong intersite repulsive interactions, accommodates these findings. When neither site is occupied by calcium, monovalent cations are bound weakly and transported. When one site is occupied by calcium, the channel is blocked. When both sites are occupied, transport of calcium is efficient and selective, and monovalent cations are excluded.

The functional properties of calcium channels are being rapidly elucidated by electrophysiological methods. Although study of the molecular properties of this physiologically important ion channel is of interest, only recently have high-affinity chemical probes for the calcium channel become available.

Organic Calcium Antagonists as Probes of Calcium Channel Structure and Function

Calcium channels are inhibited by three different classes of organic antagonists: the dihydropyridines, including nifedipine and nitrendipine; the phenylalkylamines and diphenylalkylamines, including verapamil; and the thiobenzazepine, diltiazem (Triggle, 1982). ^{3}H-labeled derivatives of nitrendipine and other dihydropyridines have been prepared, and their binding to high-affinity receptor sites in homogenates and membrane preparations from excitable tissues has been examined extensively (Janis and Scriabine, 1983). A single class of high-affinity binding sites is observed with a K_D for nitrendipine in the range of 0.1–1.0 nM. The structure–activity relationships for occupancy of these high-affinity binding sites correlate closely with the concentrations of various dihydropyridines required to block contraction of smooth muscle over a wide range of dissociation constants (Bolger et al., 1982). Similar structure–activity relationships are observed in other tissues, but the absolute concentration required to block calcium currents is often substantially greater than that required to occupy the high-affinity nitrendipine binding sites (Almers et al., 1981; Lee and Tsien, 1983). This apparent discrepancy has now been resolved by the finding that dihydropyridine binding and block of calcium channels is highly voltage-sensitive (Bean, 1984). In cardiac cells, a half-maximal block of calcium currents at the resting membrane potential requires 700 nM nitrendipine. In contrast, when cells are electrically depolarized to inactivate 70% of the calcium current, only 0.8 nM nitrendipine is required for a half-maximal block. This value is in close agreement with K_D values for high-affinity binding sites in cardiac membrane preparations, which are depolarized by tissue homogenization and cell disruption (Janis and Scriabine, 1983). These results resolve an important discrepancy between previous biochemical and physiological measurements and provide additional strong support for the view that measurements of specific binding of nitrendipine and other dihydropyridines represent drug interactions with calcium channels or a closely associated regulatory component.

The binding of nitrendipine to its receptor site is modulated via an allosteric mechanism by diltiazem and by various mono- and diphenylalkylamines such as verapamil, which interact with a separate receptor site (Murphy et al., 1983). Verapamil decreases nitrendipine binding and enhances the rate of dissociation of the nitrendipine–receptor complex, whereas diltiazem increases binding and slows the rate of dissociation of the nitrendipine-receptor complex. Thus, the calcium antagonist receptor of the calcium channel contains at least two drug binding sites, one specific for dihydropyridines and one specific for diltiazem and phenylalkylamines, which interact allosterically in modulating calcium channel function.

The development of the calcium antagonists has been important in the treatment of atrial hypertension, arrhythmia, and angina. It has allowed a clearer definition of the role of calcium channels in various physiological pathways. In addition, the development of radioactively labeled derivatives of high affinity and specificity now allows the use of these drugs as probes to identify and isolate the protein components of calcium channels and understand their molecular properties.

Molecular Size of the Calcium Antagonist Receptor of the Calcium Channel

The first estimates of the molecular size of the component(s) of the calcium channel that bind dihydropyridines have been derived from radiation inactivation measurements. Estimates of the target size for the inactivation of ^{3}H]nitrendipine binding to receptor sites are 180 kD or 210 kD for skeletal muscle (Ferry et al., 1983a; Norman et al., 1983a), 210 kD for brain (Norman et al., 1983a), and 280 kD for guinea pig ileum (Venter et al., 1983). The apparent molecular weight derived from radiation inactivation studies depends upon the radiolabeled calcium antagonist used in the receptor binding assay and on the assay and irradiation conditions, suggesting that the calcium antagonist receptor is a complex oligomeric structure (Ferry et al., 1983b).

Identification of Protein Components of the Calcium Antagonist Receptor by Covalent Labeling

The dihydropyridines are amenable to structural modification at several positions and therefore are potentially valuable tools for affinity chromatography and covalent labeling. An isothiocyanate analogue of nitrendipine covalently labels a protease-sensitive polypeptide with an apparent molecular weight of 45 kD in guinea pig ileum membrane preparations (Venter et al., 1983). Nitrendipine itself is photolabile and can be covalently incorporated into a polypeptide with an apparent molecular weight of 32 kD in cardiac sarcolemma by high-intensity irradiation (Campbell et al., 1984). A photoreactive azidobenzoyl analogue of nitrendipine has been prepared by Ferry et al. (1984). This compound labels a polypeptide with an apparent molecular weight of 145 kD in skeletal muscle transverse tubule membranes. In each case, the covalent labeling reactions described were prevented by incubation with excess, unlabeled calcium antagonist, suggesting that the polypeptides labeled are components of the calcium antagonist receptor in these different tissues. Either the calcium antagonist receptor from these different tissues has different polypeptide components or, as argued below, the receptor is an oligomer of subunits of different molecular weight that are differentially labeled by the probes used.

Characterization of the Detergent-Solubilized Calcium Anatagonist Receptor

Since it is likely to be an intrinsic membrane protein, the first essential step in the purification and biochemical characterization of the calcium antagonist receptor is solubilization from an appropriate membrane source and characterization of the solubilized protein. After a survey of several detergents, we concluded that digitonin is the most effective detergent for solubilization of a specific [^{3}H]nitrendipine–receptor complex from brain and skeletal muscle transverse tubule membranes (Curtis and Catterall, 1983, 1984). Up to 40% of the receptor–ligand complex is solubilized. The dissociation of bound [^{3}H]nitrendipine from the complex is accelerated by verapamil and slowed by diltiazem through allosteric interactions between the nitrendipine binding site and the binding site for those ligands, as observed in intact membranes. These results provide further support for the conclusion that a specific [^{3}H]nitrendipine–receptor complex has been solubilized under conditions that allow retention of the functional allosteric regulation of dihydropyridine binding.

Sedimentation of the solubilized [^{3}H]nitrendipine–receptor–digitonin complex in sucrose gradients gives a single peak of specifically bound nitrendipine with a sedimentation coefficient of 19–20 S (Curtis and Catterall, 1983). Comparison

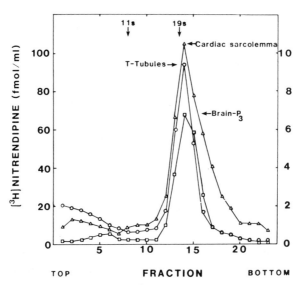

Figure 4. *Analysis of the size of the solubilized [³H]nitrendipine–calcium antagonist receptor complex by sucrose gradient sedimentation.* Crude synaptosomal membranes (*squares*), skeletal muscle transverse tubule membranes (*circles*), and cardiac sarcolemmal membranes (*triangles*) were prepared, as described previously (Rosemblatt et al., 1981; Curtis and Catterall, 1983; Flockerzi et al., 1983). The membranes were incubated for 90 min at 37°C with [³H]nitrendipine to form a specific [³H]nitrendipine–calcium antagonist receptor complex. The complex was then solubilized in the presence of 1% digitonin, undissolved membranes were removed by sedimentation at 175,000 × g for 30 min, and the supernatant was layered over a linear 5–20% sucrose gradient in 5 mM MOPS (pH 7.4), 1 mM calcium chloride, 100 mM diltiazem, and protease inhibitors. The samples were sedimented for 1.5 hours at 210,000 × g, fractions were collected, and specifically bound [³H]nitrendipine was measured by precipitation with polyethyleneglycol, as described previously (Curtis and Catterall, 1983). Values for transverse tubule membranes are shown on the *left ordinate* and for brain and cardiac membranes on the *right ordinate*.

of the sedimentation behavior of the solubilized complex from brain, heart, and skeletal muscle indicates that they have identical sizes (Figure 4). These results provide support for the view that the calcium antagonist receptor in different tissues is quite similar.

Many plasma membrane proteins are glycosylated during their synthesis and transport to the cell surface. The solubilized calcium antagonist receptor from brain or skeletal muscles is specifically adsorbed to, and eluted from, affinity columns with immobilized wheat germ agglutinin or other lectins (Curtis and Catterall, 1983, 1984; Glossmann and Ferry, 1983). Evidently, one or more of the subunits of the calcium antagonist receptor are glycoproteins.

Skeletal Muscle Transverse Tubules as a Model System for Examination of the Biochemical Properties of Calcium Channels

Skeletal muscle fibers have substantial voltage-activated calcium currents that have been measured under voltage clamp conditions (Sanchez and Stefani, 1978). These currents originate almost entirely in the transverse tubular system and are blocked by dihydropyridine calcium antagonists (Almers et al., 1981). They have been presumed to play a role in excitation–contraction coupling, although direct evidence for such a role has not been obtained. Transverse (T) tubule membranes can be extensively purified from skeletal muscle by a combination of differential and density gradient centrifugation (Rosemblatt et al., 1981). Antibodies prepared against the most highly purified fractions of T-tubule membranes stain only T-tubules, and not the sarcolemma or sarcoplasmic reticulum of intact muscle, indicating a high degree of purity of this preparation (Rosemblatt et al., 1981). Analysis of [^{3}H]nitrendipine binding to membrane fractions from skeletal muscle reveals a specific localization of the calcium antagonist receptor in the T-tubule fraction (Fosset et al., 1983; Glossmann et al., 1983). These membranes contain a 10-fold greater concentration of calcium antagonist receptor (10–50 pmol/mg) than any other membrane preparation described to date (Janis and Scriabine, 1983). Since T-tubule membranes are the most enriched source of calcium antagonist receptors and have a substantial voltage-activated calcium current that is blocked by dihydropyridines, they provide a favorable experimental preparation for examination of the molecular properties of the calcium antagonist receptor and its relationship to voltage-sensitive calcium channels. It is anticipated that the T-tubule calcium channel will resemble those of other tissues that are blocked by dihydropyridines, and that therefore information on the molecular properties of this calcium channel will give insight into others.

Purification and Characterization of the Calcium Antagonist Receptor from Skeletal Muscle Transverse Tubules

If the calcium antagonist has a molecular weight of 210 kD (Norman et al., 1983a) and has one dihydropyridine binding site per mole, the pure protein would have a specific binding capacity of 4760 pmol/mg. The specific binding capacity of purified T-tubule membranes is 10–50 pmol/mg (Fosset et al., 1983; Glossman et al., 1983; Curtis and Catterall, 1984). Thus, only 100- to 500-fold purification is required to achieve a homogeneous preparation. This degree of purification can usually be obtained by conventional procedures.

We have purified the calcium antagonist receptor solubilized from T-tubule membranes by digitonin 330-fold by affinity chromatography on wheat germ agglutinin–Sepharose, ion exchange chromatography on DEAE-Sephadex, and velocity sedimentation through sucrose gradients (Curtis and Catterall, 1984). The purified preparation contained 1950 pmol of calcium antagonist receptor per milligram of protein, implying a purity of at least 42%. Analysis of the purified preparation by polyacrylamide gel electrophoresis after denaturation in SDS revealed three major protein bands, as illustrated in Figure 5. Their molecular weights are: α, 135 kD; β, 50 kD; and γ, 33 kD. All three of these polypeptides quantitatively comigrate with the [^{3}H]nitrendipine–receptor complex during velocity sedimentation in sucrose gradients (Curtis and Catterall, 1984) and therefore are likely to be subunits of the calcium antagonist receptor. The concentration of the β-subunit varies among preparations. This seems to result from both dissociation of the β-subunit and high protease sensitivity.

It is of interest to compare the apparent molecular weights of the subunits of the purified calcium antagonist receptor from T-tubules with those of the polypeptides covalently labeled by dihydropyridine derivatives. The polypeptide

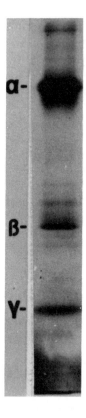

Figure 5. *Subunit composition of the calcium antagonist receptor.* The calcium antagonist receptor was solubilized and purified from skeletal muscle transverse tubule membranes, as described previously (Curtis and Catterall, 1984). The peak fraction from the final sucrose gradient was denatured in SDS and β-mercaptoethanol and analyzed by polyacrylamide gel electrophoresis. The migration positions of the α- (135 kD), β- (50 kD), and γ- (33 kD) subunits are indicated.

with an apparent molecular weight of 145 kD labeled by azidopine (Ferry et al., 1984) is similar in size to the α-subunit of the purified preparation. The polypeptide with an apparent molecular weight of 32 kD covalently labeled by nitrendipine itself (Campbell et al., 1984) is the same size as the γ-subunit of the purified preparation. The polypeptide with an apparent molecular weight of 45 kD covalently labeled with the isothiocyanate derivative of nitrendipine is somewhat smaller than the β-subunit of the purified preparation, but their protease sensitivity suggests that they may be related. Thus, the disparate results of covalent labeling experiments in different tissues may be reconciled by the hypothesis that the dihydropyridine binding site of the calcium antagonist receptor is located near the contact regions of the α-, β-, and γ-subunits, such that different dihydropyridine ligands preferentially label different subunits. These results provide further evidence that these subunits are components of the calcium antagonist receptor in intact membranes.

PHOSPHORYLATION OF SODIUM AND CALCIUM CHANNELS

The classic work of Reuter and his colleagues (Reuter, 1974, 1983) established that the positive inotropic effect of epinephrine and norepinephrine on the heart is mediated by a cAMP-dependent increase in inward calcium current. This effect is due to an increase in the number of calcium channels that are active during the cardiac action potential (Cachelin et al., 1983; Tsien et al., 1983). These effects are mimicked by intracellular injection of the catalytic subunit of cAMP-dependent protein kinase, suggesting that protein phosphorylation mediates the effects of cAMP (Brum et al., 1983). It is uncertain whether the substrate for cAMP-dependent phosphorylation is the calcium channel itself or another regulatory component. In addition to these studies on mammalian heart, calcium channels in mammalian dorsal root ganglion neurons, and both calcium channels and calcium-activated potassium ion channels in molluscan neurons, are regulated by cAMP-dependent protein phosphorylation. Thus, modulation of ion channel properties by cellular regulatory processes may be a widespread phenomenon.

Phosphorylation of the Sodium Channel *In Vitro* and *In Situ*

The availability of purified preparations of voltage-sensitive sodium and calcium channels makes possible the direct study of the phosphorylation of these ion channels by various protein kinases. This approach is complementary to the analysis of the physiological effects of cAMP and protein kinase injection, since it can define the substrates and sites for functionally significant phosphorylation. The first evidence for direct phosphorylation of a voltage-sensitive channel came from the work of Costa et al. (1982), who showed that the α-subunit of the purified sodium channel from rat brain is rapidly and specifically phosphorylated by cAMP-dependent protein kinase added *in vitro*. Up to three to four moles of phosphate were incorporated per mole of channel, and the rate of phosphorylation was comparable to that of the best substrates for this enzyme, suggesting that the α-subunit of the sodium channel is a physiological substrate for this protein kinase.

Antiserum against the sodium channel can be used to examine phosphorylation of the α-subunit in brain membrane fractions. Incubation of lysed synaptosomal plasma membranes with added catalytic subunit of cAMP-dependent protein kinase, followed by solubilization, immunoprecipitation, and analysis of phosphorylated proteins by polyacrylamide gel electrophoresis, reveals marked phosphorylation of the α-subunit of the sodium channel (Figure 6A, lane 1). Immunoprecipitation of this band is completely blocked by incubation of the antiserum with purified sodium channel, indicating that the labeled band is indeed the sodium channel (Figure 6A, lane 2). Phosphorylation of the sodium channel *in situ* in intact synaptosomes by the endogenous cAMP-dependent protein kinase was examined by a rephosphorylation method after activation of the protein kinase by 8-BrcAMP (Costa and Catterall, 1984a). Phosphorylation of the α-subunit *in situ* reached 80% of maximum within 15 sec of the addition of 8-BrcAMP (Figure 7). Four of the tryptic peptides phosphorylated *in vitro* were also phosphorylated *in situ*. This rapid rate of *in situ* phosphorylation confirms that the α-subunit of the sodium channel is modified by phosphorylation–dephosphorylation *in situ*.

Several protein kinases have been described in mammalian brain. Among these, the calcium- and phospholipid-dependent protein kinase, protein kinase C, is present in brain at higher concentrations than in other tissues (Kikkawa et al., 1982). Incubation of lysed synaptosomal membranes with protein kinase C also results in specific phosphorylation of the α-subunit of the sodium channel,

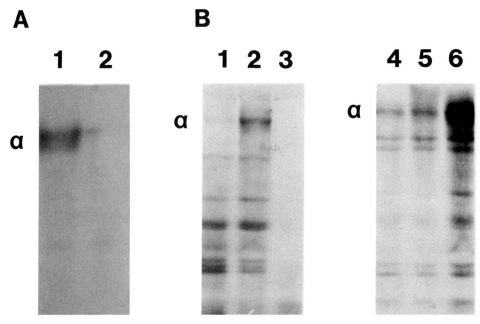

Figure 6. *Specific phosphorylation of the α-subunit of the sodium channel in synaptosomal membranes by cAMP-dependent protein kinase and protein kinase C. A:* Synaptosomes were prepared, lysed, and reacted with [^{32}P]ATP and the catalytic subunit of cAMP-dependent protein kinase (Costa and Catterall, 1984a). *Lane 1:* The labeled membranes were solubilized, and sodium channels were isolated by specific immunoprecipitation. *Lane 2:* Antiserum blocked with 700 fmol of pure sodium channel was used for immunoprecipitation. *B:* A similar experiment was carried out with protein kinase C, as described previously (Costa and Catterall, 1984b). *Lane 1:* Immunoprecipitation with blocked antiserum. *Lane 2:* Immunoprecipitation with specific antiserum. *Lane 3:* Preimmune serum. *Lane 4:* Calcium-free medium. *Lane 5:* Calcium-free medium plus phosphatidylserine and phosphatidylethanolamine. *Lane 6:* 10 μM calcium chloride.

as detected by immunoprecipitation and gel electrophoresis (Figure 6B). Phosphorylation is dependent upon added calcium (Costa and Catterall, 1984b). Both common and unique tryptic peptides were phosphorylated in comparison with the cAMP-dependent protein kinase. Evidently, multiple regulatory pathways of protein phosphorylation converge on the α-subunit of the sodium channel as a substrate.

Sodium channel function has not yet been clearly shown to be modulated by altering intracellular cAMP or calcium concentrations, although some suggestive results have been described. Windisch and Tritthart (1982) found that isoproterenol, norepinephrine, and phosphodiesterase inhibitors increased inactivation of sodium channels in ventricular muscle fibers. Ribeiro and Sebastião (1984) report that dibutyryl cAMP enhances conduction block in sciatic nerve. We found that phosphorylation of sodium channels in synaptosomes is accompanied by a reduction in neurotoxin-activated sodium-22 influx mediated by the sodium channel (Costa and Catterall, 1984a). Thus, while cAMP and protein phosphorylation do not have as marked effects on sodium channel function as have been reported

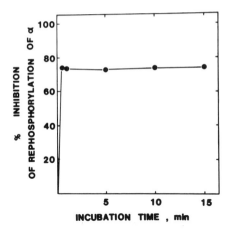

Figure 7. *Time course of phosphorylation of the α-subunit of the sodium channel by endogenous cAMP-dependent protein kinase in synaptosomes.* Intact synaptosomes were incubated with 8-BrcAMP for the indicated times at 36°C. The incubation was terminated by boiling in the presence of SDS. The level of endogenous phosphorylation of the α-subunit of the sodium channel was then measured by rephosphorylation, immunoprecipitation, and polyacrylamide gel electrophoresis in SDS, as described previously (Costa and Catterall, 1984a).

for calcium and calcium-activated potassium ion channels, subtle effects on physiological properties may be revealed by more detailed investigations.

Phosphorylation of the Calcium Channel

The purified calcium antagonist receptor of the voltage-sensitive calcium channel is also a good substrate for cAMP-dependent protein kinase (Curtis and Catterall, 1985). Both the α- and β-subunits are phosphorylated, whereas the γ-subunit is not. Analysis of the phosphorylation of the proteins in T-tubule membranes indicates that the β-subunit is also a preferred substrate *in situ*, while phosphorylation of the α-subunit becomes less prominent (Curtis and Catterall, 1985). Therefore, phosphorylation of the β-subunit by cAMP-dependent protein kinase is a likely mechanism for the mediation of the action of norepinephrine and cAMP on the calcium channel and ultimately on the regulation of calcium-dependent electrical excitability and contractility in the heart and other tissues.

CONCLUSION

The voltage-sensitive ion channels are critical components of the nervous system that are intimately involved in information processing and signal transduction within and between neurons. Molecular analysis of the properties of this unique class of membrane proteins has come of age in the past few years with the development of patch voltage clamp methods for the measurement of single ion channel currents and of biochemical methods for the purification and structural and functional analysis of the protein components of ion channels. The studies reviewed in this chapter have provided the first identification and purification of the protein components of voltage-sensitive ion channels, an analysis of the functional properties of the purified components, and a delineation of the possible sites of long-term modulation by protein phosphorylation. There is little doubt that these approaches will continue to yield valuable information concerning the molecular basis of electrical excitability and its role in information processing in the nervous system.

REFERENCES

Agnew, W. S., S. R. Levinson, J. S. Brabson, and M. A. Raftery (1978) Purification of the tetrodotoxin-binding component associated with the voltage-sensitive sodium channel from *Electrophorus electricus* electroplax membranes. *Proc. Natl. Acad. Sci. USA* **75**:2606–2610.

Agnew, W. S., A. C. Moore, S. R. Levinson, and M. A. Raftery (1980) Identification of a large molecular weight peptide associated with a tetrodotoxin binding protein from the electroplax of *Electrophorus electricus. Biochem. Biophys. Res. Commun.* **92**:860–866.

Albuquerque, E. X., and J. W. Daly (1976) Batrachotoxin, a selective probe for channels modulating sodium conductances in electrogenic membranes. In *The Specificity and Action of Animal, Bacterial and Plant Toxins* (*Receptors and Recognition*, Series B, Volume 1), P. Cuatrecasas, ed., pp. 299–338, Chapman and Hall, London.

Aldrich, R. W., D. P. Corey, and C. F. Stevens (1983) A reinterpretation of mammalian sodium channel gating based on single channel recording. *Nature* **306**:436–441.

Almers, W., and E. W. McCleskey (1984) Non-selective conductance in calcium channels of frog muscle: Calcium-selectivity in a single file pore. *J. Physiol. (Lond.)* **353**:585–608.

Almers, W., R. Fink, and P. T. Palade (1981) Calcium depletion in frog muscle tubules: The decline of calcium current under maintained depolarization. *J. Physiol. (Lond.)* **312**:177–207.

Almers, W., E. W. McCleskey, and P. T. Palade (1984) A non-selective cation conductance in frog-muscle membrane blocked by micromolar external calcium-ions. *J. Physiol. (Lond.)* **353**:565–583.

Armstrong, C. M., and F. Bezanilla (1974) Charge movement associated with the opening and closing of the activation gates of the Na channels. *J. Gen. Physiol.* **63**:533–552.

Armstrong, C. M., and F. Bezanilla (1977) Inactivation of the sodium channel. II. Gating current experiments. *J. Gen. Physiol.* **70**:567–590.

Barchi, R. L. (1983) Protein components of the purified sodium channel from rat skeletal muscle sarcolemma. *J. Neurochem.* **40**:1377–1385.

Barchi, R. L., S. A. Cohen, and L. E. Murphy (1980) Purification from rat sarcolemma of the saxitoxin-binding component of the excitable membrane sodium channel. *Proc. Natl. Acad. Sci. USA* **77**:1306–1310.

Barhanin, J., J. R. Giglio, P. Leopold, A. Schmid, S. V. Sampaio, and M. Lazdunski (1982) *Tityus serrulatus* venom contains two classes of toxins. *J. Biol. Chem.* **257**:12553–12558.

Barhanin, J., A. Schmid, A. Lombet, K. P. Wheeler, M. Lazdunski, and J. C. Ellory (1983) Molecular size of different neurotoxin receptors on the voltage-sensitive Na$^+$ channel. *J. Biol. Chem.* **258**:700–702.

Bean, B. P. (1984) Nitrendipine block of cardiac calcium channels: High-affinity binding to the inactivated state. *Proc. Natl. Acad. Sci. USA* **81**:6388–6392.

Beneski, A. A., and W. A. Catterall (1980) Covalent labeling of protein components of the sodium channel with a photoactivable derivative of scorpion toxin. *Proc. Natl. Acad. Sci. USA* **77**:639–643.

Benzer, T. I., and M. A. Raftery (1973) Solubilization and partial characterization of the tetrodotoxin binding component from nerve axons. *Biochem. Biophys. Res. Commun.* **51**:939–944.

Blaustein, M. P. (1975) Effects of potassium, veratridine and scorpion venom on calcium accumulation and transmitter release by nerve terminals *in vitro. J. Physiol. (Lond.)* **247**:617–655.

Bolger, G. T., P. J. Gengo, E. M. Luchowski, H. Siegel, D. J. Triggle, and R. A. Janis (1982) High affinity binding of a calcium channel antagonist to smooth and cardiac muscle. *Biochem. Biophys. Res. Commun.* **104**:1604–1609.

Brum, G., V. Flockerzi, F. Hofmann, W. Osterrieder, and W. Trautwein (1983) Injection of catalytic subunit of cAMP-dependent protein kinase into isolated cardiac myocytes. *Pflügers Arch.* **398**:147–154.

Cachelin, A. B., J. E. de Peyer, S. Kokubun, and H. Reuter (1983) Ca^{2+} channel modulation by 8-bromocyclic AMP in cultured heart cells. *Nature* **304**:462–464.

Cahalan, M. D. (1975) Modification of sodium channel gating in frog myelinated nerve fibres by *Centruroides sculpturatus* scorpion venom. *J. Physiol. (Lond.)* **244**:511–534.

Campbell, K. P., G. M. Lipschutz, and G. H. Denney (1984) Direct photoaffinity labeling of the high affinity nitrendipine-binding site in subcellular membrane fractions isolated from canine myocardium. *J. Biol. Chem.* **259**:5384–5387.

Catterall, W. A. (1980) Neurotoxins that act on voltage-sensitive sodium channels in excitable membranes. *Annu. Rev. Pharmacol. Toxicol.* **20**:15–43.

Catterall, W. A., C. S. Morrow, and R. P. Hartshorne (1979) Neurotoxin binding to receptor sites associated with voltage-sensitive sodium channels in intact, lysed, and detergent-solubilized brain membranes. *J. Biol. Chem.* **254**:11379–11387.

Catterall, W. A., C. S. Morrow, J. W. Daly, and G. B. Brown (1981) Binding of batrachotoxinin A 20-α-benzoate to a receptor site associated with sodium channels in synaptic nerve ending particles. *J. Biol. Chem.* **256**:8922–8927.

Costa, M. R. C., and W. A. Catterall (1984a) Cyclic AMP-dependent phosphorylation of the α subunit of the sodium channel in synaptic nerve ending particles. *J. Biol. Chem.* **259**:8210–8218.

Costa, M. R. C., and W. A. Catterall (1984b) Phosphorylation of the α subunit of the sodium channel by protein kinase-C. *Cell Mol. Neurobiol.* **4**:291–297.

Costa, M. R. C., J. E. Casnellie, and W. A. Catterall (1982) Selective phosphorylation of the α subunit of the sodium channel by cAMP-dependent protein kinase. *J. Biol. Chem.* **257**:7918–7921.

Couraud, F., E. Jover, J. M. Dubois, and H. Rochat (1982) Two types of scorpion toxin receptor sites, one related to the activation, the other to the inactivation, of the action potential sodium channel. *Toxicon* **20**:9–16.

Curtis, B. M., and W. A. Catterall (1983) Solubilization of the calcium antagonist receptor from rat brain. *J. Biol. Chem.* **258**:7280–7283.

Curtis, B. M., and W. A. Catterall (1984) Purification of the calcium antagonist receptor of the voltage-sensitive calcium channel from skeletal muscle transverse tubules. *Biochemistry* **23**:2113–2118.

Curtis, B. M., and W. A. Catterall (1985) Phosphorylation of the calcium antagonist receptor of the voltage-sensitive calcium channel by cAMP-dependent protein kinase. *Proc. Natl. Acad. Sci. USA* **82**:2528–2532.

Darbon, H., E. Jover, F. Couraud, and H. Rochat (1983) Photoaffinity labeling of α- and β-scorpion toxin receptors associated with rat brain sodium channel. *Biochem. Biophys. Res. Commun.* **115**:415–422.

Feller, D., J. Talvenheimo, and W. A. Catterall (1985) The sodium channel from rat brain: Reconstitution of voltage-dependent scorpion toxin binding in vesicles of defined lipid composition. *J. Biol. Chem.* **260**:1542–1547.

Ferry, D. R., A. Goll, and H. Glossmann (1983a) Putative calcium channel molecular weight determination by target size analysis. *Naunyn Schmiedebergs Arch. Pharmacol.* **323**:292–297.

Ferry, D. R., A. Goll, and H. Glossmann (1983b) Calcium channels: Evidence for oligomeric nature by target size analysis. *EMBO J.* **2**:1729–1732.

Ferry, D. R., M. Rombusch, A. Goll, and H. Glossmann (1984) Photoaffinity labelling of Ca^{2+} channels with [^{3}H]azidopine. *FEBS Lett.* **169**:112–167.

Flockerzi, U., R. Mewes, P. Ruth, and F. Hofmann (1983) Phosphorylation of purified bovine cardiac sarcolemma and potassium-stimulated calcium uptake. *Eur. J. Biochem.* **135**:131–142.

Fosset, M., E. Jaimovich, E. Delpont, and M. Lazdunski (1983) [³H]Nitrendipine receptors in skeletal muscle. *J. Biol. Chem.* **258**:6086–6092.

Glossmann, H., and D. R. Ferry (1983) Solubilization and partial purification of putative calcium channels labelled with [³H]-nimodipine. *Naunyn Schmiedebergs Arch. Pharmacol.* **323**:279–291.

Glossmann, H., D. R. Ferry, and C. B. Boschek (1983) Purification of the putative calcium channel from skeletal muscle with the aid of [³H]-nimodipine binding. *Naunyn Schmiedebergs Arch. Pharmacol.* **323**:1–11.

Hagiwara, S., and L. Byerly (1981) Calcium channel. *Annu. Rev. Neurosci.* **4**:69–125.

Hartshorne, R. P., and W. A. Catterall (1981) Purification of the saxitoxin receptor of the sodium channel from rat brain. *Proc. Natl. Acad. Sci. USA* **78**:2620–2624.

Hartshorne, R. P., and W. A. Catterall (1984) The sodium channel from rat brain. Purification and subunit composition. *J. Biol. Chem.* **259**:1667–1675.

Hartshorne, R. P., J. Coppersmith, and W. A. Catterall (1980) Size characteristics of the solubilized saxitoxin receptor of the voltage-sensitive sodium channel from rat brain. *J. Biol. Chem.* **255**:10572–10575.

Hartshorne, R. P., D. J. Messner, J. C. Coppersmith, and W. A. Catterall (1982) The saxitoxin receptor of the sodium channel from rat brain. Evidence for two nonidentical β subunits. *J. Biol. Chem.* **257**:13888–13891.

Hartshorne, R. P., B. U. Keller, J. A. Talvenheimo, W. A. Catterall, and M. Montal (1985) Functional reconstitution of the purified brain sodium channel in planar lipid bilayers. *Proc. Natl. Acad. Sci. USA* **82**:240–244.

Henderson, R., and J. H. Wang (1972) Solubilization of a specific tetrodotoxin-binding component from garfish olfactory nerve membrane. *Biochemistry* **11**:4565–4569.

Hess, P., and R. W. Tsien (1984) Mechanism of ion permeation through calcium channels. *Nature* **309**:453–456.

Hille, B. (1971) The permeability of the sodium channel to organic cations in myelinated nerve. *J. Gen. Physiol.* **58**:599–619.

Hille, B. (1972) The permeability of the sodium channel to metal cations in myelinated nerve. *J. Gen. Physiol.* **59**:637–658.

Hodgkin, A. L., and A. F. Huxley (1952) A quantitative description of membrane current and its application to conduction and excitation in nerve. *J. Physiol. (Lond.)* **117**:500–544.

Janis, R. A., and A. Scriabine (1983) Sites of action of Ca^{2+} channel inhibitors. *Biochem. Pharmacol.* **32**:3499–3507.

Jover, E., F. Couraud, and H. Rochat (1980) Two types of scorpion neurotoxins characterized by their binding to two separate receptor sites on rat brain synaptosomes. *Biochem. Biophys. Res. Commun.* **95**:1607–1614.

Katz, B., and R. Miledi (1969) Tetrodotoxin-resistant electric activity in presynaptic terminals. *J. Physiol. (Lond.)* **203**:459–487.

Kikkawa, U., Y. Takai, R. Minakuchi, S. Inohara, and Y. Nishizuka (1982) Calcium-activated, phospholipid-dependent protein kinase from rat brain. *J. Biol. Chem.* **257**:13341–13348.

Kraner, S. D., J. Tanaka, and R. L. Barchi (1985) Purification and functional reconstitution of the voltage-sensitive sodium channel from rabbit T-tubular membranes. *J. Cell Biol.* **260**:6341–6347.

Krueger, B. K., R. W. Ratzlaff, G. R. Strichartz, and M. P. Blaustein (1979) Saxitoxin binding to synaptosomes, membranes, and solubilized binding sites from rat brain. *J. Membr. Biol.* **50**:287–310.

Krueger, B. K., J. F. Worley, III, and R. J. French (1983) Single sodium channels from rat brain incorporated into planar bilayers. *Nature* **303**:172–175.

Lee, K. S., and R. W. Tsien (1983) Mechanism of calcium channel blockade by verapamil, D600, diltiazem and nitrendipine in single dialysed heart cells. *Nature* **302**:790–794.

Levinson, S. R., and J. C. Ellory (1973) Molecular size of the tetrodotoxin binding site estimated by irradiation inactivation. *Nature New Biol.* **245**:122–123.

Llinás, R., Y. Yarom, and M. Sugimori (1981) Isolated mammalian brain *in vitro*: New technique for analysis of electrical activity of neuronal circuit function. *Fed. Proc.* **40**:2240–2245.

Messner, D. J., and W. A. Catterall (1985) The sodium channel from rat brain: Separation and characterization of subunits. *J. Biol. Chem.* **260**:597–604.

Meves, H., N. Rubly, and D. D. Watt (1982) Effect of toxins isolated from the venom of the scorpion *Centruroides sculpturatus* on the Na currents of the node of Ranvier. *Pflügers Arch.* **393**:56–62.

Miller, J. A., W. S. Agnew, and S. R. Levinson (1983) Principal glycopeptide of the tetrodotoxin/ saxitoxin binding protein from *Electrophorus electricus*: Isolation and partial chemical and physical characterization. *Biochemistry* **22**:462–470.

Montal, M. (1974) Formation of bimolecular membranes from lipid monolayers. *Methods Enzymol.* **32**:545–554.

Murphy, K. M. M., R. J. Gould, B. L. Largent, and S. H. Snyder (1983) A unitary mechanism of calcium antagonist drug action. *Proc. Natl. Acad. Sci. USA* **80**:860–864.

Nakayama, H., R. M. Withy, and M. A. Raftery (1982) Use of a monoclonal antibody to purify the tetrodotoxin binding component from the electroplax of *Electrophorus electricus*. *Proc. Natl. Acad. Sci. USA* **79**:7575–7579.

Narahashi, T. (1974) Chemicals as tools in the study of excitable membranes. *Physiol. Rev.* **54**:813–889.

Norman, R. I., M. Borsotto, M. Fosset, M. Lazdunski, and J. C. Ellory (1983a) Determination of the molecular size of the nitrendipine-sensitive Ca^{2+} channel by radiation inactivation. *Biochem. Biophys. Res. Commun.* **111**:878–883.

Norman, R. I., A. Schmid, A. Lombet, J. Barhanin, and M. Lazdunski (1983b) Purification of binding protein for *Tityus* γ toxin identified with the gating component of the voltage-sensitive Na^{+} channel. *Proc. Natl. Acad. Sci. USA* **80**:4164–4168.

Reuter, H. (1974) Localization of beta adrenergic receptors, and effects of noradrenaline and cyclic nucleotides on action potentials, ionic currents and tension in mammalian cardiac muscle. *J. Physiol. (Lond.)* **242**:429–451.

Reuter, H. (1979) Properties of two inward membrane currents in the heart. *Annu. Rev. Physiol.* **41**:413–424.

Reuter, H. (1983) Calcium channel modulation by neurotransmitters, enzymes and drugs. *Nature* **301**:569–574.

Ribeiro, J. A., and A. M. Sebastião (1984) Enhancement of tetrodotoxin-induced axonal blockade by adenosine, adenosine analogues, dibutyryl cyclic AMP and methylxanthines in the frog sciatic nerve. *Br. J. Pharmacol.* **83**:485–492.

Ritchie, J. M., and R. B. Rogart (1977) The binding of saxitoxin and tetrodotoxin to excitable tissue. *Rev. Physiol. Biochem. Pharmacol.* **79**:1–49.

Rosemblatt, M., C. Hidalgo, C. Vergara, and N. Ikemoto (1981) Immunological and biochemical properties of transverse tubule membranes isolated from rabbit skeletal muscle. *J. Biol. Chem.* **256**:8140–8148.

Rosenberg, R. L., S. A. Tomiko, and W. S. Agnew (1984) Reconstitution of neurotoxin-modulated ion transport by the voltage-regulated sodium channel isolated from the electroplax of *Electrophorus electricus*. *Proc. Natl. Acad. Sci. USA* **81**:1239–1243.

Sanchez, J. A., and E. Stefani (1978) Inward calcium current in twitch muscle fibres of the frog. *J. Physiol. (Lond.)* **283**:197–209.

Schwartzkroin, P. A., and M. Slawsky (1977) Probable calcium spikes in hippocampal neurons. *Brain Res.* **135**:157–161.

Sharkey, R. G., D. A. Beneski, and W. A. Catterall (1984) Differential labeling of the α and β1 subunits of the sodium channel by photoreactive derivatives of scorpion toxin. *Biochemistry* **23**:6078–6086.

Talvenheimo, J. A., M. M. Tamkun, and W. A. Catterall (1982) Reconstitution of neurotoxin-stimulated sodium transport by the voltage-sensitive sodium channel purified from rat brain. *J. Biol. Chem.* **257**:11868–11871.

Tamkun, M. M., J. A. Talvenheimo, and W. A. Catterall (1984) The sodium channel from rat brain: Reconstitution of neurotoxin-activated ion flux and scorpion toxin binding from purified components. *J. Biol. Chem.* **259**:1676–1688.

Tanaka, J. C., J. F. Eccleston, and R. L. Barchi (1983) Cation selectivity characteristics of the reconstituted voltage-dependent sodium channel purified from rat skeletal muscle sarcolemma. *J. Biol. Chem.* **258**:7519–7526.

Triggle, D. J. (1982) Biochemical pharmacology of calcium blockers. In *Calcium Blockers: Mechanisms of Action and Clinical Applications*, S. F. Flaim and R. Zelis, eds., pp. 121–134, Urban and Schwarzenberg, Baltimore.

Tsien, R. W. (1983) Calcium channels in excitable cell membranes. *Annu. Rev. Physiol.* **45**:341–358.

Tsien, R. W., B. P. Bean, P. Hess, and M. Nowycky (1983) Calcium channels: Mechanisms of β-adrenergic modulation and ion permeation. *Cold Spring Harbor Symp. Quant. Biol.* **48**:201–212.

Venter, J. C., C. M. Fraser, J. S. Schaber, C. Y. Jung, G. Bolger, and D. J. Triggle (1983) Molecular properties of the slow inward calcium channel. *J. Biol. Chem.* **258**:9344–9348.

Wang, G. K., and G. Strichartz (1982) Simultaneous modifications of sodium channel gating by two scorpion toxins. *Biophys. J.* **40**:175–179.

Weigele, J. B., and R. L. Barchi (1982) Functional reconstitution of the purified sodium channel protein from rat sarcolemma. *Proc. Natl. Acad. Sci. USA* **79**:3651–3655.

Windisch, H., and H. A. Tritthart (1982) Isoproterenol, norepinephrine and phosphodiesterase inhibitors are blockers of the depressed fast Na^+-system in ventricular muscle fibers. *J. Mol. Cell. Cardiol.* **14**:431–434.

Chapter 6

Evolutionary Origins of Voltage-Gated Channels and Synaptic Transmission

BERTIL HILLE

ABSTRACT

A literature survey reveals two major periods of diversification in the origin of excitation and transmission: (1) at the transition from prokaryotic to eukaryotic cellular architecture, and (2) at the transition from protozoa to metazoan animals. Voltage-gated potassium channels and calcium channels arose in the first transitional period, perhaps in concert with the calmodulin-based control of cellular activities. Sodium channels and synaptic transmission arose in the second transitional period. The sodium channel solved the problem of rapid, long-distance communication in a multicellular organism without using the second-messenger calcium ion in the conducting cell. Chemical synaptic transmission permitted both excitatory and inhibitory messages to be received by excitable cells in a multicellular system.

Most of our knowledge of membrane excitability comes from a few well-studied electrophysiological preparations, including the giant axon and giant synapse of the squid, the node of Ranvier, the neuromuscular junction and twitch muscle fiber of the frog, vertebrate electric organs, molluscan ganglion cells, and the crustacean neuromuscular junction and muscle. One clear conclusion from studies of the higher animal phyla is that excitability mechanisms have changed little in the half-billion years since the chordates, mollusks, and arthropods last had a common ancestor. All known axons make their propagated action potentials by means of an electrical duet played between tetrodotoxin-sensitive sodium channels and delayed rectifier potassium channels, as was first shown by Hodgkin and Huxley (1952) for the squid giant axon. Excitability in other parts of neurons, and in muscles and gland cells, involves a much larger repertoire of channel types working in concert. However, even this expanded repertoire seems to be common across the higher animal phyla.

This chapter explores when and how electrical excitability and synaptic transmission arose in phylogeny. The basic material is taken from my recent book (Hille, 1984). Many arguments are based on the absence of certain properties in lower organisms. Such arguments are not always secure, since my reading is limited and some phyla simply have not been as easy or as interesting to study as others. Finally, evolutionary arguments are limited by the vastness of time separating us from the actual events. Some of the relationships proposed here should soon be testable by using the RNA and DNA sequences corresponding to channel proteins.

Living organisms may be classified into two major groups, the prokaryotes and the eukaryotes, which differ profoundly in their cellular architecture. The single-celled prokaryotes arose about 3200 million years ago as self-reproducing, membrane-bound bags of cytoplasm and genetic material—a group that includes the archaebacteria, cyanobacteria, and eubacteria. They each have but one chromosome, which is circular, lacks histones, and segregates into daughter cells without the benefit of a spindle apparatus. Although they may have some infoldings of the cytoplasmic membranes, prokaryotes have no membrane-bound internal organelles. Thus, energy metabolism using electron transport chains must occur in the cytoplasmic membrane, and the primary energy storage—the chemosmotic proton motive force—develops across this membrane.

Eukaryotes are believed to have evolved from prokaryotes about 1400 million years ago. They did not evolve in a single step but after a radical sequence of innovative modifications of virtually every aspect of cellular function. The intermediate forms of this restructuring have presumably long since been exterminated by the successful eukaryotes—the protists, fungi, plants, and animals.

As the name implies, all eukaryotes have a true nucleus with a nuclear envelope, several chromosomes containing histones, and a nucleolus; their chromosomes segregate by mitosis or meiosis, organized by spindle fibers and centrioles, at cell division. But many other aspects of their physiology are different as well. The cytoplasm contains new organelles—mitochondria, endoplasmic reticulum, Golgi apparatus, and lysosomes—and new proteins such as tubulin, actin, myosin, and calmodulin. These developments, found in all eukaryotes, free the surface membrane from the task of primary energy storage, permit sorting and packaging of membrane proteins in vesicles and secretion by exocytosis, give cells an internal skeleton that can change shape and generate movements, and introduce the ability to control cellular activities through the calcium ion as an internal second messenger.

By 700 million years ago, the single-celled eukaryotes (protists) gave rise to three multicellular kingdoms—fungi, plants, and animals—and by 500 million years ago, the differentiation of the major animal phyla had been accomplished (Figure 1). An obvious special feature of most *animals* is that they make more rapid and coordinated movements than do fungi or plants, a property conferred by the early evolution of distinct conducting and contractile tissues. (See Bullock and Horridge (1965) and Shelton (1982) for excellent reviews of early nervous systems.) Sponges, the most primitive surviving animal experiment, have diffusely arrayed body-wall cells and aggregated choanocytes but lack axons or muscle fibers. The organism is sessile and may show a long-lasting local or general contraction in response to irritation (Lawn, 1982). By contrast, at the next level of animal evolution, the coelenterates show many coordinated muscular responses. The graceful, rhythmic swimming of a jellyfish or the closing of the sea anemone on its prey is a consequence of the evolution of axons, synapses, and neuroepithelial and myoepithelial cells. Proceeding to the primitive worms (platyhelminths, nemerteans, and nematodes), we find that neurons have become organized in ganglia, distinct muscle fibers appear, and the nervous and muscular systems

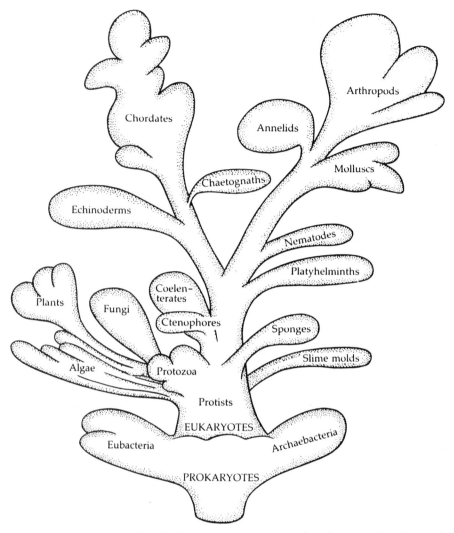

Figure 1. *Phylogenetic tree of life*. The drawing emphasizes animal phyla whose channels have been studied. (From Hille, 1984.)

separate permanently. Although both systems become increasingly complex with subsequent evolution, most of the membrane excitability mechanisms seem to be in place at this time—a stage reached nearly 700 million years ago.

REQUIREMENTS FOR EXCITATION AND TRANSMISSION

Electrical excitability, as we know it, requires conditions that are present in every eukaryotic cell. Namely, there must be a cell membrane, ionic gradients, gated permeability changes, and an effector system capable of responding to the resulting signals.

Even prokaryotes have cell membranes and ionic gradients, features that may be as old as life itself; however, they have no known gated ionic channels to use for signaling. Like eukaryotes, bacteria use the potassium ion as the major intracellular cation and keep the internal free calcium ion concentration low, but many bacteria will grow perfectly well in the complete absence of sodium or chloride ions. Their ionic gradients are usually established by cotransport and exchange mechanisms powered directly by the proton motive force across the cytoplasmic membrane. (See Ingraham et al., 1983, for a recent discussion of bacterial physiology.)

The four eukaryote kingdoms have several potassium ion transport mechanisms, most of which are not well understood, and a variety of extracellular fluids ranging from the osmolarity of pond water to that of seawater. All cells in the animal kingdom seem to have a ouabain-sensitive sodium–potassium ATPase in the cytoplasmic membrane and an extracellular tissue fluid with a stable tonicity and a high sodium ion content (except in phytophagous insects). All eukaryotes have effector systems sensitive to membrane-potential changes or to changes of internal free calcium ion concentration.

Synaptic transmission has additional requirements. The first is multicellularity. For electrical synapses, two cells need only have a conductive pathway joining them, a simple condition known in the multicellular algae and fungi, the higher plants, and the animals. Except in the animals, such connections are accomplished by protoplasmic bridges (forming a true syncytium), and only in the animals are the connections made through conventional gap junctions.

For chemical synapses in the "modern" form the list is longer. There must be pathways for producing and packaging a neurotransmitter into secretory vesicles. There must be a regulated method for phasic exocytosis of the contents. Finally, there must be chemosensitive channels. None of these prerequisites is known to be available in prokaryotes, with the exception that they can synthesize some of the relevant molecules, such as glutamate and glycine, and they do have chemosensory mechanisms (which are not thought to operate through ionic channels). In prokaryotes, the export proteins are synthesized directly into the extracellular space by ribosomes bound to the inner surface of the cytoplasmic membrane. There is no Golgi apparatus, endoplasmic reticulum, or secretory vesicle.

Exocytosis enters with the eukaryotes. *Euglena* (protozoa) and yeast (fungi) have a Golgi apparatus resembling our own. Euglenoids and *Tetrahymena* (protozoa) secrete mucilage and are covered by slime, as are the slime molds. Yeast secrete invertase, enzyme components of cell walls, and even peptide pheromones. Their secretory pathway has been particularly well described and is remarkably similar to that in our pancreatic acinar cells (Novick et al., 1981). As in the pancreas, yeast secretory proteins are synthesized in the rough endoplasmic reticulum, where the glycosylation reactions also transfer the same oligosaccharide core to asparagine residues. Processing continues in the Golgi apparatus, and then secretory vesicles pinch off and move up to the region of a forming cell bud, where they fuse with the surface membrane. One possible difference is that exocytosis is not yet known to be regulated in yeast as it is in all animals. Indeed, complete documentation for calcium-controlled exocytosis is available only for animal cells. However, some evidence has appeared for calcium control of secretion of trichocysts from *Paramecium*. The calcium ionophore A23187 induces trichocyst release in calcium-containing media, but not when magnesium is substituted for calcium (Satir and Oberg, 1978). As in the active zone of a presynaptic terminal, there is a collection of membrane particles—the "fusion rosette"—organized in the membrane of the release zone above each trichocyst. If this is a collection of calcium channels ready to admit activator calcium ions in the immediate vicinity of calcium receptors for exocytosis, then the protozoa already have developed one of the major physiological components of chemical synapses. There is also some evidence for calcium control of secretion in algae and higher plants (Marmé and Dieter, 1983).

The biosynthesis of neurotransmitters is not remarkable and could in principle be achieved in any of the eukaryote kindgoms. Plants make GABA, amino acids, and even acetylcholine and acetylcholinesterase, while yeast make the 13-amino-acid peptide pheromone, α-factor, from a polyprotein precursor (Julius et al., 1984). Probably the unique aspects of chemical synapses in animals are the close apposition and organization of the release sites with respect to postsynaptic receptors and the extent and speed of the modulation of release by presynaptic calcium ion entry.

EVOLUTION OF ELECTRICAL EXCITABILITY

Distribution of Voltage-Gated Channels

We can now summarize the known occurrences of electrical excitability. As we have already remarked, the higher animal phyla, such as chordates, arthropods, and mollusks apparently have the same repertoire of voltage-dependent ionic channels. They all have at least one kind of tetrodotoxin-sensitive sodium channel, several calcium channels, and a large number of potassium channels: delayed rectifiers, an inward rectifier, at least two calcium-activated potassium channels [K(Ca) channels], a transient A-current channel, and so forth (see Hille, 1984).

How far back can these distinct channel types be traced? Table 1 and Figure 2 list clear reports of some of the well-known voltage-gated channels in lower phyla. Except where noted, the identification is based on voltage clamp experiments with sufficient observation of ionic preference, gating kinetics, and pharmacology for a reliable identification of the channel. Before examining this listing in detail, we can note that the continuous presence of such channels through long stretches of phylogeny, and their invariant properties, suggest an early origin and refinement with little subsequent modification. I do not favor the alternative possibility of multiple origins through convergent evolution to explain why the voltage-dependent sodium, calcium, and potassium channels of chordates, arthropods, and mollusks are so similar.

Consider first the significance of the missing entries on the table. Several common channels have not been reported in some higher animal phyla, notably in the annelids (e.g., earthworm and *Myxicola*), the echinoderms (sea urchin and starfish), and the lower chordates (tunicates and *Amphioxus*). This probably reflects on the difficulty of, and perhaps lesser interest in, using the cells of these animals rather than on the absence of the channels. For example, the

Table 1. Evidence for Ionic Channels in Animal Phyla[a,b]

| | | | Type of Ionic Channel | | | | | |
Phylum	Na	K	A	IR	K(Ca)	Ca	Nicotinic AChR[1]	GABA Cl[1]
		Potassium Channels						
Chordata	++	++	++	++	++	++	++	++
Vertebrata	++	++	++	++	++	++	++	++
Cephalochordata[2]	++					++	+	
Urochordata[3]	(a)	+		++		++	+	
Echinodermata[4]		+		++		++	++	
Chaetognatha[5]	++	+				+		
Mollusca	++	++	++	++	++	++	++	++
Arthropoda	++	++	++		++	++	++	++
Annelida	++	++		+		++	++	++
Nematoda[6]						++	++	++
Platyhelminthes[7]	+						+	+
Ctenophora[8]	(b)	+			+	++		
Coelenterata[9]	(b)	++	++	+	+	+	+	
Porifera								
Protozoa[10]		++	+		+	++		

Source: Hille, 1984.

[a] ++, convincing electrical and pharmacological evidence; +, some evidence; K and IR, delayed rectifier and inward rectifier potassium channels, respectively; AChR, acetylcholine receptor (nicotinic); (a), the sodium channel of tunicate eggs binds *Leiurus* scorpion toxin, which modifies its inactivation gating, but the channel is insensitive to 15 μM tetrodotoxin; (b), coelenterate axons and ctenophore smooth muscles have brief sodium-dependent action potentials that are insensitive to 10 μM tetrodotoxin.

[b] *References:* [1]Gerschenfeld, 1973; [2]Hagiwara and Kidokoro, 1971; [3]Ohmori and Yoshii, 1977; Ohmori, 1978; [4]Hagiwara and Takahashi, 1974; Hagiwara, 1983; [5]Schwartz and Stühmer, 1984; [6]Byerly and Masuda, 1979; [7]Koopowitz, 1982; Koopowitz and Keenan, 1982; [8]Stein and Anderson, 1984; [9]Hagiwara et al., 1981; Anderson and Schwab, 1982; [10]Eckert and Brehm, 1979; Naitoh, 1982; Deitmer, 1984.

"giant" axons of starfish reach only 4 μm in diameter, and the typical axons are 0.3 μm; they have not been recorded from intracellularly (Pentreath and Cobb, 1982). Thus, the absence of reports of sodium channels in echinoderms is understandable. The echinoderm egg, which has clear calcium and inward rectifier potassium channels (for a review, see Hagiwara, 1983), is the only robust preparation for voltage clamp study. Similarly, for many of the lower animal phyla, suitable preparations are only now being developed. Intracellular recordings from the lowest animal phylum, the porifera (sponges), are altogether lacking (Lawn, 1982).

Of the common voltage-gated channels, the sodium channel has the shortest pedigree. There is no evidence for the conventional sodium channel outside the animal kingdom. Platyhelminths (e.g., *Planaria*) have tetrodotoxin-sensitive spikes (Koopowitz and Keenan, 1982), while ctenophores (comb jellies) and coelenterates (jellyfish) have sodium-dependent spikes without known tetrodotoxin sensitivity (Anderson and Schwab, 1982). These are the earliest known voltage-gated sodium channels. They coincide with the first evolution of axons, perhaps 700 million years ago.

Evidence for potassium channels and calcium channels goes back much further. Voltage-dependent potassium channels and calcium channels are certainly present in protozoa, algae, and higher plants, as well as in animals (Sibaoka, 1966; Simons, 1981; Naitoh, 1982). In many cases, however, the resolution of the experiments has not been sufficient to sort out which of the several types of potassium channels are present. Delayed rectifier, K(Ca), and transient A-current channels have been suggested in the ciliate protozoa, *Paramecium* and *Stylonychia*. The evidence for a tetraethylammonium-sensitive delayed rectifier in *Paramecium* is strong (Eckert and Brehm, 1979; Naitoh, 1982). Further evidence is needed to be sure of the other two. Voltage clamp studies of the giant green algae *Nitella*, *Chara*, and *Hydrodictyon* show a clear, outward potassium current that activates with a delay and is 95% blocked by 10 mM tetraethylammonium (Findlay and Coleman, 1983). This is probably a delayed rectifier potassium channel but could possibly be a K(Ca) channel. *Paramecium*, *Stylonychia*, and *Nitella* also have voltage-dependent calcium channels permeable to calcium, strontium, and barium ions (Eckert and Brehm, 1979; Lunevsky et al., 1983; Deitmer, 1984). In *Stylonychia*, as in the animal kingdom, there are even two types of calcium channels with different voltage ranges of activation and different kinetics of inactivation. The trap-lobe plant, *Aldrovanda*, has action potentials whose peak height depends on the bathing concentration of calcium ions and are accompanied by a calcium influx (Iijima and Sibaoka, 1985). This higher plant, whose insect trap can be snapped shut in tens of milliseconds, therefore probably has calcium channels.

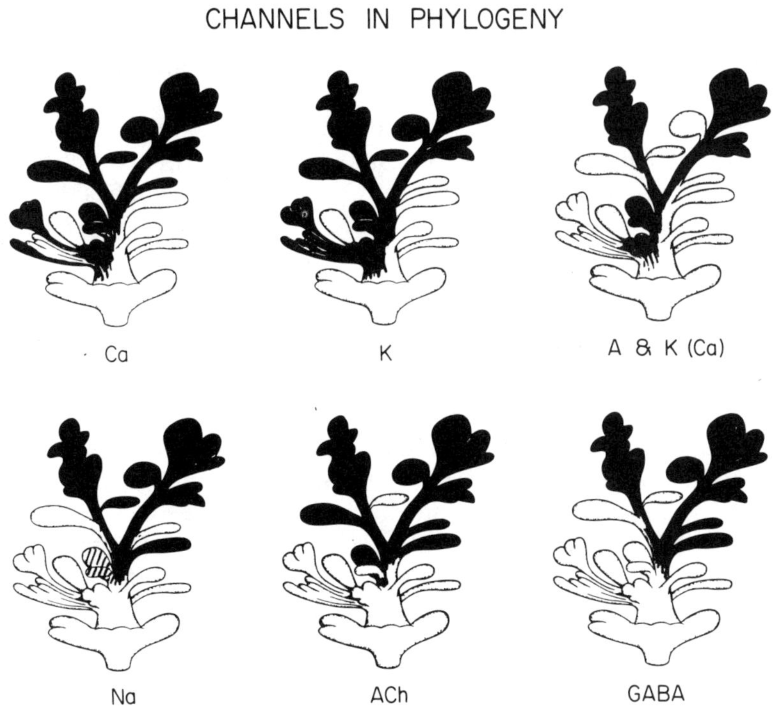

CHANNELS IN PHYLOGENY

Figure 2. *Reports of ionic channels in phylogeny.* The phylogenetic trees are arranged as in Figure 1 and shaded to represent reported occurrences of specific channel types given in Table 1.

Speculations on the Origins of Voltage-Gated Channels

Neglecting some missing entries in our phylogeny, the foregoing can be summarized. Voltage-dependent potassium and calcium channels appeared and diversified in stem eukaryotes by the time the modern protozoa evolved. They were passed on to the animals and probably also to all other modern unicellular and multicellular eukaryotes. Voltage-dependent sodium channels came later, coinciding with the appearance of axons in lower animals, and underlie the action potentials of axons in all animal phyla from the coelenterates and ctenophores up.

We generally focus on the *electrical* signals coming from channels because they are easiest to measure, but we should remember that, except in the special case of electric organs, the nervous system would serve no purpose if it made only electricity. The interesting outputs, namely secretion and movement, are calcium-controlled processes. Electrical signals in the nervous system seem always to be transduced into actions through their effect on the movements of calcium ions.

In animals, ionic channels transduce sensory inputs, propagate messages, sum positive and negative influences, generate rhythms, and ultimately control and coordinate activities in a wide variety of organs. Nonanimal eukaryotes also require appropriate responses to the environment. The avoidance response of *Paramecium* (backing away from obstacles; Figure 3A) is controlled by a calcium action potential (Figure 3B). The touch-sensitive leaf closures of *Mimosa*, Venus's-flytrap, or the trap-lobe plant are also controlled by action potentials (Figure 4). Hence, the coordination of activities through ionic channels and electrical signals is probably an early role rather than one evolved in conjunction with nervous systems.

As a working hypothesis, I propose that voltage-dependent channels are an essential component of the revolution that led to the appearance of the eukaryote style of cellular architecture. One of the eukaryotic innovations is the control of cellular functions through variations in the intracellular free calcium ion concentration. The control is exerted through the calcium-binding protein, calmodulin, found throughout the eukaryotes with very little sequence variation, and its homologous family of derived proteins: myosin light chains, troponin C, parvalbumin, and others (Goodman et al., 1979). The control also requires a regulated delivery of calcium ions to the cytoplasm from the extracellular space or from intracellular stores. This is accomplished by voltage-gated calcium channels that deliver calcium ions during membrane depolarizations and by voltage-gated potassium channels that define a resting potential and terminate periods of depolarization. Finally, the calcium regulating system has to respond to external stimuli. This might have required membrane-potential changes from "sensory" channels such as the potassium-permeable channels and the calcium-permeable channels of the mechanoreceptors of protozoa. I propose that all of these mechanisms were improvised and coadapted 1.4 billion years ago during the emergence of the eukaryotic way of life.

Voltage-dependent sodium channels apparently did not evolve until early animal evolution. One might imagine that there was no need for a new channel to make action potentials when there already were calcium channels that could

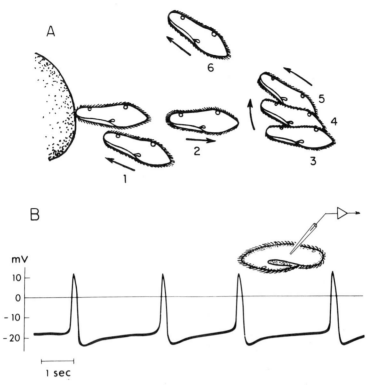

Figure 3. *Excitability in* Paramecium. *A:* The classical avoidance reaction showing a period of ciliary reversal and backward locomotion after collision with an obstacle. Reversal occurs when mechanoreceptors in the anterior end of the cell depolarize the membrane and initiate a calcium action potential. (After Grell, 1956.) *B:* Spontaneous repetitive "calcium spikes" induced by exposing *P. caudatum* to a medium containing only 2 mM barium chloride, 1 mM calcium chloride, and 1 mM Tris buffer. Rapid ciliary reversal occurs during each spike. (From Kinosita et al., 1964.)

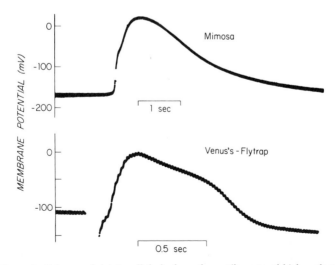

Figure 4. *Action potentials recorded intracellularly from the motile parts of higher plants.* Propagated responses are normally triggered by the bending of sensory hairs. (From Sibaoka, 1966.)

propagate regenerative impulses. However, sodium channels offer special advantages that make possible the rapidly conducting axons essential for nervous system function as we know it. Typical cells making calcium spikes have maximum calcium current densities of 100 μA/cm^2, have slow rates of rise and propagation velocities of the action potential, and turn on calcium-regulated processes fully by raising the internal free calcium concentration to 10 μM. Axons achieve a high conduction velocity by switching on a much higher density of inward sodium current (approximately 4 mA/cm^2) in the rising phase of the action potential, which during periods of intense repetitive firing may raise their internal sodium concentration by as much as 10 mM. Were the axon to use calcium ions instead, such an internal concentration rise would constitute an intolerable calcium overload. Hence, sodium channels are a specialization for making powerful currents without a flood of internal messengers. They permit the specialization of conducting—as opposed to contractile and secretory—tissue.

A possible evolutionary tree for voltage-gated channels is given in Figure 5. Potassium, calcium, and sodium channels are viewed as descending from each other because of their many biophysical similarities (Hille, 1984). Each has a sigmoid time course of activation during a depolarization, with a steep voltage dependence equivalent to a gating process controlled by 4–6 electronic charges. Each has a narrow pore and is highly ion selective. Each has gates that open from the inner end to reveal a wide, hydrophobic vestibule where blocking drugs may bind. There is no clear prokaryote antecedent of such channels, but prokaryotes do have a narrow, proton-selective pore, F$_o$, as one component of the energy-coupling proton ATPase, and gram-negative bacteria have the wide-mouthed porins and colicins, which could conceivably be precursors. In addition, the voltage-dependent anion channel of eukaryote mitochondria is a candidate precursor.

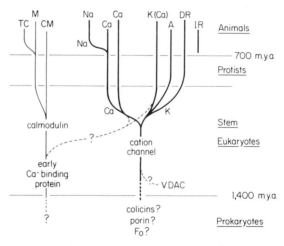

Figure 5. *Proposed descent of voltage-gated channels from a stem eukaryote cation channel.* Possible introduction of calcium-binding sites from a calmodulin precursor is shown. Abbreviations of channels as in Table 1. Other abbreviations: TC, troponin C; M, myosin light chains; CM, calmodulin; VDAC, voltage-dependent anion channel; m.y.a., million years ago.

Several authors have suggested that the calcium-binding sites within the calcium channel have binding properties analogous to those of the calmodulin family (Kostyuk et al., 1983; Almers and McCleskey, 1984; Hess and Tsien, 1984). Hence calcium channels, and K(Ca) channels as well, may have differentiated through inclusion of some parts of the amino-acid sequence of an early calcium-binding protein. The tree shows sodium channels descending from calcium channels only because both carry inward currents and have less high ionic selectivity than do potassium channels. The inward rectifier, which so far is known only in animals, has ionic selectivity like that of other potassium channels but such completely different gating properties that it is difficult to guess which one it might be descended from.

ORIGIN OF SYNAPSES

If we believe that multicellularity arose independently in the plant, fungus, and animal kingdoms, then we conclude that synaptic transmission in animals could not be inherited from other multicellular forms. At the same time, synaptic transmission must appear as soon as there is a nervous system with differentiated neurons. Electrical synapses would suffice to transmit excitatory messages, but chemical transmission seems necessary to permit the type of inhibitory influences that have become an essential feature of even simple motor patterns.

Little can be said now about the lowest modern animals, the sponges, because of the difficulty of doing electron microscopy on an organism that is mostly spicules, and because there are no clearly differentiated nerve or muscle cells from which to make intracellular recordings (Lawn, 1982). However, coelenterates and ctenophores, the first animals with neurons and myoid tissue, already show many of the features of chemical and electrical synapses seen in higher animals (Mackie, 1970; Anderson and Schwab, 1982). They are the first animals to be made up of columnar epithelia standing on basement membranes. In hydrozoan coelenterates, these cells are electrically coupled by conventional-looking gap junctions and in some cases conduct action potentials from cell to cell. In addition, there are differentiated neurons that make morphological electrical and chemical synapses with each other and with other cell types. Electrical and dye coupling can be demonstrated. The chemical synapses show synaptic vesicles at a narrow synaptic cleft (sometimes on both sides), and transmission can be blocked by elevating the magnesium ion concentration and by cadmium or nickel ions. There is evidence for catecholaminergic transmission in anthozoan coelenterates and nicotinic cholinergic transmission in hydrozoans. Undoubtedly there are other transmitters, but the search is still in its early stages. Behavioral experiments are interpreted to mean that there are both excitatory and inhibitory junctions.

Evidently, major problems of synaptic transmission were resolved by the first successful animals with neurons. Formation of the junction, packaging and organization of the vesicles, a rapid calcium-dependent release, and sensitively responsive postsynaptic channels are all in hand. Also, many neurotransmitters appear in simple animals. The soil nematode *Caenorhabditis elegans* has been especially well studied (Chalfie, 1984). It has a little over 300 neurons forming 7000 chemical synapses and 600 gap junctions. Behavioral mutants have been found for acetylcholine, dopamine, 5-hydroxytryptamine, and octopamine. In other nematodes, there is evidence for excitatory nicotinic transmission and inhibitory GABAergic transmission (Gerschenfeld, 1973). Hence, lower invertebrates have the conventional molecular elements of synaptic transmission.

There is no evidence that synaptic channels have an evolutionary relationship to voltage-gated channels. Synaptic channels usually have wide, poorly selective pores and are only weakly influenced by membrane potential. In addition, there is no obvious structural similarity between the five modest-sized protein subunits of the acetylcholine receptor (Raftery et al., 1980; Changeux and Heidmann, this volume) and the one very large plus several smaller subunits of the sodium channel (Miller et al., 1983; Catterall et al., this volume). I would favor an origin of transmitter-sensitive channels from a poorly ion-selective mechanosensor or other sensory channel.

CONCLUSION

Ionic channels used for signaling may be absent in prokaryotes but are universal and essential aspects of eukaryotic life. Their origin greatly precedes the origin of animal nervous systems, but nevertheless they probably arose for an analogous purpose, namely to coordinate cellular responses to external stimuli. As it still is today, the earliest use for electrical signals would have been to control the concentration of calcium ions in the cytoplasm as an internal second messenger. Voltage-gated calcium and potassium channels arose in these early eukaryotes, and together with "sensory" ionic channels probably were passed along to all eukaryote phyla. Hence, study of any eukaryote could help us understand the basic mechanisms of voltage sensitivity and ionic selectivity.

Sodium channels and synaptic transmission arose much later, in the first animals, enabling them to produce nervous systems. The molecular elements of axonal excitation and synaptic transmission seem to have been developed, diversified, and refined, quite early in animal evolution. Subsequent nervous system evolution apparently concerned more the problems of nerve cell connections—wiring—and may not have required much change in the ionic channels.

ACKNOWLEDGMENTS

I thank Ms. Lea Miller for valuable secretarial help. My research is supported by grant NS-08174 from the National Institutes of Health.

REFERENCES

Almers, W., and E. W. McCleskey (1984) The nonselective conductance due to calcium channels in frog muscle: Calcium selectivity in a single-file pore. *J. Physiol. (Lond.)* **353**:585–608.

Anderson, P. A. V., and W. E. Schwab (1982) Recent advances and model systems in coelenterate neurobiology. *Prog. Neurobiol.* **19**:213–236.

Bullock, T. H., and G. A. Horridge (1965) *Structure and Function of the Nervous Systems of Invertebrates*, W. H. Freeman, San Francisco.

Byerly, L., and M. O. Masuda (1979) Voltage-clamp analysis of the potassium current that produces a negative-going action potential in *Ascaris* muscle. *J. Physiol. (Lond.)* **288**:263–284.

Chalfie, M. (1984) Neural development in *Caenorhabditis elegans*. *Trends Neurosci.* **7**:197–202.

Deitmer, J. W. (1984) Evidence for two voltage-dependent calcium currents in the membrane of the ciliate *Stylonychia*. *J. Physiol. (Lond.)* **355**:137–159.

Eckert, R., and P. Brehm (1979) Ionic mechanisms of excitation in *Paramecium*. *Annu. Rev. Biophys. Bioeng.* **8**:353–383.

Findlay, G. P., and H. A. Coleman (1983) Potassium channels in the membrane of *Hydrodictyon africanum*. *J. Membr. Biol.* **75**:241–251.

Gerschenfeld, H. M. (1973) Chemical transmission in invertebrate central nervous systems and neuromuscular junctions. *Physiol. Rev.* **53**:1–119.

Goodman, M., J.-F. Pechère, J. Haiech, and J. G. Demaille (1979) Evolutionary diversification of structure and function in the family of intracellular calcium-binding proteins. *J. Mol. Evol.* **13**:331–352.

Grell, K. G. (1956) *Protozoologie*, Springer-Verlag, Berlin.

Hagiwara, S. (1983) *Membrane Potential-Dependent Ion Channels in Cell Membrane. Phylogenetic and Developmental Approaches*, Raven, New York.

Hagiwara, S., and Y. Kidokoro (1971) Na and Ca components of action potential *Amphioxus* muscle cells. *J. Physiol. (Lond.)* **219**:217–232.

Hagiwara, S., and K. Takahashi (1974) The anomalous rectification and cation selectivity of the membrane of a starfish egg cell. *J. Membr. Biol.* **18**:61–80.

Hagiwara, S., S. Yoshida, and M. Yoshii (1981) Transient and delayed potassium currents in the egg cell membrane of the coelenterate, *Renilla koellikeri*. *J. Physiol. (Lond.)* **318**:123–141.

Hess, P., and R. W. Tsien (1984) Mechanism of ion permeation through calcium channels. *Nature* **309**:453–456.

Hille, B. (1984) *Ionic Channels in Excitable Membranes*, Sinauer, Sunderland, Massachusetts.

Hodgkin, A. L., and A. F. Huxley (1952) A quantitative description of membrane current and its application to conduction and excitation in nerve. *J. Physiol. (Lond.)* **117**:500–544.

Iijima, T., and T. Sibaoka (1985) Membrane potentials in the excitable cells of *Aldrovanda vesiculosa* trap-lobes. *Plant Cell Physiol.* **26**:1–14.

Ingraham, J. L., O. Maaloe, and F. C. Neidhardt (1983) *Growth of the Bacterial Cell*, Sinauer, Sunderland, Massachusetts.

Julius, D., R. Schekman, and J. Thorner (1984) Glycosylation and processing of prepro-α-factor through the yeast secretory pathway. *Cell* **36**:309–318.

Kinosita, H., S. Dryl, and Y. Naitoh (1964) Changes in membrane potential and the responses to stimuli in *Paramecium*. *J. Fac. Sci. Univ. Tokyo IV* **10**:291–301.

Koopowitz, H. (1982) Free-living platyhelminthes. In *Electrical Conduction and Behaviour in "Simple" Invertebrates*, G. A. B. Shelton, ed., pp. 359–392, Clarendon, Oxford.

Koopowitz, H., and L. Keenan (1982) The primitive brains of platyhelminthes. *Trends Neurosci.* **5**:77–79.

Kostyuk, P. G., S. L. Mironov, and Y. M. Shuba (1983) Two ion-selecting filters in the calcium channel of the somatic membrane of mollusc neurons. *J. Membr. Biol.* **76**:83–93.

Lawn, I. D. (1982) Porifera. In *Electrical Conduction and Behaviour in "Simple" Invertebrates*, G. A. B. Shelton, ed., pp. 49–72, Clarendon, Oxford.

Lunevsky, V. Z., O. M. Zherelova, I. Y. Vostrikov, and G. N. Berestovsky (1983) Excitation of *Characeae* cell membranes as result of activation of calcium and chloride channels. *J. Membr. Biol.* **72**:43–58.

Mackie, G. O. (1970) Neuroid conduction and the evolution of conducting tissues. *Q. Rev. Biol.* **45**:319–332.

Marmé, D., and P. Dieter (1983) Role of Ca^{2+} and calmodulin in plants. In *Calcium and Cell Function*, Vol. IV, W. Y. Cheung, ed., pp. 263–311, Academic, New York.

Miller, J. A., W. S. Agnew, and S. R. Levinson (1983) Principal glycopeptide of the tetrodotoxin/saxitoxin binding protein from *Electrophorus electricus*: Isolation and partial chemical and physical characterization. *Biochemistry* **22**:462–470.

Naitoh, Y. (1982) Protozoa. In *Electrical Conduction and Behaviour in "Simple" Invertebrates*, G. A. B. Shelton, ed., pp. 1–48, Clarendon, Oxford.

Novick, P., S. Ferro, and R. Schekman (1981) Order of events in yeast secretory pathway. *Cell* **25**:461–469.

Ohmori, H. (1978) Inactivation kinetics and steady-state current noise in the anomalous rectifier of tunicate egg cell membranes. *J. Physiol. (Lond.)* **281**:77–99.

Ohmori, H., and M. Yoshii (1977) Surface potential reflected in both gating and permeation mechanisms of sodium and calcium channels of the tunicate egg cell membrane. *J. Physiol. (Lond.)* **267**:429–463.

Pentreath, V. W., and J. L. S. Cobb (1982) In *Electrical Conduction and Behaviour in "Simple" Invertebrates*, G. A. B. Shelton, ed., pp. 440–472, Clarendon, Oxford.

Raftery, M. A., M. W. Hunkapiller, C. D. Strader, and L. E. Hood (1980) Acetylcholine receptor: Complex of homologous subunits. *Science* **208**:1454–1457.

Satir, B. H., and S. G. Oberg (1978) *Paramecium* fusion rosettes: Possible function as Ca^{2+} gates. *Science* **199**:536–538.

Schwartz, L. M., and W. Stühmer (1984) Voltage-dependent sodium channels in invertebrate striated muscle. *Science* **225**:523–525.

Shelton, G. A. B., ed. (1982) *Electrical Conduction and Behaviour in "Simple" Invertebrates*, Clarendon, Oxford.

Sibaoka, T. (1966) Action potentials in plant organs. *Symp. Soc. Exp. Biol.* **20**:49–74.

Simons, P. J. (1981) The role of electricity in plant movements. *New Phytol.* **87**:11–37.

Stein, P. G., and P. A. V. Anderson (1984) The physiology of single giant smooth muscle cells isolated from the ctenophore *Mnemiopsis*. *Biophys. J.* **45**:233a.

Section 2

Neurotransmitters and Synaptic Function

Since the demonstration of the chemical nature of synaptic transmission, an explosion of research has opened fields of investigation concerned with the stereochemistry of transmitters, their categorization in chemical families, their relation to channels, their modulation by second messengers, and their relation to drug action. These subjects are richly represented in this section.

Hökfelt, using the paradigm of examining the distribution patterns and cellular localization of transmitters and neuropeptides in various brain regions, addresses the question of their coexistence in a single neuron. Since the first demonstration of the coexistence of the peptide somatostatin and a classical transmitter in peripheral noradrenergic neurons, many examples of coexistence have been found. Neurons may release more than one compound at their synapses, and responses may be the result of the integration of multiple signals emerging from the interaction of several messengers. This may increase the capacity to use the huge but nonetheless finite wiring of neuronal networks and enhance the capacity for information transfer, particularly over time.

Transmitter action is subtle, and it operates by means of a series of biochemical regulatory pathways which it in turn regulates. One of the most important of these pathways is subserved by protein phosphorylation mediated by a variety of protein kinases. Hemmings et al. explore the significance of such regulation in their illustrative example of the effects of a phosphoprotein, DARPP-32. This protein is found on D1-dopamine-positive neurons and is regulated by dopamine acting through cAMP. Phosphorylated DARPP-32 inhibits protein phosphatase, thus inhibiting the dephosphorylation of other specific phosphoproteins; in turn, DARPP-32 is dephosphorylated by protein phosphatase 2B. There is thus a rich regulatory loop mediated by this protein, connecting the synergistic and antagonistic actions of cAMP and calcium second messenger systems. A link between transmitter level and response regulation is suggested, and the subtlety of the chemical transmission network is revealed particularly well by this example.

Snyder, in his contribution, shows how neurotransmitters, drug receptors, and associations between channels and second messenger systems can be characterized through the use of ligand binding techniques. This approach has shown that certain drug receptors are enzymes: Phorbol ester receptors are protein kinase C; receptors for the neurotoxin MPTP are likely to be monoamine oxidase type B. Snyder also reviews the use of the ligand binding approach to elucidate the molecular processes governing neurotransmitter uptake. This work represents the modern vanguard in support of the classical pharmacologic idea of cellular receptors, and it promises to link enzymic regulation to drug and transmitter binding in a satisfyingly precise way.

Transmitters can be excitatory or inhibitory. In his chapter, Olsen takes up an important receptor mediating the action of a major inhibitory neurotransmitter, γ-aminobutyric acid (GABA). The most common GABAergic synapse involves regulation of postsynaptic membrane chloride ion permeability on a short time scale, inhibiting the target cell. Olsen reviews evidence based on assays with agonists and antagonists that suggests that the GABA receptor may represent a three-receptor–ion channel complex with modulatory sites for various drugs, which acts to increase or decrease the activity of the receptor-regulated chloride channels. The complex can be purified, and its various activities and allosteric interactions are being studied.

A rich and large class of peptides mediating various responses in synaptic systems has been subjected to intense study in the last decade. Many of the neuropeptides are cleaved from large precursors (polyproteins) and must be posttranslationally modified to acquire activity. Specific endoproteolytic cleavage at flanking basic amino acids occurs in many cases, followed by trimming with carboxypeptidases. Herbert and Douglas have characterized kallikrein endoproteases by using recombinant DNA technology to identify an RNA species coding for enzymes that process pro-opiomelanocortin. While not identified as the key enzymes in processing neuropeptides, kallikreins, which are known to be important for processing growth hormones, provide a valuable model for the understanding of neuropeptide processing.

Bloom et al., in the concluding chapter of this section, provide several examples of transmitter synergism using the relationship between norepinephrine and vasoactive intestinal polypeptide as a key example. A second example involves somatostatin and acetylcholine in the hippocampus. In the anticipation that many such interactions will be found, these authors describe their strategy to discover new neuropeptides and brain-specific molecules by means of molecular genetic techniques. A brain-specific protein, 1B236, has been found by these methods to be present in olfactory, limbic, somatosensory, and extrapyramidal systems. These data are being coupled with those from various assays to test whether this protein may represent a neurotransmitter precursor. While it remains to be demonstrated whether molecular genetic approaches will allow the discovery as well as the complete characterization of new neurotransmitters, it is already clear that they provide an excellent opportunity to isolate brain-specific proteins in a first-pass survey.

Given the richness of synaptic types and neurotransmitter types, their effects in different neural networks become a major interest, one that is taken up in Section 3.

Chapter 7

Neuronal Communication Through Multiple Coexisting Messengers

TOMAS HÖKFELT

ABSTRACT

Comparison of the distribution patterns and the cellular localization of neurotransmitters and neuropeptides has revealed that in many cases a classical transmitter occurs together with a peptide in the same neuron. There are also many examples of neurons containing several peptides, each of which apparently arises from a different precursor molecule. This topic is discussed, and an attempt is made to analyze the possible physiological significance of such coexistence situations.

Studying the action of epinephrine in peripheral tissues, Elliott (1905) suggested that neurons may communicate with effector cells in the periphery via chemical messengers (see Stjärne et al., 1981). The chemical compounds known to be involved in chemical transmission were for a long time fairly small in number and included the catecholamines [dopamine (DA), norepinephrine (NE), and epinephrine (E)], 5-hydroxytryptamine (5-HT), acetylcholine (ACh), and a group of amino acids such as glutamate and γ-aminobutyric acid (GABA). More recent evidence suggests that certain peptides may also be present in neurons and may in fact be involved in the transmission processes at synapses (see Otsuka and Takahashi, 1977; Snyder, 1980), thus notably increasing the number of putative messenger substances (see Snyder, 1980).

This development is based on progress in peptide and protein biochemistry, which has led to the discovery of numerous new peptides in, for example, the laboratories of Erspamer, Guillemin, Leeman, Mutt, Schally, and Vale. Recombinant DNA technology has also provided evidence for additional biologically active peptides, including new members of the tachykinin family (Kangawa et al., 1983; Kimura et al., 1983; Nawa et al., 1983), a calcitonin gene-related peptide (CGRP) (Amara et al., 1982; Rosenfeld et al., 1983), and a PHI-27-like peptide (PHM-27) with a structure similar to that of vasoactive intestinal polypeptide (VIP) (Itoh et al., 1983). Both radioimmunological and immunohistochemical studies have shown that most of these peptides are present in an immunoreactive form in both peripheral and central nervous system neurons.

In view of the large number of compounds present in neurons, the question of whether or not there are neurons available to host all of them individually has arisen. Immunohistochemical experiments carried out mainly during the last 10 years have come up with a partial answer to this problem; there is now evidence that neurons may contain both a classical transmitter and one or more biologically active peptides (Hökfelt et al., 1980a,b, 1982, 1984b; Lundberg et al., 1982a; Lundberg and Hökfelt, 1983; see also Cuello, 1982; Chan-Palay and Palay, 1984). The first demonstration of the coexistence of a peptide and a classical transmitter was the observation of somatostatinlike immunoreactivity in some peripheral noradrenergic neurons (Hökfelt et al., 1977). Subsequently, many such coexistence situations have been encountered, and there is at least one example of the coexistence with a peptide for each of the transmitters—DA, NE, E, 5-HT, GABA, and ACh (Table 1). Thus, the coexistence of multiple messengers may be a rule rather than a rare exception. Neurons may release more than one compound at their synapses, and the response(s) seen upon synaptic activation may be a result of the interaction of several messengers and of the integration of multiple signals.

In this chapter, I summarize some studies dealing with this topic. First, some experiments carried out on the peripheral nervous system are described, in which some tissues were shown to contain well-defined neuronal inputs that are favorable for experimental analysis of the significance of classical transmitters and peptides. Then some work on the central nervous system that may have some bearing on the functional significance of central coexistence is described: (1) 5-HT neurons in the medulla oblongata containing substance P- and thyrotropin-releasing hormone (TRH)-like immunoreactivities; (2) DA neurons in the ventral mesencephalon containing a cholecystokinin (CCK)-like peptide; (3) primary sensory neurons containing substance P and a CGRP-like peptide; and finally, (4) luteinizing hormone-releasing hormone (LHRH) neurons possibly containing leukotriene C_4 (LTC$_4$)-like immunoreactivity.

COMMENTS ON METHODOLOGY

The findings from our laboratory discussed in the present chapter are based mainly on results obtained with the immunohistochemical technique originally developed by Coons and collaborators more than 40 years ago (see Coons, 1958). With this method, a novel principle was introduced into histochemistry: the use of antisera to characterize chemical components in tissue sections. This pioneering technique has only recently emerged as a powerful tool in neurobiological research. Geffen et al. (1969) applied immunohistochemistry to demonstrate the enzyme dopamine-β-hydroxylase in tissue sections. Thanks to the explosive development in biochemistry that has resulted in the purification of numerous peptides, enzymes, and other proteins, antisera could be raised against these compounds and used both in radioimmunoassays and immunohistochemistry.

Immunohistochemistry is often considered to have a high degree of specificity and sensitivity when compared to many other histochemical approaches. There are, however, considerable problems, both with regard to specificity and to sensitivity. It must be emphasized that the staining patterns observed can not be attributed to a specific substance, since it is impossible to exclude the occurrence of cross-reactivity with compounds that bear structural similarities to the im-

Table 1. Some Examples of the Coexistence of Classical Transmitters and Peptides in the Central Nervous System

Classical Transmitter	Peptide	Brain Region and Species	References
Dopamine	Neurotensin	Ventral mesencephalon (humans, rat)	Hökfelt et al., 1984a
	CCK	Ventral mesencephalon (humans, rat)	Hökfelt et al., 1980c,d, 1985
Norepinephrine	Enkephalin	Locus coeruleus (cat)	Charnay et al., 1982
	NPY	Medulla oblongata (humans, rat)	Hökfelt et al., 1983a; Everitt et al., 1984
		Locus coeruleus (rat)	Everitt et al., 1984
Epinephrine	Neurotensin	Medulla oblongata (rat)	Hökfelt et al., 1984a
	NPY	Medulla oblongata (rat)	Everitt et al., 1984
5-HT	Substance P	Medulla oblongata (rat, cat)	Chan-Palay et al., 1978; Hökfelt et al., 1978; Johansson et al., 1981; Lovick and Hunt, 1983
	TRH	Medulla oblongata (rat)	Johansson et al., 1981
	Enkephalin	Medulla oblongata, pons (cat)	Glazer et al., 1981; Hunt and Lovick, 1982
ACh	VIP	Cortex (rat)	Eckenstein and Baughman, 1984
	Substance P	Pons (rat)	Vincent et al., 1983
GABA	Somatostatin	Thalamus (cat)	Oertel et al., 1983

munogens. It is, therefore, only possible to state, for example, that "substance P-like immunoreactivity" is present in a tissue section.

The need for such caution has been repeatedly underlined with regard to this technique. For example, it has been discovered that neurons may contain several similar peptides produced from the same precursor. Recent observations have shown that the gene for substance P also codes for a structurally similar peptide, substance K (Nawa et al., 1983). Since the sensitivity problem is also important, negative findings should be interpreted with great caution. Lack of immuno-reactivity in neurons may merely mean that the histochemical technique may not be sufficiently sensitive to detect very low levels of a certain compound.

Our immunohistochemical protocol for indirect immunofluorescence (see Coons, 1958) includes fixation of animals by perfusion with formalin (Pease, 1962) or a formalin–picric acid mixture (Zamboni and De Martino, 1967), followed by sectioning in a cryostat. Incubation with primary antisera is carried out overnight at 4°C, followed by rinsing and incubation with fluorescein isothiocyanate (FITC)- or rhodamine isothiocyanate (RITC)-labeled secondary antibodies. The sections are mounted with a glycerol buffer solution containing, for example, p-phenyl-enediamine, an agent recently introduced to prevent the fading of fluorescence upon ultraviolet exposure (Johnson and de C Nogueira Araujo, 1981; Platt and Michael, 1983). The sections are examined in a fluorescence microscope equipped with proper filter combinations. To analyze the possible occurrence of more than one compound in a neuron, we have either stained adjacent thin sections with two different antisera or carried out sequential staining of the same section by using the elution–restaining method of Tramu et al. (1978). This procedure includes photographing the first staining pattern, treating the sections with acid potassium permanganate, rinsing and incubating the sections with FITC-conjugated antibodies, and analyzing them in the fluorescence microscope. If no specific fluorescence can be seen, the sections are incubated with a new primary antibody, followed by incubation with FITC-conjugated antibodies. The staining patterns are compared, and the coexistence of compounds can be established or, under certain conditions, excluded.

To analyze the projections of transmitter-identified neurons, a combination of immunofluorescence and retrograde tracing with fluorescent compounds is used (see Hökfelt et al., 1983b; Skirboll et al., 1984). Dyes such as True Blue, Fast Blue, or Propidium Iodide (see Kuypers and Huisman, 1984) are injected into a certain brain area and taken up by nerve terminals (and occasionally by axons). The dyes are transported retrogradely to the cell bodies and after two to ten days the animals are perfused with fixative (as above) and the brains are cut in a cryostat. Dye-labeled cell bodies are searched for and photographed, and the sections are subsequently processed immunohistochemically (as above). The sections are then screened for double-labeled cell bodies, those containing both the retrograde tracer and the immunoreactivity.

COEXISTENCE OF CLASSICAL TRANSMITTERS AND PEPTIDES IN THE CAT SALIVARY GLAND

Analysis of secretory mechanisms in the cat salivary gland has been conducted for more than a century (Ludwig, 1851; Bernard, 1858; Heidenhain, 1872). The gland receives sympathetic and parasympathetic innervation (Figure 1), and stimulation of the latter causes secretion and an increase in blood flow. Early on it was discovered that only salivary secretion could be completely blocked by atropine, whereas vasodilation, at least when induced with high-stimulation frequencies, was atropine-resistant (Heidenhain, 1872). Stimulation of the sympathetic nerves causes vasoconstriction and, to a smaller degree, secretion (Emmelin, 1967, 1972).

Immunohistochemical analysis has revealed a small biologically active peptide in both sympathetic and parasympathetic neurons—VIP (Said and Mutt, 1970; Mutt and Said, 1974)—that coexists with ACh in parasympathetic fibers (Lundberg et al., 1979, 1981, 1982a); neuropeptide Y (NPY) (Tatemoto, 1982; Tatemoto et al., 1982) occurs together with NE in sympathetic fibers (Lundberg et al., 1982c; Figure 1). Virtually all cholinergic fibers seem to contain VIP, whereas NPY-like immunoreactivity is present in a subpopulation of noradrenergic fibers with a preferential location around blood vessels. In contrast, the secretory elements seem to be surrounded by noradrenergic fibers without the peptide.

The cat submandibular gland offers a favorable experimental model for the analysis of the functional significance of the presence of these peptides in the autonomic neurons controlling secretion and blood flow through the gland, as has been shown by Lundberg, Änggård, and their collaborators (see Lundberg et al., 1982a). These studies have shown that stimulation of the parasympathetic neurons causes the release of both VIP and ACh. The release of VIP is well correlated with an increase in blood flow. The infusion of ACh induces secretion and an increase in blood flow, both of which are atropine-sensitive. ACh is about 100 times less potent than VIP, on a molar basis, with regard to vasodilatory action. The infusion of VIP alone causes only an increase in blood flow. When ACh and VIP are infused together, additive blood flow effects are observed. Furthermore, VIP causes a potentiation of the ACh-induced secretion. *In vitro* studies on isolated membranes from the cat submandibular gland have shown that VIP in low concentrations (5×10^{-9} M) causes an increase in the association

INNERVATION OF THE SUBMANDIBULAR GLAND OF THE CAT

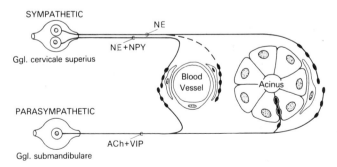

Figure 1. *Schematic representation of the sympathetic and parasympathetic innervation of the submandibular gland of the cat.* The sympathetic noradrenergic neurons innervating blood vessels contain neuropeptide Y (NPY), whereas the noradrenergic neurons around secretory elements seem to lack this compound. The parasympathetic cholinergic neurons innervating blood vessels and secretory elements contain vasoactive intestinal polypeptide (VIP). (From Lundberg and Hökfelt, 1983).

rate of receptor binding for the muscarinic antagonist N-methyl-4-piperidinyl benzilate (NMPB) (Lundberg et al., 1982b).

NE and the NPY-like peptide present in sympathetic neurons innervating the submandibular gland have also been shown to interact. NPY causes a slowly developing, long-lasting vasoconstriction (Lundberg and Tatemoto, 1982), whereas NE has a short-lasting vasoconstrictory effect with a rapid onset. NE, but not NPY, causes secretion. When infused together, NE and NPY induce a blood flow response similar to the one seen after electrical stimulation of sympathetic neurons. This suggests that the compounds are working together in a complementary fashion to induce a full physiological response.

In the rat vas deferens, where NE and NPY coexist in the sympathetic neurons, a second type of interaction has been observed that differs from the one described above (Lundberg et al., 1982c). *In vitro* experiments show that NPY, in a dose-dependent manner, inhibits electrically induced contraction of the vas deferens, in all probability because of an inhibition of norepinephrine release (Allen et al., 1982; Lundberg et al., 1982c; Stjärne and Lundberg, 1984). Such a mechanism may serve to prevent an excessive release of NE.

If classical transmitters and peptides are able to produce differential effects, it should be possible to release these compounds separately. This could be achieved if, for example, they have different subcellular storage sites within the neuron. In fact, subcellular fractionation studies on the cat submandibular gland (Lundberg et al., 1981) and rat vas deferens (Fried et al., 1985) have provided evidence that the peptides (VIP and NPY) are stored exclusively in large granular vesicles, whereas the classical transmitters (ACh and NE) are present both in these vesicles and in small vesicles in the two systems (Figure 2).

In conclusion, two types of interactions between coexisting classical transmitters and peptides have been observed in studies on peripheral neurons: (1) The two types of compounds act synergistically in a complementary fashion; and (2) the peptides counteract the action of the classical transmitters by inhibiting their release.

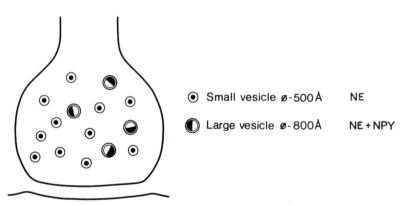

Figure 2. *Schematic representation of a noradrenergic nerve ending in the vas deferens of the rat.* The small vesicles contain only norepinephrine (NE), whereas the large vesicles contain both the amine and neuropeptide Y (NPY).

5-HT/SUBSTANCE P/TRH COEXISTENCE

Several 5-HT neurons in the medulla oblongata contain a substance P-like peptide (Chan-Palay et al., 1978; Hökfelt et al., 1978). They were observed in the midline raphe nuclei and extending laterally over the pyramidal tract into the adjacent pars α of the gigantocellular reticular nucleus, as well as underlying the pyramidal tract close to the ventral surface of the brain (Figure 3; Hökfelt et al., 1978). No evidence for the coexistence of 5-HT and substance P could be obtained in the dorsal raphe nuclei (Hökfelt et al., 1978). Early studies by Dahlström and Fuxe (1965) showed that medullary raphe neurons, at least in part, project to the spinal cord, in agreement with results from classical neuroanatomical studies (Figure 3; Brodal et al., 1960). In rats treated with 5-HT neurotoxins, an almost complete disappearance of substance P-immunoreactive fibers was observed in the ventral horn, a finding which was paralleled by the disappearance of 5-HT fibers (Hökfelt et al., 1978). Similar results have been obtained with biochemical techniques (Björklund et al., 1979; Singer et al., 1979; Gilbert et al., 1982). Gilbert et al. (1981) have demonstrated that reserpine not only depletes 5-HT but also substance P and TRH, further supporting the costorage of these compounds in the same neurons. With electron microscope immunohistochemistry, Pelletier et al. (1981) have shown that 5-HT and substance P are present in the same nerve endings in the ventral horn of the spinal cord, probably stored in the same large dense core vesicles. Biochemical analysis has also revealed a slight drop in substance P immunoreactivity in the dorsal horn after neurotoxin treatment, suggesting that some neurons containing both 5-HT and substance P project to the dorsal horn (Gilbert et al., 1982).

Subsequently, numerous TRH-immunoreactive cell bodies were found in the medullary raphe nuclei and adjacent areas (Johansson and Hökfelt, 1980), and this immunoreactivity could often be observed in 5-HT cell bodies (Hökfelt et al., 1980b). An analysis, including experiments with neurotoxins as above, revealed that the medullary 5-HT neurons seem to contain in some cases both substance P- and TRH-like immunoreactivity, in other cases only one of the peptides, and finally, some 5-HT neurons may not contain either peptide (Johansson et al., 1981). TRH neurons project to the ventral horn of the spinal cord, where TRH-immunoreactive fibers were observed several years ago (Hökfelt et al., 1975). It has been firmly established that spinal cord TRH does not originate in the paraventricular nucleus, as revealed in lesion experiments (Lechan et al., 1983). This nucleus contains TRH cell bodies (Hökfelt et al., 1978; Johansson and Hökfelt, 1980; Lechan and Jackson, 1982) but only other types of peptide-containing neurons in this nucleus do in fact project to the spinal cord (Saper et al., 1976; Swanson, 1977). For a more detailed account of descending 5-HT neurons that contain peptides, I refer the reader to recent analyses using retrograde tracing and immunohistochemical techniques (see, e.g., Bowker et al., 1983). TRH-immunoreactive fibers have so far been observed only in the ventral horn. It is therefore possible that, in contrast to 5-HT and substance P, descending neurons containing TRH project only to the ventral horn.

The possible presence of supraspinal descending 5-HT neurons containing TRH and/or substance P offers a favorable experimental situation for the analysis of a possible functional role of coexisting transmitter candidates. Several studies

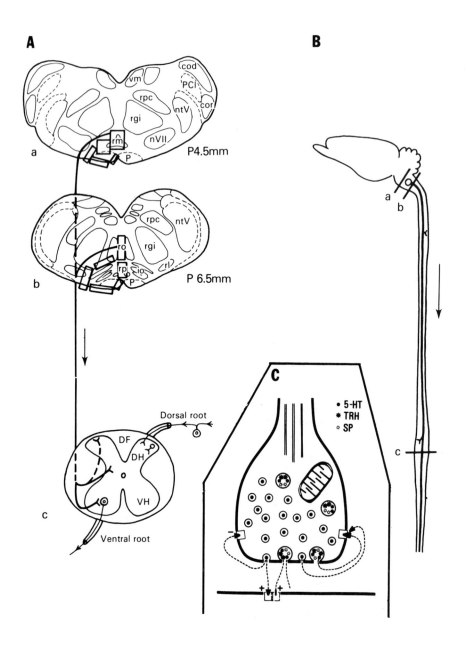

A

vm

cod

PCi

rpc

ntV

cor

rgi

rm

nVII

a

P

P4.5mm

rpc

ntV

ro

rgi

rp

io

rl

b

P

P 6.5mm

Dorsal root

DF

DH

VH

c

Ventral root

B

a

b

c

C

• 5-HT
✳ TRH
○ SP

in the literature provide interesting results, which may be related to the coexistence of these three compounds. The effect of intravenously administered TRH on the stretch reflex in chronically spinalized or 5-HT neurotoxin-treated rats has been studied by Barbeau and Bédard (1981). They observed a marked activation of the stretch reflex, similar to the effect seen after administration of the 5-HT precursor 5-hydroxytryptophan (5-HTP) (see also Andén et al., 1964). Interestingly, the effect of TRH could be blocked by previous administration of a 5-HT antagonist. Barbeau and Bédard (1981) suggested that TRH may act at a site closely associated with the 5-HT receptor. Peripheral administration of TRH may exert effects centrally, since Mitsuma and Nogimori (1983) have provided evidence that intravenous, intraperitoneal, and intramuscular injection of TRH results in the penetration of about 0.2% of the total dose administered into the mouse brain.

The findings of Barbeau and Bédard (1981) suggest that TRH and 5-HT cooperate at synapses in the ventral horn of the spinal cord, either directly or indirectly influencing motoneurons and the muscles involved in the stretch reflex. The experiments of Sharif et al. (1983) indicate that a postsynaptic receptor may be involved. Thus, after destruction of 5-HT/TRH nerve endings by the 5-HT neurotoxin 5,7-dihydroxytryptamine, there was no loss of binding.

Experiments carried out by Mitchell and Fleetwood-Walker (1981) are also of interest. The effect of peptides on the potassium-induced release of 5-HT in spinal cord slices was studied. The addition of substance P or TRH did not influence the potassium-induced tritium outflow from the slices. However, if cold 5-HT was added to the bath in a concentration of 1 mM, a concentration that is known to activate the inhibitory 5-HT presynaptic receptor, substance P, but not TRH, exerted a marked influence on tritium outflow. These experiments were interpreted as indicating that substance P blocks the 5-HT presynaptic receptor and thus 5-HT-induced inhibition of release. Taken together, these results suggest that two compounds, TRH and substance P, may cooperate with the main transmitter (5-HT) to enhance 5-HT transmission. However, the two peptides cause these effects by different mechanisms: substance P by preventing activation of the inhibitory presynaptic 5-HT receptor and TRH by an action closely related to the postsynaptic 5-HT receptor (Figure 3).

Figure 3.   *5-Hydroxytryptamine (5-HT)-containing cell bodies are present in the ventral medulla oblongata including the raphe nuclei as indicated in $A_{a,b}$ and project to the spinal cord as shown in A_c and B. Many* of these 5-HT neurons contain substance P or TRH or both. *Inset C is a schematic representation* of a 5-HT/TRH/substance P synapse in the ventral horn of the spinal cord. According to our hypothesis, 5-HT is present in small and large vesicles, whereas the peptides are found exclusively in large vesicles. 5-HT acts at both post- and presynaptic receptors, substance P at presynaptic receptors, and TRH at postsynaptic receptors. Abbreviations (according to Palkovits and Jacobowitz, 1974): cod, nucleus cochlearis dorsalis; cor, nucleus cochlearis ventralis; DF, dorsal funiculus; DH, dorsal horn; io, nucleus olivaris inferior; ip, nucleus interpenduncularis; ncu, nucleus cuneiformis; ntV, nucleus tractus spinalis nervi trigemini; nIII, nucleus originis nervi oculomotorii; nVII, nucleus originis nervi facialis; P, tractus corticospinalis; PCI, pedunculus cerebellaris inferior; rgi, nucleus reticularis gigantocellularis; rl, nucleus reticularis lateralis; rm, nucleus raphe magnus; ro, nucleus raphe obscurus; rp, nucleus raphe pallidus; rpc, nucleus reticularis parvocellularis; VH, ventral horn; vm, nucleus vestibularis medialis.

This hypothesis has been tested in a behavioral model. Recently, Svensson and Hansen (1984) have demonstrated that descending 5-HT neurons may be involved in the control of certain aspects of sexual behavior. Using this paradigm and intrathecal application of various compounds, several parameters, such as the number of mounts and intromissions, latencies (mount, intromission, and ejaculation), as well as postejaculatory intervals were analyzed in male rats. 5-HT (50 µg), TRH (10 µg), substance P (10 µg), or combinations of these compounds were administered intrathecally via a catheter introduced according to the technique of Yaksh and Rudy (1976). When given alone, no effects of 5-HT were observed at this dose. The effects described earlier by Svensson and Hansen (1984) were obtained with higher doses of 5-HT (200 µg) and involved the number of mounts. A small increase in mount and intromission latencies was observed with 50 µg of 5-HT or 10 µg of TRH. No effects were observed with substance P alone (L. Svensson and S. Hansen, unpublished observations). However, when 5-HT and TRH were given together, a marked increase in both the mount and intromission latencies was observed, from about 0.2 min to more than 7 min. None of the other parameters studied was affected by the combined administration of 5-HT and TRH (Hansen et al., 1983). These results are compatible with the findings obtained in the *in vitro* models described above, suggesting an interaction of 5-HT and TRH at the postsynaptic level.

These findings indicate powerful intrinsic mechanisms for the enhancement of transmission at a particular synapse, in this case the 5-HT synapses in the ventral horn of the spinal cord. The purpose of such hypothetical mechanisms is unknown, but some speculative ideas may be offered. It is well known that certain transmitter–neuron systems are quantitatively small. For example, norepinephrine fibers in the cerebral cortex constitute less than 1% of its total fibers (Descarries and Baudet, 1983) as compared to, for example, GABA synapses, which constitute more than 30% of the synapses in this brain area (Iversen and Bloom, 1972). It may be estimated that 5-HT synapses constitute less than 1% of the synapses on motoneurons in the ventral horn. It is also well known that motoneurons are innervated by a large number of boutons. Thus, a single motoneuron may have up to 10,000 synapses of many different types impinging upon its dendrites and soma (S. Conradi, personal communication). As a result, there is only a small possibility that a restricted system such as the descending 5-HT system can influence the impulse activity in motoneurons in competition with all other systems in a decisive way. Enhancement of 5-HT transmission by coexisting peptides, as shown schematically in Figure 4, may help to convey a message of high priority by overriding other neuronal inputs to the motoneurons.

Other interesting 5-HT/TRH/substance P system interactions have been reported. Sharif et al. (1983) have demonstrated an increase in the binding of TRH analogues to spinal cord membranes after the depletion of 5-HT and TRH from the spinal cord by neurotoxins. This may indicate that spinal cord TRH receptors become supersensitive after the depletion of TRH. Mueller et al. (1984) have also demonstrated supersensitivity to TRH after neurotoxin destruction of 5-HT (and TRH) neurons in a respiratory experimental paradigm. Furthermore, Sharif and Burt (1983) have shown that substance P in micromolar concentrations reduces receptor binding for TRH in the spinal cord.

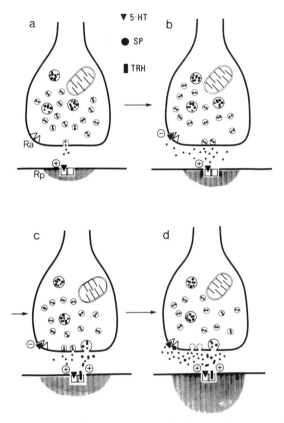

Figure 4. *Schematic representation of hypothetical events leading to enhancement of 5-HT transmission at nerve endings in the ventral horn of the spinal cord. a*: At low impulse activity, only 5-HT is released, activating the postsynaptic receptor (Rp). *b*: With increased activity, additional amounts of 5-HT are released, activating the inhibitory presynaptic receptor (Ra) and causing inhibition of further 5-HT release. *c* and *d*: With a further increase in impulse traffic, the peptides are released—TRH activates a postsynaptic receptor, resulting in an enhanced response (*c*), and substance P acts on a presynaptic receptor, leading to a blockade of 5-HT inhibition of 5-HT release. In this way a maximal response is obtained (*d*).

Some 5-HT/substance P neurons may project to the dorsal horn of the spinal cord. Fasmer and Post (1983) observed scratching and biting of hind parts of the body after intrathecal injection of 5-HT and substance P. Interestingly, substance P antagonists reduced not only the effect of substance P but also that of 5-HT in this model. This may indicate a close proximity of the substance P and 5-HT receptors involved in this behavior, similar to the 5-HT/TRH interaction described above in the studies of spinal reflexes by Barbeau and Bédard (1981).

Finally, pharmacological experiments have revealed complex changes. Savard et al. (1983) demonstrated that neonatal thyroidectomy caused an increase in TRH levels in the ventral horn of the spinal cord. Inhibition of 5-HT synthesis with parachlorophenylalanine abolished this effect, suggesting a relationship between 5-HT and TRH in these spinal systems. Pradhan et al. (1981) analyzed the effects of cocaine and 5-HTP on substance P-like and 5-HT immunoreactivities in various brain nuclei. No effects were seen in the medullary raphe areas, but significant changes in levels were observed in the dorsal medullary nuclei. As discussed above, the dorsal medullary nuclei do not exhibit the coexistence of substance P and 5-HT, whereas coexistence is observed in the medullary raphe areas. Barden et al. (1983) showed that the 5-HT neurotoxin parachloramphetamine and the 5-HT synthesis inhibitor parachlorophenylalanine caused changes in the substance P content of many areas, as did administration of the 5-HT receptor antagonist methysergide. An important aspect of these findings is that the majority of interactions between peptides and amines may reflect an interaction between two compounds that are stored in separate systems and that are either directly or indirectly in functional contact, rather than reflecting the coexistence of the two compounds in one system.

DA/CCK COEXISTENCE

Vanderhaeghen and his collaborators (Vanderhaeghen et al., 1975) first provided evidence for the occurrence of a gastrin/CCK-like peptide in the central nervous system of the rat. Subsequently, several groups initiated work in this area, and it could be established that the peptide present in the brain was mainly the carboxy-terminal octapeptide of the CCK molecule (CCK-8) (Dockray, 1976; Müller et al., 1977; Dockray et al., 1978; Rehfeld, 1978; Robberbrecht et al., 1978; Larsson and Rehfeld, 1979; Beinfeld, 1981; Beinfeld and Palkovits, 1981).

Biochemical and immunohistochemical studies revealed a wide distribution of CCK in most brain areas, with particularly high concentrations in cortical regions (Innis et al., 1979; Larsson and Rehfeld, 1979; Lorén et al., 1979; Vanderhaeghen et al., 1980). Numerous CCK-immunoreactive cell bodies were observed in the ventral mesencephalon (Hökfelt et al., 1980c,d; Vanderhaeghen et al., 1980). It was established that many of these CCK cell bodies were identical to DA cell bodies by using tyrosine hydroxylase (TH) antiserum in the elution–restaining technique (Hökfelt et al., 1980c,d; Figure 5). The distribution of DA/CCK cell bodies exhibits marked regional variations (Figure 6). Virtually all DA cell bodies contain CCK-like immunoreactivity in the pars compacta of the anterior substantia nigra and in the pars lateralis of the substantia nigra. In the ventral tegmental area (A10 cell group; nomenclature according to Dahlström and Fuxe, 1964), it has been calculated that about 40% of all DA cell bodies have CCK-like immunoreactivity. In addition, there is a small number (about 5%) of CCK-immunoreactive neurons in the A10 area that lack TH-like immunoreactivity. No DA/CCK neurons have so far been observed in the pars reticulata of the substantia nigra.

These findings suggest that not all DA neurons contain a CCK-like peptide. Furthermore, DA/CCK neurons may project to specific brain regions. In fact, in certain forebrain areas CCK-immunoreactive fibers have a distribution closely overlapping that of DA fibers: the posterior medial nucleus accumbens, the posterior medial tuberculum olfactorium, the bed nucleus of the stria terminalis, the periventricular region, the cauda of the caudate nucleus, and the central amygdaloid nucleus (Figure 7; Hökfelt et al., 1980d). The main part of the caudate

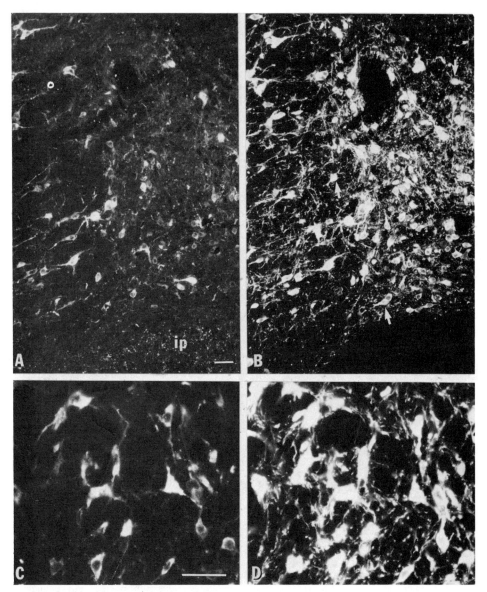

Figure 5. *Immunofluorescence micrographs of the ventral tegmental area (A10 cell group) after incubation with antiserum to cholecystokinin (CCK) (A and C).* Numerous cell bodies and some fibers are seen in the interpeduncular nucleus (ip). After $KMnO_4$ elution, the same section was restained with tyrosine hydroxylase (TH) antiserum (*B* and *D*). Virtually all CCK-positive cell bodies are also TH-immunoreactive, but there are also TH-positive/CCK-negative cell bodies (*arrows*). Note the lack of TH-positive nerve endings in the ip. *Calibration bars = 50 μm.*

191

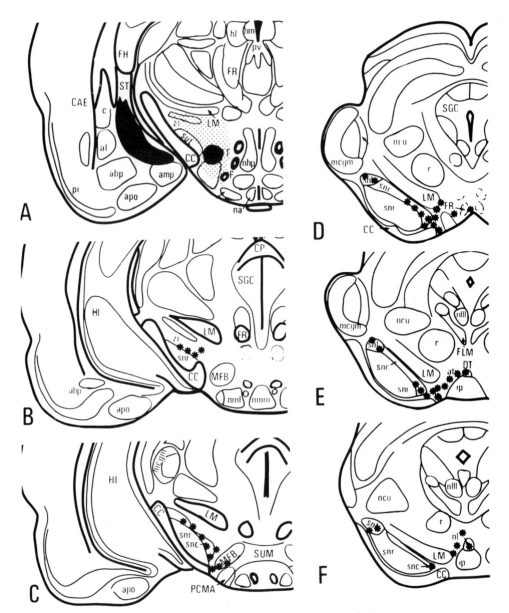

Figure 6. *Schematic representation of the distribution of dopamine (DA)/CCK cell bodies* (asterisks) *at various frontal levels of the mesencephalon of the rat.* Abbreviations: abp, nucleus amygdaloideus basalis posterior; al, nucleus amygdaloideus lateralis; amp, nucleus amygdaloideus medialis posterior; apo, nucleus amygdaloideus posterior; atv, area tegmentalis ventralis Tsai; c, cingulum; CAE, capsula externa; CC, crus cerebri; CP, commissura posterior; DT, decussationes tegmenti; FH, fimbria hippocampi; FLM, fasciculus longitudinalis medialis; FMT, fasciculus mamillo-thalamicus; FR, fasciculus retroflexus; HI, hippocampus; hl, nucleus habenulae lateralis; hm, nucleus habenulae medialis; ip, nucleus interpeduncularis; LM, lemniscus medialis; mcgm, nucleus marginalis corporis geniculati medialis; MFB, fasciculus medialis prosencephali (medial forebrain bundle); na, nucleus arcuatus; ncu, nucleus cuneiformis; nhp, nucleus hypothalamicus posterior; nl, nucleus linearis pars caudalis; nml, nucleus mamillaris lateralis; nmm, nucleus mamillaris medialis; nIII, nucleus originis nervi oculomotorii; PCMA, pedunculus corporis mamillaris; pi, cortex piriformis; pv, nucleus periventricularis thalami; r, nucleus ruber; SGC, substantia grisea centralis; snc, substantia nigra zona compacta; snl, substantia nigra pars lateralis; snr, substantia nigra zona reticularis; ST, stria terminalis; SUM, decussatio supramamillaris; sut, nucleus subthalamicus; zi, zona incerta. (From Hökfelt et al., 1980d.)

192

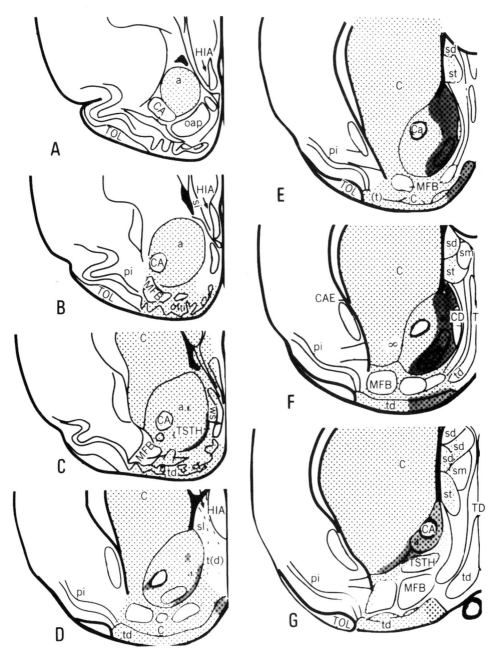

Figure 7. *Schematic representation of the distribution of DA fibers* (dotted area) *and DA and CCK fibers with overlapping distribution* (shaded area) *at various frontal levels of the ventral forebrain of the rat.* At these levels, note that DA/CCK coexistence is in all probability confined mainly to caudal medial areas of the nucleus accumbens and the tuberculum olfactorium. Abbreviations: a, nucleus accumbens; C, nucleus caudatus putamen; CA, commissura anterior; HIA, hippocampus anterior; iC, insulae Callejae; iCm, insula Callejae magna; oap, nucleus olfactorius anterior pars posterior; sd, nucleus dorsalis septi; sl, nucleus lateralis septi; sm, nucleus medialis septi; TD, tractus diagonalis Broca; td, nucleus tractus diagonalis Broca; TOL, tractus olfactorius lateralis; TSTH, tractus striohypothalamicus; tu, tuberculum olfactorium. Other abbreviations as in Figure 6. (From Hökfelt et al., 1980d.)

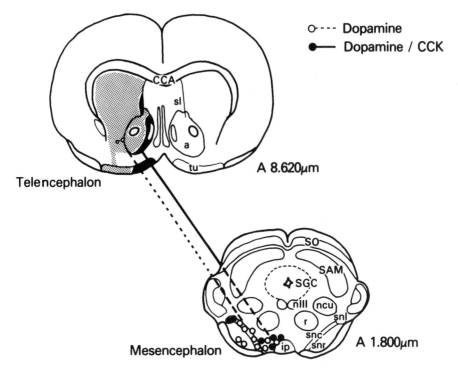

Figure 8. *Schematic representation of DA and DA/CCK neurons in the ventral mesencephalon projecting to the telencephalic areas.* Abbreviations (according to Jacobowitz and Palkovits, 1974): a, nucleus accumbens; CCA, corpus callosum; sl, nucleus lateralis sept; tu, tuberculum olfactorium. Other abbreviations as in Figure 3.

nucleus seems, however, to receive its CCK innervation from cortical regions (Meyer et al., 1982).

By combining the technique of retrograde tracing with immunohistochemistry (see Hökfelt et al., 1983b; Skirboll et al., 1984), it was established that neurons containing both CCK- and TH-like immunoreactivities located in the ventral tegmental area (A10 DA cell bodies) project to the medial accumbens (Hökfelt et al., 1980d; Figure 8). The retrograde tracer True Blue (Bentivoglio et al., 1979) was injected into the medial posterior nucleus accumbens. Two days later, the rats received an intraventricular injection of colchicine to increase the cell body levels of CCK and after 24 hours the brains were cut on a cryostat. The sections were analyzed in the fluorescence microscope and True Blue-stained cells in the ventral mesencephalon were photographed. The sections were then incubated with CCK antiserum and the immunoreactive cells were photographed. The CCK staining was subsequently eluted with acid potassium permanganate (Tramu et al., 1978), and the sections were incubated with TH antiserum (for control, see above). The TH-positive patterns were photographed and compared to the CCK-immunoreactive and True Blue-positive cell bodies. Several cells in the A10 area were observed to contain True Blue and both CCK- and TH-like immunoreactivities (Hökfelt et al., 1980d). The origin of the CCK/TH-positive fibers in the central amygdaloid nucleus has also been analyzed with this combined technique. It was found that they originate, in part, in the pars lateralis of substantia nigra (L. R. Skirboll and T. Hökfelt, unpublished observations).

The coexistence of a CCK-like peptide and DA in forebrain synapses was supported by neurotoxin experiments. The number of both CCK- and TH-positive fibers in, for example, the bed nucleus of the stria terminalis was reduced after intraventricular injection of 6-hydroxydopamine (Hökfelt et al., 1980d). This is in agreement with biochemical studies based on 6-hydroxydopamine treatment, as well as with lesion experiments (Studler et al., 1981; Williams et al., 1981; Marley et al., 1982; Gilles et al., 1983). These studies showed decreases in CCK levels in, for example, the medial nucleus accumbens, whereas no effects were observed in the head of the caudate nucleus, suggesting a heterogeneity of the DA systems. Furthermore, pharmacological experiments showed that reserpine treatment causes a decrease in CCK-8 in the posterior but not in the anterior part of the nucleus accumbens (Studler et al., 1984), further supporting the coexistence of dopamine and CCK peptides.

Immunohistochemical analysis of some other species has revealed interesting similarities and differences (Hökfelt et al., 1985). In the cat, a much larger proportion of nigral DA neurons seems to contain a CCK-like peptide. Virtually all DA neurons in the zona compacta and pars lateralis contain CCK-like immunoreactivity, whereas many neurons in the medial aspects (A10 area) seem to lack the peptide. The distribution of DA and CCK fiber systems in the forebrain are in agreement with these findings, with overlapping fields of densely packed TH- and CCK-positive terminals in the nucleus caudatus putamen. Preliminary observations suggest that the situation in the monkey is more similar to the one seen in the rat, with cell bodies containing both TH- and CCK-like immunoreactivity in the medial aspects of the ventral mesencephalon, that is, in the A10 area.

The question of the functional significance of the coexistence of DA and a CCK-like peptide has been approached in several studies. Some attempts have been made to investigate possible interactions between DA and CCK at the level of the cell bodies in the ventral mesencephalon, whereas others have focused on terminal areas, that is, the presumptive synapses at which DA and CCK-like peptides are released.

Skirboll et al. (1981) analyzed the effects of iontophoretically applied sulfated (S) and nonsulfated (NS) CCK-7 on DA neurons by using extracellular single unit recording techniques. CCK-7S, but not CCK-7NS, increased the activity of the neurons present in areas with CCK/TH-immunoreactive cell bodies. This effect can be blocked by proglumide (Chiodo and Bunney, 1983), a CCK antagonist (Hahne et al., 1981). In contrast, no such activation could be observed in areas where DA neurons that apparently lacked CCK-like immunoreactivity were present. These results were obtained by analyzing the localization of the extracellular recording site by using the immunohistochemical technique subsequent to the electrophysiological experiments (Skirboll et al., 1981). In some cases, the increase in firing rate induced by CCK was so strong that the neurons were driven into apparent depolarization inactivation.

One possible explanation for these findings is that DA/CCK neurons contain autoreceptors for CCK, and that CCK may exert a direct depolarizing action. Other mechanisms of action may also be considered. CCK may (1) increase the release of an endogenous excitatory transmitter; (2) cause a potentiation of the action of an excitatory agent; or (3) cause a decrease in the release or in the effectiveness of an endogenous inhibitory transmitter such as GABA (Skirboll et al., 1981). More recently, Hommer and Skirboll (1983) have analyzed the effect of intravenously administered CCK-7S (and ceruletide) on the apomorphine-induced inhibition of DA neurons. A significant shift to the left of the apomorphine dose–response curve was observed, suggesting that the peptides induce supersensitivity of the DA autoreceptor. Thus, these findings also support the idea that CCK may act on a receptor located on the DA neurons. In this connection, it may be mentioned that there are nondopamine CCK fibers mainly in the lateral part of the pars compacta of the substantia nigra; it cannot be excluded that iontophoretically applied CCK may act on receptors for CCK released from nondopamine neurons.

Possible interactions between DA and CCK have also been recorded in the forebrain. An increase in the firing rate of neurons after local microiontophoretic administration of CCK-8S into the dorsomedial nucleus accumbens has been observed (White and Wang, 1984). This increase, but not glutamate-induced excitation, can be blocked by proglumide. Initial studies in the rat suggested a possible inhibitory effect of CCK on DA release in the medial nucleus accumbens (Hökfelt et al., 1980a). However, in vitro experiments in which more advanced methodology was used indicate that CCK-7S and CCK-8S, but not their unsulphated forms, enhance electrically induced DA release in slices of the medial nucleus accumbens and medial tuberculum olfactorium (Markstein et al., 1986). Only minor effects were obtained when the same experiments were carried out on slices from the caudate nucleus. In contrast, Hamilton et al. (1984) have recently been unable to observe any effects of cerulein in concentrations of 10^{-9} to 10^{-4} M on the potassium-evoked release of carbon-labeled DA from the nucleus accumbens in vitro. However, in another recent study Voigt and Wang (1984) have demonstrated that CCK-8S suppresses the release of endogenous DA induced by high potassium. In this in vivo push–pull cannula model, the tip was positioned in the medial caudal part of nucleus accumbens which, as described above, contains overlapping CCK- and TH-immunoreactive terminal fields.

The diverse results obtained above may indicate that the rat DA/CCK coexistence system may not be ideal for the analysis of possible interactions between the two compounds. The areas exhibiting coexistence are limited, and it may not always be possible to confine the analysis to this particular area. Therefore, we have studied the cat in which, as described above, most nigral DA neurons and their terminals in the forebrain contain CCK-like immunoreactivity. Thus, the entire nucleus caudatus putamen is available for experiments in this species. In in vitro superfusion experiments, small tissue cylinders (3 mm in diameter) of cat neostriatum were incubated with tritiated DA, and both the electrically induced and the basal outflow of radioactive DA were analyzed (Markstein and Hökfelt, 1984). The outflow was shown to be calcium-dependent and could be abolished by tetrodotoxin, suggesting that the release is induced by action potentials. CCK-8S, but not its unsulfated form, inhibited both the basal and electrically induced tritium outflow at concentrations as low as 10^{-14} M, with the maximum at 10^{-11} M. These effects were observed when bovine serum albumin (BSA) and bacitracin were present in the media. In contrast, without these two agents in the buffer, an enhancement of tritium outflow was seen at concentrations of 10^{-7} M. The different effects, apparently depending on the incubation medium, are at present difficult to explain. The present findings, which are basically in agreement with the results of Voigt and Wang (1984), suggest the possibility that CCK released from DA terminals at very low concentrations may exert an inhibitory action on DA release. A local feedback inhibition mediated by presynaptic DA receptors has been also described in striatal tissues (see Langer and Shepperson, 1982; Starke, 1982).

Possible interactions of CCK and DA have been studied in behavioral models. In rats implanted with a cannula in the A10 ventral tegmental area, a reduction in the number and in the duration of rearing was seen after infusions into the ventral tegmental area (Schneider et al., 1983). A reduction in rearing behavior was also observed after injections into the nucleus accumbens. The effects were seen only when amphetamine was used to stimulate behavior and only when CCK-8S was administered. Crawley et al. (1985) observed potentiation of DA-induced hyperlocomotion and apomorphine-induced stereotypy when DA and CCK were injected directly into the nucleus accumbens. CCK alone, however, had no effects on these behavioral parameters, and no potentiation of these behaviors could be seen when CCK and DA were injected together into the caudate nucleus. No consistent effects of CCK-8 on amphetamine-induced locomotion and apomorphine-induced stereotypies could be observed after intraventricular administration of the peptide, according to Widerlöv et al. (1983a,b). CCK peptides have been demonstrated to exert neurolepticlike effects (Zetler, 1981, 1983a,b; Van Ree et al., 1983; Fekete et al., 1984), which represents another link to dopaminergic mechanisms. Finally, it should be noted that other types of peptide–amine interactions may occur. For example, Hole et al. (1984) have provided evidence that CCK-8 can reduce brain TH activity.

The existence of CCK receptors in the central nervous system has been demonstrated with biochemical and autoradiographic methods (Hays et al., 1980, 1981; Innis and Snyder 1980a,b; Saito et al., 1980, 1981; Zarbin et al., 1981, 1983; Van Dijk et al., 1984). Interesting effects of CCK peptides on the binding of DA agonists and antagonists have been reported, suggesting that such peptides may modulate DA receptors (Fuxe et al., 1981a,b; Murphy and Schuster, 1982; Agnati et al., 1983a,b; Mashal et al., 1983; Mishra, 1983). For example, CCK-8 in a concentration of 10^{-8} M reduces both the B_{max} and K_D values of striatal [^{3}H]spiperone binding sites (Agnati et al., 1983b). In binding studies, effects of the shorter peptide fragment, the carboxy-terminal tetrapeptide of CCK (CCK-4), have been recorded (Agnati et al., 1983a,b). Murphy and Schuster (1982) have observed the modulation of [^{3}H]dopamine binding by the CCK-8S peptide in striatal homogenates. A reduction in the number of [^{3}H]spiperone binding sites in the striatum after the intraventricular administration of CCK-8 was shown by Mashal et al. (1983). One further example of an interesting interaction is the regional changes in DA turnover in the caudate nucleus observed after intraventricular administration of CCK-8S (Fuxe et al., 1980, 1981b; Fekete et al., 1981a,b). In these studies, however, the effects have been analyzed in rat striatal tissues, that is, in an area where DA and CCK peptides in all probability do not coexist but occur in anatomically separate systems (see above).

The occurrence of a CCK-like peptide in certain DA neurons (particularly in the limbic system) in the rat, monkey, and possibly humans may be of interest with regard to the DA hypothesis of schizophrenia (see Randrup and Munkvad, 1972; Matthysse and Kety, 1975; Crow, 1978; Stevens, 1979). In recent studies, Moroji et al. (1982), Nair et al. (1982, 1983), and Van Ree et al. (1985) have presented results suggesting that peripherally administered CCK or CCK-like peptides (ceruletide) may cause a beneficial effect in schizophrenic patients. According to the DA hypothesis, at least some of the symptoms manifested may be related to overactivity in the limbic DA neurons. The results of these clinical investigations could be explained if CCK-like peptides exert an inhibitory influence on DA release, as is indicated in some of the studies discussed above. Because very low concentrations (as little as 10^{-14} M) seem to be able to inhibit dopamine release in the cat striatum (Markstein and Hökfelt, 1984), it is not impossible that a peripherally administered peptide can reach the brain in sufficient concentrations to cause such effects. It should also be mentioned again that several groups have demonstrated that CCK-8 and related peptides may produce behavioral effects in animal experiments that are similar to those observed after neuroleptic treatment (Zetler 1981, 1983a,b; Van Ree et al., 1983; Fekete et al., 1984).

So far only a few studies have been carried out to investigate CCK levels in the cerebrospinal fluid of patients or in postmortem brains. Verbanck et al. (1984) have reported a significant decrease in CCK immunoreactivity in the cerebrospinal fluid of patients with untreated schizophrenia. However, it is not possible to relate this decrease in CCK to a specific system in the brain. Roberts et al. (1983) have observed decreases in CCK-like immunoreactivity in the hippocampus, amygdala, and temporal cortex of schizophrenic patients.

SUBSTANCE P AND CGRP

Alternative processing of RNA transcripts from the calcitonin gene can result in the production of two different messenger RNAs encoding, respectively, the hormone calcitonin and the neuropeptide CGRP (Amara et al., 1982; Rosenfeld et al., 1983). Whereas processing to calcitonin is the major pathway in the thyroid gland, the production of CGRP occurs mainly in neuronal tissues (Amara et al., 1982; Rosenfeld et al., 1983). On the basis of the structural analysis of calcitonin gene expression, a synthetic polypeptide corresponding to a portion of the predicted carboxy-terminal sequence was synthesized, and antiserum was raised against it (Rosenfeld et al., 1983). The antiserum was used for both immunohistochemistry and radioimmunoassay. The immunohistochemical analysis revealed widespread distribution of CGRP-immunoreactive neurons in the central and peripheral nervous system, for example, in the cell bodies of such central motor nuclei as the facial nucleus and the hypoglossal nucleus, as well as in primary sensory ganglia (Rosenfeld et al., 1983). It has also been demonstrated that CGRP can be released by potassium from cultured rat trigeminal ganglion cells (Mason et al., 1984).

The characteristic distribution of CGRP in primary sensory ganglion cells, as well as in fibers in the dorsal horn of the spinal cord (Figure 9A, B) and in the spinal trigeminal nucleus (Rosenfeld et al., 1983), raised the question of the relation of these neurons to earlier subclasses of primary sensory neurons identified

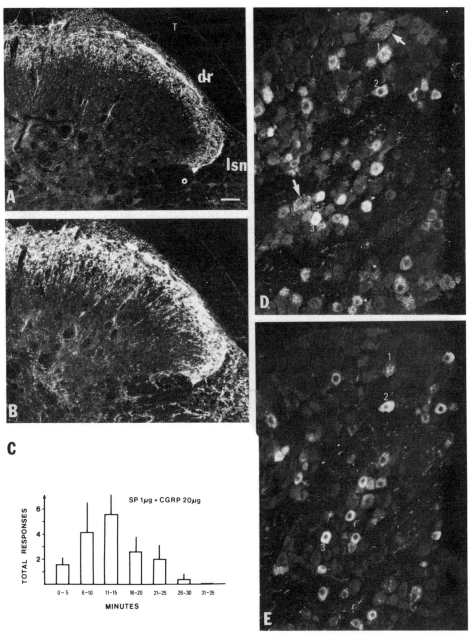

Figure 9. *Immunofluorescence micrographs of the dorsal horn of the spinal cord* (A *and* B) *and spinal ganglion* (D *and* E) *of the rat after incubation with antiserum to CGRP* (A *and* D) *and substance P* (B *and* E). *A and B, as well as D and E, represent adjacent sections, respectively.* A *and* B: Note the distribution overlap of CGRP- and substance P-like immunoreactivities in the superficial layers of the dorsal horn. No CGRP-, but numerous substance P-positive, fibers are seen in the lateral spinal nucleus (lsn). In the deeper layers of the dorsal horn, there are more substance P- than CGRP-positive fibers. D *and* E: Virtually all substance P-positive cell bodies contain CGRP-like immunoreactivity (1–3 indicate some examples). In addition, many CGRP-positive/substance P-negative cell bodies (*big arrows*) can be seen. Note that substance P-positive/CGRP-positive cells are often smaller than substance P-negative/CGRP-positive cells. C: A long-lasting biting and scratching response can be seen after intrathecal administration of 1 μg substance P + 20 μg CGRP. *Calibration bar* = 50 μm. All micrographs are of the same magnification. (From Wiesenfeld-Hallin et al., 1984.)

199

on the basis of their peptide content. For example, substance P- and somatostatinlike immunoreactivities occur in two different populations of small-sized primary sensory neurons (Hökfelt et al., 1976). A recent analysis has revealed that virtually all substance P-immunoreactive neurons in spinal ganglia seem to contain CGRP-like immunoreactivity, but that there is in addition a population of neurons that exhibits only CGRP-like immunoreactivity (Figure 9D, E; Wiesenfeld-Hallin et al., 1984).

Previous studies have shown that CGRP exerts certain effects in the central nervous system. Thus, intraventricularly administered CGRP causes a rise in plasma norepinephrine levels as well as a dose-related elevation of mean arterial pressure and heart rate (Fisher et al., 1983). In contrast, intravenously injected CGRP evokes a rapid decrease in mean arterial pressure (Fisher et al., 1983). In view of this biological activity, we have studied whether coexisting CGRP and substance P may exert any interactive effects on primary sensory neuron function. It had been shown that intraspinally or intrathecally administered substance P causes a characteristic behavior consisting of caudally directed biting and scratching (CBS) of the flanks and hind limbs when it is injected at lumbar levels (Hylden and Wilcox, 1981; Piercey et al., 1981; Seybold et al., 1982). In agreement, our experiments showed a dose-dependent CBS lasting for a few minutes after intrathecal administration of substance P (Wiesenfeld-Hallin et al., 1984). In doses up to 20 µg, CGRP alone did not cause any observable response. However, when the two compounds were administered together, a long-lasting CBS response was seen. 10 µg of substance P plus 20 µg of CGRP induced CBS behavior lasting up to 40 min (Wiesenfeld-Hallin et al., 1984). Even 1 µg of substance P plus 20 µg of CGRP caused a long-lasting response (Figure 9C). These results indicate an interaction of the two peptides, culminating in a marked prolongation of this particular behavior. Further studies are needed to clarify the mechanism behind this response, but the findings suggest interesting interactions between two compounds stored in and possibly released from the same primary sensory synapses. Studies are now in progress to elucidate whether similar interactions occur at the peripheral branches of primary sensory neurons.

LEUKOTRIENES AND LHRH NEURONS

Leukotrienes (LT) represent a new group of bioactive compounds belonging to the arachidonic acid family (see Samuelsson, 1983). They have been found in the cells of certain peripheral tissues (for example, as their name would suggest, in leukocytes) and are assumed to be mediators of inflammatory and allergic reactions (see Samuelsson, 1983). They are formed from arachidonic acid via 5-lipoxygenation to an unstable epoxide, LTA_4, which can be enzymatically hydrolyzed to LTB_4 or LTC_4 by the addition of the tripeptide glutathione (Murphy et al., 1979; Morris et al., 1980). Successive enzymatic elimination of glutamic acid and glycine from the glutathione molecule results in conversion to LTD_4 and LTE_4, respectively (Örning and Hammarström, 1980; Bernström and Hammarström, 1981).

The possible occurrence of leukotrienes in other tissues has been investigated. Using high-performance liquid chromatography, radioimmunoassays, and bioassays, evidence was obtained that LTC_4, LTD_4, and LTE_4 can be formed in brain tissue after the incubation of slices with an ionophore and arachidonic acid (Lindgren et al., 1984). *In vitro* biosynthesis of LTC_4 occurred in most regions of the brain, with the highest production occurring in the hypothalamus and the median eminence. Immunohistochemical methods employing an antiserum raised to LTC_4 (Aehringhaus et al., 1982) revealed LTC_4-like immunoreactivity in fiber networks in the median eminence, located mainly in the lateral parts of its external layer. In control experiments, these fibers were not seen after incubation with LTC_4 antiserum pretreated with LTC_4–BSA conjugate (Lindgren et al., 1984). Preabsorption with glutathione in concentrations about 10 times higher also prevented fiber staining in the median eminence, but preabsorption with LTC_4 alone did not reduce staining intensity. Thus, the nature of the compound in the external layer of the median eminence reacting with our LTC_4 antiserum is still unclear but may represent an LTC_4-like or glutathionelike compound.

The distribution patterns of LTC_4-like immunoreactivity in the median eminence resembled staining patterns observed earlier with LHRH antiserum (see Barry, 1979). Elution–restaining experiments undertaken according to Tramu et al. (1978) clearly indicated that the vast majority of LTC_4-positive boutons also contained an LHRH-like peptide (Hulting et al., 1985).

The identity of LTC_4- and LHRH-positive synapses in the median eminence suggested a possible role for LTC_4 in the regulation of LH secretion. Dispersed cultures of anterior pituitary cells were therefore incubated with LTC_4 in various concentrations, and the LH released into the incubation medium was measured with radioimmunoassays (Hulting et al., 1984, 1985). A stimulatory effect of LTC_4 could be seen after 15 min of incubation. This effect was seen at concentrations as low as 10^{-14} M, with a maximum at 10^{-12} M. No effects were observed with LTB_4 in a similar concentration range, and LTC_4 (or LTB_4) did not seem to affect the release of growth hormone. The time course for LH release was considerably more rapid for LTC_4 than for LHRH (Hulting et al., 1985). We have therefore speculated that LH release may be under the control of two factors—LHRH and an LTC_4 (or glutathione)-like compound—possibly stored in and released from the same nerve endings in the median eminence. The second compound may be responsible for rapid and short-lasting LH release, whereas LHRH induces a response with a slower onset and of a longer duration.

CONCLUSIONS

In this chapter, I have focused attention on some neuronal systems that contain more than one messenger (for example, a classical transmitter and a peptide or several peptides) and have discussed the present status of the functional significance of this coexistence phenomenon. On the basis of a peripheral system, the cat salivary gland, in which parasympathetic and sympathetic innervation represent coexistence systems, evidence is presented that a classical transmitter and a peptide act postsynaptically in a cooperative manner to induce a certain physiological response. Other modes of interaction may also occur—a peptide may inhibit the release of a classical transmitter, as seems to be the case in the vas deferens of the rat (Figure 10). In the central nervous system, bulbospinal neurons

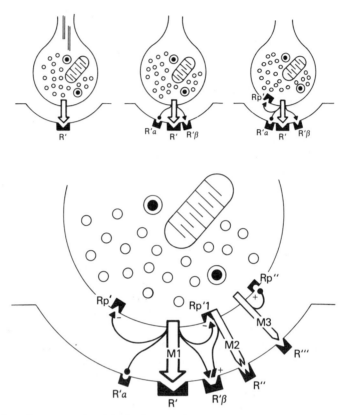

Figure 10. *Schematic representation of the development of the concept of chemical transmission. Top:* Various phases of the "one neuron–one transmitter" concept are shown, in which the transmitter affects one postsynaptic receptor (R'), multiple postsynaptic receptors (R', R'α, R'β), and a presynaptic receptor (autoreceptor, Rp'). *Bottom:* The release of several messengers (M1–M3) and how they may interact at pre- and postsynaptic levels is depicted. (From Lundberg and Hökfelt, 1983.)

containing substance P- and TRH-like immunoreactivities and DA neurons containing a CCK-like peptide were discussed. In central systems, multiple messengers may also strengthen transmission at synaptic (and nonsynaptic) sites or, alternatively, the peptide may inhibit transmitter release. Clearly, there is no single type of interaction characteristic for all systems, but a variety of mechanisms may operate.

In general terms, multiple messengers may serve the purpose of increasing the capacity for information transfer in a given system. Although the redundancy in the nervous system is often pointed out, it may also be relevant to consider the idea that there is a need to utilize the huge but still finite number of neurons in the most efficient way—to achieve the tremendous operational capacity of our brains. Perhaps transmission via multiple messengers is needed to accomplish this performance with the neuronal machinery available. On the other hand, it should be emphasized that, at present, the correlation of coexistence and the possible co-release of several messengers at synapses with certain pharmacological, physiological, or behavioral effects remains to be shown. It cannot be excluded that the coexistence of multiple messengers is a paraphenomenon, perhaps representing sequelae in evolution. During one phase, peptides may have been important messenger molecules but subsequently were functionally replaced by more efficient small molecule transmitters and are now perhaps carried on as more or less "silent passengers." Future work using more sophisticated experimental models will be needed to establish the significance of the coexistence of multiple messengers in the nervous system.

ACKNOWLEDGMENTS

This research was supported by grants from the Swedish Medical Research Council (04X-2887), Knut and Alice Wallenbergs Stiftelse, and Magnus Bergvalls Stiftelse. We thank Mrs. W. Hiort, Miss A. Peters, and Miss S. Kleinau for excellent technical assistance and Mrs. E. Björklund for skillful help in preparing the manuscript. Figures 1, 3, 8, and 10 were produced by the medical illustration department of the National Institutes of Health while T.H. was a Fogarty Scholar. The scholarship and support of Dr. M. Brownstein of the National Institute of Mental Health and Dr. P. Condliffe of the National Institutes of Health are gratefully acknowledged.

REFERENCES

Aehringhaus, U., R. H. Wölbling, W. König, C. Patrono, B. M. Peskar, and B. Peskar (1982) Release of leukotriene C_4 from human polymorphonuclear leucocytes as determined by radioimmunoassay. FEBS Lett. **146**:111–114.

Agnati, L. F., M. F. Celani, and K. Fuxe (1983a) Cholecystokinin peptides in vitro modulate the characteristics of the striatal ³H-N-propylnorapomorphine sites. Acta Physiol. Scand. **118**:79–81.

Agnati, L. F., K. Fuxe, F. Benfenati, B. M. F. Celani, N. Battistini, V. Mutt, L. Cavicchioli, G. Galli, and T. Hökfelt (1983b) Differential modulation by CCK-8 and CCK-4 of [³H]spiperone binding sites linked to dopamine and 5-hydroxytryptamine receptors in the brain of the rat. Neurosci. Lett. **35**:179–183.

Allen, J. M., K. Tatemoto, J. M. Polak, J. Hughes, and S. R. Bloom (1982) Two novel related peptides, neuropeptide Y (NPY) and peptide YY (PYY), inhibit the contraction of the electrically stimulated mouse vas deferens. Neuropeptides **3**:71–77.

Amara, S. G., V. Jonas, M. G. Rosenfeld, E. S. Ong, and R. M. Evans (1982) Alternative RNA-processing in calcitonin gene expression generates mRNAs encoding different polypeptide products. Nature **298**:240–244.

Andén, N.-E., M. Jukes, and A. Lundberg (1964) Spinal reflexes and monoamine liberation. Nature **202**:1222–1223.

Barbeau, H., and P. Bédard (1981) Similar motor effects of 5-HT and TRH in rats following chronical spinal transection and 5,7-dihydroxytryptamine injection. Neuropharmacology **20**:477–481.

Barden, N., M. Daigle, V. Picard, and T. Di Paolo (1983) Perturbation of rat brain serotonergic systems results in an inverse relation between substance P and serotonin concentrations measured in discrete nuclei. J. Neurochem. **41**:834–840.

Barry, J. (1979) Immunohistochemistry of luteinizing hormone-releasing hormone produced in neurons of the vertebrates. Int. Rev. Cytol. **60**:179–221.

Beinfeld, M. C. (1981) An HPLC and RIA analysis of the cholecystokinin peptide in rat brain. *Neuropeptides* 1:203–209.

Beinfeld, M. C., and M. Palkovits (1981) Distribution of cholecystokinin (CCK) in the hypothalamus and limbic system of the rat. *Neuropeptides* 2:123–129.

Bentivoglio, M., H. G. J. M. Kuypers, C. Catsman-Berrevoets, and O. Dann (1979) Fluorescent retrograde neuronal labeling in rat by means of substances binding specifically to adenine–thymine rich DNA. *Neurosci. Lett.* 12:235–240.

Bernard, C. (1858) De l'influence de deux ordres de nerfs qui déterminent les variations de couleur du sang veineux dans les organes glandulaires. *C. R. Seances Acad. Sci.* 47:245–253.

Bernström, K., and S. Hammarström (1981) Metabolism of leukotriene D by porcine kidney. *J. Biol. Chem.* 256:9579–9582.

Björklund, A., P. C. Emson, R. T. F. Gilbert, and G. Skagerberg (1979) Further evidence for the possible coexistence of 5-hydroxytryptamine and substance P in medullary raphe neurones of rat brain. *Br. J. Pharmacol.* 66:112–113.

Bowker, R. M., K. N. Westlund, M. C. Sullivan, J. F. Wilber, and J. D. Coulter (1983) Descending serotonergic, peptidergic and cholinergic pathways from the raphe nuclei: A multiple transmitter complex. *Brain Res.* 288:33–48.

Brodal, A., E. Taber, and F. Walberg (1960) The raphe nuclei of the brain stem in the cat. II. Efferent connections. *J. Comp. Neurol.* 114:239–259.

Chan-Palay, V., and S. L. Palay (1984) *Coexistence of Neuroactive Substances in Neurons*, Wiley, New York.

Chan-Palay, V., G. Jonsson, and S. L. Palay (1978) Serotonin and substance P coexist in neurons of the rat's central nervous system. *Proc. Natl. Acad. Sci. USA* 75:1582–1586.

Charnay, Y., L. Léger, F. Dray, A. Bérod, M. Jouvet, J. F. Pujol, and P. M. Dubois (1982) Evidence for the presence of enkephalin in catecholaminergic neurons of cat locus coeruleus. *Neurosci. Lett.* 30:147–151.

Chiodo, L. A., and B. S. Bunney (1983) Proglumide: Selective antagonism of excitatory effects of cholecystokinin in central nervous system. *Science* 219:1449–1451.

Coons, A. H. (1958) Fluorescent antibody methods. In *General Cytochemical Methods*, J. F. Danielli, ed., pp. 399–422, Academic, New York.

Crawley, J. N., J. A. Stivers, L. K. Blumstein, and S. M. Paul (1985) Cholecystokinin potentiates dopamine-mediated behaviors—Evidence for modulation specific to a site of coexistence. *J. Neurosci.* 5:1972–1983.

Crow, T. J. (1978) An evaluation of the dopamine hypothesis of schizophrenia. In *The Biological Basis of Schizophrenia*, G. Hemmings and W. A. Hemmings, eds., pp. 63–78, MTP Press, Lancaster, England.

Cuello, A. C. (1982) *Co-Transmission*, MacMillan, London.

Dahlström, A., and K. Fuxe (1964) Evidence of the existence of monoamine-containing neurons in the central nervous system. I. Demonstration of monoamines in the cell bodies of brain stem neurons. *Acta Physiol. Scand. (Suppl.)* 62:1–55.

Dahlström, A., and K. Fuxe (1965) Evidence for the existence of monoamine-containing neurons in the central nervous system. II. Experimentally induced changes in the intraneuronal levels of bulbospinal neuron system. *Acta Physiol Scand. (Suppl.)* 64:5–36.

Descarries, L., and A. Baudet (1983) The use of radioautography for investigating transmitter-specific neurons. *Handb. Chem. Neuroanat., Methods in Chemical Neuroanatomy* 1:286–364.

Dockray, G. J. (1976) Immunochemical evidence of cholecystokinin-like peptides in brain. *Nature* 264:568–570.

Dockray, G. J., R. A. Gregory, J. B. Hutchinson, J. J. Harris, and M. J. Runswick (1978) Isolation, structure and biological activity of two cholecystokinin octapeptides from sheep brain. *Nature* 274:711–713.

Eckenstein, F., and R. W. Baughman (1984) Two types of cholinergic innervation in cortex, one co-localized with vasoactive intestinal polypeptide. *Nature* 309:153–155.

Elliott, T. R. (1905) The action of adrenalin. *J. Physiol. (Lond.)* 32:401–407.

Emmelin, N. (1967) Nervous control of salivary glands. *Handb. Physiol., Alimentary Canal* **2**:595–632.

Emmelin, N. (1972) Control of salivary glands. In *Oral Physiology*, N. Emmelin and Y. Zotterman, eds., pp. 1–16, Pergamon, Oxford.

Everitt, B. J., T. Hökfelt, L. Terenius, K. Tatemoto, V. Mutt, and M. Goldstein (1984) Differential co-existence of neuropeptide Y (NPY)-like immunoreactivity with catecholamines in the central nervous system of the rat. *Neuroscience* **11**:443–462.

Fasmer, O. B., and C. Post (1983) Behavioral responses induced by intrathecal injection of 5-hydroxytryptamine in mice are inhibited by a substance P antagonist, D-Pro^2, D-Trp^{7,9}-substance P. *Neuropharmacology* **22**:1397–1400.

Fekete, M., T. Kádár, B. Penke, K. Kovács, and G. Telegdy (1981a) Influence of cholecystokinin octapeptide sulphate ester on brain monoamine metabolism in rats. *J. Neural Transm.* **50**:81–88.

Fekete, M., M. Várszegi, T. Kádár, B. Penke, K. Kovács, and G. Telegdy (1981b) Effects of cholecystokinin octapeptide sulfate ester on brain monoamines in rats. *Acta Physiol. Acad. Sci. Hung.* **56**:37–46.

Fekete, M., Á. Lengyel, B. Hegedüs, B. Penke, M. Zarándy, G. K. Tóth, and G. Telegdy (1984) Further analysis of the effects of cholecystokinin octapeptides on avoidance behaviour in rats. *Eur. J. Pharmacol.* **98**:79–91.

Fisher, L. A., D. O. Kikkawa, J. E. Rivier, S. G. Amara, R. M. Evans, M. G. Rosenfeld, W. W. Vale, and M. R. Brown (1983) Stimulation of noradrenergic sympathetic outflow by calcitonin gene-related peptide. *Nature* **305**:534–536.

Fried, G., L. Terenius, T. Hökfelt, and M. Goldstein (1985) Evidence for differential localization of noradrenaline and neuropeptide Y (NPY) in neuronal storage vesicles isolated from vas deferens. *J. Neurosci.* **5**:437–442.

Fuxe, K., K. Andersson, V. Locatelli, L. F. Agnati, T. Hökfelt, L. Skirboll, and V. Mutt (1980) Cholecystokinin in peptides produces marked reduction of dopamine turnover in discrete areas in the rat brain following intraventricular injection. *Eur. J. Pharmacol.* **67**:329–331.

Fuxe, K., L. F. Agnati, F. Benfenati, M. Cimmino, S. Algeri, T. Hökfelt, and V. Mutt (1981a) Modulation by cholecystokinins of ^{3}H-spiroperidol binding in rat striatum: Evidence for increased affinity and reduction in the number of binding sites. *Acta Physiol. Scand.* **113**:567–569.

Fuxe, K., L. F. Agnati, C. Köhler, D. Kuonen, S.-O. Ögren, K. Andersson, and T. Hökfelt (1981b) Characterization of normal and supersensitive dopamine receptors: Effects of ergot drugs and neuropeptides. *J. Neural Transm.* **51**:3–37.

Geffen, L. B., D. G. Livett, and R. A. Rush (1969) Immunohistochemical localization of protein component of catecholamine storage vesicles. *J. Physiol. (Lond.)* **204**:593–605.

Gilbert, R. F. T., G. W. Bennett, C. A. Marsden, and P. C. Emson (1981) The effects of 5-hydroxytryptamine-depleting drugs on peptides in the ventral spinal cord. *Eur. J. Pharmacol.* **76**:203–210.

Gilbert, R. F. T., P. C. Emson, S. P. Hunt, G. W. Bennett, C. A. Marsden, B. E. B. Sandberg, H. Steinbusch, and A. A. J. Verhofstad (1982) The effects of monoamine neurotoxins on peptides in the rat spinal cord. *Neuroscience* **7**:69–88.

Gilles, C., F. Lotstra, and J. J. Vanderhaeghen (1983) CCK nerve terminals in the rat striatal and limbic areas originate partly in the brain stem and partly in telencephalic structures. *Life Sci.* **32**:1683–1690.

Glazer, E. J., H. Steinbusch, A. Verhofstad, and A. T. Basbaum (1981) Serotonin neurons in nucleus raphe dorsalis and paragigantocellularis of the cat contain enkephalin. *J. Physiol. (Paris)* **77**:241–245.

Hahne, W. F., R. T. Jensen, G. F. Lemp, and J. D. Gardner (1981) Proglumide and benzotript: Members of a different class of cholecystokinin receptor antagonists. *Proc. Natl. Acad. Sci. USA* **78**:6304–6308.

Hamilton, M., M. J. Sheehan, J. de Belleroche, and L. J. Herberg (1984) The cholecystokinin analogue, caerulein, does not modulate dopamine release or dopamine-induced locomotor activity in the nucleus accumbens of rat. *Neurosci. Lett.* **44**:77–82.

Hansen, S., L. Svensson, T. Hökfelt, and B. J. Everitt (1983) 5-hydroxytryptamine–thyrotropin releasing hormone interactions in the spinal cord: Effects on parameters of sexual behaviour in the male rat. *Neurosci. Lett.* **42**:299–304.

Hays, S. E., M. C. Beinfeld, R. T. Jensen, F. K. Goodwin, and S. M. Paul (1980) Demonstration of a putative receptor site for cholecystokinin in rat brain. *Neuropeptides* **1**:53–62.

Hays, S. E., F. K. Goodwin, and S. M. Paul (1981) Cholecystokinin receptors in brain: Effects of obesity, drug treatment and lesion. *Peptides* **2**:21–26.

Heidenhain, R. (1872) Ueber die Wirkung einiger Gifte auf die Nerven der glandula submaxillaris. *Pflügers Arch.* **5**:309–318.

Hökfelt, T., K. Fuxe, O. Johansson, S. Jeffcoate, and N. White (1975) Thyrotropin-releasing hormone (TRH)-containing nerve terminals in certain brain stem nuclei and in the spinal cord. *Neurosci. Lett.* **9**:133–139.

Hökfelt, T., R. Elde, O. Johansson, R. Luft, G. Nilsson, and A. Arimura (1976) Immunohistochemical evidence for separate populations of somatostatin-containing and substance P-containing primary afferent neurons in the rat. *Neuroscience* **1**:131–136.

Hökfelt, T., L. G. Elfvin, R. Elde, M. Schultzberg, M. Goldstein, and R. Luft (1977) Occurrence of somatostatin-like immunoreactivity in some peripheral sympathetic noradrenergic neurons. *Proc. Natl. Acad. Sci. USA* **74**:3587–3591.

Hökfelt, T., Å. Ljungdahl, H. Steinbusch, A. Verhofstad, G. Nilsson, E. Brodin, B. Pernow, and M. Goldstein (1978) Immunohistochemical evidence of substance P-like immunoreactivity in some 5-hydroxytryptamine-containing neurons in the rat central nervous system. *Neuroscience* **3**:517–538.

Hökfelt, T., O. Johansson, Å. Ljungdahl, J. M. Lundberg, and M. Schultzberg (1980a) Peptidergic neurons. *Nature* **284**:515–521.

Hökfelt, T., J. M. Lundberg, M. Schultzberg, O. Johansson, Å. Ljungdahl, and J. Rehfeld (1980b) Coexistence of peptides and putative transmitters in neurons. In *Neural Peptides and Neuronal Communication*, E. Costa and M. Trabucchi, eds., pp. 1–23, Raven, New York.

Hökfelt, T., J. F. Rehfeld, L. Skirboll, B. Ivemark, M. Goldstein, and K. Markey (1980c) Evidence for coexistence of dopamine and CCK in mesolimbic neurones. *Nature* **285**:476–478.

Hökfelt, T., L. Skirboll, J. F. Rehfeld, M. Goldstein, K. Markey, and O. Dann (1980d) A subpopulation of mesencephalic dopamine neurons projecting to limbic areas contains a cholecystokinin-like peptide: Evidence from immunohistochemistry combined with retrograde tracing. *Neuroscience* **5**:2093–2124.

Hökfelt, T., J. M. Lundberg, L. Skirboll, O. Johansson, M. Schultzberg, and S. R. Vincent (1982) Coexistence of classical transmitters and peptides in neurons. In *Co-Transmission*, A. C. Cuello, ed., pp. 77–126, MacMillan, London.

Hökfelt, T., J. M. Lundberg, H. Lagercrantz, K. Tatemoto, V. Mutt, L. Terenius, B. J. Everitt, K. Fuxe, L. F. Agnati, and M. Goldstein (1983a) Occurrence of neuropeptide Y (NPY)-like immunoreactivity in catecholamine neurones in the human medulla oblongata. *Neurosci. Lett.* **36**:217–222.

Hökfelt, T., G. Skagerberg, L. Skirboll, and A. Björklund (1983b) Combination of retrograde tracing and neurotransmitter histochemistry. *Handb. Chem. Neuroanat.*, *Methods in Chemical Neuroanatomy* **1**:228–285.

Hökfelt, T., B. J. Everitt, E. Theodorsson-Norheim, and M. Goldstein (1984a) Occurrence of neurotensinlike immunoreactivity in subpopulations of hypothalamic, mesencephalic, and medullary catecholamine neurons. *J. Comp. Neurol.* **222**:543–559.

Hökfelt, T., O. Johansson, and M. Goldstein (1984b) Chemical anatomy of the brain. *Science* **225**:1326–1334.

Hökfelt, T., L. Skirboll, B. J. Everitt, B. Meister, M. Brownstein, T. Jacobs, A. Faden, S. Kuga, M. Goldstein, R. Markstein, G. Dockray, and J. Rehfeld (1985) Distribution of cholecystokinin-like immunoreactivity in the nervous system with special reference to coexistence with classical neurotransmitters and other neuropeptides. *Ann. N.Y. Acad. Sci.* **448**:255–274.

Hole, K., P. V. Russo, and A. J. Mandell (1984) Neuropeptide influence on amines: Cholecystokinin-8 and neurotensin reduce brain tyrosine hydroxylase activity. *Prog. Neuropsychopharmacol. Biol. Psychiatry (Suppl.)* **8**:171.

Hommer, D. W., and L. R. Skirboll (1983) Cholecystokinin-like peptides potentiate apomorphine-induced inhibition of dopamine neurons. *Eur. J. Pharmacol.* **91**:151–152.

Hulting, A.-L., J.-Å. Lindgren, T. Hökfelt, K. Heidvall, P. Eneroth, S. Werner, C. Patrono, and B. Samuelsson (1984) Leukotriene C_4 stimulates LH secretion from rat pituitary cells *in vitro. Eur. J. Pharmacol.* **106**:459–460.

Hulting, A.-L., J.-Å. Lindgren, T. Hökfelt, P. Eneroth, S. Werner, C. Patrono, and B. Samuelsson (1985) Leukotriene C_4 as a mediator of LH release from rat anterior pituitary cells. *Proc. Natl. Acad. Sci. USA* **82**:3834–3838.

Hunt, S. P., and T. A. Lovick (1982) The distribution of serotonin, metenkephalin and β-lipotropin-like immunoreactivity in neuronal perikarya of the cat brain stem. *Neurosci. Lett.* **30**:139–145.

Hylden, J. L. K., and G. L. Wilcox (1981) Intrathecal substance P elicits a caudally-directed biting and scratching behavior in mice. *Brain Res.* **217**:212–215.

Innis, R. B., and S. H. Snyder (1980a) Distinct cholecystokinin receptors in brain and pancreas. *Proc. Natl. Acad. Sci. USA* **77**:6917–6921.

Innis, R. B., and S. H. Snyder (1980b) Cholecystokinin receptor binding in brain and pancreas: Regulation of pancreatic binding by cyclic and acyclic guanyl nucleotides. *Eur. J. Pharmacol.* **65**:123–124.

Innis, R. B., F. M. A. Correa, G. R. Uhl, B. Schneider, and S. H. Snyder (1979) Cholecystokinin octapeptide-like immunoreactivity: Histochemical localization in rat brain. *Proc. Natl. Acad. Sci. USA* **76**:521–525.

Itoh, N., K. Obata, N. Yanaihara, and H. Okamoto (1983) Human prepro-vasoactive intestinal polypeptide contains a novel PHI-27-like peptide, PHM-27. *Nature* **304**:547–549.

Iversen, L. L., and F. E. Bloom (1972) Studies of the uptake of ^{3}H-GABA and ^{3}H-glycine in slices and homogenates of rat brain and spinal cord by electron microscopic autoradiography. *Brain Res.* **41**:131–143.

Jacobowitz, D. M., and M. Palkovits (1974) Topographic atlas of catecholamine- and acetylcholinesterase-containing neurons in the rat brain. I. Forebrain (Telencephalon, Diencephalon). *J. Comp. Neurol.* **157**:13–28.

Johansson, O., and T. Hökfelt (1980) Thyrotropin-releasing hormone, somatostatin, and enkephalin: Distribution studies using immunohistochemical techniques. *J. Histochem. Cytochem.* **28**:364–366.

Johansson, O., T. Hökfelt, B. Pernow, S. L. Jeffcoate, N. White, H. W. M. Steinbusch, A. A. J. Verhofstad, P. C. Emson, and E. Spindel (1981) Immunohistochemical support for three putative transmitters in one neuron: Coexistence of 5-hydroxytryptamine-, substance P-, and thyrotropin-releasing hormone-like immunoreactivity in medullary neurons projecting to the spinal cord. *Neuroscience* **6**:1857–1881.

Johnson, D. G., and G. M. de C Nogueira Araujo (1981) A simple method of reducing the fading of immunofluorescence during microscopy. *J. Immunol. Methods* **43**:349.

Kangawa, K., N. Minamoto, A. Fukuda, and H. Matsuo (1983) Neuromedin K: A novel mammalian tachykinin identified in porcine spinal cord. *Biochem. Biophys. Res. Comm.* **114**:533–540.

Kimura, S., M. Okada, Y. Sugita, I. Kanazawa, and E. Munekata (1983) Novel neuropeptides, neurokinin α and β, isolated from porcine spinal cord. *Proc. Jpn. Acad.* **59**:101.

Kuypers, H. G. J. M., and A. M. Huisman (1984) Fluorescent retrograde tracers. *Adv. Cell. Neurobiol.* **5**:307–340.

Langer, S. Z., and N. B. Shepperson (1982) The role of presynaptic receptors in the modulation of neurotransmission. *Proc. Int. Congr. Pharmacol.* **2**:81–91.

Larsson, L.-I., and J. F. Rehfeld (1979) Localization and molecular heterogeneity of cholecystokinin in the central and peripheral nervous system. *Brain Res.* **165**:201–218.

Lechan, R. M., and I. M. D. Jackson (1982) Immunohistochemical localization of thyrotropin-releasing hormone in the rat hypothalamus and pituitary. *Endocrinology* **111**:55–65.

Lechan, R. M., S. B. Snapper, and I. M. D. Jackson (1983) Evidence that spinal cord thyrotropin-releasing hormone is independent of the paraventricular nucleus. *Neurosci. Lett.* **43**:61–65.

Lindgren, J. Å., T. Hökfelt, S.-E. Dahlén, C. Patrono, and B. Samuelsson (1984) Leukotrienes in the rat central nervous system. *Proc. Natl. Acad. Sci. USA* **81**:6212–6216.

Lorén, I., J. Alumets, R. H. Håkanson, and F. Sundler (1979) Distribution of gastrin- and cholecystokinin-like peptides in rat brain. *Histochemistry* **59**:249–257.

Lovick, T. A., and S. P. Hunt (1983) Substance P-immunoreactive and serotonin-containing neurones in the ventral brainstem of the cat. *Neurosci. Lett.* **36**:223–228.

Ludwig, C. (1851) Neue Versuche über die Beihilfe der Nerven zur Speichelabsonderung. *Z. Med. Rationelle* **1**:255–277.

Lundberg, J. M., and T. Hökfelt (1983) Coexistence of peptides and classical neurotransmitters. *Trends Neurosci.* **6**:325–333.

Lundberg, J. M., and K. Tatemoto (1982) Pancreatic polypeptide family (APP, BPP, NPY and PYY) in relation to sympathetic vasoconstriction resistant to α-adrenoceptor blockade. *Acta Physiol. Scand.* **116**:393–402.

Lundberg, J. M., T. Hökfelt, M. Schultzberg, K. Uvnäs-Wallensten, C. Köhler, and S. I. Said (1979) Occurrence of vasoactive intestinal polypeptide (VIP)-like immunoreactivity in certain cholinergic neurons of the cat: Evidence from combined immunohistochemistry and acetylcholine esterase staining. *Neuroscience* **4**:1539–1559.

Lundberg, J. M., G. Fried, J. Fahrenkrug, B. Holmstedt, T. Hökfelt, H. Lagercrantz, G. Lundgren, and A. Änggård (1981) Subcellular fractionation of cat submandibular gland: Comparative studies on the distribution of acetylcholine and vasoactive intestinal polypeptide (VIP). *Neuroscience* **6**:1001–1010.

Lundberg, J. M., B. Hedlund, A. Änggård, J. Fahrenkrug, T. Hökfelt, K. Tatemoto, and T. Bartfai (1982a) Costorage of peptides and classical transmitters in neurons. In *Systemic Role of Regulatory Peptides*, S. R. Bloom, J. M. Polak, and E. Lindenlaub, eds., pp. 93–119, Schottauer, Stuttgart.

Lundberg, J. M., B. Hedlund, and T. Bartfai (1982b) Vasoactive intestinal polypeptide (VIP) enhances muscarinic ligand binding in the cat submandibular salivary gland. *Nature* **295**:147–149.

Lundberg, J. M., L. Terenius, T. Hökfelt, C. R. Martling, K. Tatemoto, V. Mutt, J. Polak, S. R. Bloom, and M. Goldstein (1982c) Neuropeptide Y (NPY)-like immunoreactivity in peripheral noradrenergic neurons and effects of NPY on sympathetic function. *Acta Physiol. Scand.* **116**:477–480.

Markstein, R., and T. Hökfelt (1984) Effect of cholecystokinin-octapeptide on dopamine release from slices of cat caudate nucleus. *J. Neurosci.* **4**:570–575.

Markstein, R., L. Skirboll, and T. Hökfelt (1986) Cholecystokinin-like peptides increase dopamine release from brain slices. *Eur. J. Pharmacol.* (submitted).

Marley, P. D., P. C. Emson, and J. F. Rehfeld (1982) Effect of 6-hydroxydopamine lesions of the medial forebrain bundle on the distribution of cholecystokinin in rat forebrain. *Brain Res.* **252**:382–385.

Mashal, R. D., F. Owen, J. F. W. Deakin, and M. Poulter (1983) The effects of cholecystokinin on dopaminergic mechanisms in rat striatum. *Brain Res.* **277**:375–376.

Mason, R. T., R. A. Peterfreund, P. E. Sawchenko, A. Z. Corrigan, J. E. Rivier, and W. W. Vale (1984) Release of the predicted calcitonin gene-related peptide from cultured rat trigeminal ganglion cells. *Nature* **308**:653–655.

Matthysse, S., and S. S. Kety, eds. (1975) *Catecholamines and Schizophrenia*, Pergamon, Oxford.

Meyer, D. K., M. C. Beinfeld, W. H. Oertel, and M. J. Brownstein (1982) Origin of the cholecystokinin-containing fibers in the rat caudatoputamen. *Science* **215**:187–188.

Mishra, R. K. (1983) Modulation of CNS dopamine receptors by peptides. *Prog. Neuro-Psychopharmacol. Biol. Psychiatry* **7**:437–442.

Mitchell, R., and S. Fleetwood-Walker (1981) Substance P, but not TRH, modulates the 5-HT autoreceptor in ventral lumbar spinal cord. *Eur. J. Pharmacol.* **76**:119–120.

Mitsuma, T., and T. Nogimori (1983) Influence of the route of administration on thyrotropin-releasing hormone concentration in the mouse brain. *Experientia (Basel)* **39**:620–622.

Moroji, T., N. Watanabe, N. Aoki, and S. Ito (1982) Antipsychotic effects of ceruletide (coerulein) on chronic schizophrenia. *Arch. Gen. Psychiatry* **39**:485–486.

Morris, H. R., G. W. Taylor, P. J. Piper, and J. R. Tippins (1980) Structure of slow-reacting substance of anaphylaxis from guinea-pig lung. *Nature* **285**:104–106.

Mueller, R. A., A. C. Towle, and G. R. Breese (1984) Supersensitivity to the respiratory stimulatory effect of TRH in 5,7-dihydroxytryptamine-treated rats. *Brain Res.* **298**:370–373.

Müller, J. E., E. Straus, and R. W. Yalow (1977) Cholecystokinin and its COOH-terminal octapeptide in the pig brain. *Proc. Natl. Acad. Sci. USA* **74**:3035–3037.

Murphy, R. B., and D. I. Schuster (1982) Modulation of [^{3}H]dopamine binding by cholecystokinin octapeptide (CCK-8). *Peptides* **3**:539–543.

Murphy, R. C., S. Hammarström, and B. Samuelsson (1979) Leukotriene C: A slow-reacting substance from murine mastocytoma cells. *Proc. Natl. Acad. Sci. USA* **76**:4275–4279.

Mutt, V., and S. I. Said (1974) Structure of the porcine vasoactive intestinal octacosapeptide. The amino-acid sequence. Use of kallikrein in its determination. *Eur. J. Biochem.* **42**:581–589.

Nair, N. P. V., D. M. Bloom, and J. N. Nestoros (1982) Cholecystokinin appears to have antipsychotic properties. *Prog. Neuropsychopharmacol. Biol. Psychiatry* **6**:509–512.

Nair, N. P. V., D. M. Bloom, J. N. Nestoros, and G. Schwarz (1983) Therapeutic efficacy of cholecystokinin in neuroleptic-resistant schizophrenic subjects. *Psychopharmacol. Bull.* **19**:134–136.

Nawa, H., T. Hirose, H. Takashima, S. Inayama, and S. Nakanishi (1983) Nucleotide sequences of cloned cDNAs for two types of bovine brain substance P precursor. *Nature* **306**:32–36.

Oertel, W. H., A. M. Graybiel, E. Mugnaini, R. P. Elde, D. E. Schmechel, and E. J. Kopin (1983) Coexistence of glutamic acid decarboxylase- and somatostatin-like immunoreactivity in neurons of the feline nucleus reticularis thalami. *J. Neurosci.* **3**:1322–1332.

Örning, L., and S. Hammarström (1980) Inhibition of leukotriene C$_4$ and leukotriene D$_4$ synthesis. *J. Biol. Chem.* **255**:8023–8026.

Otsuka, M., and T. Takahashi (1977) Putative peptide neurotransmitters. *Annu. Rev. Pharmacol. Toxiocol.* **17**:425–439.

Palkovits, M., and D. M. Jacobowitz (1974) Topographic atlas of catecholamine- and acetylcholinesterase-containing neurons in the rat brain. II. Hindbrain (Mesencephalon, Rhombencephalon). *J. Comp. Neurol.* **157**:29–41.

Pease, P. C. (1962) Buffered formaldehyde as a killing agent and primary fixative for electron microscopy. *Anat. Rec.* **142**:342.

Pelletier, G., H. W. Steinbusch, and A. Verhofstad (1981) Immunoreactive substance P and serotonin present in the same dense core vesicles. *Nature* **293**:71–72.

Piercey, M. F., P. J. K. Dobry, L. A. Schroeder, and F. J. Einspahr (1981) Behavioral evidence that substance P may be a spinal cord sensory neurotransmitter. *Brain Res.* **210**:407–412.

Platt, J. L., and A. F. Michael (1983) Retardation of fading and enhancement of intensity of immunofluorescence by *p*-phenylenediamine. *J. Histochem. Cytochem.* **31**:840–842.

Pradhan, S., G. Hanson, and W. Lovenberg (1981) Inverse relation of substance P-like immunoreactivity in dorsal raphe nucleus to serotonin levels in pons–medulla following administration of cocaine and 5-hydroxytryptophan. *Biochem. Pharmacol.* **30**:1071–1076.

Randrup, A., and I. Munkvad (1972) Evidence indicating an association between schizophrenia and dopaminergic hyperactivity in the brain. *Orthomol. Psychiat.* **1**:2–7.

Rehfeld, J. F. (1978) Immunohistochemical studies on cholecystokinin. II. Distribution and molecular heterogeneity in the central nervous system and small intestine of man and hog. *J. Biol. Chem.* **253**:4022–4030.

Robberbrecht, P., M. Deschodt-Lanckman, and J. J. Vanderhaeghen (1978) Demonstration of biological activity of brain gastrin-like peptidic material in the human: Its relationship with the COOH-terminal octapeptide of cholecystokinin. *Proc. Natl. Acad. Sci. USA* **75**:524–528.

Roberts, G. W., I. N. Ferrier, Y. Lee, T. J. Crow, E. C. Johnstone, D. G. C. Owens, A. J. Bacarese-Hamilton, G. McGregor, D. O'Shaughnessey, J. M. Polak, and S. R. Bloom (1983) Peptides, the limbic lobe and schizophrenia. *Brain Res.* **288**:199–211.

Rosenfeld, M. G., J.-J. Mermod, S. G. Amara, L. W. Swanson, P. E. Sawchenko, J. Rivier, W. W. Vale, and R. M. Evans (1983) Production of a novel neuropeptide encoded by the calcitonin gene via tissue-specific RNA processing. *Nature* **304**:129–135.

Said, S. I., and V. Mutt (1970) Polypeptide with broad biological activity. Isolation from small intestine. *Science* **169**:1217–1218.

Saito, A., H. Sankaran, I. D. Goldfine, J. A. Williams (1980) Cholecystokinin receptors in the brain: Characterization and distribution. *Science* **208**:1155–1156.

Saito, A., I. D. Goldfine, and J. A. Williams (1981) Characterization of receptors for cholecystokinin and related peptides in mouse cerebral cortex. *J. Neurochem.* **37**:483–490.

Samuelsson, B. (1983) Leukotrienes: Mediators of immediate hypersensitivity reactions and inflammation. *Science* **220**:568–575.

Saper, C. B., A. D. Loewy, L. W. Swanson, and W. M. Cowan (1976) Direct hypothalamo-autonomic connections. *Brain Res.* **117**:305–312.

Savard, P., Y. Mérand, P. Bédard, J. H. Dussault, and A. Dupont (1983) Comparative effects of neonatal hypothyroidism and euthyroidism on TRH and substance P content of lumbar spinal cord in saline and PCPA-treated rats. *Brain Res.* **277**:263–268.

Schneider, L. H., J. E. Alpert, and S. D. Iversen (1983) CCK-8 modulation of mesolimbic dopamine: Antagonism of amphetamine-stimulated behaviours. *Peptides* **4**:749–753.

Seybold, V. S., J. L. K. Hylden, and G. L. Wilcox (1982) Intrathecal substance P and somatostatin in rats: Behaviors indicative of sensation. *Peptides* **3**:49–54.

Sharif, N. A., and D. R. Burt (1983) Micromolar substance P reduces spinal receptor binding for thyrotropin-releasing hormone—Possible relevance to neuropeptide coexistence. *Neurosci. Lett.* **43**:245–251.

Sharif, N. S., D. R. Burt, A. C. Towle, R. A. Mueller, and G. R. Breese (1983) Codepletion of serotonin and TRH induces apparent supersensitivity of spinal TRH receptors. *Eur. J. Pharmacol.* **95**:301–304.

Singer, E., G. Sperk, P. Placheta, and S. E. Leeman (1979) Reduction of substance P levels in the cervical spinal cord of the rat after intracisternal 5,7-dihydroxytryptamine injection. *Brain Res.* **174**:362–365.

Skirboll, L., A. A. Grace, D. W. Hommer, J. Rehfeld, M. Goldstein, T. Hökfelt, and S. Bunney (1981) Peptide monoamine coexistence: Studies of the actions of a cholecystokinin-like peptide on the electrical activity of midbrain dopamine neurons. *Neuroscience* **6**:2111–2124.

Skirboll, L., T. Hökfelt, G. Norell, O. Phillipson, H. G. J. M. Kuypers, M. Bentivoglio, C. E. Catsman-Berrevoets, T. J. Visser, H. Steinbusch, A. Verhofstad, A. C. Cuello, M. Goldstein, and M. Brownstein (1984) A method for specific transmitter identification of retrogradely labeled neurons: Immunofluorescence combined with fluorescence tracing. *Brain Res. Rev.* **8**:99–127.

Snyder, S. H. (1980) Brain peptides as neurotransmitters. *Science* **209**:976–983.

Starke, K. (1982) Presynaptic autoreceptors. *Proc. Int. Congr. Pharmacol.* **2**:81–91.

Stevens, J. R. (1979) Schizophrenia and dopamine regulation in the mesolimbic system. *Trends Neurosci.* **2**:102–105.

Stjärne, L., and J. M. Lundberg (1984) Neuropeptide Y (NPY) depresses the secretion of ^{3}H-noradrenaline and the contractile response evoked by field stimulation in rat vas deferens. *Acta Physiol. Scand.* **120**:477–479.

Stjärne, L., P. Hedqvist, H. Lagercrantz, and Å. Wennmalm (1981) *Chemical Neurotransmission*, Academic, London.

Studler, J. M., H. Simon, F. Cesselin, J. C. Legrand, J. Glowinski, and J. P. Tassin (1981) Biochemical investigation of the localisation of the cholecystokinin octapeptide in dopaminergic neurons originating from the ventral tegmental area of the rat. *Neuropeptides* **2**:131–139.

Studler, J. M., M. Reibaud, G. Tramu, G. Blanc, J. Glowinski, and P. Tassin (1984) Pharmacological study on the mixed CCK8/DA mesonucleus accumbens pathway: Evidence for the existence of storage sites containing the two transmitters. *Brain Res.* **298**:91–97.

Svensson, L., and S. Hansen (1984) Spinal monoaminergic modulation of masculine copulatory behavior in the rat. *Brain Res.* **302**:315–321.

Swanson, L. W. (1977) Immunohistochemical evidence for a neurophysin-containing autonomic pathway arising in the paraventricular nucleus of the hypothalamus. *Brain Res.* **128**:356–363.

Tatemoto, K. (1982) Neuropeptide Y: Complete amino acid sequence of the brain peptide. *Proc. Natl. Acad. Sci. USA* **79**:5485–5489.

Tatemoto, K., M. Carlquist, and V. Mutt (1982) Neuropeptide Y—A novel brain peptide with structural similarities to peptide YY and pancreatic polypeptide. *Nature* **296**:659–660.

Tramu, G., A. Pillez, and J. Leonardelli (1978) An efficient method of antibody elution for the successive or simultaneous location of two antigens by immunocytochemistry. *J. Histochem. Cytochem.* **26**:322–324.

Vanderhaeghen, J. J., J. C. Signeau, and W. Gepts (1975) New peptide in the vertebrate CNS reacting with antigastrin antibodies. *Nature* **257**:604–605.

Vanderhaeghen, J. J., F. Lotstra, J. De May, and C. Gilles (1980) Immunohistochemical localization of cholecystokinin- and gastrin-like peptides in the brain and hypophysis of the rat. *Proc. Natl. Acad. Sci. USA* **77**:1190–1194.

Van Dijk, A., J. G. Richards, A. Trzeciak, D. Gillessen, and H. Möhler (1984) Cholecystokinin receptors: Biochemical demonstration and autoradiographical localization in rat brain and pancreas using [^{3}H]cholecystokinin-8 as radioligand. *J. Neurosci.* **4**:1021–1033.

Van Ree, J. M., O. Gaffori, and D. de Wied (1983) In rats, the behavioural profile of CCK-8 related peptides resembles that of antipsychotic agents. *Eur. J. Pharmacol.* **93**:63–78.

Van Ree, J. M., W. M. B. Verhoeven, G. J. Brouwer, and D. de Wied (1985) Ceruletide resembles antipsychotics in rats and schizophrenic patients. *Neuropsychobiology* **12**:4–8.

Verbanck, P. M. P., F. Lotstra, C. Gilles, P. Linkowski, J. Mendlewicz, and J. J. Vanderhaeghen (1984) Reduced cholecystokinin immunoreactivity in the cerebrospinal fluid of patients with psychiatric disorders. *Life Sci.* **34**:67–72.

Vincent, S. R., K. Satoh, D. M. Armstrong, and H. C. Fibiger (1983) Substance P in the ascending cholinergic reticular system. *Nature* **306**:688–691.

Voigt, M. M., and R. Y. Wang (1984) *In vivo* release of dopamine in the nucleus accumbens of the rat: Modulation by cholecystokinin. *Brain Res.* **296**:189–193.

White, F. J., and R. Y. Wang (1984) Interactions of cholecystokinin octapeptide and dopamine on nucleus accumbens neurons. *Brain Res.* **300**:161–166.

Widerlöv, E., H. Ågren, A. Wahström, J. F. Rehfeld, and G. R. Breese (1983a) Lack of interactions between cholecystokinin and dopamine in the central nervous system of rats and humans. *Psychopharmacol. Bull.* **19**:355–360.

Widerlöv, E., P. W. Kalivas, M. H. Lewis, A. J. Prange, Jr., and G. R. Breese (1983b) Influence of cholecystokinin on central monoaminergic pathways. *Reg. Pep.* **6**:99–109.

Wiesenfeld-Hallin, Z., T. Hökfelt, J. M. Lundberg, W. G. Forssmann, M. Reinecke, F. A. Tschopp, and J. Fischer (1984) Immunoreactive calcitonin gene-related peptide and substance P coexist in sensory neurons and interact in spinal behavioural responses. *Neurosci. Lett.* **52**:199–204.

Williams, R. G., R. J. Gayton, W-Y. Zhu, and G. J. Dockray (1981) Changes in brain cholecystokinin octapeptide following lesions of the medial forebrain bundle. *Brain Res.* **213**:227–230.

Yaksh, T. L., and T. A. Rudy (1976) Chronic catheterization of the spinal subarachnoid space. *Physiol. Behav.* **17**:1031–1036.

Zamboni, L., and C. De Martino (1967) Buffered picric-acid formaldehyde: A new rapid fixative for electron-microscopy. *J. Cell Biol.* **35**:148A.

Zarbin, M. A., R. B. Innis, J. K. Wamsley, S. H. Snyder, and M. J. Kuhar (1981) Autoradiographical localisation of CCK receptors in guinea pig brain. *Eur. J. Pharmacol.* **71**:349–350.

Zarbin, M. A., R. B. Innis, J. K. Wamsley, S. H. Snyder, and M. J. Kuhar (1983) Autoradiographic localization of cholecystokinin receptors in rodent brain. *J. Neurosci.* **3**:877–906.

Zetler, G. (1981) Central depressant effects of caerulein and cholecystokinin octapeptide (CCK-8) differ from those of diazepam and haloperidol. *Neuropharmacology* **20**:227–283.

Zetler, G. (1983a) Cholecystokinin octapeptide (CCK-8), ceruletide and ceruletide analogues: Effects on tremors induced by oxotremorine, harmine and ibogaine. A comparison with prolyl-leucyl-glycine amide (MIF), anti-Parkinsonian drugs and clonazepam. *Neuropharmacology* **22**:757–766.

Zetler, G. (1983b) Neuroleptic-like effects of ceruletide and cholecystokinin octapeptide: Interactions with apomorphine, methylphenidate and picrotoxin. *Eur. J. Pharmacol.* **94**:261–270.

Chapter 8

Protein Phosphorylation and Neuronal Function: DARPP-32, an Illustrative Example

HUGH C. HEMMINGS, JR.
ERIC J. NESTLER
S. IVAR WALAAS
CHARLES C. OUIMET
PAUL GREENGARD

ABSTRACT

Protein phosphorylation is a general regulatory mechanism involved in the control of many physiological processes and appears to be particularly important in the nervous system. Several protein kinases regulated by the second messengers cAMP, cGMP, and calcium have been identified in brain, and their physiological importance has been demonstrated by microinjection studies. A great variety of neuron-specific phosphoproteins has been found in nervous tissue, supporting the view that protein phosphorylation plays many roles in neuronal function. One of these phosphoproteins, DARPP-32, is localized to neurons that possess D_1-dopamine receptors and is regulated by dopamine acting through cAMP. The phosphorylated form of DARPP-32 acts as a potent inhibitor of the enzyme protein phosphatase-1. Regulation of the phosphorylation of DARPP-32 by dopamine in dopaminoceptive neurons represents a molecular mechanism for carrying out the intracellular actions of dopamine by inhibiting the dephosphorylation of specific phosphoproteins. Furthermore, DARPP-32 is dephosphorylated and inactivated by protein phosphatase-2B, a calcium/calmodulin-dependent protein phosphatase. These findings indicate the potential for positive feedback within the cAMP second messenger system and for both synergistic and antagonistic interactions between the cAMP and calcium second messenger systems mediated by the phosphorylation of DARPP-32 and its inhibition of protein phosphatase-1.

A major focus of biomedical research for many years has been the elucidation of the molecular mechanisms by which extracellular signals such as hormones and neurotransmitters produce their biological responses in specific target cells. Recent work in numerous laboratories has provided strong evidence that a wide variety of extracellular signals, both inside and outside the nervous system, produce many of their metabolic and physiological responses through protein phosphorylation—that is, by regulating the state of phosphorylation of specific substrate proteins in target tissues. The individual molecular pathways involving

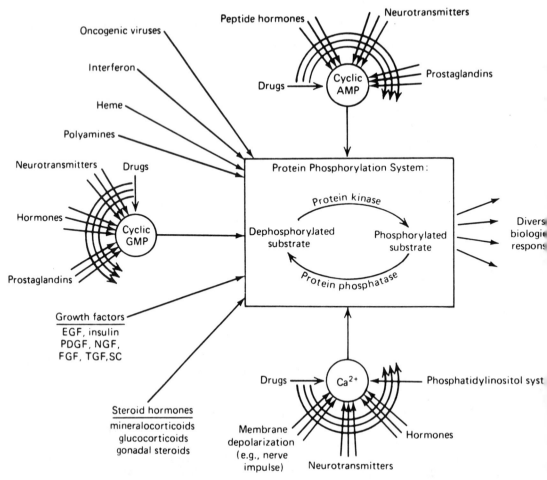

Figure 1. *Schematic diagram of the postulated role played by protein phosphorylation in mediating some of the biological effects of a variety of regulatory agents.* Many of these agents regulate protein phosphorylation by altering intracellular levels of the second messengers cAMP, cGMP, or calcium. Other agents appear to regulate protein phosphorylation through mechanisms that do not involve these second messengers. Most drugs regulate protein phosphorylation by affecting the ability of first messengers to alter second messenger levels (*curved arrows*). A small number of drugs (e.g., phosphodiesterase inhibitors, calcium channel blockers) regulate protein phosphorylation by directly altering second messenger levels (*straight arrows*). Abbreviations: EGF, epidermal growth factor; PDGF, platelet-derived growth factor; NGF, nerve growth factor; FGF, fibroblast growth factor; TGF, transforming growth factor; SC, somatomedin C. (From Nestler and Greengard, 1984.)

protein phosphorylation that have been elucidated in animal tissues over the past several years are shown schematically in Figure 1 (for a review, see Nestler and Greengard, 1984). The existence of a large number of such pathways supports the view that protein phosphorylation is a final common pathway of fundamental importance in biological regulation. In this chapter, we summarize recent evidence for such a vital role of protein phosphorylation in neuronal function.

PROTEIN PHOSPHORYLATION SYSTEMS IN BRAIN

The scheme shown in Figure 2 summarizes current concepts about the individual steps in the molecular pathways by which protein phosphorylation mediates certain of the effects of extracellular signals on neuronal function. Extracellular signals, or first messengers, in the nervous system include a variety of neurotransmitters and hormones, as well as photons and the nerve impulse itself. Many of these first messengers produce biological responses by regulating the intracellular concentration of specific second messengers in their target neurons. Prominent second messengers in the nervous system include cAMP, cGMP, and calcium.

Much evidence suggests that most, and possibly all, of the second messenger actions of cAMP and cGMP, as well as many of those of calcium, are achieved through the activation of specific cAMP-dependent, cGMP-dependent, and calcium-dependent protein kinases. Brain contains virtually one type of cAMP-dependent protein kinase and one type of cGMP-dependent protein kinase, but multiple types of calcium-dependent protein kinases (Rosen and Krebs, 1981; Corbin and Hardman, 1984; Nestler and Greengard, 1984; Nishizuka, 1984; Nairn et al., 1985). Two subclasses of calcium-dependent protein kinases are known. One is activated by calcium in conjunction with the calcium-binding protein calmodulin and is referred to as calcium/calmodulin-dependent protein kinase. The other subclass is activated by calcium in conjunction with diacylglycerol and phosphatidylserine, and is referred to as calcium/phosphatidylserine-dependent protein kinase or protein kinase C (Nishizuka, 1984). Brain contains four known types of calcium/calmodulin-dependent protein kinase, but only one known type of calcium/phosphatidylserine-dependent protein kinase. One of the calcium/calmodulin-dependent protein kinases, namely calcium/calmodulin-dependent protein kinase II, as well as calcium/phosphatidylserine-dependent protein kinase, has broad substrate specificities. They represent multifunctional enzymes that probably mediate many of the diverse second messenger actions of calcium in the nervous system. The other calcium/calmodulin-dependent protein kinases, namely calcium/calmodulin-dependent protein kinase I, myosin light chain kinase, and phosphorylase kinase, on the other hand, have more limited substrate specificities and appear to mediate a more limited number of the second messenger actions of calcium. An important goal is to determine which of these calcium-dependent protein kinases is responsible for each of the physiological actions of calcium that is mediated through protein phosphorylation.

Activation of these protein kinases by their respective second messengers results in the phosphorylation of specific substrate proteins ("third messengers"), leading, through one or more steps, to the production of specific biological responses. Protein phosphorylation in brain may be involved in carrying out or regulating such diverse processes as neurotransmitter biosynthesis, axoplasmic transport, neurotransmitter release, generation of postsynaptic potentials, ion channel conductance, neuronal shape and motility, elaboration of dendritic and axonal processes, and development and maintenance of the differentiated characteristics of neurons (for reviews, see Nestler and Greengard, 1983, 1984). In addition, some of the effects of protein phosphorylation on neuronal function

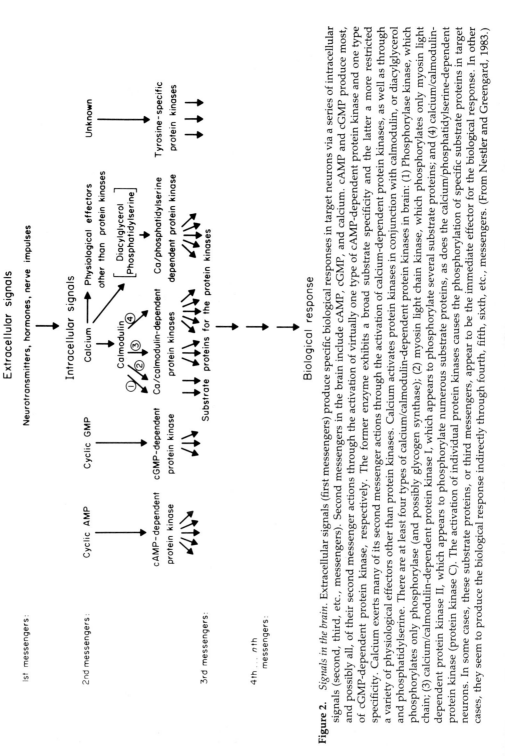

Figure 2. *Signals in the brain.* Extracellular signals (first messengers) produce specific biological responses in target neurons via a series of intracellular signals (second, third, etc., messengers). Second messengers in the brain include cAMP, cGMP, and calcium. cAMP and cGMP produce most, and possibly all, of their second messenger actions through the activation of virtually one type of cAMP-dependent protein kinase and one type of cGMP-dependent protein kinase, respectively. The former enzyme exhibits a broad substrate specificity and the latter a more restricted specificity. Calcium exerts many of its second messenger actions through the activation of calcium-dependent protein kinases, as well as through a variety of physiological effectors other than protein kinases. Calcium activates protein kinases in conjunction with calmodulin, or diacylglycerol and phosphatidylserine. There are at least four types of calcium/calmodulin-dependent protein kinases in brain: (1) Phosphorylase kinase, which phosphorylates only phosphorylase (and possibly glycogen synthase); (2) myosin light chain kinase, which phosphorylates only myosin light chain; (3) calcium/calmodulin-dependent protein kinase I, which appears to phosphorylate several substrate proteins; and (4) calcium/calmodulin-dependent protein kinase II (protein kinase II), which appears to phosphorylate numerous substrate proteins, as does the calcium/phosphatidylserine-dependent protein kinase (protein kinase C). The activation of individual protein kinases causes the phosphorylation of specific substrate proteins in target neurons. In some cases, these substrate proteins, or third messengers, appear to be the immediate effector for the biological response. In other cases, they seem to produce the biological response indirectly through fourth, fifth, sixth, etc., messengers. (From Nestler and Greengard, 1983.)

may include the biochemical events that underlie short-term and long-term memory (Greengard and Kuo, 1970; Kandel and Schwartz, 1982).

DIRECT EVIDENCE FOR A ROLE OF PROTEIN PHOSPHORYLATION IN NEURONAL FUNCTION

Over the past several years, the validity of the scheme shown in Figure 2 has been confirmed in a variety of neuronal systems. These studies, summarized below and in Table 1, have demonstrated an obligatory role in the regulation of neuronal function for members of each major class of protein kinase (for reviews, see Kandel and Schwartz, 1982; Kennedy, 1983; Levitan et al., 1983; Nestler and Greengard, 1983, 1984).

cAMP-Dependent Protein Kinase

Direct evidence for a role of cAMP-dependent protein kinase in neuronal function has been obtained in a number of laboratories (see Table 1). In these studies, intracellular injection of the catalytic subunit of cAMP-dependent protein kinase has been shown to mimic the ability of first messengers to elicit specific physiological responses in certain neurons. Conversely, injection of inhibitors of the protein kinase into the neurons has been shown to block the ability of the first messengers to elicit those responses. More specifically, such studies have demonstrated a role for cAMP-dependent protein kinase in the physiological regulation of voltage-dependent calcium channels and in the regulation of several types of potassium channels. Activation of cAMP-dependent protein kinase also appears to be a step in the sequence of events through which epinephrine and cAMP increase the conductance of voltage-dependent calcium channels in mammalian heart muscle cells (Osterrieder et al., 1982; Reuter, 1983). These findings indicate that the regulation of ion channel function by cAMP-dependent protein phosphorylation represents a common and physiologically important property of many ion channels.

Calcium-Dependent Protein Kinases

Recent studies have provided direct evidence for a role of calcium-dependent protein kinases in the regulation of nervous system function. DeRiemer et al. (1985) have shown that injection of purified calcium/phosphatidylserine-dependent protein kinase into cultured bag cell neurons of *Aplysia* increases the height, but not the width, of action potentials evoked by depolarizing current pulses. Exposure of the cells to tumor-promoting phorbol esters, compounds that activate calcium/phosphatidylserine-dependent protein kinase in many cell types (Nishizuka, 1984), produced similar changes in bag cell neuron action potentials. These effects on the action potential appear to be achieved through increases in the conductance of calcium channels. The results suggest that this protein kinase plays a role in the physiological regulation of the electrical excitability of bag cell neurons *in vivo*.

Other workers (Llinás et al., 1985) have injected purified calcium/calmodulin-dependent protein kinase II into terminal digits of the squid giant synapse and

Table 1. Systems in which Direct Evidence Has Been Obtained for a Role of Protein Phosphorylation in Neuronal Function

Cell (Genus)	Kinase Injected[a]	Inhibitor Injected[b]	Conclusion of Studies	References
Bag cell neurons (*Aplysia*)	cAMP	PKI	Kinase mediates effect of synaptic activation and of exogenous cAMP in producing the afterdischarge; this action appears to be achieved through decreases in the conductance of up to three distinct voltage-dependent potassium channels	Kaczmarek et al., 1980, 1984, 1985; Kaczmarek and Strumwasser, 1984
Sensory neurons (*Aplysia*)	cAMP	PKI	Kinase mediates effect of synaptic activation and of exogenous serotonin and cAMP in facilitating neurotransmitter release in response to nerve impulses; this action appears to be achieved through increases in the conductance of novel serotonin-regulated potassium channels	Castellucci et al., 1980, 1982; Siegelbaum et al., 1982
Neuron R15 (*Aplysia*)	PKI		Kinase mediates effect of exogenous serotonin and of cAMP in inhibiting bursting activity and enhancing interburst hyperpolarization; this action appears to be achieved through increases in the conductance of novel serotonin-regulated,	Adams and Levitan, 1982; Benson and Levitan, 1983

anomalously rectifying
potassium channels

Cell type	Kinase	Inhibitor	Action	Reference
Unidentified neurons (*Helix*)	cAMP		Kinase increases the conductance of calcium-dependent potassium channels	de Peyer et al., 1982
Unidentified neurons (*Helix*)	cAMP	Tolbutamide[c]	Kinase increases the conductance of voltage-dependent calcium channels	Doroshenko et al., 1984; Chad and Eckert, 1984
Photoreceptor cells (*Hermissenda*)	cAMP		Kinase decreases the conductance of early (I_A) and late (I_B) voltage-dependent potassium channels	Alkon et al., 1983
Hippocampal (CA$_1$) pyramidal neurons (*Rattus*)	cAMP	PKI	Kinase mediates effect of dopamine and of cAMP in producing a long-lasting increase in input resistance	Gribkoff et al., 1984
Bag cell neurons (*Aplysia*)	calcium/ phosphatidylserine		Kinase increases the height of action potentials; this action appears to be achieved through increases in the conductance of calcium channels	DeRiemer et al., 1985
Terminal digits of giant synapse (*Loligo*)	calcium/ calmodulin II		Kinase facilitates neurotransmitter release	Llinás et al., 1985

Source: Modified from Nestler and Greengard, 1983.

[a]Protein kinase abbreviations: cAMP, catalytic subunit of cyclic AMP-dependent protein kinase; calcium/phosphatidylserine, calcium/phosphatidylserine-dependent protein kinase holoenzyme; calcium/calmodulin II, calcium/calmodulin-dependent protein kinase II holoenzyme.

[b]PKI, specific protein inhibitor of cAMP-dependent protein kinase.

[c]The authors claim that tolbutamide is a specific inhibitor of cAMP-dependent protein kinase *in vitro*.

measured the effect of such injections on both the amount of neurotransmitter released from, and on presynaptic calcium currents in, the injected terminal. They found that injection of this protein kinase increased neurotransmitter release but had no effect on presynaptic calcium currents. These and other results support the hypothesis that the mechanism by which calcium/calmodulin-dependent protein kinase II facilitates neurotransmitter release includes the phosphorylation of synapsin I, a neuron-specific, synaptic vesicle-associated phosphoprotein that is a prominent substrate for this protein kinase (see also Nestler and Greengard, 1983, 1984).

The results of the studies summarized in Table 1 provide direct evidence for a causal relationship between protein phosphorylation and physiological responses in the nervous system. The results also support the view that, through the detection and characterization of neuronal substrate proteins for a variety of protein kinases and through the elucidation of the physiological roles of these neuronal substrate proteins, a detailed understanding will be achieved of many of the molecular mechanisms underlying the diverse types of physiological responses in neurons.

NEURONAL PHOSPHOPROTEINS

Experimental Approaches

Since many of the second messenger actions of cAMP, cGMP, and calcium are mediated via the activation of specific protein kinases, identification of the specific substrate protein(s) involved in a particular biological response to a first messenger is crucial to the elucidation of the molecular pathway through which that response is achieved. There are two conceptually distinct experimental approaches to the identification of protein kinase substrates. One is to investigate the possible phosphorylation of known proteins with established functions, such as enzymes, neurotransmitter receptors, and ion channels, or with no established functions, such as cytoskeletal proteins and myelin basic protein. The first approach has yielded much important information, but is limited to the small number of cellular proteins so far characterized, to physiological processes with known molecular bases, and to regulatory mechanisms in which known proteins are implicated.

The second approach, not limited in these ways, is to search for previously unknown proteins by virtue of their phosphorylation in response to appropriate stimuli and then to characterize these proteins with respect to their physiological, anatomical, and biochemical properties. This approach is unconventional in that it involves the extensive characterization of proteins whose biological functions are not yet known. Its unique power lies in its potential for leading to the discovery of new proteins and new molecular steps by which diverse physiological processes are regulated.

Classes of Neuronal Proteins Regulated by Phosphorylation

Through the use of these two approaches, a large number of neuronal proteins have been shown to be regulated by phosphorylation. Analysis of the patterns of protein phosphorylation in different brain regions revealed by one-dimensional SDS-polyacrylamide gel electrophoresis has led to the identification of more than 70 proteins that are substrates for cAMP-dependent, cGMP-dependent, or calcium-dependent protein kinases and that appear to be specific to nervous tissue (Walaas et al., 1983a,b). Analysis of brain protein phosphorylation by two-dimensional SDS-polyacrylamide gel electrophoresis has revealed the existence of an even larger number of neuron-specific phosphoproteins (S. I. Walaas and P. Greengard, unpublished observations).

Proteins found to undergo phosphorylation in the brain exhibit a great diversity in many of their properties. The phosphoproteins differ in their regional, cellular, and subcellular distribution in nervous tissue. Some are not restricted to nervous tissue and are probably involved in general cellular functions, while others appear to be specific to nervous tissue and are probably involved in neuron-specific functions. Some appear to be present in every neuron, while others are present in only a single type or class of neuron. Moreover, some of the phosphoproteins are presynaptic, while others are postsynaptic; some are cytosolic, while others are particulate. Among the particulate substrate proteins, some are associated with synaptic vesicles, and others are associated with nuclei, plasma membranes, or the cytoskeleton. In addition, these phosphoproteins differ in their protein kinase specificity, in that they are specifically phosphorylated by one or more types of protein kinase, as well as in the number and types of amino acid residues that undergo phosphorylation. The phosphoproteins also differ in a variety of their physicochemical properties. For example, they exhibit differences in molecular weight, isoelectric point, acid solubility, and conformation. Finally, the proteins differ in their biological functions and in the mechanisms by which they produce physiological responses. Some of the phosphoproteins may be directly involved in producing physiological responses, while others may be several steps away from the physiological response under regulation.

The large number and diversity of neuronal proteins that undergo phosphorylation support the view that protein phosphorylation has numerous and varied roles in the nervous system. Those neuronal phosphoproteins that have been most intensively studied fall into certain categories. These categories are listed in Table 2 and include enzymes involved in neurotransmitter biosynthesis, enzymes involved in cyclic nucleotide metabolism, autophosphorylated protein kinases, protein phosphatase inhibitors, proteins involved in the regulation of transcription and translation, cytoskeletal proteins, synaptic vesicle-associated proteins, neurotransmitter and hormone receptors, and ion channels. In several cases, the functional roles of the phosphorylation reactions have already been established. Regulation of many of these neuronal proteins by phosphorylation has been reviewed recently (Nestler and Greengard, 1983, 1984; Nestler et al., 1984).

As an illustration of the discovery and characterization of a new neuronal phosphoprotein, it is worth considering in detail a dopamine- and cAMP-regulated phosphoprotein with a molecular weight of 32 kD, DARPP-32. A discussion of DARPP-32 demonstrates the power of the study of protein phosphorylation as an experimental framework within which to elucidate the molecular basis of neuronal function and to contribute to aspects of neuroscience not related primarily to the study of protein phosphorylation.

Table 2. Neuronal Proteins Regulated by Phosphorylation[a]

Enzymes involved in neurotransmitter biosynthesis
    Tyrosine hydroxylase
    Tryptophan hydroxylase
Enzymes involved in cyclic nucleotide metabolism
    Adenylate cyclase
    Guanylate cyclase
    Ca^{2+}/calmodulin-dependent cyclic nucleotide phosphodiesterase
Autophosphorylated protein kinases
    cAMP-dependent protein kinase, regulatory subunit
    cGMP-dependent protein kinase
    Calcium/calmodulin-dependent protein kinases
    Calcium/phosphatidylserine-dependent protein kinase (protein kinase C)
    Casein kinases
    Tyrosine-specific protein kinases
    Double-stranded RNA-dependent protein kinase
    Rhodopsin kinase
Protein phosphatase inhibitors
    Phosphatase inhibitor-1
    Phosphatase inhibitor-2
    DARPP-32
    G-substrate
Proteins involved in transcription and translation regulation
    RNA polymerase
    Histones
    Nonhistone nuclear proteins
    Eukaryotic initiation factor, EIF-2
    Ribosomal protein S6
    Other ribosomal proteins
Cytoskeletal proteins
    MAP-2
    Tau
    Other microtubule-associated proteins
    Neurofilaments
    Calspectin
    Myosin light chain
    Actin
Synaptic vesicle-associated proteins
    Synapsin I
    Protein III
    Clathrin
Neurotransmitter and hormone receptors
    Nicotinic acetylcholine receptor
    Muscarinic acetylcholine receptor
    β-Adrenergic receptor
    GABA receptor (GABAmodulin)
    Insulin receptor
Ion channels[b]
    Voltage-dependent
        Sodium channel
        Potassium channel

Ion channels (*continued*)[b]
   Calcium channel
  Calcium-dependent
   Potassium channel
Neurotransmitter-dependent
  Nicotinic acetylcholine receptor
  Serotonin-regulated potassium channel in *Aplysia* sensory neurons
  Serotonin-regulated (anomalously rectifying) potassium channel in *Aplysia* neuron R15
Other
  Sodium channel in rod outer segments

Source: Nestler et al., 1984.
[a]Some of the proteins included are specific to neurons. The others are present in many cell types, in addition to being present in neurons, and are included because the regulation of neuron-specific phenomena is among their multiple functions in the nervous system. Not included are many phosphoproteins present in diverse tissues (including brain) that play roles in generalized cellular processes, such as intermediary metabolism, and that do not appear to play roles in neuron-specific phenomena.
[b]Several of the ion channels listed have been shown to be physiologically regulated by protein phosphorylation reactions, although it is not yet known whether such regulation is achieved directly through the phosphorylation of the ion channel, or indirectly through the phosphorylation of a modulatory protein that is not a constituent of the ion channel molecule.

DARPP-32, A DOPAMINE- AND cAMP-REGULATED PHOSPHOPROTEIN

Identification

DARPP-32 was originally observed during the examination of the regional distribution of cAMP- and calcium-regulated protein phosphorylation systems in rat brain (Walaas et al., 1983a,b). Some of the cAMP-regulated phosphoproteins, one of which was DARPP-32, were found to have restricted regional distributions in the brain that paralleled the gross anatomical distribution of dopaminergic innervation. A detailed biochemical analysis of the distribution of DARPP-32 in rat brain revealed that it was specifically enriched in the basal ganglia (Walaas and Greengard, 1984). High concentrations were found in the caudatoputamen, nucleus accumbens, and olfactory tubercle (the main dopamine-innervated regions of the forebrain basal ganglia), and in the main targets of the output neurons of these three regions, the globus pallidus and substantia nigra. DARPP-32 was shown to be contained within intrinsic neurons of the caudatoputamen by use of the neurotoxin kainic acid. Injection into the caudatoputamen of kainic acid, which destroys intrinsic striatal neurons while sparing nerve terminals and glia (Schwarcz and Coyle, 1977), produced a considerable decrease in the amount of striatal DARPP-32 (Walaas and Greengard, 1984) present. Further studies, employing lesioning techniques that eliminated specific neuronal populations in these regions, demonstrated that DARPP-32 was absent from the nigrostriatal dopaminergic neurons themselves but was present throughout the striatonigral dopaminoceptive neurons, specifically those dopaminoceptive neurons possessing D_1-dopamine receptors (Walaas and Greengard, 1984).

Regulation of Phosphorylation

The mammalian brain appears to contain at least two types of dopamine receptors, designated D_1- and D_2-dopamine receptors (Kebabian and Calne, 1979). The D_1-dopamine receptor is linked to the activation of adenylate cyclase, while at least some D_2-dopamine receptors appear to be linked to inhibition of adenylate cyclase (Kebabian and Calne, 1979; Kebabian and Cote, 1981; Stoof and Kebabian, 1981). The striking correlation between dopaminergic innervation and DARPP-32 localization, and the localization of DARPP-32 to the subclass of dopaminoceptive neurons possessing D_1-dopamine receptors, suggested that dopamine, acting through D_1-dopamine receptors, might regulate the phosphorylation of DARPP-32 by cAMP-dependent protein kinase in these dopaminoceptive cells. Using techniques that allowed analysis of the state of phosphorylation of DARPP-32 in brain slice preparations containing intact cells (Walaas et al., 1983c), it was found that either dopamine or the 8-bromo analog of cAMP could convert 40–50% of DARPP-32 from the dephosphorylated to the phosphorylated form (Walaas and Greengard, 1984). Phosphorylation of DARPP-32 was observed at concentrations of dopamine that have previously been found to activate specific dopamine receptors linked to the activation of adenylate cyclase (Forn et al., 1974). The effect of dopamine could be inhibited by the dopamine receptor blocker fluphenazine (Walaas et al., 1983c) and was specific for dopamine insofar as other neurotransmitter candidates (norepinephrine, serotonin, and adenosine) were without effect. These studies, which established a physiological link between DARPP-32 phosphorylation and dopaminergic neurotransmission, made it important to undertake further anatomical and biochemical studies of this phosphoprotein.

Regional, Cellular, and Subcellular Distribution in Brain

The tissue, cellular, and subcellular distribution of DARPP-32 has been investigated by several immunochemical techniques involving the use of both monoclonal and polyclonal antibodies prepared against purified bovine DARPP-32 (see below). The regional and cellular distribution of DARPP-32 in the central nervous system of the rat has been determined by a detailed immunocytochemical study (Ouimet et al., 1984). In general, the results of this study are supported by results obtained in a similar study of the distribution of DARPP-32 in the central nervous system of the rhesus monkey (C. C. Ouimet, A. LaMantia, H. C. Hemmings, Jr., P. Rakic, P. Goldman-Rakic, and P. Greengard, manuscript in preparation).

Figures 3 and 4 illustrate the localization of DARPP-32 in parasagittal and coronal sections of rat brain, as determined by an indirect immunoperoxidase method. The distribution of DARPP-32 exhibits large regional variations, with particularly strong labeling occurring in most of the brain regions that are heavily innervated by dopamine fibers, including the basal ganglia. Strong DARPP-32 immunoreactivity in neuronal cell bodies and dendrites was found within the caudatoputamen (Figure 5), nucleus accumbens, and olfactory tubercle (the forebrain basal ganglia), all of which receive dense dopamine inputs. Immunoreactive puncta, which represent nerve terminals as determined by electron microscopy (see below), were observed in the globus pallidus (Figure 5), ventral pallidum,

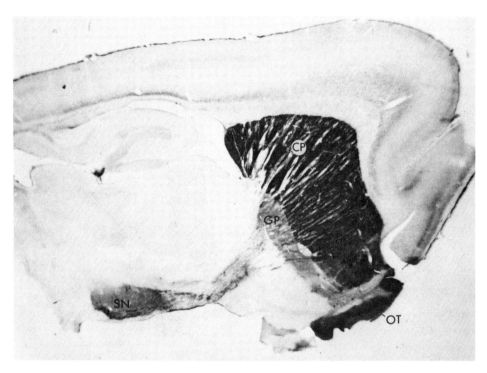

Figure 3. *Low-power light micrograph illustrating the distribution of DARPP-32 in a parasagittal section of rat brain.* DARPP-32 was stained through an indirect immunoperoxidase method by using mouse monoclonal antibodies prepared against purified bovine DARPP-32. Strong immunoreactivity can be seen throughout the caudatoputamen (CP), and in the olfactory tubercle (OT), globus pallidus (GP), and substantia nigra (SN). Weak immunoreactivity can be seen in layers III and IV of the neocortex. At higher magnification, and through the use of electron microscopy, it was found that DARPP-32 immunoreactivity is located predominantly in neuronal cell bodies and dendrites in the caudatoputamen, olfactory tubercle, and neocortex, and in axon terminals in the globus pallidus and pars reticulata of the substantia nigra. (C. C. Ouimet, H. C. Hemmings, Jr., and P. Greengard, unpublished observations.)

and pars reticulata of the substantia nigra, brain regions known to receive projections from the forebrain basal ganglia. Strong neuronal immunoreactivity was also found in the central, lateral, and cortical amygdaloid nuclei, in the dorsolateral bed nucleus of the stria terminalis, and in the massa intercalata, while strong glial immunoreactivity was found in tanycytes in the arcuate nucleus and median eminence of the mediobasal hypothalamus. All of these regions receive dense dopaminergic innervation (Lindvall and Björklund, 1978).

Studies employing high-resolution light and electron microscopy have shown that DARPP-32 is present in the cytosol of the somata, dendrites, dendritic spines, axons, and axon terminals of the medium-sized spiny neurons of the caudatoputamen and nucleus accumbens (Figure 6) but not in the giant cholinergic striatal interneurons (C. C. Ouimet, H. C. Hemmings, Jr., and P. Greengard, manuscript in preparation). The medium-sized spiny neurons receive most of the dopamine input to the neostriatum (Groves, 1983) and represent more than 90% of the Golgi-impregnated neurons in this brain region (Pasik et al., 1979;

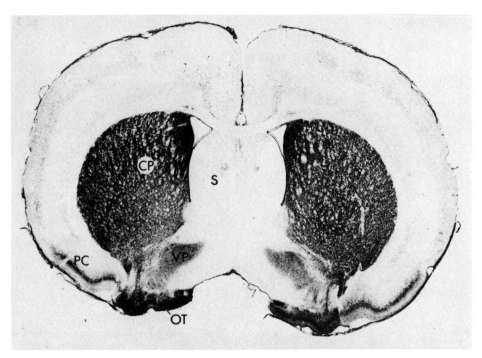

Figure 4. *Low-power light micrograph illustrating the distribution of DARPP-32 in a coronal section of rat brain.* DARPP-32 was stained through an indirect immunoperoxidase method by using mouse monoclonal antibodies prepared against purified bovine DARPP-32. Strong immunoreactivity can be seen throughout the caudatoputamen (CP), and in the ventral pallidum, olfactory tubercle (OT), and in layers III and IV of the pyriform cortex (PC). At higher magnification, and through the use of electron microscopy, it was found that DARPP-32 immunoreactivity is located predominantly in neuronal cell bodies and dendrites in the caudatoputamen, olfactory tubercle, and pyriform cortex, and in axon terminals in the ventral pallidum (which is defined with exceptional clarity and definition by DARPP-32 immunolabeling). (C. C. Ouimet, H. C. Hemmings, Jr., and P. Greengard, unpublished observations.)

Dimova et al., 1980). DARPP-32 immunoreactivity is absent from corticostriatal fibers and the dopaminergic nigrostriatal neurons.

Weak immunoreactivity was observed in cells of the deep layers of the medial prefrontal cortex and in cell clusters in the entorhinal cortex, regions with well-defined dopamine inputs (Lindvall and Björklund, 1978). Weak immunoreactivity was also found in several regions in which dopamine innervation is believed to be less important. Thus, some neurons were weakly labeled in the medial habenula, the cerebellum, and layers II, III, and VI of the neocortex, while the thalamus and hippocampus showed a weak nerve terminal staining pattern. A restricted number of astrocytes, located throughout the neuroaxis, were also found to be weakly immunoreactive.

The results obtained by immunocytochemical methods are supported by quantitative analyses employing both a biochemical assay (Walaas and Greengard, 1984) and a specific radioimmunoassay (Hemmings and Greengard, 1986) of the distribution of DARPP-32 in the rat central nervous system. The highest concentrations of DARPP-32 were found in the caudatoputamen, the globus pallidus,

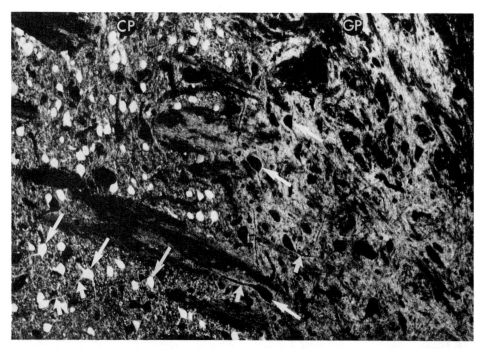

Figure 5. *Fluorescence photomicrograph of DARPP-32 immunoreactivity in a coronal section through the border between the caudatoputamen (CP) and the globus pallidus (GP) of rat brain.* DARPP-32 was stained through an indirect immunofluorescence method by using mouse monoclonal antibodies prepared against purified bovine DARPP-32. In the caudatoputamen, neuronal cell bodies and dendrites are labeled. In the globus pallidus, in contrast, neuronal cell bodies and dendrites are unlabeled, but are surrounded by labeled puncta representing nerve terminals. *Long arrows,* cell bodies; *short arrows,* dendrites. (From Ouimet et al., 1984.)

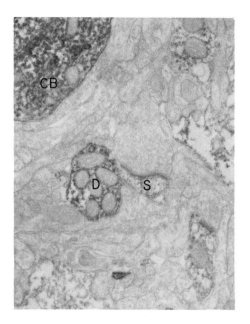

Figure 6. *Electron micrograph illustrating the ultrastructural localization of DARPP-32 in the rat caudatoputamen.* DARPP-32 was stained through an indirect immunoperoxidase method by using mouse monoclonal antibodies prepared against purified bovine DARPP-32. Reaction product can be seen in a neuronal cell body (CB), a dendritic shaft (D), and a dendritic spine (S). A nerve terminal can be seen making a synaptic contact on the labeled spine. (C. C. Ouimet, H. C. Hemmings, Jr., and P. Greengard, unpublished observations.)

and the substantia nigra. Intermediate concentrations were found in the nucleus accumbens and the olfactory tubercle, and low concentrations in the frontal cortex, neocortex, hippocampus, amygdala, thalamus, cerebellum, and retina.

   The levels of DARPP-32 in subcellular fractions prepared from the rat caudatoputamen have also been analyzed with the biochemical phosphorylation assay and the radioimmunoassay. These studies demonstrated that the soluble fraction of this brain region is highly enriched with DARPP-32, consistent with its localization within cell bodies and dendrites. A significant amount of DARPP-32 was also found in the crude synaptosomal fraction that could be released by hypotonic lysis, suggesting that a fraction of DARPP-32 is also present in nerve terminals. This observation is supported by the finding that, in the substantia nigra, DARPP-32 is enriched in the particulate fraction and can be released by hypotonic lysis (Walaas and Greengard, 1984). In this brain region, evidence obtained by immunocytochemistry at both the light and electron microscope levels indicates that DARPP-32 is contained within nerve terminals. Thus, the results of studies of the subcellular localization of DARPP-32 determined by the analysis of subcellular fractions are consistent with those of ultrastructural studies employing immunocytochemical techniques in which cell bodies, dendrites, axons, and nerve terminals were all immunoreactive for DARPP-32. Furthermore, DARPP-32 immunoreactivity was evenly distributed throughout the cytoplasm, suggesting that DARPP-32 is not primarily associated with any subcellular organelles (Ouimet et al., 1984).

   The nature of the neurotransmitter(s) in DARPP-32-containing neurons has not been established. The vast majority of the medium-sized spiny neurons in the rat caudatoputamen and nucleus accumbens contain γ-aminobutyric acid (GABA), as revealed by immunocytochemical staining for glutamic acid decarboxylase (Oertel and Mugnaini, 1984). It is likely that most, if not all, of these neurons also contain DARPP-32 (Ouimet et al., 1984). However, GABAergic neurons are much more widely distributed throughout the brain than are neurons immunoreactive for DARPP-32, so not all GABAergic neurons in the brain contain DARPP-32 (see Ouimet et al., 1984). Furthermore, since DARPP-32 is present in a variety of other nerve cell types that are not GABAergic, the general distribution of neurons immunoreactive for DARPP-32 is not identical to that of GABAergic neurons. Many striatal medium-sized spiny neurons are also immunoreactive for substance P (Ljungdahl et al., 1978) and enkephalin (Pickel et al., 1980). Thus, it is possible that DARPP-32 is also present in neurons that contain substance P and/or enkephalin.

Species and Tissue Distribution

Immunochemical methods have also been used to identify DARPP-32 in various vertebrate species and to study its distribution in peripheral nervous and nonnervous tissues. DARPP-32 has been detected in brain tissue from the mouse, rat, guinea pig, rabbit, cat, cow, rhesus monkey, human, canary, and turtle by phosphorylation, radioimmunoprecipitation, radioimmunoassay, and antibody labeling of nitrocellulose blots of SDS-polyacrylamide gels (H. C. Hemmings, Jr., S. I. Walaas, G. Burd, C. C. Ouimet, and P. Greengard, unpublished observations). Studies of peripheral nervous tissues employing the same techniques have shown that DARPP-32 is present in the posterior pituitary, which has both D_1- and D_2-dopamine receptors, but is absent from the anterior pituitary, which has only D_2-dopamine receptors (Kebabian and Calne, 1979). DARPP-32 has also been detected in bovine and rabbit superior cervical sympathetic ganglia, which contain dopaminergic neurons and dopamine receptors coupled to adenylate cyclase (Kebabian and Greengard, 1971); in bovine parathyroid cells, which contain D_1-dopamine receptors (Brown et al., 1977); and in the chromaffin cells of the bovine adrenal medulla (Hemmings and Greengard, 1986). DARPP-32 has not been detected in any of the peripheral nonnervous tissues tested other than the parathyroid gland.

Recently, immunochemical methods have been used to carry out a phylogenetic survey of DARPP-32 localization. In the basal forebrain of the turtle, strong immunoreactivity was detected by radioimmunoprecipitation, radioimmunoassay, and antibody labeling of nitrocellulose blots of SDS-polyacrylamide gels (H. C. Hemmings, Jr., C. C. Ouimet, and P. Greengard, unpublished observations) and in the paleostriatum of the canary (H. C. Hemmings, Jr., G. Burd, and P. Greengard, unpublished observations). In the canary, these findings have been confirmed by immunocytochemical studies (G. Burd, H. C. Hemmings, Jr., J. Heintz, P. Greengard, and F. Nottebohm, unpublished observations). In the turtle and in the canary (as in the rat), the brain regions that contain DARPP-32 are the regions that receive major dopaminergic inputs, and that are thought to be homologous to the neostriatum of mammals (Reiner et al., 1984). Further studies of the immunocytochemical localization of DARPP-32 in these species should yield valuable information concerning the phylogenetic development of dopaminoceptive neurons, particularly within the basal ganglia. From these studies, it appears that the regional distribution of DARPP-32 in the brains of several mammalian and nonmammalian vertebrates corresponds to that of dopamine innervation, and probably reflects the different locations of dopaminoceptive neurons possessing D_1-dopamine receptors in these species. Immunoreactive DARPP-32 could not be detected in the brains of two other vertebrate classes, the fish and the frog (Hemmings and Greengard, 1986).

DARPP-32 as a Marker for Dopaminoceptive Neurons

Results obtained by a variety of techniques indicate a close association between DARPP-32 localization and the subclass of dopaminoceptive neurons containing D_1-dopamine receptors. However, several cell types that appear to be weakly immunoreactive for DARPP-32 are not known to receive dopaminergic innervation (e.g., neurons in layers II and III of the cerebral cortex, the cerebellar Purkinje cells, various astrocytes and tanycytes). There are several possible explanations for these apparent discrepancies. First, the distribution of D_1-dopamine receptors may be wider than that of dopaminergic nerve terminals. Second, a minor dopaminergic input may have escaped detection by the currently available methods in some brain regions. Third, DARPP-32 may be able to act as an effector for neurotransmitters that elevate cAMP levels other than dopamine.

In some instances of apparent discrepancy, the presence of DARPP-32 appears to be correlated with the presence of D_1-dopamine receptors. Thus, dopamine-sensitive adenylate cyclase (which indicates the presence of D_1-dopamine receptors) has been found in cat cerebellum (Dolphin et al., 1979) and in certain glial cells (Schubert et al., 1976; Henn et al., 1977). In other cases, the presence of DARPP-32 may indicate the existence of a previously unknown dopamine input, as for the tanycytes of the arcuate nucleus and median eminence (Calas, 1985). Furthermore, neurotransmitters other than dopamine that elevate cAMP may be able to regulate the phosphorylation of DARPP-32 in certain DARPP-32-containing neurons that possess receptors for these neurotransmitters. For example, in Purkinje cells, cAMP levels can be increased by norepinephrine (Kakiuchi and Rall, 1968), which could result in the phosphorylation of DARPP-32. In the rat caudatoputamen, however, the regulation of the state of phosphorylation of DARPP-32 appears to be specific for dopamine (Walaas and Greengard, 1984), although peptide neurotransmitters have not yet been tested.

Most brain regions found to contain high levels of DARPP-32 (Walaas and Greengard, 1984; Hemmings and Greengard, 1986) or to be intensely immunoreactive for DARPP-32 (Ouimet et al., 1984) have been shown to contain D_1-dopamine receptors. Conversely, DARPP-32 has been found to be absent from cells containing D_2-dopamine receptors but not containing D_1-dopamine receptors (e. g., nigrostriatal dopaminergic neurons, corticostriatal nerve terminals, and anterior pituicytes). Despite this strong correlation, it is not yet possible to conclude whether DARPP-32 is present in all dopaminoceptive neurons containing D_1-dopamine receptors, or whether it is absent from all nondopaminoceptive neurons and from dopaminoceptive neurons containing only D_2-dopamine receptors.

Purification and Biochemical Characterization

DARPP-32 was identified in bovine caudate nucleus cytosol and purified 435-fold to apparent homogeneity from this source (Hemmings et al., 1984a). Purified DARPP-32 has been extensively characterized, and some of its biochemical properties are summarized in Table 3. It is an acidic, highly elongated monomer that is both heat stable and acid soluble. It has a relative molecular mass of 32 kD, as determined by SDS-polyacrylamide gel electrophoresis (Hemmings et al., 1984a), and a molecular mass of 24 kD, as determined by high-speed sedimentation equilibrium centrifugation (Hemmings et al., 1984b). The value determined by SDS-polyacrylamide gel electrophoresis appears to be anomalously high (probably because of abnormally low detergent binding to DARPP-32), since amino acid sequencing indicates that the actual molecular mass is 22.6 kD (Williams et al., 1986).

DARPP-32 is phosphorylated at a single threonine residue by cAMP-dependent protein kinase (Hemmings et al., 1984a,c). The amino acid sequence surrounding the phosphorylated threonine of DARPP-32 (Hemmings et al., 1984d) was found to include two proline residues flanking the phosphothreonine residue and four consecutive arginine residues amino-terminal to the phosphothreonine residue (Table 4). Many of the other biochemical properties of DARPP-32 in addition to its phosphorylation site sequence were found to be remarkably similar to those of protein phosphatase inhibitor-1. Phosphatase inhibitor-1, in its phosphorylated form, is a potent and specific inhibitor of the enzyme protein phosphatase-1

Table 3. Summary of Biochemical Properties of DARPP-32[a]

Property	Method of Determination	Value
Molecular weight	SDS-polyacrylamide gel electrophoresis	32 kD
	Sedimentation equilibrium centrifugation	24 kD
Stokes radius	Gel filtration	34 Å
Sedimentation coefficient	Sucrose density gradient centrifugation	2.05 S
Frictional ratio (f/f_0)	Stokes radius and sedimentation coefficient	1.7
Axial ratio	Stokes radius and sedimentation coefficient	13.5
Isoelectric point	Isoelectric focusing	
	Phospho form	4.6
	Dephospho form	4.7
Amino acid composition		High Glu and Pro
		Low hydrophobic residues
Phosphorylatable residue	Thin-layer electrophoresis and chromatography	Threonine
K_m for cAMP-dependent protein kinase	Kinetic analysis	2.4 μM
k_{cat} for cAMP-dependent protein kinase	Kinetic analysis	2.7 sec^{-1}
K_m for cGMP-dependent protein kinase	Kinetic analysis	5.4 μM
k_{cat} for cGMP-dependent protein kinase	Kinetic analysis	2.3 sec^{-1}

[a] Data from Hemmings et al., 1984a,b,c.

(Huang and Glinsmann, 1976; Nimmo and Cohen, 1978). In order to determine whether the biochemical similarities between DARPP-32 and phosphatase inhibitor-1 were indicative of similar physiological functions, the effect of purified DARPP-32 on protein phosphatase activity was studied and compared to that of phosphatase inhibitor-1.

Interactions with Protein Phosphatases

The protein phosphatase activities involved in the dephosphorylation of most of the known proteins phosphorylated on serine or threonine residues can be accounted for by four distinct enzymes (Cohen, 1982; Ingebritsen and Cohen,

Table 4. Amino Acid Sequence Around the Phosphorylatable Threonine Residues of DARPP-32 and Phosphatase Inhibitor-1[a]

Phosphoprotein	Sequence
DARPP-32	Met-*Ile-Arg-Arg-Arg-Arg-Pro-Thr(P)-Pro-Ala*-Met-*Leu*-Phe-Arg
Phosphatase inhibitor-1	Gln-*Ile-Arg-Arg-Arg-Arg-Pro-Thr(P)-Pro-Ala*-Thr-*Leu*-Val-Leu

[a]Sequence homology between DARPP-32 and phosphatase inhibitor-1 is indicated by italics. Data for DARPP-32 from Hemmings et al., 1984c and Williams et al., 1986, and for phosphatase inhibitor-1 from Aitken et al., 1982.

1983a,b). These enzymes are grouped into two classes: type 1 protein phosphatase (protein phosphatase-1) and type 2 protein phosphatases (protein phosphatase-2A, -2B, and -2C). Type 1 protein phosphatase selectively dephosphorylates the β-subunit of phosphorylase kinase and is inhibited by nanomolar concentrations of phosphatase inhibitor-1 or phosphatase inhibitor-2 (another protein phosphatase inhibitor). Type 2 protein phosphatases selectively dephosphorylate the α-subunit of phosphorylase kinase and are insensitive to these inhibitors.

Analysis of the effect of DARPP-32 on purified preparations of these four protein phosphatases showed that the phosphorylated form of DARPP-32 inhibited protein phosphatase-1 noncompetitively, with an IC_{50} of approximately 10^{-9} M under the experimental conditions employed (Figure 7). It showed no inhibitory activity toward protein phosphatase-2A, -2B, or -2C (Hemmings et al., 1984b). The dephosphorylated form of DARPP-32 was inactive as an inhibitor of protein phosphatase-1. Phosphorylated DARPP-32 itself was not a substrate for protein phosphatase-1. Rather, it was dephosphorylated most efficiently by the calcium/

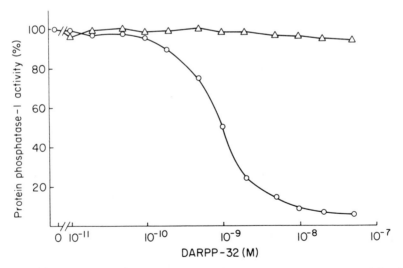

Figure 7. *Inhibition of purified rabbit muscle protein phosphatase-1 by various concentrations of phosphorylated* (circles) *or dephosphorylated* (triangles) *DARPP-32.* The activity of protein phosphatase-1 was determined by measuring the release of [^{32}P]phosphate from [^{32}P]phosphorylase *a*. (Modified from Hemmings et al., 1984b.)

calmodulin-regulated enzyme protein phosphatase-2B (Hemmings et al., 1984b; King et al., 1984). This observation is of interest, since the substrate specificity of protein phosphatase-2B (also known as calcineurin) has been reported to be quite limited (Stewart et al., 1982; Ingebritsen and Cohen, 1983b). The potency and specificity of DARPP-32 as a protein phosphatase inhibitor and as a substrate for the various protein phosphatases were very similar to those of phosphatase inhibitor-1. Thus, the basal ganglia of mammalian brain contain a region-specific neuronal phosphoprotein, namely DARPP-32, that is a potent inhibitor, in its phosphorylated form, of protein phosphatase-1 and that is regulated by dopamine. Although DARPP-32 is very similar in its biochemical and functional properties to phosphatase inhibitor-1, DARPP-32 and phosphatase inhibitor-1 are clearly distinct proteins, as determined by amino acid sequencing, peptide mapping, and sensitivity to cyanogen bromide (Williams et al., 1986).

Physiological Role

Dopamine, acting at D_1-dopamine receptors, increases the state of phosphorylation of DARPP-32 in intact nerve cells by elevating cAMP levels and thereby activating cAMP-dependent protein kinase (Walaas et al., 1983c; Walaas and Greengard, 1984). These observations suggest that DARPP-32, as an intracellular "third messenger" for dopamine, may be involved in mediating certain of the actions of dopamine acting at D_1-dopamine receptors. A molecular mechanism by which DARPP-32 may mediate some of the effects of dopamine on dopaminoceptive neurons has been discovered by studying the effects of DARPP-32 on the activity of purified preparations of protein phosphatases. According to this scheme, dopamine would produce some of its physiological effects by increasing the phosphorylation of DARPP-32, thereby inhibiting protein phosphatase-1.

Figure 8 illustrates two possible mechanisms by which the inhibition of protein phosphatase-1 could mediate some of the physiological effects produced by dopamine acting through cAMP. Regions of the brain containing DARPP-32, most notably the basal ganglia, also contain many other substrates for cAMP-dependent protein kinase (Walaas et al., 1983a,b). It is likely that many of these substrates can be dephosphorylated by protein phosphatase-1, as has been determined for other substrates of cAMP-dependent protein kinase (Ingebritsen and Cohen, 1983b). The phosphorylation and activation of DARPP-32 in these brain regions would therefore inhibit the dephosphorylation of these other substrates for cAMP-dependent protein kinase, thereby amplifying the effects of cAMP by a positive feedback mechanism (Hemmings et al., 1984b). Furthermore, phosphoproteins that are phosphorylated by protein kinases other than cAMP-dependent protein kinase are also dephosphorylated by protein phosphatase-1 (Ingebritsen and Cohen, 1983b). Thus, phosphorylation and activation of DARPP-32 may also allow dopamine, acting through cAMP, to modulate the phosphorylation state of substrates for other second messenger-regulated protein kinases. By this mechanism, dopamine and cAMP would be able to interact with other first and second messenger systems at the level of protein phosphorylation by regulating the state of phosphorylation of some of the same substrate proteins. The inhibition by dopamine, acting through the cAMP-dependent phosphorylation of DARPP-32, of the dephosphorylation by protein phosphatase-1 of substrate

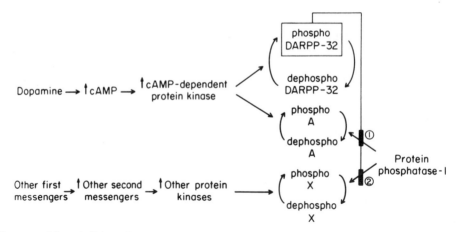

Figure 8.   *Schematic diagram illustrating two possible mechanisms by which the inhibition of protein phosphatase-1 by DARPP-32 may be involved in mediating the physiological effects of dopamine on dopaminoceptive neurons possessing D₁-dopamine receptors. The first messenger dopamine, acting through cAMP and cAMP-dependent protein kinase, stimulates the phosphorylation of DARPP-32 and of various other substrate proteins in target neurons. The phosphorylation of DARPP-32 converts it to an active inhibitor of protein phosphatase-1. Activated DARPP-32 then decreases the dephosphorylation of some of the proteins (represented by A) that are substrates for cyclic AMP-dependent protein kinase (arrow 1), and of other proteins (represented by X) that are substrates for other protein kinases (arrow 2). By increasing the phosphorylation of A, phosphorylated DARPP-32 represents a positive feedback signal through which the actions of dopamine are amplified. By increasing the phosphorylation of X, phosphorylated DARPP-32 represents a mediator through which dopamine modulates the actions of other first messengers.*

protein(s) regulated by another neurotransmitter, acting through another second messenger and protein kinase, would provide a molecular mechanism for the synergistic interaction between two neurotransmitters.

The interaction of dopamine and cAMP with other first and second messenger systems is also possible through another mechanism. DARPP-32 and protein phosphatase-2B are both highly concentrated in the basal ganglia within the medium-sized spiny neurons (Wallace et al., 1980; Wood et al., 1980; Ouimet et al., 1984; Walaas and Greengard, 1984; P. De Camilli, unpublished observations). A role for protein phosphatase-2B in the regulation of the state of phosphorylation of DARPP-32 *in vivo* is likely, since DARPP-32 is a particularly effective substrate for this protein phosphatase *in vitro* (Hemmings et al., 1984b; King et al., 1984). The dephosphorylation of DARPP-32 by protein phosphatase-2B, a calcium/calmodulin-regulated enzyme (Figure 9), provides a mechanism by which calcium, acting as a second messenger, could antagonize some of the effects of the dopamine-induced cAMP signal in dopaminoceptive neurons (Hemmings et al., 1984b).

Two potential interactions between the cAMP and calcium second messenger systems, mediated through the regulation of the state of phosphorylation of DARPP-32 and the concomitant control of protein phosphatase-1 activity, are illustrated schematically in Figure 9. These interactions provide molecular mechanisms by which a protein phosphatase inhibitor can mediate either synergistic or antagonistic effects of one first messenger on another through the second messengers cAMP and calcium. In this scheme, dopamine is shown to regulate the phosphorylation of DARPP-32 (Walaas et al., 1983c; Walaas and Greengard, 1984), while glutamate is shown as an example of a neurotransmitter that produces some of its effects through the elevation of intracellular calcium levels. Calcium may antagonize the effects of cAMP by activating a calcium/calmodulin-dependent protein phosphatase (protein phosphatase-2B), thereby leading to the dephosphorylation of DARPP-32 and possibly other substrate proteins for cAMP-dependent protein kinase. A synergistic effect of cAMP on the effects of calcium could occur by the cAMP-dependent phosphorylation of DARPP-32, leading to the inhibition of the dephosphorylation by protein phosphatase-1 of substrate proteins for calcium-dependent protein kinases. The synergistic effects produced by this latter mechanism would be reversed if the substrate protein being affected inhibited the response to glutamate by a negative feedback mechanism. This may occur in the medium-sized spiny neurons of the striatum, where dopamine, apparently acting through cAMP, antagonizes the ability of glutamate to depolarize certain dopaminoceptive neurons (Moore and Bloom, 1978; Bunney, 1979), possibly by inhibiting the dephosphorylation by protein phosphatase-1 of an "inhibitory modulator protein," which is phosphorylated and activated by glutamate acting through a calcium-dependent protein kinase, and thereby inhibits glutamate-induced depolarization by a negative feedback mechanism (see Nestler et al., 1984). From this example and the previous discussion, it is clear that many variations in the types of interactions between neurotransmitters are possible at the level of protein phosphatase inhibitors. It is likely that these interactions occur in many different types of neurons between many pairs of neurotransmitters.

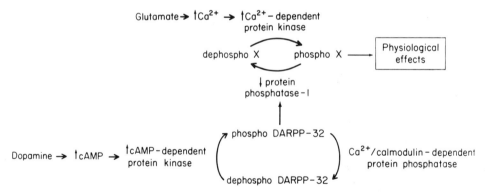

Figure 9. *Schematic diagram illustrating a possible role for DARPP-32 in mediating the interaction of dopamine with glutamate.* The first messenger glutamate, which increases intracellular calcium levels, causes the activation of a calcium-dependent protein kinase and subsequently the phosphorylation of specific substrate proteins (represented by X), which are involved in mediating the physiological effects of glutamate. The first messenger dopamine, acting through cAMP and cAMP-dependent protein kinase, stimulates the phosphorylation of DARPP-32, which converts it to an active inhibitor of protein phosphatase-1 and thereby decreases the dephosphorylation of these substrate proteins for the calcium-dependent protein kinase. In this way, dopamine may modulate the response to glutamate. Another possible interaction between the cAMP and calcium second messenger systems may occur via calcium/calmodulin-dependent protein phosphatase (protein phosphatase-2B), which can dephosphorylate and inactivate phosphorylated DARPP-32.

The regulation of protein phosphatase activity by the reversible phosphorylation of specific protein phosphatase inhibitors appears to be a particularly important mechanism of cellular regulation in the brain. In addition to phosphatase inhibitor-1, which is present in many tissues including brain (Detre et al., 1984), two cell type-specific protein phosphatase inhibitors have been identified in brain. One of these, DARPP-32, is present in dopaminoceptive neurons possessing D_1-dopamine receptors and may function as a protein phosphatase inhibitor specific for the dopamine system. The other, G-substrate, is a specific substrate protein for cGMP-dependent protein kinase that resembles phosphatase inhibitor-1 and DARPP-32 in many of its biochemical properties (Aitken et al., 1981; Aswad and Greengard, 1981a,b; King et al., 1984). It is specifically localized within the Purkinje cells of the cerebellum (Schlichter et al., 1980; Detre et al., 1984) and has been found to inhibit a protein phosphatase isolated from cerebellum (P. Simonelli, H.-C. Li, A. C. Nairn, and P. Greengard, unpublished observations). G-substrate thus appears to function as a Purkinje cell-specific protein phosphatase inhibitor. The study of these two neuronal phosphoproteins has revealed that the regulation of protein phosphatase activity by the phosphorylation and activation of specific inhibitor proteins appears to be a prominent regulatory mechanism in brain and suggests that this mechanism may be common to the action of several neurotransmitters. Further studies on the role of DARPP-32 in the control of protein phosphorylation in dopaminoceptive neurons should provide additional insights into the molecular mechanisms of the transsynaptic actions of dopamine.

CONCLUSIONS

The study of protein phosphorylation in nervous tissue has resulted in the detection of a great variety of neuronal phosphoproteins, supporting the view that this regulatory mechanism is involved in many aspects of neuronal function. Direct evidence for a role of three major classes of protein kinase in the regulation of neuronal function has been obtained in microinjection experiments. These studies have demonstrated that activation of specific protein kinases is both necessary and sufficient to produce a variety of physiological responses to neurotransmitters, depolarization, or synaptic activation in nerve cells. Therefore, the identification and characterization of the specific substrate proteins for these protein kinases is of considerable importance in establishing the molecular mechanisms involved in the regulation of a variety of neuronal functions. This has already been demonstrated for two distinct classes of neuronal phosphoproteins.

One class consists of neuronal phosphoproteins that have been detected throughout the nervous system. One member of this class, synapsin I, has recently been shown to be involved in the regulation of neurotransmitter release, a function common to all neurons. The other class consists of neuronal phosphoproteins that are localized to one or a few neuronal cell types. DARPP-32, a member of this latter class, appears to be specifically enriched in dopaminoceptive neurons possessing D_1-dopamine receptors. Biochemical studies have shown that DARPP-32 functions as a potent inhibitor of protein phosphatase-1 *in vitro*, and that it may be involved in mediating some of the transsynaptic effects of dopamine by inhibiting this enzyme *in vivo*. DARPP-32 appears to play an important role in certain dopaminoceptive neurons, given its high concentration in these cells. Regulation of the state of phosphorylation of DARPP-32 may be involved in mediating interactions between the dopamine/cAMP second messenger system and other second messenger system(s), possibly one involving calcium. Future studies of phosphoproteins in the basal ganglia, and of DARPP-32 in particular, should lead to the further elucidation of the molecular mechanisms underlying neuronal function.

REFERENCES

Adams, W. B., and I. B. Levitan (1982) Intracellular injection of protein kinase inhibitor blocks the serotonin-induced increase of K^+ conductance in *Aplysia* neuron R15. *Proc. Natl. Acad. Sci. USA* **79**:3877–3880.

Aitken, A., T. Bilham, P. Cohen, D. Aswad, and P. Greengard (1981) A specific substrate from rabbit cerebellum for guanosine 3':5'-monophosphate-dependent protein kinase. III. Amino acid sequences at the two phosphorylation sites. *J. Biol. Chem.* **256**:3501–3506.

Aitken, A., T. Bilham, and P. Cohen (1982) Complete primary structure of protein phosphatase inhibitor-1 from rabbit skeletal muscle. *Eur. J. Biochem.* **126**:235–246.

Alkon, D. L., J. Acosta-Urguidi, J. Olds, G. Kuzma, and J. T. Neary (1983) Protein kinase injection reduces voltage-dependent potassium currents. *Science* **219**:303–306.

Aswad, D. W., and P. Greengard (1981a) A specific substrate from rabbit cerebellum for guanosine 3':5'-monophosphate-dependent protein kinase. I. Purification and characterization from rabbit cerebellum. *J. Biol. Chem.* **256**:3487–3493.

Aswad, D. W., and P. Greengard (1981b) A specific substrate for guanosine 3':5'-monophosphate-dependent protein kinase. II. Kinetic studies on its phosphorylation by guanosine 3':5'-monophosphate-dependent and adenosine 3':5'-monophosphate-dependent protein kinases. *J. Biol. Chem.* **256**:3494–3500.

Benson, J. A., and I. B. Levitan (1983) Serotonin increases an anomalously rectifying K^+ current in the *Aplysia* neuron R15. *Proc. Natl. Acad. Sci. USA* **80**:3522–3525.

Brown, E. M., R. J. Carroll, and G. D. Aurbach (1977) Dopaminergic stimulation of cyclic AMP accumulation and parathyroid hormone release from dispersed bovine parathyroid cells. *Proc. Natl. Acad. Sci. USA* **74**:4210–4213.

Bunney, B. S. (1979) The electrophysiological pharmacology of midbrain dopaminergic systems. In *The Neurobiology of Dopamine*, A. S. Horn, J. Korf, and B. H. C. Westerink, eds., pp. 417–452, Academic, New York.

Calas, A. (1985) Morphological correlates of chemically specified neuronal interactions in the hypothalamo-hypophyseal area. *Neurochem. Int.* **7**:927–940.

Castellucci, V. F., E. R. Kandel, J. H. Schwartz, F. D. Wilson, A. C. Nairn, and P. Greengard (1980) Intracellular injection of the catalytic subunit of cyclic AMP-dependent protein kinase simulates facilitation of transmitter release underlying behavioral sensitization in *Aplysia*. *Proc. Natl. Acad. Sci. USA* **77**:7492–7496.

Castellucci, V. F., A. Nairn, P. Greengard, J. H. Schwartz, and E. R. Kandel (1982) Inhibitor of adenosine 3':5'-monophosphate-dependent protein kinase blocks presynaptic facilitation in *Aplysia*. *J. Neurosci.* **2**:1673–1681.

Chad, J. E., and R. Eckert (1984) Stimulation of cAMP-dependent protein phosphorylation retards both inactivation and "washout" of Ca current in dialyzed *Helix* neurons. *Soc. Neurosci. Abstr.* **10**:866.

Cohen, P. (1982) The role of protein phosphorylation in the neural and hormonal control of cellular activity. *Nature* **296**:613–620.

Corbin, J. D., and J. G. Hardman, eds. (1984) *Hormone Action, Protein Kinases, Methods Enzymology*, Vol. 99F, Academic, New York.

de Peyer, J. E., A. B. Cachelin, I. B. Levitan, and H. Reuter (1982) Ca^{2+}-activated K^+ conductance in internally perfused snail neurons is enhanced by protein phosphorylation. *Proc. Natl. Acad. Sci. USA* **79**:4207–4211.

DeRiemer, S. A., J. A. Strong, K. A. Albert, P. Greengard, and L. K. Kaczmarek (1985) Phorbol ester and protein kinase C enhance calcium current in *Aplysia* neurons. *Nature* **313**:313–316.

Detre, J. A., A. C. Nairn, D. W. Aswad, and P. Greengard (1984) Localization in mammalian brain of G-substrate, a specific substrate for cyclic GMP-dependent protein kinase. *J. Neurosci.* **4**:2843–2849.

Dimova, R., J. Vuillet, and R. Seite (1980) Study of the rat neostriatum using a combined Golgi–electron microscope technique and serial sections. *Neuroscience* **5**:1581–1596.

Dolphin, A., M. Hamont, and J. Bockaert (1979) The resolution of dopamine and β_1- and β_2-adrenergic-sensitive adenylate cyclase activities in homogenates of cat cerebellum, hippocampus and cerebral cortex. *Brain Res.* **179**:305–317.

Doroshenko, P. A., P. G. Kostyuk, A. E. Martynyuk, M. D. Kursky, and Z. D. Vorobetz (1984) Intracellular protein kinase injection and calcium inward currents in perfused neurons of the snail *Helix pomatia*. *Neuroscience* **11**:263–267.

Forn, J., B. K. Krueger, and P. Greengard (1974) Adenosine 3':5'-monophosphate content in rat caudate nucleus. Demonstration of dopaminergic and adrenergic receptors. *Science* **186**:1118–1120.

Greengard, P., and J. F. Kuo (1970) On the mechanism of action of cyclic AMP. *Adv. Biochem. Psychopharmacol.* **3**:287–306.

Gribkoff, V. K., J. H. Ashe, W. H. Fletcher, and M. E. Lekawa (1984) Dopamine, cyclic AMP, and protein kinase produce a similar long-lasting increase in input resistance in hippocampal CA_1 neurons. *Soc. Neurosci. Abstr.* **10**:898.

Groves, P. M. (1983) A theory of the functional organization of the neostriatum and the neostriatal control of voluntary movement. *Brain. Res. Rev.* **5**:109–132.

Hemmings, H. C., Jr., and P. Greengard (1986) DARPP-32, a dopamine-regulated and adenosine 3'-5'-monophosphate-regulated phosphoprotein—Regional, tissue, and phylogenetic distribution. *J. Neurosci.* **6**:1469–1481.

Hemmings, H. C., Jr., A. C. Nairn, D. W. Aswad, and P. Greengard (1984a) DARPP-32, a dopamine- and adenosine 3':5'-monophosphate-regulated phosphoprotein enriched in dopamine-innervated brain regions. II. Purification and characterization of the phosphoprotein from bovine caudate nucleus. *J. Neurosci.* **4**:99–110.

Hemmings, H. C., Jr., P. Greengard, H. Y. L. Tung, and P. Cohen (1984b) DARPP-32, a dopamine-regulated neuronal phosphoprotein, is a potent inhibitor of protein phosphatase-1. *Nature* **310**:503–505.

Hemmings, H. C., Jr., A. C. Nairn, and P. Greengard (1984c) DARPP-32, a dopamine- and adenosine 3':5'-monophosphate-regulated neuronal phosphoprotein. II. Comparison of the kinetics of phosphorylation of DARPP-32 and phosphatase inhibitor-1. *J. Biol. Chem.* **259**:14486–14490.

Hemmings, H. C., Jr., K. R. Williams, W. H. Konigsberg, and P. Greengard (1984d) DARPP-32, a dopamine- and adenosine 3':5'-monophosphate-regulated neuronal phosphoprotein. I. Amino acid sequence around the phosphorylated threonine. *J. Biol. Chem.* **259**:14491–14497.

Henn, F. A., D. J. Anderson, and A. Sellstrom (1977) Possible relationship between glial cells, dopamine and the effects of antipsychotic drugs. *Nature* **266**:637–638.

Huang, F. L., and W. H. Glinsmann (1976) Separation and characterization of two phosphorylase phosphatase inhibitors from rabbit skeletal muscle. *Eur. J. Biochem.* **70**:419–426.

Ingebritsen, T. S., and P. Cohen (1983a) Protein phosphatases: Properties and role in cellular regulation. *Science* **221**:331–338.

Ingebritsen, T. S., and P. Cohen (1983b) The protein phosphatases involved in cellular regulation. I. Classification and substrate specificities. *Eur. J. Biochem.* **132**:255–261.

Kaczmarek, L. K., K. R. Jennings, F. Strumwasser, A. C. Nairn, U. Walter, F. D. Wilson, and P. Greengard (1980) Microinjection of catalytic subunit of cyclic AMP-dependent protein kinase enhances calcium action potentials of bag cell neurons in cell culture. *Proc. Natl. Acad. Sci. USA* **77**:7487–7491.

Kaczmarek, L. K., A. C. Nairn, and P. Greengard (1984) Microinjection of protein kinase inhibitor prevents enhancement of action potentials in peptidergic neurons of *Aplysia*. *Soc. Neurosci. Abstr.* **10**:895.

Kaczmarek, L. K., and S. Strumwasser (1984) A voltage clamp analysis of currents underlying cyclic AMP-induced membrane modulation in peptidergic neurons of *Aplysia*. *J. Neurophysiol.* **52**:340–349.

Kaczmarek, L. K., J. A. Strong, and S. DeRiemer (1985) Biochemical mechanisms that modulate potassium and calcium currents in peptidergic neurons. In *Neurosecretion and the Biology of Neuropeptides*, H. Kobayashi, ed., pp. 275–282, Springer-Verlag, New York.

Kakiuchi, S., and T. W. Rall (1968) The influence of chemical agents on the accumulation of adenosine 3′:5′-monophosphate in slices of rabbit cerebellum. *Mol. Pharmacol.* **4**:367–378.

Kandel, E. R., and J. H. Schwartz (1982) Molecular biology of learning: Modulation of transmitter release. *Science* **218**:433–442.

Kebabian, J. W., and D. B. Calne (1979) Multiple receptors for dopamine. *Nature* **277**:93–96.

Kebabian, J. W., and T. E. Cote (1981) Dopamine receptors and cyclic AMP: A decade of progress. *Trends Pharmacol. Sci.* **2**:69–71.

Kebabian, J. W., and P. Greengard (1971) Dopamine-sensitive adenyl cyclase: Possible role in synaptic transmission. *Science* **174**:1346–1349.

Kennedy, M. B. (1983) Experimental approaches to understanding the role of protein phosphorylation in the regulation of neuronal function. *Annu. Rev. Neurosci.* **6**:493–525.

King, M. M., C. Y. Huang, P. B. Chock, A. C. Nairn, H. C. Hemmings, Jr., K.-F. J. Chan, and P. Greengard (1984) Mammalian brain phosphoproteins as substrates for calcineurin. *J. Biol. Chem.* **259**:8080–8083.

Levitan, I. B., J. R. Lemos, and I. Novak-Hofer (1983) Protein phosphorylation and the regulation of ion channels. *Trends Neurosci.* **6**:496–499.

Lindvall, O., and A. Björklund (1978) Organization of catecholamine neurons in the rat central nervous system. *Handb. Psychopharmacol.* **9**:139–231.

Ljungdahl, Å., T. Hökfelt, and G. Nilsson (1978) Distribution of substance P-like immunoreactivity in the central nervous system of the rat. I. Cell bodies and nerve terminals. *Neuroscience* **3**: 861–943.

Llinás, R., T. M. McGuinness, C. S. Leonard, M. Sugimori, and P. Greengard (1985) Intraterminal injection of synapsin I or of calcium/calmodulin-dependent protein kinase II alters neurotransmitter release at the squid giant synapse. *Proc. Natl. Acad. Sci. USA* **82**:3035–3039.

Moore, R. Y., and F. E. Bloom (1978) Central catecholamine neuron systems: Anatomy and physiology of the dopamine systems. *Annu. Rev. Neurosci.* **1**:129–169.

Nairn, A. C., H. C. Hemmings, Jr., and P. Greengard (1985) Protein kinases in the brain. *Annu. Rev. Biochem.* **54**:931–976.

Nestler, E. J., and P. Greengard (1983) Protein phosphorylation in the brain. *Nature* **305**:583–588.

Nestler, E. J., and P. Greengard (1984) *Protein Phosphorylation in the Nervous System*, Wiley, New York.

Nestler, E. J., S. I. Walaas, and P. Greengard (1984) Neuronal phosphoproteins: Physiological and clinical implications. *Science* **225**:1357–1364.

Nimmo, G. A., and P. Cohen (1978) The regulation of glycogen metabolism: Purification and characterization of protein phosphatase inhibitor-1 from rabbit skeletal muscle. *Eur. J. Biochem.* **87**:341–351.

Nishizuka, Y. (1984) Turnover of inositol phospholipids and signal transduction. *Science* **225**:1365–1370.

Oertel, W. H., and E. Mugnaini (1984) Immunocytochemical studies of GABAergic neurons in rat basal ganglia and their relations to other neuronal systems. *Neurosci. Lett.* **47**:233–238.

Osterrieder, W., G. Brum, J. Hescheler, W. Trautwein, V. Flockerzi, and F. Hofmann (1982) Injection of subunits of cyclic AMP-dependent protein kinase into cardiac myocytes modulates Ca^{2+} current. *Nature* **298**:576–578.

Ouimet, C. C., P. E. Miller, H. C. Hemmings, Jr., S. I. Walaas, and P. Greengard (1984) DARPP-32, a dopamine- and adenosine 3':5'-monophosphate-regulated phosphoprotein enriched in dopamine-innervated brain regions. III. Immunocytochemical localization. *J. Neurosci.* **4**:111–124.

Pasik, P., T. Pasik, and M. Di Figlia (1979) The internal organization of the neostriatum in mammals. In *The Neostriatum*, I. Divac and G. E. Oberg, eds., pp. 5–36, Pergamon, New York.

Pickel, V. M., K. K. Sumal, S. C. Beckley, R. J. Miller, and D. J. Reis (1980) Immunocytochemical localization of enkephalin in the neostriatum of rat brain: A light and electron microscopic study. *J. Comp. Neurol.* **189**:721–740.

Reiner, A., S. E. Braith, and H. J. Karten (1984) Evolution of the amniote basal ganglia. *Trends Neurosci.* **7**:320–325.

Reuter, H. (1983) Calcium channel modulation by neurotransmitters, enzymes and drugs. *Nature* **301**:569–574.

Rosen, O. M., and E. G. Krebs (1981) *Protein Phosphorylation*, Cold Spring Harbor Laboratory, Cold Spring Harbor, New York.

Schlichter, D. J., J. A. Detre, D. W. Aswad, B. Chehrazi, and P. Greengard (1980) Localization of cyclic GMP-dependent protein kinase and substrate in mammalian cerebellum. *Proc. Natl. Acad. Sci. USA* **77**:5537–5541.

Schubert, D., H. Tarikas, and M. LaCombiere (1976) Neurotransmitter regulation of adenosine 3':5'-monophosphate in clonal nerve, glia and muscle cells. *Science* **192**:471–472.

Schwarcz, R., and J. T. Coyle (1977) Striatal lesions with kainic acid: Neurochemical characteristics. *Brain Res.* **127**:235–249.

Siegelbaum, S. A., J. S. Camardo, and E. R. Kandel (1982) Serotonin and cyclic AMP close single K^+ channels in *Aplysia* sensory neurons. *Nature* **299**:413–417.

Stewart, A. A., T. S. Ingebritsen, A. Manalan, C. B. Klee, and P. Cohen (1982) Discovery of a Ca^{2+}- and calmodulin-dependent protein phosphatase. *FEBS Lett.* **137**:80–84.

Stoof, J. C., and J. W. Kebabian (1981) Opposing roles for D-1 and D-2 dopamine receptors in efflux of cyclic AMP from rat neostriatum. *Nature* **294**:366–368.

Walaas, S. I., and P. Greengard (1984) DARPP-32, a dopamine- and adenosine 3':5'-monophosphate-regulated phosphoprotein enriched in dopamine-innervated brain regions. I. Regional and cellular distribution in rat brain. *J. Neurosci.* **4**:84–98.

Walaas, S. I., A. C. Nairn, and P. Greengard (1983a) Regional distribution of calcium- and cyclic AMP-regulated protein phosphorylation systems in mammalian brain. I. Particulate systems. *J. Neurosci.* **3**:291–301.

Walaas, S. I., A. C. Nairn, and P. Greengard (1983b) Regional distribution of calcium- and cyclic AMP-regulated protein phosphorylation systems in mammalian brain. II. Soluble systems. *J. Neurosci.* **3**:302–311.

Walaas, S. I., D. W. Aswad, and P. Greengard (1983c) A dopamine- and cyclic AMP-regulated phosphoprotein enriched in dopamine-innervated brain regions. *Nature* **301**:69–71.

Wallace, R. W., E. A. Tallant, and W. Y. Cheung (1980) High levels of a heat-labile calmodulin-binding protein (CaM-BP$_{80}$) in bovine neostriatum. *Biochemistry* **19**:1831–1837.

Williams, K. R., H. C. Hemmings, Jr., M. B. Lopresti, W. H. Konigsberg, and P. Greengard (1986) DARPP-32, a dopamine-regulated and cyclic AMP-regulated neuronal phosphoprotein—Primary structure and homology with protein phosphatase inhibitor-1. *J. Biol. Chem.* **261**:1890–1903.

Wood, J. G., R. W. Wallace, J. N. Whitaker, and W. Y. Cheung (1980) Immunocytochemical localization of calmodulin and a heat-labile calmodulin-binding protein (CaM-BP$_{80}$) in basal ganglia of mouse brain. *J. Cell Biol.* **84**:66–76.

Chapter 9

Idiosyncratic Receptors in the Brain

SOLOMON H. SNYDER

ABSTRACT

Ligand binding techniques have proved to be powerful tools for characterizing neurotransmitter and drug receptors, differentiating subtypes of receptors, and monitoring associations between the recognition sites of receptors and ion channels or second messenger systems such as adenylate cyclase and the phosphoinositide cycle. Besides the characterization of conventional neurotransmitter receptors, ligand binding procedures have permitted studies of many other sites in the brain. A number of drug receptors have been found to represent specific enzymes. For instance, phorbol ester receptors are identical to protein kinase C, an enzyme of importance in conveying effects of the phosphoinositide cycle to intracellular metabolic systems. Receptor sites for the neurotoxin MPTP (N-methyl-4-phenyl-1,2,3,6-tetrahydropyridine), which causes nigrostriatal destruction similar to that of Parkinson's disease, appear to reflect monoamine oxidase type B. Well-characterized enzymes, such as enkephalin convertase and angiotensin-converting enzyme, can be elucidated in terms of their molecular properties by ligand binding with potent inhibitors. Voltage-dependent calcium channels in the brain can be labeled with calcium antagonist drugs, which appear to bind to receptor sites that may be associated with neurotransmitters whose synaptic effects involve alterations in calcium permeability. Neurotransmitter uptake sites can also be characterized by the binding of drugs that inhibit neurotransmitter uptake, thus permitting an elucidation of the molecular mechanisms that regulate neurotransmitter uptake processes.

The notion that drugs, neurotransmitters, and hormones act at specific recognition sites or receptors on the surfaces of cells dates back to the earliest part of the twentieth century. The receptor concept has been a cornerstone of pharmacological research, and drugs acting at specific receptors have been developed systematically for many years. Even the existence of receptor subtypes has been appreciated for more than 40 years.

In the past decade, the advent of receptor binding techniques has permitted a considerable escalation in our appreciation of neurotransmitter and drug receptors, especially in the brain. By utilizing appropriate ligands, it is now possible to characterize receptor binding sites for virtually every known neurotransmitter in the brain (Snyder, 1984). Even the linkage between recognition of the neurotransmitter and second messengers can be examined through binding techniques by evaluating the influence of ions, whose permeability is altered in synaptic transmission, upon receptor binding. The regulation of receptor binding by guanine nucleotides provides an indication of interactions with the N proteins that link receptors to adenylate cyclase.

As the sophistication of receptor binding techniques has increased, these approaches have been used to characterize features of synaptic function in addition to the conventional influences of neurotransmitters on postsynaptic receptors. For instance, biogenic amines and amino acid neurotransmitters are inactivated by reuptake into the nerve endings that release them. The uptake recognition sites for receptors can now be explored through radioligand binding techniques. Ion channels not generally thought to be related to neurotransmitters, such as voltage-sensitive calcium channels, have been characterized by ligand binding approaches. Enzymes that function as second messengers for synaptic transmission, such as protein kinase C, have also been elucidated by receptor-binding techniques. Finally, a number of neurotransmitter-related enzymes can be characterized through the binding of potent inhibitors, providing important information about their molecular properties and functions that cannot be elucidated by assays of catalytic activity. This chapter reviews some of these very recent themes in receptor research.

PHORBOL ESTER RECEPTORS, PROTEIN KINASE C, AND THE PHOSPHOINOSITIDE CYCLE

At some receptors, such as the nicotinic cholinergic receptor, recognition of the transmitter is "translated" immediately into an opening of an ion channel. At many other receptors, there seems to be some intervening second messenger biochemical event. Activation or inhibition of adenylate cyclase is the best known of these. Recently, there has been increased interest in alterations in phosphoinositide (PI) turnover as mediators of synaptic transmission (Nishizuka, 1984; Figure 1). A substantial number of neurotransmitters and hormones seem to act through alterations in PI turnover. Examples include acetylcholine at muscarinic cholinergic receptors, α_1-adrenergic actions, bradykinin, histamine H_1 receptors, and serotonin at certain receptor subtypes. A given neurotransmitter may utilize different second messengers at different synapses. Thus, norepinephrine activates adenylate cyclase at β-receptors, inhibits adenylate cyclase at α_2-receptors, and acts via PI turnover at α_1-receptors. Monitoring the effects of neurotransmitters on the fairly complex PI cycle is sometimes difficult. Moreover, few drugs are available that act potently and selectively to block steps in the cycle and permit inferences as to whether a given neurotransmitter or other

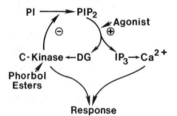

Figure 1. *The phosphoinositide cycle.* Feedback points and the role of protein kinase C are indicated.

agent is acting through the cycle. Biochemical monitors of PI turnover are not suitable for visualization by histochemical techniques, so that one cannot localize the PI cycle to particular neuronal populations in the brain and examine the influence of individual neurotransmitter systems.

The details of the PI cycle are not altogether clear, but the general pattern appears to be something like the following: Neurotransmitters activate the PI cycle by stimulating the breakdown of phosphatidylinositol-4,5-bis-phosphate (PIP_2), leading to the formation of diacylglycerol and inositol triphosphate (IP_3). IP_3 releases calcium from intracellular stores, which may be responsible in part for the effects of neurotransmitters on cellular function. Diacylglycerol stimulates the activity of protein kinase C by increasing its affinity for calcium, an ion required for maximal protein kinase C activity (Nishizuka, 1984). The identity of the key proteins phosphorylated through the action of protein kinase C is not clear. Diacylglycerol and IP_3 are thought to act synergistically.

There is evidence that lithium may exert its therapeutic effects in manic–depressive illness through actions upon the PI cycle. In low millimolar concentrations, corresponding to those that occur in plasma with therapeutic doses of lithium, the ion inhibits the phosphatase that degrades inositol monophosphate, slowing the turnover of the PI cycle. Such an effect would be expected to attenuate receptor sensitivity, which is thought to be a major action of lithium in psychiatric illness.

Recently, a new tool has become available with which to evaluate protein kinase C. Research on tumor promoters has been ongoing for many years. Phorbol esters are among the most potent of known tumor promoters, acting in nanomolar or even lower concentrations. Besides facilitating the actions of carcinogens, phorbol esters exert potent inflammatory effects. Blumberg and his colleagues (1984) pioneered in identifying and characterizing specific receptor recognition sites for phorbol esters by utilizing receptor binding techniques. Phorbol esters are extremely hydrophobic; nonspecific binding is so great with most of the esters that one cannot identify specific receptor interactions. Blumberg developed more hydrophilic derivatives of the esters, which preserved biological activity adequate enough to permit receptor labeling. The parallel characterization of phorbol ester receptors and protein kinase C, achieved largely in the laboratory of Nishizuka (1984), culminated in an appreciation that phorbol ester receptors are, in fact, identical to protein kinase C. Thus, what was thought to be a receptor for a druglike substance turned out to be a specific enzyme.

Our initial interest in phorbol esters preceded the identification of these sites as protein kinase C. We were impressed with observations that receptor binding sites were more highly concentrated in the brain than in any other tissue. We conducted whole-body autoradiographic studies in rat fetuses and found a selective association of the receptors with differentiating cellular processes, but not with cellular proliferation or DNA synthesis (Murphy et al., 1983). The association of these receptors with protein kinase C suggested that this enzyme might mediate actions of neurotransmitters and hormones. However, a number of assumptions were involved in such speculations and there seemed to be no direct evidence linking protein kinase C to neurotransmission. We felt that phorbol esters, which act in nanomolar concentrations, might be the potent and selective probes needed to evaluate a possible role of protein kinase C in synaptic transmission. Presumably, phorbol esters mimicked diacylglycerol in enhancing protein kinase C activity. One simple system in which to examine this hypothesis involves the effects of neurotransmitters on smooth-muscle contractions, and it was here that we studied the actions of phorbol esters (Baraban et al., 1985).

We utilized a variety of smooth-muscle preparations in which numerous neurotransmitters influence contractions, some via the PI cycle and some via adenylate cyclase or other mechanisms. For instance, the guinea pig ileum contracts via influences at muscarinic cholinergic, histamine H_1, serotonin, and bradykinin receptors. Nanomolar concentrations of various phorbol esters did not induce contractions of the ileum but rapidly and reversibly blocked contractions elicited by oxotremorine, muscarinic cholinergic agonists, histamine, serotonin, and bradykinin (Table 1). Serotonin contracts the ileum both directly and indirectly by releasing acetylcholine. The phorbol ester effect was exerted on the direct effects of serotonin on smooth muscle, since it persisted in the presence of atropine. The blockade of neurotransmitter effects involved pharmacologically relevant phorbol esters, since the absolute and relative potencies of several phorbol esters in blocking these effects corresponded closely to their relative affinities for receptor binding sites.

The influence of phorbol esters appeared to be exerted directly on receptor-linked events rather than on voltage-dependent ion channels or the contractile machinery of the muscle, since phorbol esters had no effect on potassium-induced contractions. Moreover, phorbol esters did not influence the relaxation of the muscle produced by catecholamines acting through adenylate cyclase. The effects of oxotremorine, bradykinin, and serotonin on contractions of the rat uterus were blocked by phorbol esters, all with the same potency and selectivity.

A rather different pattern was apparent in the rat vas deferens and in the dog basilar artery. In the vas deferens, phorbol esters alone did not have any effect upon contractions. However, they potently and selectively enhanced nor-

Table 1. Comparison of Phorbol Ester Analogues in Smooth-Muscle Systems and Receptor Binding[a]

Drug	Inhibition of Guinea Pig Ileum Contractions K_i (nM)	Contraction of Rat Vas Deferens ED_{50} (nM)	Inhibition of [^{3}H]PDBU Binding in Rat Vas Deferens K_i (nM)
PDBU	31 ± 4	16 ± 5	36 ± 6
DPB	78 ± 19	25 ± 6	180 ± 20
PDA	470 ± 160	140 ± 40	1,100 ± 100
P 13-A	20,000 ± 4,000	6,000 ± 2,100	22,000 ± 3,000
PDA 13,20	>25,000	>25,000	>25,000
Phorbol	>25,000	>25,000	>25,000

[a]K_i values in guinea pig ileum were determined for blockade of oxotremorine-induced contractions. ED_{50} values in the rat vas deferens were obtained from strips immersed in depolarizing Tyrode's buffer after the addition of 1 mM calcium chloride. Data are mean values of 3–6 determinations ± SEMs. PDBU, phorbol 12,13-dibutyrate; DPB, 12-deoxyphorbol 13-isobutyrate; PDA, phorbol diacetate; P 13-A, phorbol 13-acetate; PDA 13,20, phorbol 13,20-diacetate.

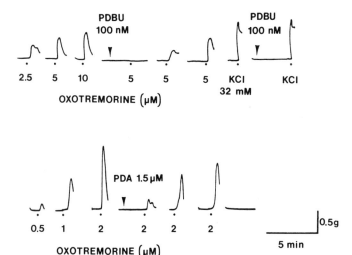

Figure 2. *Inhibition of oxotremorine-induced contraction of rat uterus.* In the record presented in the *top panel*, 100 nM phorbol 12,13-dibutyrate (PDBU) did not alter baseline muscle tension, but completely prevented the effect of 5 μM oxotremorine. In contrast, the same dose of PDBU did not influence uterine contractions initiated by bath application of 32 mM potassium chloride. Similar effects of another phorbol ester, phorbol diacetate (PDA), are shown in the *lower panel*.

epinephrine-induced contractions in a pattern indicating mediation via specific receptors (Figure 2). No facilitation of potassium-induced contractions was apparent. In the dog basilar artery, phorbol esters produced direct contractions with potencies corresponding to affinities for receptor-binding sites.

The virtually opposite effects of phorbol esters in the ileum and uterus, compared to their effects in the basilar artery and vas deferens, may not be as puzzling as they seem. The PI cycle involves complex feedback mechanisms. Thus, activation of protein kinase C may inhibit the formation of PIP$_2$. Through such a feedback system, stimulation of protein kinase C might inhibit PIP$_2$ formation in the ileum and uterus, whereas in the basilar artery and vas deferens the esters might predominantly synergize with calcium to produce physiological responses.

The influences of phorbol esters on tissue contractions fit well with the relationship of protein kinase C and calcium. The contractions of smooth muscle elicited by the transmitters investigated all involve effects on calcium. Even more direct evidence for such interactions comes from our recent neurophysiological studies in hippocampal brain slices (Baraban et al., 1985). Intracellular recordings indicate that phorbol esters inhibit a calcium-induced augmentation of potassium conductance in pyramidal cells, an effect essentially identical to that of muscarinic cholinergic stimulation.

Autoradiographic studies permit a visualization of phorbol esters, and hence protein kinase C, at the microscopic level (Blumberg et al., 1984; Worley et al., 1986). The receptors are quite discretely localized. Dense receptor clusters occur in the zona compacta of the substantia nigra, the ventral tegmental area, and in the caudate and putamen, suggesting an association with dopamine systems. Very dense localizations also occur in the periaqueductal gray. Within the cerebellum, autoradiographic grains are most concentrated in the molecular layer. The pyramidal cell layer of the hippocampus is greatly enriched in receptors. Clearly, such autoradiographic studies will permit an analysis of exact neuronal groups whose functions are regulated by the PI cycle. Conventional biochemical approaches have not yet permitted such an analysis for adenylate cyclase or any other second messenger system. Thus, the protein kinase C system represents an instance in which simple receptor binding techniques have greatly facilitated an understanding of second messenger systems.

RECEPTOR FOR THE NEUROTOXIN MPTP (N-METHYL-4-PHENYL-1,2,3,6-TETRAHYDROPYRIDINE) SHEDS LIGHT ON PARKINSON'S DISEASE AND MONOAMINE OXIDASE

Though the knowledge that Parkinson's disease involves a dopamine deficiency has permitted the development of L-dopa as a therapeutic agent, little is yet known of the reasons for the selective loss of dopamine neurons. Recent studies of the unique neurotoxin MPTP may shed light on the selective neuropathology of Parkinson's disease and may also provide new tools with which to probe synaptic function. In the late 1970s, numerous young drug abusers in California suddenly developed severe Parkinsonian symptoms, which were shown to result from the accidental self-administration of MPTP, a by-product in the synthesis of black-market opiates related to meperidine (Langston and Ballard, 1984). Administration of MPTP to monkeys and mice produces irreversible destruction of dopamine pathways in the brain, with little evidence of any other permanent neuropathology. Since MPTP and related chemicals are widely used in industry, researchers have speculated that exposure to them might initiate damage to the nigrostriatal system, with subsequent age-related degeneration of dopamine neurons ultimately attaining a threshold for the initiation of Parkinsonian symptoms.

Clearly, elucidating the molecular sites of MPTP activity was desirable. Accordingly, we evaluated the binding of [^{3}H]MPTP to brain membranes (Javitch et al., 1984b). [^{3}H]MPTP binds with high affinity (in the nanomolar range) to membranes. The relative affinity of various pyridine derivatives fits with its neurotoxic effects. Thus, the oxidized derivative of MPTP, MPP$^+$, which possesses a fully unsaturated pyridine ring, has about the same affinity for binding sites as MPTP and is also neurotoxic. Removal of the methyl group from the pyridine ring of MPTP greatly reduces neurotoxicity and affinity for binding sites. Similarly, removal of the benzene ring from MPTP abolishes neurotoxicity and affinity for binding sites. Replacement of the tetrahydropyridine ring of MPTP with a piperidine ring abolishes neurotoxicity and binding affinity altogether. Thus, the binding sites examined seem to be associated with the neurotoxic effects of MPTP.

Autoradiographic studies provide even stronger evidence of the link between sites and neurotoxicity (Table 2). In human brain, the highest density of binding sites occurs in the caudate and substantia nigra, fitting ideally with sites of maximal neurotoxicity. Interestingly, high receptor densities also occur in the locus coeruleus, which is damaged in idiopathic Parkinson's disease. The rat is

Table 2. Distribution of ([³H]MPTP) Binding Sites in Human and Rat Brain[a]

Human

Caudate	++++	Nucleus parabrachialis	+−++
Substantia nigra	+++	Red nucleus	trace
Locus coeruleus	+++	Cerebellar peduncle	trace
Cerebral cortex gray matter	++−+++	Cerebral cortex white matter	trace

Rat

Interpeduncular nucleus	++++	Medial habenula	++
Locus coeruleus	+++	Lateral septum	++
Hypothalamus		Cerebral cortex	+−++
Arcuate nucleus	+++	Hippocampus	+−++
Periventricular nucleus	+++	Cerebellum	+
Subfornical organ	+++	Nucleus accumbens	+
Ventricular ependyma	+++	Globus pallidus	+
Superior colliculus	++	Lateral habenula	+
Periaqueductal gray	++	Medial septum	+
Substantia nigra	++	Other hypothalamic nuclei	+
Corpus striatum	++	Fornix	trace
Amygdala	++	Corpus callosum	trace
Bed nucleus of stria terminalis	++	Internal capsule	trace

[a]Semiquantitative evaluation of receptor autoradiographic grain densities in human and rat brain structures (averaged estimations by two independent observers). ++++, very dense; +++, dense; ++, moderate density; +, modest density; trace, slightly greater than background.

one species in which MPTP administration fails to produce permanent nigrostriatal neuronal destruction, and the density of MPTP receptors in the substantia nigra and caudate in the rat is much less than that in the human brain. In the rat, as in humans, high densities of receptors occur in the locus coeruleus as well as in the interpeduncular nucleus.

One wonders about the nature of the MPTP binding sites. Might they be receptors for some hitherto unidentified neurotransmitter or for a known neurotransmitter? An extensive evaluation of all known neurotransmitters, as well as many drugs, failed to reveal any with selective high affinity for the binding sites.

Insight into the nature of the MPTP binding sites came initially from studies of MPTP metabolism. Incubation of MPTP with mitochondria results in the oxidative conversion of MPTP to MPP^+ (Chiba et al., 1984). This conversion is blocked by monoamine oxidase (MAO) inhibitors, especially inhibitors of MAO type B (MAO-B). To ascertain whether this metabolic conversion is involved in the neurotoxicity of MPTP, Heikkila and his colleagues (1984) examined the effect of treatment with MAO inhibitors on the neurotoxicity of MPTP in mice. MAO inhibitors abolish MPTP neurotoxicity. Thus, MPP^+ appears to be the active agent mediating MPTP neurotoxicity, and MAO plays a major role in its formation.

Parsons and Rainbow (1984) then examined the autoradiographic localization of [^{3}H]pargyline, an inhibitor of MAO with somewhat greater preference for type B than for type A isozymes. The autoradiographic patterns of [^{3}H]pargyline and [^{3}H]MPTP binding sites are virtually identical. Moreover, deprenyl, a potent inhibitor of MAO-B, has about the same affinity for [^{3}H]MPTP binding sites as for MAO. Thus, MPTP binding sites appear to represent MAO-B.

Besides shedding light on mechanisms of MPTP toxicity, the identification of MAO-B as the MPTP receptor again illustrates the role of enzymes as "receptors" for pharmacological agents. These findings suggest a more specific role of MAO in neuronal function than had been previously assumed. Since MAO is a mitochondrial enzyme and occurs in many tissues of the body, it was thought that MAO in the brain was distributed ubiquitously. However, MAO-B labeled with [^{3}H]pargyline is selectively localized to specific neuronal populations. Such localization studies have not yet been done with MAO type A (MAO-A), but one can anticipate similarly discrete patterns. Interestingly, MAO-A acts selectively upon biogenic amine neurotransmitters such as norepinephrine, serotonin, and dopamine, which display very little affinity for MAO-B. One might even speculate that some hitherto unappreciated monoamine is the physiological substrate for MAO-B, localized to neuronal systems enriched with MAO-B.

ENKEPHALIN CONVERTASE CHARACTERIZED BY RECEPTOR BINDING APPROACHES

In many ways, receptor proteins behave like enzymes, except that there is no conversion of substrate to product. Kinetic analyses of receptors display parallels to the behavior of enzymes. The "functional" way of monitoring enzymes, via their catalytic activity, has been the major approach to their characterization. Receptor binding technology may be a powerful tool for approaching the molecular properties of enzymes, even in crude tissue extracts. This is illustrated nicely by studies of enkephalin convertase labeled with radioactive ligands.

Neuropeptides are formed by cleavage from large protein precursors. Neurotransmitter and hormonal peptides are embedded in the precursors, flanked on both sides by pairs of basic amino acids. Trypsinlike enzymes cleave to the right of the basic amino acids, freeing up the biologically active peptide on its amino terminus, while a single basic amino acid remains attached to the carboxyl terminus of the peptide. A carboxypeptidase B-like enzyme activity then removes the basic amino acid. A fundamental question in the processing of hormonal and neurotransmitter peptides has been whether selective enzymes exist for the processing of each neuropeptide, or whether a few generalized enzymes deal with all of them.

Recently, we showed that enkephalin convertase, a unique carboxypeptidase B-like enzyme, exists in the chromaffin granules of the adrenal medulla (where enkephalin is stored together with epinephrine), in the pituitary gland, and in the brain (Fricker and Snyder, 1982). The regional distribution of this enzymatic activity in the brain parallels the distribution of enkephalin to a certain extent, while other carboxypeptidase activity is homogeneously distributed. Purification to homogeneity confirms that enkephalin convertase is a novel enzyme (Fricker and Snyder, 1983).

A definitive association of enkephalin convertase with the enkephalin neurons comes from the receptor binding-like labeling of the enzyme. In a screen of various chemicals for possible inhibitors, we found a series of agents that had been designed as carboxypeptidase inhibitors and displayed nanomolar affinity for enkephalin convertase but only micromolar affinity for other carboxypeptidases (Fricker et al., 1983). One of these inhibitors, guanidinoethylmercaptosuccinic acid (GEMSA), was labeled with tritium and its receptor binding was examined (Strittmatter et al., 1984b). [^{3}H]GEMSA binds with nanomolar affinity and selectivity to enkephalin convertase, so that even in crude tissue homogenates the only protein bound by the inhibitor is enkephalin convertase. As a result, one can monitor the number of enzyme protein molecules, a task that would be quite difficult to accomplish by conventional techniques. If one simultaneously measures enkephalin convertase catalytic activity, then it is also possible to monitor the turnover number of the enzyme in these crude preparations. Because enkephalin convertase catalytic activity can be readily measured, and because [^{3}H]GEMSA binding is easily detected, one can measure the turnover number of the enzyme in 500 crude tissue specimens in a day, something inconceivable by conventional protein chemistry. This permits one to assess the influence of varying physiological and pharmacological conditions on the turnover of enkephalin convertase.

Labeling with [^{3}H]GEMSA permits autoradiographic studies analogous to those performed with neurotransmitter receptors (Lynch et al., 1984; Figure 3). Monitored in this way, enkephalin convertase is localized to specific neuronal populations in the brain. In general, its localization is the same as that of enkephalin neurons. [^{3}H]GEMSA-associated silver grains are highly concentrated in the median eminence, the bed nucleus of the stria terminalis, the lateral septum, the central nucleus of the amygdala, the preoptic and magnocellular nuclei of the hypothalamus, the locus coeruleus, the nucleus of the solitary tract, and the substantia gelatinosa of the spinal trigeminal tract.

Enkephalin convertase presumably has functions other than the formation of enkephalin, since high concentrations of the enzyme occur in the anterior pituitary gland, which possesses very little enkephalin. The enzyme may also be involved in the processing of other neurotransmitter or hormonal peptides. The high density of the enzyme in the salivary gland presumably indicates an association with some peptide other than enkephalin, which is not known to occur in the salivary gland.

The fact that enkephalin convertase may be involved in the processing of other peptides does not diminish the importance of its selective association with enkephalin neurons in the brain. It is rare for any enzyme, especially a peptidase, to possess only a single function. Angiotensin-converting enzyme (ACE) is involved in the degradation of bradykinin as well as in the formation of angiotensin II. Dopa decarboxylase forms serotonin as well as dopamine.

ACE CLARIFIED BY LIGAND BINDING WITH [^{3}H]CAPTOPRIL

Enkephalin convertase is not the only peptidase that can be labeled by receptorlike ligand binding techniques. ACE is a dipeptidyl carboxypeptidase that removes the two carboxy-terminal amino acids from the decapeptide angiotensin I, giving rise to the physiologically potent angiotensin II. In the periphery, angiotensin

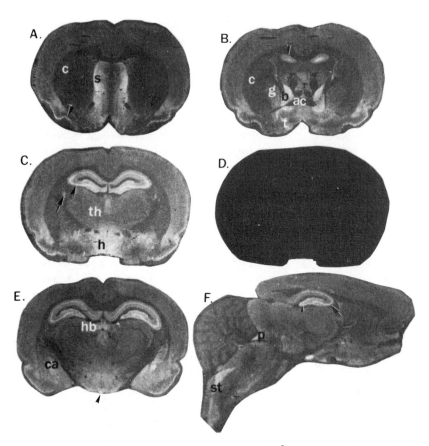

Figure 3. *Distribution of [³H]guanidinoethylmercaptosuccinic acid ([³H]GEMSA) binding in rat brain.* Rat brain sections were incubated in 4 n*M* [³H]GEMSA and apposed to LKB-Ultrafilm. Pictures were printed directly from Ultrafilm; thus white areas indicate high levels of [³H]GEMSA binding. *A*: The most densely labeled areas are the lateral septum (S) and the pyriform cortex (*arrowhead*). The caudate putamen (c) and the frontal cortex are less densely labeled. *B*: The densely labeled areas are the bed nucleus of the stria terminalis (b), olfactory tubercle (t), and the rostral hippocampus (*arrowhead*), while the globus pallidus (g) is moderately labeled. The anterior commissure (ac) is unlabeled. *C*: Labeling in the hippocampus is high in both the dentate gyrus and the area around pyramidal cell region CA3–4 (*arrowhead*). Labeling in the stria terminalis is also visible (*arrow*). The preoptic hypothalamus (h) is labeled much more densely than the thalamus (th). In the thalamus, labeling is highest in the periventricular nucleus. *D*: Binding in the presence of 10 μ*M* unlabeled GEMSA. Nonspecific binding is negligible. *E*: The area of highest binding is the median eminence (*arrowhead*). Several nuclei of the amygdala are labeled, but labeling in the central nucleus (ca) is the most intense. The habenula (hb) is also labeled. *F*: Labeling is present in the dorsal parabrachial nucleus (p) and the nucleus of the solitary tract (st). The dentate gyrus (*arrowhead*) and hippocampus (*arrow*) are distinctly labeled. Labeling is low in the cerebellum.

is a potent constrictor of blood vessels and acts selectively on the adrenal cortex to enhance the formation of aldosterone, which in turn stimulates the reabsorption of sodium. Thus, angiotensin II is thought to be involved in the maintenance of blood pressure. The development of potent and selective inhibitors of ACE that have hypotensive effects confirms the importance of ACE in blood pressure regulation (Cushman and Ondetti, 1980).

ACE also occurs in high concentrations in the brain. Catalytic assays indicate that the highest levels occur in the corpus striatum, though very little endogenous angiotensin exists in the brain and none has been demonstrated in the corpus striatum. To characterize the physiological role of brain ACE, we took advantage of the very high potency and selectivity of the ACE inhibitor captopril. We showed that [^{3}H]captopril binds potently and selectively to ACE (Strittmatter et al., 1983); in crude tissue homogenates, [^{3}H]captopril binds to ACE and to no other protein. As with enkephalin convertase, this finding permits a direct measurement of the number of enzyme molecules; combined with catalytic assays, one can estimate the turnover number for ACE in large numbers of samples. Additionally, one can readily characterize the thermodynamics of the enzyme, which is extremely difficult to do with catalytic assays alone (Strittmatter et al., 1985). Finally, direct interactions of ions and cofactors can be monitored, providing precise affinity constants.

Autoradiographic studies with [^{3}H]captopril indicate strikingly selective localizations of ACE in the brain (Strittmatter et al., 1984a). Very high densities of [^{3}H]captopril occur in the choroid plexus. There it may be involved in the production of angiotensin II, which is thought to be secreted from the choroid plexus into the ventricles and to alter thirst and blood pressure via effects on circumventricular organs. ACE labeled with [^{3}H]captopril is also highly concentrated in the subfornical organ and median preoptic areas, where application of angiotensin II regulates drinking behavior. Angiotensin occurs endogenously in the median eminence, where it probably regulates the formation of vasopressin. Localizations of [^{3}H]captopril binding in these zones may also relate to endogenous angiotensin.

The most striking localizations of ACE, however, occur in areas containing no endogenous angiotensin (Figure 4). Specifically, the greatest density of ACE labeled with [^{3}H]captopril occurs in the caudate nucleus and in a neuronal pathway descending to the substantia nigra. Lesion studies indicate that ACE is specifically localized in neurons that originate in the caudate nucleus and terminate in the substantia nigra. The adjacent cerebral cortex and other areas contain negligible ACE. The extremely high density of ACE and its selective localization in this area raise questions as to its function. Presumably ACE must be involved in the formation or destruction of some peptide in this neuronal pathway. The one known peptide contained in a descending striatonigral pathway is substance P. Because substance P contains an amide at its carboxyl terminus, it had not been thought to be a substrate for ACE. However, recent studies indicate that substance P is indeed such a substrate (Yokosawa et al., 1983; Cascieri et al., 1984). We have confirmed these findings in our own laboratory, and have shown that substance K as well as substance P is a substrate for the brain enzyme, while ACE prepared from the lung degrades substance P but not substance K.

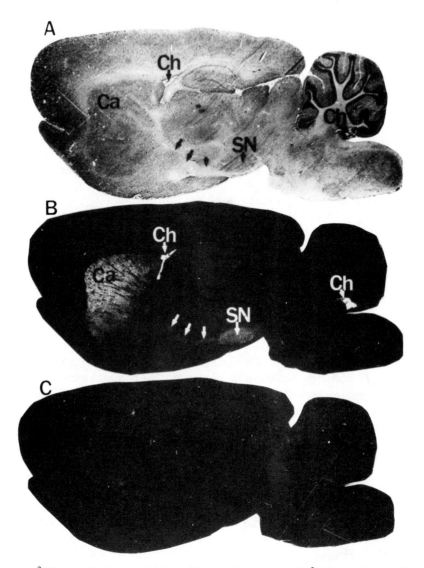

Figure 4. *[³H]Captopril binding to rat brain.* A: Toluidine blue staining. B: [³H]Captopril autoradiography. C: [³H]Captopril autoradiography in the presence of 1 μM captopril. Note the intense labeling of the choroid plexus (Ch) in B. The caudate putamen (Ca) and the substantia nigra (SN) are also visualized by autoradiography. The streaks of decreased grain density in the caudate putamen correspond to the location of white matter tracts. The *arrows* indicate the band that appears to connect the caudate putamen and the substantia nigra.

Conceivably, substance P and/or substance K are the endogenous peptides associated with ACE. However, other evidence from our laboratory suggests that there may be an unidentified peptide associated with ACE in the striatonigral pathway (Thiele et al., 1985). Screening for the endogenous substrate of an enzyme by using catalytic assays would be difficult, if not impossible. However, using ligand binding techniques, the task is much easier. We reasoned that the endogenous ACE substrate should be substantially more concentrated in the corpus striatum than in the adjacent cerebral cortex. Accordingly, we examined extracts of the corpus striatum and of the adjacent cerebral cortex for their ability to compete for [^{3}H]captopril binding. Striatal extracts are substantially more potent than are cortical extracts in inhibiting [^{3}H]captopril binding. Fractionation studies indicate that neither substance P nor substance K accounts for this activity. Thus, what appears to be a novel small peptide is an endogenous substrate for ACE in a fairly prominent neuronal pathway. It is hoped that further purification studies will result in the identification of this substance.

OTHER NOVEL SITES LABELED BY RECEPTOR BINDING TECHNIQUES

The instances cited above indicate how receptor binding techniques can shed light on neuronal mechanisms other than conventional synaptic neurotransmitter receptors. In the instance of phorbol ester receptors and [^{3}H]MPTP binding sites, what were thought to be specific drug receptors turned out to be known enzymes. For enkephalin convertase and ACE, ligand binding techniques greatly enhanced our ability to characterize the properties of unknown enzymes. In recent years, similar ligand binding techniques have been applied productively to characterize a number of other synaptic areas.

For instance, voltage-dependent calcium channels have become a focus of much research, based on the clinical importance of calcium antagonist drugs in cardiovascular medicine. At least three distinct receptor sites have been identified for dihydropyridine, verapamillike, and diltiazem calcium antagonist receptors (Snyder and Reynolds, 1985). Characterization of these receptors has indicated that the drugs do not simply bind to the pores of voltage-dependent calcium channels. Rather than being homogeneously distributed throughout the brain in association with blood vessels, where calcium antagonists often act, dihydropyridine receptors are highly localized to specific synaptic zones. The emotion-activating effects of some neuroleptics, the diphenylbutylpiperidines, may be associated with actions on calcium antagonist receptors in the brain. Indeed, it seems that these receptors may interact with some normally occurring neurotransmitter molecule that happens to exert its synaptic effects through voltage-dependent calcium channels. Thus, as in the case of opiate receptors, the calcium antagonist drug receptors may provide insight into a new neurotransmitter system.

Additional receptorlike recognition sites labeled by radioactive drugs are associated with the uptake sites for such biogenic amines as norepinephrine, serotonin, and dopamine. Uptake sites associated with serotonin neurons can be labeled with [^{3}H]imipramine (Langer et al., 1981), norepinephrine uptake sites are readily labeled with [^{3}H]desipramine (Lee et al., 1982; Rehavi et al., 1982) or the appetite suppressant [^{3}H]mazindol (Javitch et al., 1984a), while dopamine uptake sites are selectively labeled with [^{3}H]mazindol (Javitch et al., 1984a). The ability to study the recognition sites associated with these uptake mechanisms in binding paradigms has greatly facilitated their characterization. For instance, it is well known that neurotransmitter uptake is absolutely dependent upon sodium and chloride ions. It has been thought that this reflected an association with the sodium pump of cells and did not indicate anything specific about the amine uptake system itself. However, binding sites associated with the uptake are absolutely dependent upon sodium and chloride both in the membrane state and even when solubilized and partially purified. A molecular characterization of the relationship of the recognition sites for neurotransmitter uptake and ions may permit characterization of the mechanisms that control neurotransmitter uptake.

ACKNOWLEDGMENTS

This research was supported by U.S. Public Health Service grants MH-18501, NS-16375, DA-00266, Research Scientist Award DA-00074 to S.H.S., and a grant from the Laboratories for Therapeutic Research.

REFERENCES

Baraban, J. M., R. J. Gould, S. J. Peroutka, and S. H. Snyder (1985) Phorbol ester effects on neuro-transmission: Interaction with neurotransmitters and calcium in smooth muscle. *Proc. Natl. Acad. Sci. USA* **82**:604–607.

Baraban, J. M., S. H. Snyder, and B. E. Alger (1985) Protein kinase-C regulates ionic conductance in hippocampal pyramidal neurons—Electrophysiological effects of phorbol esters. *Proc. Natl. Acad. Sci. USA* **82**:2538–2542.

Blumberg, P. M., S. Jaken, B. Konig, N. A. Sharkey, K. L. Leach, A. Y. Jeng, and E. Yeh (1984) Mechanism of action of the phorbol ester tumor promoters: Specific receptors for lipophilic ligands. *Biochem. Pharmacol.* **33**:933–940.

Cascieri, M. A., H. G. Bull, R. A. Mumford, A. A. Patchett, N. A. Thornberg, and T. Liang (1984) Carboxyl-terminal tripeptidyl hydrolysis of substance P by purified rabbit lung angiotensin-converting enzyme and the potentiation of substance P activity *in vivo* by captopril and MK-422. *Mol. Pharmacol.* **25**:287–293.

Chiba, K., A. Trevor, and N. Castagnoli, Jr. (1984) Metabolism of the neurotoxic amine, MPTP, by brain monoamine oxidase. *Biochem. Biophys. Res. Comm.* **120**:574–578.

Cushman, D., and M. Ondetti (1980) Inhibitors of angiotensin-converting enzyme for treatment of hypertension. *Biochem. Pharmacol.* **29**:1871–1877.

Fricker, L. D., and S. H. Snyder (1982) Enkephalin convertase: Purification and characterization of a specific enkephalin synthesizing carboxypeptidase localized to adrenal chromaffin granules. *Proc. Natl. Acad. Sci. USA* **79**:3886–3890.

Fricker, L. D., and S. H. Snyder (1983) Purification and characterization of enkephalin convertase, an enkephalin-synthesizing carboxypeptidase. *J. Biol. Chem.* **258**:10950–10955.

Fricker, L. D., T. H. Plummer, Jr., and S. H. Snyder (1983) Enkephalin convertase: Potent, selective and irreversible inhibitors. *Biochem. Biophys. Res. Comm.* **111**:994–1000.

Heikkila, R. E., L. Manzino, F. S. Cabbat, and R. C. Duvoisin (1984) Protection against the dopaminergic neurotoxicity of 1-methyl-4-phenyl-1,2,5,6-tetrahydropyridine by monoamine oxidase inhibitors. *Nature* **311**:467–469.

Javitch, J. A., R. O. Blaustein, and S. H. Snyder (1984a) ^{3}H-mazindol binding associated with neuronal dopamine and norepinephrine uptake sites. *Mol. Pharmacol.* **26**:35–44.

Javitch, J. A., G. R. Uhl, and S. H. Snyder (1984b) Parkinsonism-inducing neurotoxin, N-methyl-4-phenyl-1,2,3,6-tetrahydropyridine: Characterization and localization of receptor binding sites in rat and human brain. *Proc. Natl. Acad. Sci. USA* **81**:4591–4595.

Langer, S., E. Zarifian, M. Briley, R. Raisman, O. Sechter (1981) High affinity binding of ^{3}H-imipramine in brain and platelets and its relevance to the biochemistry of effective disorders. *Life Sci.* **29**:211–216.

Langston, J. W., and P. Ballard (1984) Parkinsonism induced by 1-methyl-4-phenyl-1,2,3,6-tetra-hydropyridine (MPTP): Implications for treatment and the pathogenesis of Parkinson's disease. *Can. J. Neurol. Sci.* **11**:160–165.

Lee, C.-M., J. A. Javitch, and S. H. Snyder (1982) Characterization of ^{3}H-desipramine binding associated with neuronal norepinephrine uptake sites in rat brain membranes. *J. Neurosci.* **2**:1515–1525.

Lynch, D. R., S. M. Strittmatter, and S. H. Snyder (1984) Enkephalin convertase localization by [^{3}H]guanidinoethylmercaptosuccinic acid ([^{3}H]GEMSA) autoradiography: Selective association with enkephalin-containing neurons. *Proc. Natl. Acad. Sci. USA* **81**:6543–6547.

Murphy, K. M. M., R. J. Gould, M. L. Oster-Granite, J. D. Gearhart, and S. H. Snyder (1983) Phorbol ester receptors: Autoradiographic identification in the developing rat. *Science* **222**:1036–1038.

Nishizuka, Y. (1984) Turnover of inositol phospholipids and signal transduction. *Science* **225**:1365–1370.

Parsons, B., and T. C. Rainbow (1984) High affinity binding sites for [^{3}H]MPTP may correspond to monoamine oxidase. *Eur. J. Pharmacol.* **102**:375–377.

Rehavi, M., P. Skolnick, M. J. Brownstein, and S. M. Paul (1982) High affinity binding of [^{3}H]desipramine to rat brain: A presynaptic marker for noradrenergic uptake sites. *J. Neurochem.* **38**:889–895.

Snyder, S. H. (1984) Drug and neurotransmitter receptors in the brain. *Science* **224**:22–31.

Snyder, S. H., and I. J. Reynolds (1985) Calcium antagonist drugs: Receptor interactions that clarify therapeutic effects. *New Engl. J. Med.* **313**:995–1002.

Strittmatter, S. M., M. S. Kapiloff, and S. H. Snyder (1983) ^{3}H-captopril binding to membrane-associated angiotensin-converting enzyme. *Biochem. Biophys. Res. Comm.* **112**:1027–1033.

Strittmatter, S. M., M. M. S. Lo, J. A. Javitch, and S. H. Snyder (1984a) Autoradiographic visualization of angiotensin-converting enzyme in rat brain with ^{3}H-captopril: Localization to a striatonigral pathway. *Proc. Natl. Acad. Sci. USA* **81**:1599–1603.

Strittmatter, S. M., D. R. Lynch, and S. H. Snyder (1984b) [^{3}H]guanidinoethylmercaptosuccinic acid binding to tissue homogenates: Selective labeling of enkephalin convertase. *J. Biol. Chem.* **259**:1812–1817.

Strittmatter, S. M., M. S. Kapiloff, and S. H. Snyder (1985) A rat brain isozyme of angiotensin-converting enzyme: Unique specificity for amidated peptide substrates. *J. Biol. Chem.* **260**: 9825–9832.

Thiele, E. A., S. M. Strittmatter, and S. H. Snyder (1985) Substance-K and substance-P as possible endogenous substrates of angiotensin converting protein in the brain. *Biochem. Biophys. Res. Commun.* **128**:317–324.

Worley, P. F., J. M. Baraban, and S. H. Snyder (1986) Heterogeneous localization of protein kinase-C in rat brain—Autoradiographic analysis of phorbol ester receptor binding. *J. Neurosci.* **6**: 199–207.

Yokosawa, H., S. Endo, Y. Ogura, and S. Ishii (1983) A new feature of angiotensin-converting enzyme in the brain: Hydrolysis of substance P. *Biochem. Biophys. Res. Commun.* **116**:735–742.

Chapter 10

The γ-Aminobutyric Acid/Benzodiazepine/ Barbiturate Receptor–Chloride Ion Channel Complex of Mammalian Brain

RICHARD W. OLSEN

ABSTRACT

The major inhibitory neurotransmitter, γ-aminobutyric acid (GABA), plays a widespread role in the central nervous system; it is implicated in numerous functions and neuronal circuits. It is also thought to play a role in several neurological and psychiatric disorders in humans. For example, a deficit in GABA-mediated inhibition appears to occur in certain types of epilepsy, and many drugs affecting the nervous system seem to act at the level of the GABA synapses. The most commonly occurring type of GABAergic inhibitory synapse involves a receptor that regulates postsynaptic membrane chloride ion permeability on a rapid time scale. This is analogous to acetylcholine regulation of cation channels at the neuromuscular junction, but in the case of GABA-activated chloride channels, the effect is to inhibit the target cells. These major inhibitory GABA receptors are defined by sensitivity to the agonist muscimol and the antagonist bicuculline at the GABA recognition site, and to the blockade of GABA function at another site (or sites) by such convulsants as picrotoxin. Furthermore, GABA action at these receptors is enhanced by two classes of central nervous system depressant drugs: the benzodiazepines and the barbiturates. Receptor sites for GABA, benzodiazepines, and picrotoxin/convulsants can be assayed by radioactive ligand binding, and these three receptor sites show mutual, chloride-dependent allosteric interactions with one another. In addition, they are allosterically modulated by barbiturates and related depressants. The ability of a long list of barbiturates to modulate GABA, benzodiazepine, and convulsant receptor binding in vitro *correlates very well with the enhancement of GABA function at the cellular level. Therefore, we have proposed that the GABA receptor consists of a three-receptor–ion channel complex, with modulatory sites for drugs that increase or decrease the activity of GABA receptor-regulated chloride channels. This complex protein can be solubilized with mild detergents and purified to near or total homogeneity, with all binding activities, including allosteric interactions, preserved in an oligomeric structure that contains only a few peptide subunits. Studies in many laboratories are currently focused on analyzing the structure, function, localization, and molecular biology of this interesting and important brain receptor protein.*

GABA

GABA is very probably the major inhibitory neurotransmitter in the nervous systems of a wide variety of species. This simple compound is synthesized in one step from L-glutamic acid. Glutamic acid decarboxylase (GAD), the biosynthetic enzyme, is expressed only in neurons that use GABA as a neurotransmitter, and GAD activity, or antibodies raised against the purified enzyme, can be used to localize GABAergic neurons in the nervous system. In addition to the specific localization of GABA and GAD, other criteria for defining GABA as a neuro- transmitter have been met. These include: demonstrations of the calcium-de- pendent release of GABA from stimulated neurons; high-affinity, sodium-de- pendent uptake systems to remove the released GABA from the synapse; specific actions of GABA on target neurons that mimic the response to stimulation of the inhibitory innervation; and specific receptor binding sites.

GABA is catabolized via conversion to succinic acid semialdehyde (catalyzed by GABA-transaminase) and then by oxidation to succinic acid (catalyzed by succinic acid semialdehyde dehydrogenase). These enzymes are not specifically localized and do not appear to play an important role in synaptic function. However, the nervous system, unlike most tissues, shunts about 10% of its metabolic carbon through the GABA synthetic pathway instead of through the normal Krebs cycle conversion of α-ketoglutarate to succinate (Roberts et al., 1976). This is due to the widespread use of GABA as a neurotransmitter. Some estimates suggest that up to 40% of all neurons use GABA. When GABA is applied to the cell membrane, virtually all neurons show a response to GABA, with greater sensitivity at membrane regions postsynaptic to GABAergic inner- vation (Enna, 1983).

Anatomical, physiological, and pharmacological observations are consistent with an extensive utilization of GABA-mediated inhibitory transmission. Virtually every brain region and functional circuitry involve some GABA activity. For example, cerebellar Golgi, basket, and stellate cells all appear to use GABA, as well as the entire output circuitry of Purkinje cells. Inhibitory GABAergic circuits in the hippocampus, cerebral cortex, and olfactory bulb are well described, and physiological and pharmacological investigations of GABA synapses have em- ployed recordings from a variety of sources ranging from the thalamus, to the cuneate nucleus, to the substantia nigra, to the spinal cord dorsal horn. Primary cultured neurons have provided a valuable tissue source for studies of GABA mechanisms. GABA activity has been studied in invertebrate neurons, and many invertebrates also exhibit GABAergic inhibitory innervation of muscles. GABA is known to play a role in regulating the important neuroendocrine system of the hypothalamus–pituitary axis. And finally, GABA synapses are now thought to be the site of action of many excitatory and depressant drugs, including the benzodiazepines and the barbiturates (Olsen, 1981, 1982).

The connection between centrally acting drugs and GABA is consistent with a growing body of evidence that suggests a role for altered GABAergic function in neurological and psychiatric disorders in humans. The diseases most often mentioned are epilepsy and anxiety, but also include Huntington's chorea, tardive dyskinesia, depression, and schizophrenia. Taking epilepsy as an example, not only do the anticonvulsant actions of the benzodiazepines, and possibly the barbiturates, appear to involve the enhancement of GABA-mediated inhibition, but any blockade of GABA function causes seizures, while any enhancement of GABA function protects against seizures (for a review, see Olsen et al., 1986a).

Furthermore, there are now several examples of altered GABAergic synaptic markers that suggest a functional GABA deficit in animal models and human epilepsies. GAD levels and GABAergic nerve cell bodies and terminals were shown to be specifically depleted in alumina cream-induced epileptic foci in the monkey cortex. Lower GAD activity was likewise observed in cobalt-induced epileptic foci in the rat brain. Preliminary results on human temporal lobe epilepsy show lower GAD activity in surgically removed regions identified as epileptic foci by stereo depth electrodes (Morselli et al., 1981). In results from our laboratory, an animal model for generalized seizures was shown to have a deficit of GABA-associated benzodiazepine receptor binding sites in the midbrain. A strain of seizure-susceptible gerbils developed at the University of California at Los Angeles was found to have lower benzodiazepine receptor binding in membrane homogenates of midbrain but not in other areas, as compared to nonseizing gerbil controls. Receptor binding to tissue slices measured by quantitative autoradiography revealed a deficit in the number of benzodiazepine binding sites without a change in affinity for the substantia nigra and the periaqueductal gray areas of the seizure-susceptible gerbils (Olsen et al., 1986a).

Examination of the animals at various ages revealed that a significant difference in benzodiazepine receptor binding was present at 60 days of age, prior to or at the same age at which seizures developed (50–100 days). This suggests that the receptor deficit could be part of the phenotypic expression of this genetic susceptibility to seizures, rather than the result of seizures, which is a potential complication in many epilepsy studies.

THE GABA RECEPTOR–CHLORIDE ION CHANNEL

The action of GABA, like that of other neurotransmitters such as acetylcholine and norepinephrine, is not limited to one type of synaptic mechanism. At present, at least two types of GABA receptor have been defined: one insensitive to the agonist bicuculline and activated by the agonist baclofen; and one sensitive to bicuculline and activated by the agonist muscimol. The latter is the major receptor type and dominates the literature; it is also the subject of this chapter. As in the case of acetylcholine action at the neuromuscular junction, the occupancy of this GABA receptor by the neurotransmitter results in a rapid and brief increase in membrane conductance. This appears to involve a ligand-induced conformational change in the ion channel protein, without the breakage or formation of any chemical bond. The difference from acetylcholine is that the GABA-regulated ion channel is specific for chloride. Because the chloride equilibrium potential is near the resting membrane potential, the opening of chloride channels stabilizes the membrane potential near resting, prevents the depolarizing response to excitatory neurotransmitters, and inhibits the tonic firing that is typical of neurons in the central nervous system.

Fluctuation analysis of chloride conductances activated by GABA ($> 1 \mu M$) in cultured neurons revealed two channel lifetimes of about 5 msec and 35 msec, with the latter carrying almost all of the current. The channels had a mean conductance state of about 21 pS (Jackson et al., 1982). Voltage clamp analysis of GABA channels on membrane patches from cultured neurons revealed similar properties, with conductance states of 30 pS and 19 pS corresponding to exponential decay constants of 29 msec and 2.4 msec, respectively (Hamill et al., 1983).

In attempting to study the GABA receptor–ion channel at the molecular level, radioactive ligand binding assay data obtained *in vitro* can be compared to that obtained at the cellular level by electrophysiology. We have also attempted to develop biochemical assays of GABA function so that comparisons with binding could be made on the same tissue and in the same laboratory. We have used the radioactive tracer chlorine-36 to measure increased membrane permeability of chloride ions induced by GABA in crayfish muscle fibers (Ticku and Olsen, 1977) and in slices of rat brain (Olsen et al., 1984b). Such assays provide a somewhat insensitive analysis of GABA function but can be used to determine the relative pharmacological activity of agonists, antagonists, and enhancing agents. A modification of the crayfish assay has been employed successfully on cultured chick cortical neurons (Thampy and Barnes, 1984). We are using this method to study the action of GABA and drugs, as well as receptor binding in membrane homogenates and in living cells, and are using the same type of cultured mouse spinal neurons that were used in the elegant electrophysiology studies just described.

GABA RECEPTOR BINDING SITES

GABA receptor sites can be assayed by radioactive ligand binding, provided that appropriate membrane preparation and assay conditions are employed (Enna, 1983). Radioactive [3H]GABA that has a high specific radioactivity is available. Its binding is generally assayed in a sodium-free buffer to prevent association of the ligand with sodium-dependent uptake sites. Calcium and magnesium are also excluded to prevent binding to baclofen-sensitive receptors. Several other agonists with reasonably high affinity for the receptor sites and little affinity for the uptake sites and baclofen sites are available. The most useful is [3H]muscimol, a high-affinity ligand that is a natural product of the hallucinogenic mushroom *Amanita muscaria*. One radioactive antagonist, the quaternary methyl derivative of bicuculline, has been employed (Olsen and Snowman, 1983). Because of rapid dissociation kinetics, the use of filtration assay methods underestimates GABA receptor binding, and optimal results require the use of centrifugation methods. Brain membranes must be washed thoroughly to remove endogeneous GABA before being assayed. Freezing and thawing the membranes or treating them with low levels of detergent (0.5% Triton X-100, 37°, 30 min) improves the binding. This is due to the removal of GABA, but could also involve a shift of the receptor protein to a high-affinity conformational state (that may or may not occur *in situ*) (Olsen et al., 1984b), or to the removal of other endogenous modulators or ligands that are not GABA (Guidotti et al., 1983).

The binding of [3H]GABA (under sodium- and calcium-free conditions), [3H]muscimol, [3H]isoguvacine, [3H]piperidine-4-sulfonic acid, [3H]4,5,6,7-tetrahydro-isoxazolo-[5,4-c]-pyridin-3-ol (THIP), and [3H]bicuculline methochloride (BMC) is inhibited by those compounds and only those compounds that are active at muscimol–bicuculline-type GABA receptors. These GABA receptor sites are insensitive to the uptake-specific GABA analogues nipecotic acid and 2,4-diaminobutyric acid (DABA). Furthermore, they are not inhibited by benzodiazepines, barbiturates, picrotoxin, or the other amino acid neurotransmitters, glutamic acid and glycine. They are inhibited by high concentrations of strychnine (a glycine antagonist) and D-tubocurarine (an acetylcholine antagonist), by the weak GABA agonists β-alanine and taurine, and by baclofen (Olsen et al., 1984b).

All of these ligands show heterogeneity in binding affinity, with significant binding over a ligand concentration range of 0.1 nM to 10 μM that is displaceable by the muscimol–bicuculline compounds. Curvilinear Scatchard plots are obtained; this is true for different membrane fractions, brain regions, ages of animals, and mammalian species, including human. Computer-assisted, nonlinear regression analyses suggested a best fit of more than one affinity, with two or three independent sites (e.g., for GABA, K_D values of 0.01 μM, 0.1 μM, and possibly 1 μM). Such a fit could not be distinguished from negative cooperativity. However, several lines of evidence suggest that most of the binding sites could involve interconvertible states of a single receptor site (Olsen et al., 1981; Olsen and Snowman, 1982, 1983; Olsen et al., 1984b). It should also be noted that all reports on physiological responses to GABA show a concentration requirement of more than 1 μM GABA to activate chloride channels. Thus, the presence of submicromolar binding affinities needs to be explained.

All the affinity subpopulations show the same chemical and stereochemical specificity expected of the GABA receptors, and they are remarkably similar to each other. We can differentiate three components by examining the dissociation kinetics of [³H]GABA or [³H]muscimol binding. One component with a half-life of dissociation and association on the order of minutes corresponds to that fraction of the binding sites with highest affinity (nanomolar). By adding excess nonradioactive GABA just prior to centrifugation, radioactive ligand bound to rapidly dissociating sites will be lost and only ligand bound to this slowly dissociating population will remain. The potency of GABA analogues to inhibit just this high-affinity subpopulation can then be determined independently. Binding to the rapidly dissociating, low-affinity sites, and inhibition of those sites by analogues, can be calculated by subtraction. Examination of a series of GABA analogues shows that the rapidly dissociating and slowly dissociating sites have the same rank order of potencies, but the agonists all show a slightly (1–10 times) greater affinity for the slowly dissociating, high-affinity GABA sites. The antagonist bicuculline, however, shows a *lower* affinity for that population than it does for the rapidly dissociating, low-affinity GABA sites.

Several other treatments cause shifts in the binding curves that may be due to subpopulation interconversion, and the affinities of GABA agonists and the antagonist bicuculline are differentially affected. The freeze–thaw and mild detergent treatments, for example, increase agonist binding and decrease antagonist binding; silver ion has a similar effect. On the other hand, physiological levels of chloride ions, or certain other anions such as bromide or thiocyanate, as well as physiological temperatures, inhibit agonist binding and potentiate antagonist binding. Barbiturates and related depressant drugs cause an increase in GABA agonist binding and a decrease in antagonist binding that appear to involve an increase in affinity for micromolar affinity GABA agonist sites. The higher affinity submicromolar affinity sites observed may correspond to those sites seen in the absence of barbiturates, that is, an interconversion of populations may occur. The barbiturate effect is reversed by picrotoxin and is chloride dependent. These shifts in binding affinity caused by various agents suggest that the GABA receptor is an allosteric membrane protein capable of adapting numerous conformational states of differing ligand affinity that may play a role in its mechanism of action.

MODULATORY DRUG RECEPTOR SITES

The bicuculline- and muscimol-sensitive GABA receptors that regulate chloride channels are also sensitive to functional antagonism by the convulsant picrotoxin and related compounds. These drugs show no chemical similarity to GABA and appear to block the coupling between the GABA receptor site and the chloride ion channel. Binding studies show that these sites are distinct from, but allosterically coupled to, the GABA receptor sites (Olsen, 1982).

Two distinct classes of depressant drugs act at two additional receptor sites to enhance the function of GABA. Benzodiazepines, such as diazepam (Valium), increase the frequency of chloride channel openings that have been activated by GABA. Barbiturates, such as pentobarbital (Nembutal), increase the channel lifetime of GABA-activated chloride channels and can even open the channels themselves in the absence of GABA (Barker et al., 1984).

Benzodiazepine binding sites in mammalian brain show the specificity for a series of benzodiazepines expected for receptor sites mediating the anticonvulsant, anxiolytic, muscle relaxant, and sedative actions of these clinically important drugs (Usdin et al., 1982). These sites are coupled to the GABA, barbiturate, and picrotoxin–convulsant receptor sites, as shown by reciprocal allosteric interactions among them. GABA receptor agonists enhance the binding of depressant benzodiazepine receptor ligands and inhibit the binding of excitatory ligands, the inverse agonists (Braestrup et al., 1983). GABA receptor ligands protect benzodiazepine receptor binding activity from inactivation by heat in an ion-sensitive manner (Squires and Saederup, 1982). As described below, GABA and benzodiazepine receptor binding activities can be solubilized with mild detergent and copurified as a single protein complex by several protein separation schemes (Gavish and Snyder, 1981; Sigel et al., 1983; Olsen et al., 1984a). Benzodiazepine receptor binding is also allosterically enhanced by barbiturates and related depressants in a chloride-dependent and picrotoxin-sensitive manner (Olsen, 1981).

The picrotoxin sites can be assayed with a radioactive ligand developed in our laboratory, [3H]α-dihydropicrotoxin (DHP). [3H]DHP binding sites are present in tissues that show GABA synapses, such as mammalian brain and crayfish muscle. They are inhibited by biologically active analogues of picrotoxin and by a series of cage convulsant drugs that also inhibit GABA synapses. [3H]DHP binding is also inhibited by convulsant barbiturates, depressant barbiturates, and related substances. Unfortunately, [3H]DHP does not have a very high affinity for its binding sites ($K_D = 1$ μM), and therefore the signal-to-noise ratio in centrifugation assays is limited to about 20% displaceable binding in the best tissue sources (Olsen, 1981, 1982). Fortunately, a higher affinity radioactive ligand has been developed for these sites: the cage convulsant [35S]t-butylbicyclophosphorothionate (TBPS; Squires et al., 1983). We have used this ligand to determine the structure–activity relationships for a series of picrotoxinlike convulsants and barbituratelike depressants. Some representative structures of active compounds are shown in Figure 1.

The second link between barbiturates and the GABA receptor was provided by the observation that the pyrazolopyridine anxiolytics, such as SQ20,009 (etazolate), did not inhibit benzodiazepine receptor binding but enhanced it in a picrotoxin-sensitive, chloride-dependent manner (Supavilai and Karobath, 1981). We found that etazolate and related compounds inhibited [³H]DHP binding at the same concentrations at which they enhanced benzodiazepine receptor binding. Picrotoxin and related convulsants blocked the latter enhancement at the same concentrations at which they inhibited [³H]DHP binding (Leeb-Lundberg et al., 1981). Furthermore, other depressants, such as barbiturates, that inhibited [³H]DHP binding were able to enhance benzodiazepine binding (Leeb-Lundberg et al., 1980). This effect was not only blocked by picrotoxinlike compounds, but was dependent on the presence of certain anions. These anions were exactly those that are able to carry inhibitory postsynaptic currents in mammalian neurons

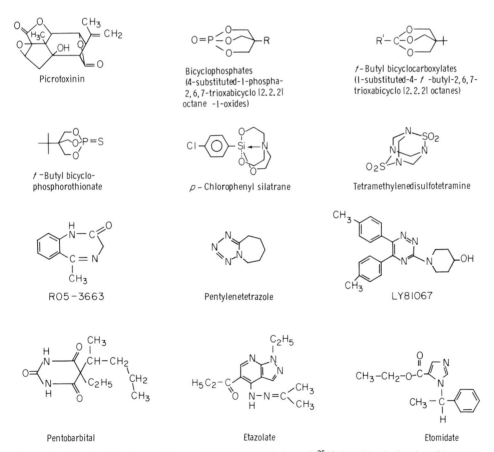

Figure 1. *Chemical structures of drugs that inhibit the binding of [³⁵S]t-butylbicyclophosphorothionate to rat brain membranes.*

now known to involve barbiturate-enhanced GABAergic chloride channels (Olsen, 1981, 1982).

Once the chloride dependence of the barbiturate enhancement of benzodiazepine binding became appreciated, a similar enhancement of GABA receptor binding by the same barbiturates was observed (Olsen and Snowman, 1982). The increased affinity of GABA binding seen in the presence of such compounds as pentobarbital (100–200 μM) may explain the ability of barbiturates to increase the lifetime of GABA-activated chloride channels.

The structures of the barbiturates that have been investigated are shown in Figure 2. There is an excellent correlation between the ability to enhance GABA and benzodiazepine agonist binding *in vitro*, to inhibit GABA antagonist and benzodiazepine inverse agonist binding, and to inhibit [^{35}S]TBPS binding (Table 1), and the ability of these drugs to enhance GABA function at the cellular level. The order of activity is 1,3-dimethylbutyl barbituric acid (DMBB) > secobarbital > pentobarbital > (+)hexobarbital > amobarbital > (−)hexobarbital = phenobarbital. A mild stereospecificity is observed for compounds of the pentobarbital type—(−)DMBB, secobarbital, and pentobarbital are more potent than the (+)isomers. A more marked stereospecificity is observed for N^1-alkylated barbiturate isomers, where (+)hexobarbital is more potent than the (−)isomer, and (−)isomers of N^1-methyl,5-phenyl,5-propyl barbituric acid (MPPB) and N^1-ethyl,5-methyl,5-piperidino barbituric acid (EMPB) are more potent than their (+)isomers. No exception has been found to the rule that all compounds that

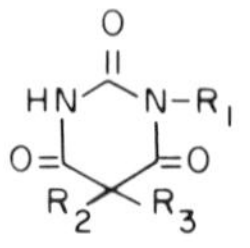

BARBITURATE	RING SUBSTITUTION		
	R_1	R_2	R_3
DMBB	H	$-CH_2CH_3$	$-CH(CH_3)CH_2CH(CH_3)_2$
SECOBARBITAL	H	$-CH_2-CH{=}CH_2$	$-CH(CH_3)CH_2CH_2CH_3$
PENTOBARBITAL	H	$-CH_2CH_3$	$-CH(CH_3)CH_2CH_2CH_3$
MEPHOBARBITAL	CH_3	$-CH_2CH_3$	(phenyl)
HEXOBARBITAL	CH_3	$-CH_3$	(cyclohexenyl)
AMOBARBITAL	H	$-CH_2CH_3$	$-CH_2CH_2CH(CH_3)_2$
MPPB	CH_3	$-CH_2CH_2CH_3$	(phenyl)
CHEB	H	$-CH_2CH_3$	$-CH_2-CH{=}$(cyclohexenyl) 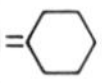
PHENOBARBITAL	H	$-CH_2CH_3$	(phenyl)
METHARBITAL	CH_3	$-CH_2CH_3$	$-CH_2CH_3$
BARBITAL	H	$-CH_2CH_3$	$-CH_2CH_3$
EMPB	C_2H_5	$-CH_3$	$-N$(piperidino)

Figure 2.   *Chemical structures of barbiturates discussed in the text.*

Table 1. Relative Potencies of Barbiturates to Allosterically Modulate Cage Convulsants, Benzodiazepine, and GABA Receptors

Compound[a]	$IC_{50}(\mu M)$ [35S]TBPS	$EC_{50}(\mu M)$			$EC_{20}(\mu M)$ [3H]βCCM
		[3H]GABA	[3H]BMC	[3H]Diazepam	
(−)DMBB	ND[b]	ND	ND	50	ND
(±)DMBB	50	150	50	80	40
(±)Secobarbital	15	300	200	100	110
(−)Pentobarbital	90	200	ND	100	ND
(±)Pentobarbital	100	300	210	130	170
(+)Pentobarbital	130	400	ND	250	ND
(+)Hexobarbital	460	300	260	150	250
Amobarbital	ND	450	ND	350	ND
(−)MPPB	300	400	280	100	800
(−)Mephobarbital	140	400	310	50	220
CHEB	210	ND	300	500	ND
(−)EMPB	600	2000	ND	2000	ND
(+)EMPB	230	>5000	ND	>5000	ND
Phenobarbital	4000	>1000	550	(200)[c]	2000
(+)Mephobarbital	200	>1000	950	>1000	440
(−)Hexobarbital	840	>1000	>1000	>1000	>1000
(+)MPPB	2200	>1000	>1000	>1000	2000

[a] For structures, see Figure 2.
[b] ND, not determined.
[c] Phenobarbital at 1 mM does not enhance equilibrium binding but alters the kinetics of [3H]diazepam binding ($EC_{50} = 200$ μM) and reverses pentobarbital enhancement.

modulate GABA/benzodiazepine receptor binding *in vitro* enhance GABA function at the cellular level, as revealed by electrophysiological assays of cultured neurons (Schulz and Macdonald, 1981; Barnes et al., 1983; Harrison and Simmonds, 1983; Barker et al., 1984), of hippocampal slices, or by chlorine-36 flux measurements of brain slices (Olsen et al., 1986b). The nonbarbiturate depressants, such as etazolate, etomidate, and LY81067, also enhance binding and function—in a stereospecific manner in the case of etomidate: (+)isomer > (−)isomer.

Some of the barbiturates that inhibit [35S]TBPS binding and enhance GABA and benzodiazepine binding, such as DMBB, (+)pentobarbital, and CHEB, are convulsant compounds that excite neurons. However, they do enhance GABA function *in addition* to their excitatory actions: we consider the latter to involve a separate, nonGABA mechanism. Some of the compounds that inhibit [35S]TBPS binding, such as phenobarbital and the anticonvulsant chlormethiazole, enhance GABA function only weakly but are not inactive. They show virtually no enhancement of equilibrium GABA and benzodiazepine receptor binding, but here too they are not inactive. They slow down the kinetics of benzodiazepine binding with an equal effect on the association and dissociation rates such that the equilibrium constant is not altered. This action of phenobarbital ($EC_{50} = 200$ μM) involves the same site as that of pentobarbital, since excess phenobarbital can reverse the equilibrium enhancement by pentobarbital (Leeb-Lundberg and

Olsen, 1982). Thus, we have defined a modulatory receptor site for barbiturates that is coupled to the GABA/benzodiazepine receptor–chloride ion channel complex and mediates the action of barbiturates to enhance GABA function. This barbiturate receptor site is likely to be involved in some of the pharmacological actions of barbiturates *in vivo*.

The hypothetical model of this GABA receptor complex is shown in Figure 3. Although there are a few differences between the binding of [³H]DHP and [³⁵S]TBPS, the similarities are more striking and probably involve the same sites. [³⁵S]TBPS binding is enhanced by chloride ions and higher temperatures (20–37°C > 0°) and inhibited by GABA; binding of [³H]DHP is not. Some convulsants (the benzodiazepine Ro5-3663, and the barbiturates DMBB and CHEB) appear to inhibit [³H]DHP binding more potently. Some of these differences appear real, while others may have been exaggerated by the poor accuracy of the [³H]DHP binding assay—albeit the assay was valuable at the time.

The relative potencies of the depressants to inhibit [³⁵S]TBPS binding agree very well with the activity of enhancing GABA receptor binding and function. Recent evidence suggests that the barbiturate binding site is distinct from that of picrotoxin and the cage convulsants. Thus, the inhibition of [³⁵S]TBPS binding by pentobarbital and etazolate appears to be allosteric because it is reversed by GABA receptor site antagonists (Squires et al., 1983), is biphasic under some conditions, and involves a change in dissociation *rate* of the labeled ligand, which does not occur with competitive, active site-directed inhibitors (Ticku and Rastogi, 1986). Thus, the "new doughnut model" in Figure 3 includes four separate drug receptor sites.

Finally, in discussing this model, one might ask why these receptor sites exist. Is there an endogenous substrate for any of them? At this point in time, no such substance has been convincingly demonstrated to play such a role for any of the sites. However, a 10-kD protein, and some fragments therefrom, has been reported to inhibit benzodiazepine receptor binding and to have some phar-macological activity opposite to that of diazepam (Guidotti et al., 1983). Recently, some GABA receptor activity has been observed for two steroids. An amidine

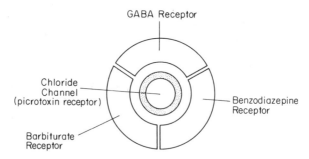

Figure 3. *The GABA receptor–ion channel complex is hypothesized to consist of four receptor sites: The GABA receptor; the benzodiazepine receptor; the barbiturate receptor; and the chloride channel (picrotoxin receptor). Chloride ion permeability may be potentiated (by central nervous system depressant drugs) or reduced (by central nervous system excitatory drugs). Endogenous or exogenous compounds may modulate the receptor complex. (For further details, see the text and Olsen, 1981.)*

steroid, 3α-hydroxy,16-imino,5β-17-androstan-11-one (RU5135; Hunt and Clements-Jewery, 1981), has bicucullinelike GABA antagonist activity, although it is not clear whether it acts at the GABA recognition site. An anesthetic steroid, 3α-hydroxy,5α-pregnane,11,20-dione (alphaxolone; Harrison and Simmonds, 1984), behaves just like pentobarbital in enhancing GABA function and binding. This opens the possibility that a steroid hormone may act specifically (as opposed to physical membrane perturbation) to modulate GABA function at one of the associated drug receptor sites.

SOLUBILIZATION AND PURIFICATION OF THE COMPLEX

GABA receptor activity assayed by [^{3}H]muscimol binding (using a mini-Sephadex column method) could be solubilized in high yield with the mild detergent deoxycholate, producing a monodisperse, protein–lipid detergent micelle with an apparent molecular weight of 900 kD (Greenlee and Olsen, 1979). Following the demonstration that benzodiazepine receptor sites could be measured in brain membranes, they were shown to be allosterically enhanced in affinity by GABA receptor agonists (Usdin et al., 1982). The effective concentration of GABA is about 1 μM. Solubilized benzodiazepine binding activity assayed by polyethylene glycol precipitation–filtration was then shown to be enhanced by GABA (1 μM) and to comigrate with GABA receptor binding activity (K_D = 20 nM) during several column chromatographic procedures (Gavish and Snyder, 1981). We observed similar results and measured an apparent molecular weight for the GABA/benzodiazepine receptor protein complex of about 355 kD in Triton X-100 (Stephenson et al., 1982). The allosteric enhancement of GABA and benzodiazepine binding by barbiturates was found to be unstable in deoxycholate- and Triton X-100-solubilized extracts, nor could we detect any binding of [^{3}H]DHP to the picrotoxin–convulsant sites. However, chloride-dependent barbiturate enhancement was retained when the GABA/benzodiazepine receptor binding activity was solubilized with the zwitterionic bile salt detergent, CHAPS (Stephenson and Olsen, 1982). CHAPS was also suitable for the solubilization of the [^{35}S]TBPS binding activity that was inhibited by picrotoxin, barbiturates, and GABA, and enhanced by chloride ions and physiological temperature. This activity comigrated with [^{3}H]flunitrazepam binding activity on a gel filtration column with an apparent molecular weight of 900 kD (King and Olsen, 1984). Thus the barbiturate, convulsant, and benzodiazepine binding sites appear to reside on the same macromolecular complex as the GABA receptor–ionophore.

Indeed, all of these activities can be retained on a benzodiazepine-derived affinity column and coeluted by unattached benzodiazepine ligands, with resulting significant purification (Olsen et al., 1984a). About 70% of the [^{3}H]muscimol binding activity in a deoxycholate extract of rat or cow brain, and 90% of the [^{3}H]flunitrazepam binding, were retained on the affinity column. After extensive washing with high salt and 1 M urea in Triton X-100, the [^{3}H]muscimol binding was recovered in a 40% yield (60% of the sample on the column) by elution with free flurazepam. Protein assays revealed that the specific activity of different prepartions varied from 410–10,000 pmol of binding sites per milligram of protein, as summarized in Table 2.

Table 2.   Properties of Purified Rat Brain GABA/Benzodiazepine/Barbiturate Receptor Complex

Binds [^{3}H]muscimol: Specific activity is greater than 410 pmol/mg; K_D = 20 nM. Inhibited by muscimol, GABA, bicuculline, and 3-aminopropane sulfonate, but not by 2,4-diaminobutyric acid (DABA) (10 μM). Enhanced by pentobarbital (1 mM) by 47–56%.

Binds [^{35}S]TBPS: K_D = 30 nM. Inhibited by ethylbicyclophosphate, picrotoxinin, pentobarbital, and GABA.

Binds [^{3}H]flunitrazepam: K_D = 8 nM. Inhibited by flunitrazepam and clonazepam, but inhibited less than 30% by Ro5-4864 (all at 300 nM). Photoaffinity-labeled in the 49-kD band.

Subunit composition: 49 kD, 56 kD, and 60 kD (iodine-125, silver stain), with some minor bands above and below.

Native molecular weight: Stokes radius approximately that of catalase.

The purified [^{3}H]muscimol binding activity (K_D = 20 nM) showed receptorlike specificity and was enhanced about 50% by pentobarbital (sometimes observed in Triton X-100 but more reproducible when assayed in CHAPS). In CHAPS, [^{35}S]TBPS binding was quantitatively absorbed to the column and detectable binding was observed in the flurazepam eluant after dialysis to lower the flurazepam concentration. After DEAE column chromatography and dialysis of the flurazepam eluant to remove the free drug, brain-specific benzodiazepine receptor ([^{3}H]flunitrazepam) binding activity was detected with a stoichiometry 0.2–0.5 that of [^{3}H]muscimol binding and was enhanced by muscimol at 200 nM. This [^{3}H]flunitrazepam binding activity allowed us to photoaffinity label the receptor on the benzodiazepine binding subunit (Möhler et al., 1980). SDS-polyacrylamide gel electrophoresis revealed a single radioactive band at 49 kD, corresponding to a peptide of the same size that both Möhler et al. (1980) and our group obtained when crude membrane homogenates were photoaffinity-labeled.

Silver staining or autoradiography of ^{125}I-labeled purified receptor revealed three major peptide bands at 49 kD, 56 kD, and 60 kD; the 49-kD band corresponded to that of the [^{3}H]flunitrazepam-labeled subunit. Three to six minor bands above and below the major bands were also visible. This nearly homogeneous material contains not only the GABA receptor activity but also the associated modulatory drug receptor sites and in all likelihood the chloride channel as well. Additional biochemical characterization, reconstitution of the protein into membranes, and production of antibodies for use as biochemical and anatomical probes are the current studies being undertaken with regard to this interesting protein.

Sigel et al. (1983) have reported a similar purification of the GABA/benzodiazepine receptor protein on a benzodiazepine affinity column, and they found only two bands at 53 kD and 57 kD on SDS-polyacrylamide gels for the purified material. Subsequently, they employed CHAPS detergent (Sigel and Barnard, 1984) to show the concomitant purification of [^{35}S]TBPS binding activity and barbiturate allosteric effects in preparations containing only these two peptide subunits; the purified material had an apparent native molecular weight of 220 kD. While it is not yet clear whether all of the functions of the GABA receptor complex are contained in this relatively simple oligomeric protein, it does appear that many properties are intact and that the complete structure of this complex will soon be known. Laying the foundation for attempts to clone the gene for the GABA/benzodiazepine receptor complex, Barnard and his collaborators (Smart et al., 1983) have demonstrated the expression of functional, drug-modulated GABA receptors in *Xenopus* oocytes injected with RNA from chick and rat brain; additionally, Schoch et al. (1985) have reported the production of monoclonal antibodies against the benzodiazepine/GABA receptor protein. Thus, rapid progress in the characterization of its structure and function is taking place.

ACKNOWLEDGMENTS

Supported by National Science Foundation grant BNS-83-18001 and National Institutes of Health grant NS-20704. I thank Drs. E. Wong, J. Fischer, and G. Stauber, J. Y. Ransom, and R. King for participating in the research described here.

REFERENCES

Barker, J. C., E. Gratz, D. G. Owen, and R. E. Study (1984) Pharmacological effects of clinically important drugs on the excitability of cultured mouse spinal neurons. In *Actions and Interactions of GABA and Benzodiazepines*, N. G. Bowery, ed., pp. 203–216, Raven, New York.

Barnes, D. M., W. F. White, and M. S. Dichter (1983) Etazolate (SQ-20009): Electrophysiology and effects on [³H]-flunitrazepam binding in cultured cortical neurons. *J. Neurosci.* 3:762–772.

Braestrup, C., M. Nielsen, T. Honoré, L. H. Jensen, and E. N. Petersen (1983) Benzodiazepine receptor ligands with positive and negative efficacy. *Neuropharmacology* 22:1451–1457.

Enna, S. J., ed. (1983) *The GABA Receptors*, Humana Press, Clifton, New Jersey.

Gavish, M., and S. H. Snyder (1981) γ-Aminobutyric acid and benzodiazepine receptors: Copurification and characterization. *Proc. Natl. Acad. Sci. USA* 78:1939–1942.

Greenlee, D. V., and R. W. Olsen (1979) Solubilization of gamma-aminobutyric acid receptor protein from mammalian brain. *Biochem. Biophys. Res. Comm.* 88:380–387.

Guidotti, A., M. G. Corda, B. C. Wise, F. Vaccarino, and E. Costa (1983) GABAergic synapses. Supramolecular organization and biochemical regulation. *Neuropharmacology* 22:1471–1479.

Hamill, O. P., J. Bormann, and B. Sakmann (1983) Activation of multiple-conductance state chloride channels in spinal neurones by glycine and GABA. *Nature* 305:805–808.

Harrison, N. L., and M. A. Simmonds (1983) Two distinct interactions of barbiturates and chlormethiazole with the $GABA_A$ receptor complex in rat cuneate nucleus *in vitro*. *Br. J. Pharmacol.* 80:387–394.

Harrison, N. L., and M. A. Simmonds (1984) Modulation of the GABA receptor complex by a steroid anaesthetic. *Brain Res.* 323:287–292.

Hunt, P., and S. Clements-Jewery (1981) A steroid derivative, R 5135, antagonizes the GABA–benzodiazepine receptor interaction. *Neuropharmacology* 20:357–361.

Jackson, M. B., H. Lecar, D. A. Mathers, and J. L. Barker (1982) Single channel currents activated by γ-aminobutyric acid, muscimol, and (−)-pentobarbital in cultured mouse spinal neurons. *J. Neurosci.* 2:889–894.

King, R. G., and R. W. Olsen (1984) Solubilization of convulsant/barbiturate binding activity on the GABA/benzodiazepine receptor complex. *Biochem. Biophys. Res. Comm.* 119:530–536.

Leeb-Lundberg, F., and R. W. Olsen (1982) Interactions of barbiturates of various pharmacological categories with benzodiazepine receptors. *Mol. Pharmacol.* 21:320–328.

Leeb-Lundberg, F., A. Snowman, and R. W. Olsen (1980) Barbiturate receptors are coupled to benzodiazepine receptors. *Proc. Natl. Acad. Sci. USA* **77**:7468–7472.

Leeb-Lundberg, F., A. Snowman, and R. W. Olsen (1981) Perturbation of benzodiazepine receptor binding by pyrazolopyridines involves picrotoxin/barbiturate receptor sites. *J. Neurosci.* **1**:471–477.

Möhler, H., M. K. Battersby, and J. G. Richards (1980) Benzodiazepine receptor protein identified and visualized in brain tissue by a photoaffinity label. *Proc. Natl. Acad. Sci. USA* **77**:1666–1670.

Morselli, P. L., K. G. Lloyd, W. Löscher, B. Meldrum, and E. H. Reynolds, eds. (1981) *Neurotransmitters, Seizures and Epilepsy*, Raven, New York.

Olsen, R. W. (1981) GABA–benzodiazepine–barbiturate receptor interactions. *J. Neurochem.* **37**:1–13.

Olsen, R. W. (1982) Drug interactions at the GABA receptor ionophore complex. *Annu. Rev. Pharmacol. Toxicol.* **22**:245–277.

Olsen, R. W., and A. M. Snowman (1982) Chloride-dependent enhancement by barbiturates of GABA receptor binding. *J. Neurosci.* **2**:1812–1823.

Olsen, R. W., and A. M. Snowman (1983) [^{3}H]Bicuculline methochloride binding to low-affinity γ-aminobutyric acid receptor sites. *J. Neurochem.* **41**:1653–1663.

Olsen, R. W., M. O. Bergman, P. C. Van Ness, S. C. Lummis, A. E. Watkins, C. Napias, and D. V. Greenlee (1981) γ-Aminobutyric acid receptor binding in mammalian brain: Heterogeneity of binding sites. *Mol. Pharmacol.* **19**:217–227.

Olsen, R. W., E. H. F. Wong, G. B. Stauber, D. Murakami, R. G. King, and J. B. Fischer (1984a) Biochemical properties of the GABA barbiturate/benzodiazepine receptor–chloride ion channel complex. In *Neurotransmitter Receptors: Mechanisms of Action and Regulation*, S. Kito, T. Segawa, K. Kuriyama, H. I. Yamamura, and R. W. Olsen, eds., pp. 205–219, Plenum, New York.

Olsen, R. W., E. H. F. Wong, G. B. Stauber, and R. G. King (1984b) Biochemical pharmacology of the GABA receptor/ionophore protein. *Fed. Proc.* **43**:2773–2778.

Olsen, R. W., J. K. Wamsley, R. Lee, and P. Lomax (1986a) The benzodiazepine/barbiturate/GABA receptor–chloride ionophore complex in a genetic model for generalized epilepsy. In *Basic Mechanisms of the Epilepsies: Molecular and Cellular Approaches*, A. V. Delgado-Escueta, A. A. Ward, and D. M. Woodbury, eds., pp. 365–378, Raven, New York.

Olsen, R. W., J. B. Fischer, and T. V. Dunwiddie (1986b) Barbiturate enhancement of γ-aminobutyric acid receptor binding and function as a mechanism of anesthesia. In *Molecular and Cellular Mechanisms of Anesthetics*, S. H. Roth and K. W. Miller, eds., pp. 165–178, Plenum, New York.

Roberts, E., T. N. Chase, and D. B. Tower (1976) *GABA in Nervous System Function*, Raven, New York.

Schoch, P., J. G. Richards, P. Häring, B. Takacs, C. Stähli, T. Staehelin, W. Haefely, and H. Möhler (1985) Co-localisation of GABA$_A$ receptors and benzodiazepine receptors in the brain shown by monoclonal antibodies. *Nature* **314**:168–171.

Schulz, D. W., and R. L. Macdonald (1981) Barbiturate enhancement of GABA-modulated inhibition and activation of chloride ion conductance: Correlation with anticonvulsants and anesthetic actions. *Brain Res.* **209**:177–188.

Sigel, E., and E. A. Barnard (1984) A γ-aminobutyric acid/benzodiazepine receptor complex from bovine cerebral cortex. Improved purification with preservation of regulatory sites and their interactions. *J. Biol. Chem.* **259**:7219–7223.

Sigel, E., F. A. Stephenson, C. Mamalaki, and E. A. Barnard (1983) A γ-aminobutyric acid/benzodiazepine receptor complex of bovine cerebral cortex. Purification and partial characterization. *J. Biol. Chem.* **258**:6965–6971.

Smart, T. G., A. Constanti, G. Bilbe, D. A. Brown, and E. A. Barnard (1983) Synthesis of functional chick brain GABA–benzodiazepine–barbiturate/receptor complexes in mRNA-injected *Xenopus* oocytes. *Neurosci. Lett.* **40**:55–59.

Squires, R. F., and E. Saederup (1982) γ-Aminobutyric acid receptors modulate cation binding sites coupled to independent benzodiazepine, picrotoxin, and anion binding sites. *Mol. Pharmacol.* **22**:327–334.

Squires, R. F., J. E. Casida, M. Richardson, and E. Saederup (1983) [^{35}S]*t*-Butyl bicyclophosphorothionate binds with high affinity to brain-specific sites coupled to γ-aminobutyric acid-A and ion recognition sites. *Mol. Pharmacol.* **23**:326–336.

Stephenson, F. A., and R. W. Olsen (1982) Solubilization by CHAPS detergent of barbiturate-enhanced benzodiazepine–GABA receptor complex. *J. Neurochem.* **39**:1579–1586.

Stephenson, F. A., A. E. Watkins, and R. W. Olsen (1982) Physicochemical characterization of detergent-solubilized γ-aminobutyric acid and benzodiazepine receptor proteins from bovine brain. *Eur. J. Biochem.* **123**:291–298.

Supavilai, P., and M. Karobath (1981) Action of pyrazolopyridines as modulators of [³H]flunitrazepam binding to the GABA/benzodiazepine receptor complex of the cerebellum. *Eur. J. Pharmacol.* **70**:183–193.

Thampy, K. G., and E. M. Barnes (1984) γ-Aminobutyric acid-gated chloride channels in cultured cerebral neurons. *J. Biol. Chem.* **259**:1753–1757.

Ticku, M. K., and R. W. Olsen (1977) γ-Aminobutyric acid-stimulated chloride permeability in crayfish muscle. *Biochim. Biophys. Acta* **464**:519–529.

Ticku, M. K., and S. K. Rastogi (1986) Barbiturate-sensitive sites in the benzodiazepine–GABA receptor–ionophore complex. In *Molecular and Cellular Mechanisms of Anesthetics*, S. H. Roth and K. W. Miller, eds., pp. 179–190, Plenum, New York.

Usdin, E., P. Skolnick, J. F. Tallman, Jr., D. Greenblatt, and S. M. Paul, eds. (1982) *Pharmacology of Benzodiazepines*, Macmillan, London.

Chapter 11

Possible Involvement of Kallikrein Enzymes in the Processing of Neuropeptide Precursors

EDWARD HERBERT
JAMES DOUGLASS

ABSTRACT

Over the past two decades, a great variety of small peptides that mediate specific behavioral responses in animals has been discovered. Many of these peptides are synthesized from large precursor proteins that contain more than one kind of neuroactive peptide. The peptides must be cleaved from these precursors (called polyproteins) and undergo posttranslational modifications to acquire activity. Production of bioactive peptides from polyproteins involves endoproteolytic cleavage at pairs of basic amino acid residues flanking the peptides, after which the basic amino acids are trimmed from the peptides with carboxypeptidases. Very little is known about these enzymes. We have attempted to identify mRNA species that code for enzymes that process pro-opiomelanocortin (POMC) by using recombinant DNA techniques. We have used cDNA clones that code for a family of endoproteolytic enzymes known as kallikreins (kindly provided by Dr. J. Shine). The kallikrein enzymes are known to be involved in the processing of growth factors. We have been able to identify a cDNA clone that codes for a kallikrein enzyme in AtT-20-D_{16v} cells (mouse pituitary tumor cells that produce large quantities of pro-opiomelanocortin). Northern blot analysis reveals that the mRNA that codes for this species of kallikrein is present at very high levels in these cells (10–20% of the level of POMC mRNA) and in the neurointermediate lobe of mouse pituitary. Furthermore, sequencing of a number of cDNA clones in the library indicates that there is only one species of kallikrein enzyme in these cells.

Over the past two decades, many small peptides that mediate diverse functions in animals have been discovered. Some of these peptides may serve both as neurotransmitters or neuromodulators and as hormones. It is not surprising, therefore, to find them in a wide variety of tissues. For example, the adrenocorticotropic hormone (ACTH)/endorphin family of peptides is found in the anterior and neurointermediate lobes of the pituitary, several sites in the brain, in the placenta, in the intestine, and in the immune system (Douglass et al., 1984a).

Small neuropeptides are synthesized initially as large precursor proteins that undergo specific proteolytic cleavage and posttranslational modifications to produce bioactive peptides. A number of precursor proteins that contain sequences of more than one bioactive peptide have recently been discovered. A striking example of this type of precursor (known as a polyprotein) is the family of proteins that contain the sequences of the opioid peptides. The opioid family of peptides consists of the pentapeptides met- and leu-enkephalin, endorphins (carboxy-terminal extensions of met-enkephalin), and dynorphins (carboxy-terminal extensions of leu-enkephalin). All of the 15 opioid peptides reported to date are derived from three different precursors: pro-opiomelanocortin (POMC), which gives rise to endorphins; proenkephalin A (proenkephalin); and proenkephalin B (prodynorphin) (Figure 1). Pro-opiomelanocortin gives rise to β-endorphin, $ACTH_{1-39}$, and three melanocyte-stimulating hormones (MSH). Proenkephalin A contains six copies of met-enkephalin and one copy of leu-enkephalin. Prodynorphin contains three copies of leu-enkephalin and gives rise to several dynorphin peptides and rimorphin.

The opioid peptide repertoire can be further diversified by tissue-specific processing of the precursor (Douglass et al., 1984a). POMC, for example, is processed to ACTH and β-lipotropin (LPH) in the anterior pituitary, whereas in the neurointermediate lobe, these peptides are further cleaved to form α-MSH, corticotropinlike intermediate lobe peptide, β-endorphin, and derivatives of β-endorphin (Figure 2). Molecular genetic studies indicate that there is only one POMC gene and one POMC mRNA expressed in mouse (Uhler et al., 1983) and rat pituitary (J. Drouin, personal communication). Therefore, it appears likely that differences in the activity or specificity of processing enzymes, or differences in the intracellular environment at the site of enzyme action, account for tissue-specific processing of POMC, rather than alternate modes of RNA splicing, or selective expression of different POMC genes in different tissues.

The major products of proenkephalin processing in the bovine adrenal medulla appear to be the higher molecular weight peptides (> 1000 D), some of which are potent opioids (Kilpatrick et al., 1981). The free pentapeptides, met- and leu-enkephalin, make up less than 5% of the total enkephalin-containing peptide pool in the adrenal gland (Udenfriend and Kilpatrick, 1983). However, in the brain (caudate nucleus), the major products of proenkephalin processing are free enkephalins and synenkephalin, the amino-terminal fragment of proenkephalin (Liston et al., 1983, 1984a). Proenkephalin-processing intermediates in

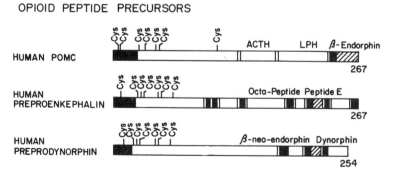

Figure 1. *Structure of the precursors to the opioid peptides.*

DIFFERENTIAL PROCESSING OF POMC IN ANTERIOR
AND INTERMEDIATE LOBES OF THE PITUITARY

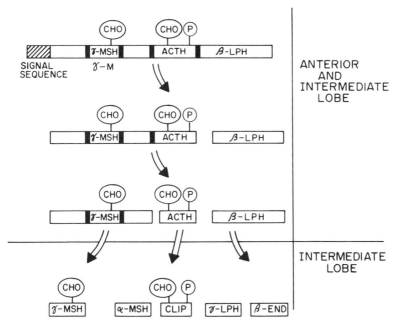

Figure 2. *Processing of pro-opiomelanocortin in the anterior and neurointermediate lobes of rodent pituitary.*

the brain are also different from those in adrenal chromaffin cells (Liston et al., 1984b). The presence of a single proenkephalin gene in several species (Comb et al., 1983) suggests that the tissue-specific products described above are a result of differences in proteolytic processing pathways, although the possibility that more than one species of proenkephalin is produced from a single gene by alternate modes of RNA splicing cannot be ruled out at this time.

Regional differences in the immunohistochemical (Weber and Barchas, 1983) and biochemical (Weber et al., 1982) distribution of the peptides derived from prodynorphin indicate that the proteolytic processing of this precursor is also regulated in a tissue-specific manner. Thus, there is strong evidence that all three precursors of the opioid peptides undergo tissue-specific processing. The resulting products may be particularly well suited to meet the demands of each tissue.

The bioactive peptide domains within neuropeptide precursors are flanked by pairs of basic amino acid residues, which are thought to be sites of cleavage by trypsinlike endopeptidases (Docherty and Steiner, 1982). The exposed carboxy-terminal lysine or arginine of the resulting peptides would then be cleaved by a carboxypeptidase B-like exopeptidase to produce bioactive peptides. In some instances, the peptides are further modified by glycosylation, phosphorylation, amidation, sulfation, or methylation.

Since most neuropeptides become active only after they are cleaved out of their precursors, it is critical to understand how cleavage is controlled. Yet our knowledge of the enzymes that carry out these proteolytic cleavage reactions is rudimentary, compared to our knowlege of the structure of the precursors and the sites of modification. Studies that have been done to date indicate that the intracellular processing enzymes are located in secretory granules. These enzymes also have a higher specificity for substrate structure and different requirements for optimal activity than do pancreatic proteases like trypsin (Docherty and Steiner, 1982). However, attempts to further characterize these enzymes in granule preparations have not been very successful. One reason is that it is difficult to separate completely the secretory granules from other cell components (such as lysosomes) that contain high levels of several types of proteolytic enzymes.

Although no definitive identification of a POMC or proenkephalin protease has yet been made, trypsinlike serine endopeptidase activities have been observed in the pituitary (Orlowski, 1983) and adrenal glands. A serine protease that converts β-LPH to β-endorphin by specific cleavage of the bond between Arg_{60} and Tyr_{61} of β-LPH has been detected in extracts of the anterior and neurointermediate lobes of the rat pituitary (Graf and Kenessey, 1976; Kenessey and Graf, 1977). This enzyme is active at pH 8.0, whereas at lower pH values the activity of other endopeptidases becomes apparent. Changes in the levels of activity of a trypsinlike enzyme in the anterior pituitary of the rat parallel those of ACTH following dexamethasone treatment, ovariectomy, and adrenalectomy (Kenessey et al., 1979). This correlation, together with the subcellular localization and biochemical properties of the trypsinlike enzyme, suggests that it may play a role in precursor processing (Kenessey et al., 1979).

Rat pituitary also has been found to contain a kininogenase enzyme highly concentrated in the neurointermediate lobe (Powers and Nasjletti, 1983). This enzyme, which belongs to a large subclass of serine proteases (trypsinlike) known as the kallikreins (Eisen and Vogt, 1970; Fiedler, 1979), is capable of converting kininogen to peptides (kinins) that regulate blood pressure in the kidney and other tissues (Eisen and Vogt, 1970). The presence of high levels of this enzyme in a gland in which over 30% of the protein present is derived from POMC, and all of the cells are engaged in synthesizing and processing POMC, strongly suggests that the enzyme is involved in processing POMC. However, POMC-producing cells in the pituitary of some species are also known to contain progastrin (or procholecystokinin) and to process this precursor to various forms of gastrin (Rehfield, 1980; Rehfield and Larsson, 1981). Because a kallikrein enzyme is believed to be involved in gastrin processing (Rehfield, 1980), the pituitary kallikrein might play a role in processing progastrin as well as POMC in the rat neurointermediate lobe. Urinary and pancreatic kallikreins have been shown to be capable of processing proenkephalin fragments from the bovine adrenal medulla (Prado et al., 1983).

The kallikrein enzymes form a distinct subgroup of mammalian serine proteases (Schachter, 1980). These enzymes, which are glycoproteins, have a molecular weight range of 25–40 kD, exhibit strict substrate specificity (Schachter, 1969), and are characterized by their ability to release kinins from kininogens. The diversity of action of these enzymes is consistent with their presence in a wide variety of tissues. The ability of kallikreins to generate biologically active growth factors from inactive precursor forms has also been demonstrated. Epidermal growth factor binding protein and nerve growth factor subunits are members of the family of specific kallikreins (Server and Shooter, 1976; Bothwell et al., 1979; Frey et al., 1979; Lazure et al., 1981) that release growth factors from their respective precursors (Frey et al., 1979; Lazure et al., 1981).

Shine and his coworkers have shown that there are at least 35 different kallikrein genes in the mouse and rat that exhibit a high degree of homology (Mason et al., 1983). In the mouse, all of the members of this gene family are closely linked on chromosome seven (Mason et al., 1983). Sequencing of mouse genomic DNA clones and cDNA clones isolated from submaxillary gland and pancreas has revealed that the limited variability in the coding region of the kallikrein genes lies in the amino acid sequences involving the active sites of the enzymes. This implies that kallikrein enzymes differ from one another in the type of substrate sequences that serve as recognition and cleavage sites (Mason et al., 1983).

The following studies represent our initial attempts to determine if a kallikrein enzyme is involved in the processing of POMC. We have used recombinant DNA techniques to characterize a kallikrein mRNA in mouse pituitary tumor cells (AtT-20-D_{16v} cells). Sequencing of the cDNA copied from the mRNA has established the existence of a new species of kallikrein enzyme in these cells, and the cloned cDNA has provided a new tool for investigating the role of this enzyme in processing and metabolism of POMC and other neuropeptide precursors.

NORTHERN BLOT ANALYSIS OF AtT-20 CELL RNA

AtT-20 tumor cells have been used as a model system in which to study the expression and proteolytic processing of POMC (Eipper and Mains, 1980). This cell line, which is derived from anterior pituitary corticotrophs of the mouse, is highly specialized for the production and processing of POMC. More than 3% of the protein made by these cells is POMC. The processing of POMC, which has been studied in great detail in several laboratories (for a review, see Douglass et al., 1984a), proceeds according to the pathway shown in the upper part of Figure 2 (in both the anterior and the neurointermediate lobes). Thus, if a kallikrein enzyme is involved in the formation of ACTH and β-LPH from POMC, it would be expected to be present in AtT-20 cells. To determine if a kallikrein enzyme is present in these cells, we analyzed AtT-20 cell RNA by the Northern blot procedure (data not shown). In the blot, we detected an mRNA band that hybridizes to a mouse kallikrein cDNA probe derived from mouse submaxillary gland RNA (kindly provided by Drs. R. Richards and J. Shine). From these data, we estimated that approximately 0.5% of the total AtT-20 poly(A)$^+$ mRNA population codes for kallikrein enzymes. These values are approximately one-sixth the level of POMC mRNA present in the same cell type.

We then constructed an AtT-20 cDNA library by using the poly(A)$^+$ mRNA isolated from AtT-20 cells. Approximately 0.1% of the cDNA clones hybridized with this cDNA probe, suggesting that kallikrein mRNA is present at high levels in AtT-20 cells. Approximately 3% of the total poly(A)$^+$ mRNA population in AtT-20 cells code for POMC, while 0.6% of the cDNA clones from the identical AtT-20 cDNA library contain POMC inserts. Thus, both POMC and kallikrein mRNA are present in relatively high levels in AtT-20 cells.

NUMBER OF SPECIES OF KALLIKREIN mRNA IN AtT-20 CELLS

In order to determine how many species of kallikrein mRNA are synthesized in AtT-20 cells, 42 individual kallikrein-positive cDNA clones were isolated. The plasmid DNA was purified and subjected to restriction analysis, while the cDNA inserts were subcloned into M13-RF DNA for full nucleotide sequence analysis. Figure 3 shows that five different classes of cDNA clones were revealed by restriction analysis. However, DNA sequencing revealed that each clone type contained a cDNA insert that was generated from the same species of kallikrein mRNA (nucleotide sequence analysis to be published elsewhere). Thus, AtT-20 cells contain relatively high levels of a unique species of kallikrein mRNA, the sequence of which is different from those of previously published mouse kallikrein cDNAs. This conclusion is more clearly illustrated in Figure 4. Here, the predicted amino acid sequence of the AtT-20 kallikrein (as determined from the nucleotide sequence of the pMAK3 insert) is compared to the primary amino acid sequence of other mouse kallikreins. Some of these amino acid sequences were deduced from the nucleotide sequence of mouse kallikrein genomic DNA clones (mGK-1 and mGK-2 from Mason et al., 1983), while others were deduced from the nucleotide sequence of kallikrein cDNA clones isolated from mouse submaxillary gland cDNA libraries (pMK-2 from Nordeen et al., 1982; pMK-1 from Richards et al., 1982; EGF-BP from Ronne et al., 1983; γ-NGF from Ullrich et al., 1984).

Although the AtT-20 kallikrein exhibits a great deal of amino acid sequence homology (approximately 80%) when compared with other mouse kallikreins, there are localized regions of sequence heterogeneity. Some of these regions

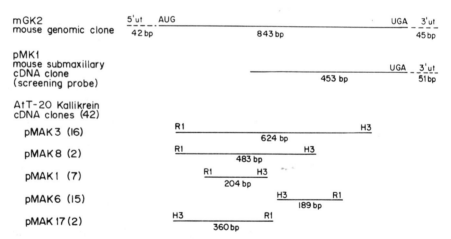

Figure 3. *Schematic diagram of AtT-20 kallikrein cDNA clones.* The structure of a full-length kallikrein mRNA is represented by mGK2 (Mason et al., 1983). The *solid line* represents the coding region, while the *dotted lines* represent untranslated regions (ut). The partial kallikrein cDNA clone used to screen an AtT-20 cDNA library is designated pMAK1 (Richards et al., 1982). The classes of AtT-20 kallikrein cDNA clones and the numbers of types in each isolated class are shown. The restriction sites present at the termini of these clones are designated R1 (Eco R1) or H3 (Hind III). .

COMPARISON OF MOUSE KALLIKREIN SEQUENCES
DETERMINED BY cDNA CLONING

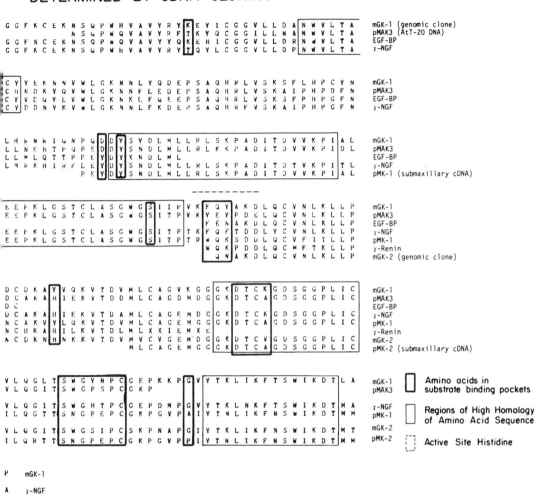

Figure 4. *Comparison of mouse kallikrein amino acid sequences, as determined by cDNA cloning*. The cDNA sequences from which these amino acid sequences were deduced are noted and referenced in the text. Regions boxed by *bold solid lines* represent amino acids believed to line the substrate binding pocket of serine proteases (Mason et al., 1983). Other regions boxed by *solid lines* represent portions of the kallikrein exhibiting a high degree of amino acid sequence homology. The *dashed box* denotes the position of a highly conserved histidine residue present in the active site of the molecules (Schachter, 1980). The *dashed line* is over a region of pronounced amino acid sequence heterogeneity.

comprise amino acid residues that are believed to constitute the substrate-binding pocket of serine proteases (Mason et al., 1983). Indeed, it may be that these regions of the protein are involved in determining the substrate specificity of the kallikrein because there is clearly less homology in these regions than in the remainder of the sequence. The regions that are highly homologous between AtT-20 kallikrein and those listed may be necessary for the formation of a proper three-dimensional structure. Thus, AtT-20 cells contain high levels of a species of mRNA that codes for a member of the kallikrein family. This kallikrein is different from those previously identified, and amino acid sequence comparison suggests that it may also have a unique substrate specificity.

SYNTHESIS OF SPECIFIC DNA PROBES FOR DETECTING AtT-20 KALLIKREIN mRNA

The high degree of homology seen at the nucleotide level is compatible with the finding that a single kallikrein cDNA probe can hybridize to numerous species of kallikrein mRNA. Therefore, cDNA probes cannot be used to study the distribution and expression of this particular species of kallikrein mRNA (to be referred to as AtT-20 kallikrein mRNA). For this reason, a synthetic oligonucleotide was designed that could be used to distinguish AtT-20 kallikrein mRNA from other species of kallikrein mRNA (Figure 5). A segment of seven amino acid residues showing a high degree of heterogeneity (boxed in bold in Figure 4) was chosen, and the nucleotide sequence coding for these residues

Strategy for Selecting AtT-20 Kallikrein mRNA...
Oligonucleotide Probe Design

pMAK3/AtT-20 Kallikrein	5' AA TAT GAA TAC CCA GAT G	3'
pMK3/pancreatic Kallikrein	GA TTG GAA TTT AGT GAT G	
mGK1/genomic clone	AG TCA CAA TAT GCA AAA G	
pMK1/submaxillary Kallikrein	GA TGG CAA AAG TCA GAT G	
pGK2/genomic clone	AA TTC CAA AAT GCA AAA G	
pmɣN/submaxillary Kallikrein (ɣ subunit of nerve growth factor)	AA TTC CAA TTC ACA GAT G	
pMAK3 oliogonucleotide (AtT-20 Kallikrein mRNA specific probe)	3' TT ATA CTT ATG GGT CTA C	5'

Mismatches are underlined
Average mismatch is 40%

Figure 5. *Strategy for selectively monitoring AtT-20 kallikrein mRNA oligonucleotide probe design.* An 18-base nucleotide sequence (5' to 3') coding for the amino acid residues highlighted by the *dashed line* in Figure 4 is shown for four species of mouse kallikrein cDNA and two different mouse kallikrein genes. The cDNA or genomic DNA fragments from which these sequences were obtained are noted in Figure 4 and in the text. The synthetic oligonucleotide, 18 bases long, which is capable of distinguishing AtT-20 kallikrein mRNA from other species of kallikrein mRNA is designated pMAK3 oligonucleotide (3' to 5'). Mismatches to this complementary probe are underlined and averaged 40%.

STRINGENCY OF HYBRIDIZATION OF AtT-20 KALLIKREIN
cDNA CLONE TO SPECIFIC DNA OLIGOMER

DOT BLOT

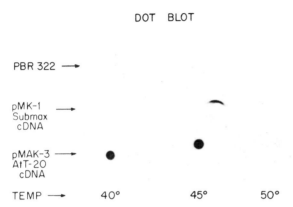

Figure 6.   Hybridization of ³²P-labeled oligomer to pBR322, pMK1, and pMAK3 plasmid DNA. Dot blot analysis was performed, as described previously (Douglass et al., 1984b). The temperatures at which hybridization was carried out are noted.

was analyzed. Over an 18-base region, there is an average 40% mismatch of bases between AtT-20 kallikrein mRNA and five other species of mouse kallikrein mRNA. Thus, an oligonucleotide 18 bases long with the sequence 5′ CATCTGGGTATTCATATT 3′ was synthesized. This oligomer should be capable of distinguishing AtT-20 kallikrein mRNA from other species of kallikrein mRNA when hybridization is carried out under the proper conditions. Plasmid dot blot analysis (Figure 6) shows that when hybridization is carried out at 40°C or 45°C, the oligomer hybridizes with complementary sequences present in pMAK3 (AtT-20 kallikrein cDNA) but gives no hybridization signal with pMK1 (mouse submaxillary kallikrein cDNA) or the plasmid vector pBR322. At 50°C, the oligomer can no longer hybridize with pMAK3 cDNA, as this temperature is above the optimal one for base pairing (based on calculated values). Thus, the oligomer is capable of distinguishing AtT-20 kallikrein mRNA from other species of kallikrein mRNA when hybridization is carried out in the 40–45°C range.

DETECTION OF AtT-20 KALLIKREIN mRNA IN THE NEUROINTERMEDIATE LOBE OF MOUSE PITUITARY

If the kallikrein coded for by AtT-20 kallikrein mRNA is involved in the proteolytic processing of POMC, tissues containing POMC may also be expected to contain AtT-20 kallikrein. In the mouse, the neurointermediate lobe of the pituitary contains high levels of POMC mRNA, while little, if any, POMC mRNA is observed in the pancreas (E. Herbert and J. Douglass, unpublished observations). The Northern blot analysis shown in Figure 7 reveals that while kallikrein mRNA is present in both mouse neurointermediate lobe and pancreas, only the neurointermediate lobe appears to contain the species of kallikrein mRNA present in AtT-20 cells.

When the cDNA insert from pMK1 was used as a hybridization probe, a radioactive band representing kallikrein mRNA was observed in the neurointermediate lobe. A relatively small amount of neurointermediate lobe total RNA was present on this blot, suggesting that the neurointermediate lobe contains high levels of kallikrein mRNA, perhaps higher than the levels seen in AtT-20 cells. Northern blot analysis also reveals the presence of kallikrein mRNA in the mouse pancreas. A kallikrein mRNA of similar size is observed in this tissue, along with one or more smaller species of RNA. These smaller species may represent degradation products of the larger form. The intensity of the hybridization signal for pancreas is much lower than that seen for the neurointermediate lobe, even though more poly(A)$^+$ mRNA is present in the pancreas sample, suggesting again that the neurointermediate lobe contains high levels of kallikrein mRNA.

When the oligomer specific for AtT-20 kallikrein mRNA was used as a hybridization probe on the same Northern blot in place of the cDNA probe, a strong hybridization signal was seen in the neurointermediate lobe RNA lane of the blot. The intensity of the signal was reduced as the hybridization temperature was raised from 35 to 45°C. This loss of signal upon raising the temperature was not observed when the oligomer was hybridized to a complementary pMAK3 cDNA sequence (Figure 6), indicating that the oligomer–DNA hybrid is more stable than the oligomer–RNA hybrid. The size of the neurointermediate lobe mRNA that hybridizes to the oligomer is identical to that which hybridizes to the cDNA probe. These data suggest that AtT-20 kallikrein mRNA is present in the mouse neurointermediate lobe. At both hybridization temperatures, no signal was apparent in the lane that contained pancreas mRNA with the oligomer, even when the autoradiograph was overexposed. Thus, although pancreas contains kallikrein mRNA, it does not contain detectable levels of AtT-20 kallikrein mRNA.

CONCLUSIONS

In mammals, many enzymes have been implicated in neuropeptide precursor processing, but only two processing enzymes have actually been identified to date [epidermal growth factor (EGF)-binding protein and the subunit of the 7S–nerve growth factor (NGF) complex]. Several candidate processing enzymes have been localized in mature secretory granules and have been shown to be active under conditions believed to exist in these granules. However, processing by the endopeptidases may occur at other sites in the cell where conditions are different from those in mature secretory granules. POMC, for example, undergoes a series of cleavages and modifications that occur in a specific order as the polyprotein moves through the secretory pathway. Some of the cleavage reactions may occur in the endoplasmic reticulum, others in the Golgi apparatus or in immature secretory granules. Since we do not know the conditions that exist at

COMPARISON OF HYBRIDIZATION OF pMK-1 KALLIKREIN
cDNA and SYNTHETIC OLIGOMER WITH RNA FROM
NEUROINTERMEDIATE LOBE (NIL) and PANCREAS (PAN)

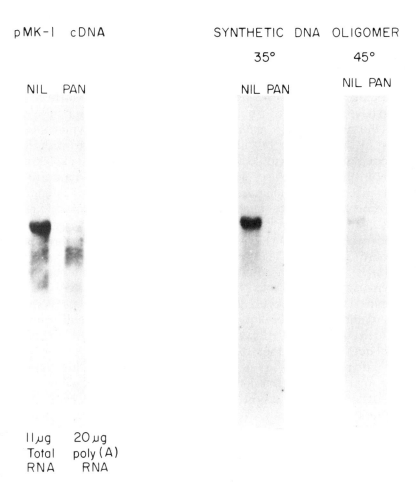

Figure 7. *Northern blot analysis of mouse neurointermediate lobe and pancreas RNA.* RNA samples [total or poly(A)+] were prepared, electrophoresed on a 1.5% agarose gel, and transferred to nitrocellulose paper, as described previously (Douglass et al., 1984b). The filter was hybridized with 10[7] cpm of either nick-translated pMK1 insert (cDNA) or 32P-labeled oligomer. Hybridization with the oligomer was performed overnight at 35°C and 45°C.

all of these sites in the cell, it is difficult to develop strict criteria for identifying processing enzymes on this basis.

The occurrence of a kallikreinlike activity in highly concentrated form in the neurointermediate lobe of rat pituitary (a major site of POMC synthesis) suggests that this enzyme is involved in POMC processing (Powers and Nasjletti, 1983). The isolation of a kallikrein cDNA clone from an AtT-20 cDNA library is consistent with this hypothesis. The level of kallikrein mRNA in AtT-20 cells is quite high. Up to 0.5% of the total poly(A)$^+$ mRNA population may code for kallikrein. This value is about one-sixth the level of POMC mRNA in the same cell line. Assuming that the translational efficiencies of these mRNAs are similar, for every six molecules of POMC there would be one kallikrein molecule. This is a high ratio of enzyme to substrate. However, this observation is not surprising in view of the finding that the kallikrein involved in NGF processing is present at the same level as the precursor or in the form of a complex with the precursor.

The finding that 42 out of 42 randomly picked kallikrein-positive cDNA clones appear to have been derived from the same species of kallikrein mRNA strongly supports the view that there is only one major kallikrein enzyme in AtT-20 cells. However, by analyzing more kallikrein-positive cDNA clones with both cDNA and oligomer probes, we should be able to determine if another kallikrein mRNA is present in these cells. Also, more nucleotide sequence data on the 20 or so uncharacterized mouse kallikrein genes is needed to determine unambiguously if our oligonucleotide probe is recognizing only one species of kallikrein mRNA (AtT-20 kallikrein mRNA). This seems likely, because the average mismatch of bases between our oligonucleotide probe and the complementary region of six other mouse kallikrein genes is nearly 40%.

Hence, we have sequenced an mRNA that codes for a potential POMC processing enzyme in AtT-20 cells. The next step will be to isolate the enzyme and to determine its specificity with natural and synthetic substrates. We would also like to determine if the subcellular distribution and the tissue distribution of the enzyme are compatible with its postulated role in processing of POMC. Another important question is whether this enzyme is involved in the processing of other neuropeptide precursors such as proenkephalin. To answer these questions, we are using immunocytochemical approaches to localize the kallikrein enzyme in various cells and tissues and synthetic oligonucleotides to determine the distribution of the kallikrein mRNA. However, even if we are able to determine the tissue distribution of the enzyme and its mRNA, we would still be faced with the critical question of precisely what role this enzyme plays in POMC processing. To date the only organism in which the specific steps catalyzed by a processing enzyme has been determined unequivocally is yeast (Julius et al., 1983). A dipeptidylaminopeptidase has been shown by mutational analysis to be required for the maturation of α-factor, a mating pheromone of yeast.

Since we do not have genetic tools available for identifying processing enzymes in mammals, we have turned to new approaches to obtain the same information. We will attempt to delete the kallikrein enzyme from the cellular protein pool of AtT-20 cells by an elegant new gene transfer technique (Izant and Weintraub, 1984). The cDNA for the kallikrein is inserted into an expression vector in such an orientation that its transcription leads to production of an anti-sense kallikrein mRNA. If enough of this anti-sense mRNA can be produced in the recipient cell, it will hybridize to the normal AtT-20 kallikrein mRNA and inactivate it. After a number of cell divisions, the kallikrein enzyme will be diluted out of the cellular protein pool. One can then determine what effect the deletion of the kallikrein protein has on the processing of POMC. This method of deleting proteins from the cellular protein pool has been used successfully to delete thymidine kinase from a cell line (Izant and Weintraub, 1984). If this method is successful with the kallikrein enzyme, it could then be used to assess the role of other putative processing enzymes, such as carboxypeptidase and other endopeptidases, in the maturation of POMC.

Many neuroendocrine peptide precursor molecules are synthesized in the brain. In the future, it will be extremely interesting to study the variety of kallikreins that may be present in this highly complex tissue. We have already isolated several cDNA clones from a rat preoptic cDNA library (courtesy of P. Seeburg) that hybridize strongly with the AtT-20 kallikrein cDNA clone. Thus, it appears that one or more kallikrein genes are expressed in the rat brain. The use of recombinant DNA techniques such as those described in this chapter should help us to identify these enzymes and to determine their role in the regulation of the production of neuropeptides.

ACKNOWLEDGMENTS

J.D. was supported by American Cancer Society postdoctoral fellowship PF-2051 and National Institutes of Health research grant F32-GM09807-01. E.H. (principal investigator) is supported by National Institutes of Health grants NIDA-DA02736, NIADDK-AM16879, and NIADDK-AM30155. The authors would also like to thank Drs. R. Richards and J. Shine for their generous gift of pMK1, and S. Engbretson and N. Gay for expert manuscript preparation.

REFERENCES

Bothwell, M. A., W. H. Wilson, and E. M. Shooter (1979) The relationship between glandular kallikrein and growth factor-processing proteases of mouse submaxillary gland. *J. Biol. Chem.* **254**:7287–7294.

Comb, M., H. Rosen, P. Seeburg, J. Adelman, and E. Herbert (1983) Primary structure of the human proenkephalin gene. *DNA* **2**:213–229.

Docherty, K., and D. Steiner (1982) Post-translational proteolysis in polypeptide hormone biosynthesis. *Annu. Rev. Physiol.* **44**:625–638.

Douglass, J., O. Civelli, and E. Herbert (1984a) Polyprotein gene expression: Generation of diversity of neuroendocrine peptides. *Annu. Rev. Biochem.* **53**:665–715.

Douglass, J., K. Ranney, M. Uhler, G. Little, and E. Herbert (1984b) Isolation of a cDNA clone coding for a kallikrein enzyme in mouse anterior pituitary tumor cells. *UCLA Symp. Mol. Cell. Biol. (New Series)* **19**:573–588.

Eipper, B. A., and R. E. Mains (1980) Structure and biosynthesis of pro-ACTH/endorphin and related peptides. *Endocr. Rev.* **1**:1–27.

Eisen, V., and W. Vogt (1970) Plasma kininogenases and their activators. *Handb. Exp. Pharmacol.* **25**:82–109.

Fiedler, F. (1979) Enzymology of glandular kallikreins. *Handb. Exp. Pharmacol.* **25**:102–161.

Frey, P., R. Forand, T. Maciag, and E. M. Shooter (1979) The biosynthesis precursor of epidermal growth factor and the mechanism of its processing. *Proc. Natl. Acad. Sci. USA* **76**:6294–6298.

Graf, L., and A. Kenessey (1976) Specific cleavage of a single peptide bond (residues 77–78) in β-lipotropin by a pituitary endopeptidase. *FEBS Lett.* **69**:255–260.

Izant, J. G., and H. Weintraub (1984) Inhibition of thymidine kinase gene expression by anti-sense RNA: A molecular approach to genetic analysis. *Cell* **36**:1007–1015.

Julius, D., L. Blair, A. Brake, G. Sprague, and J. Thorner (1983) Yeast α-factor is processed from a larger precursor polypeptide: The essential role of a membrane-bound dipeptidyl aminopeptidase. *Cell* **32**:839–852.

Kenessey, A., and L. Graf (1977) Regional distribution of β-lipotropin converting enzymes in rat pituitary and brain. *Brain Res. Bull.* **2**:247–250.

Kenessey, A., P. Paldi-Haris, G. B. Makara, and L. Graf (1979) Trypsin-like activity of rat anterior pituitary in relation to secretory activity. *Life Sci.* **25**:437–443.

Kilpatrick, D. L., T. Taniguchi, B. N. Jones, A. S. Stern, J. E. Shively, J. Hullihan, S. Kimura, S. Stein, and S. Udenfriend (1981) A highly potent 3200-dalton adrenal opioid peptide that contains both a [Met]- and [Leu]-enkephalin sequence. *Proc. Natl. Acad. Sci. USA* **78**:3265–3268.

Lazure, C., N. G. Seidah, G. Thibault, R. Boucher, J. Grant, and M. Chrétien (1981) Sequence homologies between tonin, nerve growth factor-binding protein and serine proteases. *Nature* **292**:383–384.

Liston, D. R., J.-J. Vanderhaeghen, and R. Rossier (1983) Presence in brain of synenkephalin, a proenkephalin-immunoreactive protein which does not contain enkephalin. *Nature* **302**:62–65.

Liston, D. R., P. Bohlen, and J. Rossier (1984a) Purification from brain of synenkephalin, the N-terminal fragment of proenkephalin. *J. Neurochem.* **43**:335–341.

Liston, D. R., G. Patey, J. Rossier, P. Verbanck, and J.-J. Vanderhaeghen (1984b) Processing of proenkephalin is tissue-specific. *Science* **225**:734–737.

Mason, A. J., B. A. Evans, D. R. Cox, J. Shine, and R. I. Richards (1983) Structure of mouse kallikrein gene family suggests a role in specific processing of biologically active peptides. *Nature* **303**:300–307.

Nordeen, S. K., A. J. Mason, R. I. Richards, J. D. Baxter, and J. Shine (1982) Mouse kallikrein arginyl-esteropeptidase genes: Analysis of cloned cDNA's suggests rapid functional divergence from a common ancestral sequence. *DNA* **1**:309–311.

Orlowski, M. (1983) Pituitary endopeptidases. *Mol. Cell. Biochem.* **52**:49–74.

Powers, C. A., and A. Nasjletti (1983) A kininogenase resembling glandular kallikrein in the rat pituitary pars intermedia. *Endocrinology* **112**:1194–1200.

Prado, E. S., L. Prado de Carvalho, M. S. Araujo-Viel, N. Ling, and J. Rossier (1983) A met-enkephalin-containing-peptide, BAM 22P, as a novel substrate for glandular kallikreins. *Biochem. Biophys. Res. Comm.* **112**:366–371.

Rehfield, J. F. (1980) Heterogeneity of gastrointestinal hormones. In *Gastrointestinal Hormones*, G. B. J. Glass, ed., pp. 433–449, Raven, New York.

Rehfield, J. F., and L. I. Larsson (1981) Pituitary gastrins: Different processing in corticotrophs and melanotrophs. *J. Biol. Chem.* **256**:10426–10429.

Richards, R. E., D. F. Catanzara, A. J. Mason, B. J. Morris, J. D. Baxter, and J. Shine (1982) Nucleotide sequence of cloned cDNA coding for a member of the kallikrein arginyl esteropeptidase group of serine proteases. *J. Biol. Chem.* **257**:2758–2761.

Ronne, H., S. Lundgren, L. Severinsson, L. Rask, and P. A. Peterson (1983) Growth factor-binding proteases in the murine submaxillary gland: Isolation of a cDNA clone. *EMBO J.* **2**:1561–1564.

Schachter, M. (1969) Kallikreins and kinins. *Physiol. Rev.* **49**:509–547.

Schachter, M. (1980) Kallikreins (kininogenases)—A group of serine proteases with bioregulatory actions. *Pharmacol. Rev.* **37**:1–17.

Server, A. C., and E. M. Shooter (1976) Comparison of the arginine esteropeptidases associated with the nerve and epidermal growth factors. *J. Biol. Chem.* **251**:165–173.

Udenfriend, S., and D. Kilpatrick (1983) Biochemistry of the enkephalin and enkephalin-containing peptides. *Arch. Biochem. Biophys.* **221**:309–323.

Uhler, M., E. Herbert, P. D'Eustachio, and F. D. Ruddle (1983) The mouse genome contains two nonallelic pro-opiomelanocortin genes. *J. Biol. Chem.* **258**:9444–9453.

Ullrich, A., A. Gray, W. I. Wood, J. Hayflick, and P. H. Seeburg (1984) Isolation of a cDNA clone coding for the γ-subunit of mouse nerve growth factor using a high stringency selection procedure. *DNA* **3**:387–392.

Weber, E., C. Evans, and J. Barchas (1982) Predominance of the amino-terminal octapeptide fragment of dynorphin in rat brain regions. *Nature* **299**:77–79.

Weber, E., and J. D. Barchas (1983) Immunohistochemical distribution of dynorphin B in rat brain: Relation to dynorphin A and β-neo-endorphin systems. *Proc. Natl. Acad. Sci. USA* **80**:1125–1129.

Chapter 12

Transmitter Synergism and Diversity

FLOYD E. BLOOM
ELENA BATTENBERG
ANDRE FERRON
JORGE MANCILLAS
ROBERT J. MILNER
GEORGE R. SIGGINS
J. GREGOR SUTCLIFFE

ABSTRACT

Our laboratories have concentrated on the use of multidisciplinary methods to combine knowledge based on transmitter localization, transmitter circuitry, and transmitter mechanisms (see Siggins and Bloom, 1981; Foote et al., 1983; Bloom, 1984). This chapter highlights two areas of recent investigation: First, we describe interactions between the transmitters of convergent synaptic inputs on their presumed common target cells, focusing on interactions between norepinephrine, the transmitter of the globally directed coeruleocortical projection, and vasoactive intestinal polypeptide, one of the peptides attributed to the intrinsic local interneurons of the rodent cerebral cortex, the bipolar neurons. In a similar manner, we describe interactions in the hippocampus between somatostatin, a peptide found within several neuronal elements of the limbic system, and acetylcholine, long a presumptive transmitter for the septohippocampal pathway. Second, we summarize recent work in which molecular genetic approaches have begun to define as yet undiscovered neuropeptides. Toward this end, we briefly summarize our strategy to identify brain-specific molecules. We interpret our early findings with this strategy to exemplify some potentially important new directions in the quest to unravel more completely the chemical and functional organization of the nervous system. Although the nature and number of neurotransmitters are still incompletely defined, a limited repertoire of response mechanisms is postulated. Interactions among these response mechanisms may provide a rich array of signaling possibilities.

INTERACTIONS BETWEEN VASOACTIVE INTESTINAL POLYPEPTIDE AND NOREPINEPHRINE IN RAT CEREBRAL CORTEX

Several lines of evidence support a role for vasoactive intestinal polypeptide (VIP) as a neuronal messenger in the cerebral cortex. Biochemical data support its presence, release, binding, and at best one possible action (for references, see Morrison and Magistretti, 1983). Immunocytochemical data have localized VIP to cortical bipolar neurons (Morrison et al., 1984). Single-unit recording studies show that iontophoretically applied VIP excites some cortical neurons (Phillis et al., 1979) but in an inconsistent manner. Other cellular actions reported for VIP include the ability to stimulate cAMP formation (Quik et al., 1979; Etgen and Browning, 1983; Magistretti and Schorderet, 1984) and glycogenolysis (Magistretti et al., 1981) in cortical slices. VIP is somewhat more potent in these actions than is norepinephrine.

Cytochemically, VIP- and norepinephrine-containing circuits show a contrasting but complementary cortical anatomy (see Morrison and Magistretti, 1983): VIP neurons are intrinsic, bipolar, radially oriented, intracortical neurons; the norepinephrine innervation arises only from the locus coeruleus and innervates a broad expanse of cortex in a horizontal plane. Both fiber systems may have the same targets—the pyramidal cells. The spontaneous firing of identified cortical pyramidal neurons is depressed by iontophoresis of either norepinephrine or cAMP (Stone et al., 1975; see also Foote et al., 1983). The findings of Magistretti and Schorderet (1984) suggest that VIP and norepinephrine can act synergistically to increase cAMP in the cerebral cortex. Therefore, we tested both on rat cortical neurons to evaluate this interaction at the cellular level through the use of iontophoresis. Analysis of more than 100 cortical neurons suggests definitively that there are significant interactions: Application of VIP during subthreshold norepinephrine administration causes pronounced inhibition of cellular discharge regardless of the effect of VIP prior to norepinephrine administration (Ferron et al., 1985).

In our hands, the direct effects of VIP on the spontaneous firing rate of sensorimotor cortical neurons were not very impressive. VIP depressed 24%, excited 20%, and had biphasic effects on 2%; maximal currents (200 nA) passed through the VIP barrel had no effect on 54% of these cells. The direction of the response and the proportion of responding neurons were similar for identified pyramidal neurons and for all cortical neurons. The direct effects of norepinephrine were predominantly depressant actions in the cortex, as previously reported (Siggins and Bloom, 1981; Foote et al., 1983). Therefore, in order to examine possible interactions between the effects of VIP and norepinephrine on single neurons, ejection currents of norepinephrine were reduced until they had little or no direct effect on neuronal firing (1–5 µA). After testing a cell for direct effects (if any) of VIP, subthreshold currents of norepinephrine were applied continuously for several minutes while VIP was repeatedly retested. Tests on approximately 50 neurons studied in this manner revealed that ejection of VIP during subthreshold norepinephrine administration produced consistent inhibition of firing. Such synergistic inhibitions were seen in more than half the cells, regardless of whether VIP alone had elicited excitatory, inhibitory, or negligible effects on the test neuron (Ferron et al., 1985). When VIP alone had a depressant action, administration of subthreshold norepinephrine markedly enhanced this depressant effect. Even in cases in which VIP alone produced excitatory effects, concurrent subthreshold norepinephrine treatment reversed the VIP effect from excitation to inhibition (six of nine cells).

Magistretti and Schorderet (1984) showed that the synergism of VIP by norepinephrine was blocked by phentolamine, an α-adrenergic receptor antagonist, and mimicked by phenylephrine, an α-receptor agonist. Therefore, we examined the effect of phenylephrine, as well as norepinephrine pretreatment, on neuronal responses to VIP. In 10 cells showing an interaction between VIP and norepinephrine, nine revealed equivalent interactive synergisms of depressant responses with phenylephrine (Ferron et al., 1985). Thus, the interaction of VIP and norepinephrine at the cellular level may also involve α-receptor activation, although further testing is required.

Our electrophysiological indications of a VIP–norepinephrine interaction at the cellular level may arise from their biochemical effects *in vitro* on cAMP generation. Such parallel findings strengthen suggestions that cAMP may mediate both norepinephrine- and VIP-evoked depressions of neuronal firing in the cortex. The reported enhancement of synaptic and other transmitter responses (including inhibitory ones) by norepinephrine may be related phenomena (see Foote et al., 1983; Bloom, 1984). An apparently similar cAMP-mediated enhancement by β-receptors of noradrenergic target cell responsiveness to α-adrenergic agonists has been reported in the pineal gland (Klein et al., 1983). Furthermore, in rat hepatocytes, increased cAMP levels induced by glucagon enhance binding of α-adrenergic agonists to these cells (Morgan et al., 1984). Two modes of indirect amplification of postsynaptic target cell mechanisms may be involved in these interactions, namely, a cAMP-mediated activation of protein kinases (as with β-adrenergic and other responses) and a calcium activation of protein kinases (as with α_1-adrenergic and other transmitter or hormone responses; see Nestler and Greengard, 1984). However, it is not yet clear how these metabolic and electrophysiologic events actually interact. If norepinephrine- and VIP-containing fibers do indeed converge on the same cortical target cell, it is feasible that cAMP is the intracellular mediator of their synergistic interaction.

INTERACTIONS BETWEEN SOMATOSTATIN AND ACETYLCHOLINE ACTIONS IN RAT HIPPOCAMPUS

Although the oligopeptide somatostatin was discovered and named for its ability to impair the release of growth hormone from somatotropes (see Guillemin, 1978), the same peptide is ubiquitous throughout the central, peripheral, and diffuse gastrointestinal nervous systems and the endocrine pancreas. Among the nonendocrine regions of the rat and primate central nervous system in which this peptide has been localized to large numbers of neurons are the hippocampus and the cerebral cortex (for references, see Morrison et al., 1982, 1983). In the rat hippocampus, tests on neurons *in vitro* (Pittman and Siggins, 1981) and *in vivo* (Siggins and French, 1984) suggest that the peptide has many of the qualities of action of so-called "classical" inhibitory messenger molecules, depressing spontaneous discharge rate, hyperpolarizing the postsynaptic membrane, and increasing membrane conductance (for different results and interpretations, see Dodd and Kelly, 1978; Olpe et al., 1980; Sillito, this volume).

We recently began additional studies on hippocampal neuronal responses to somatostatin when we observed some unexpected interactions between the effects of systemic ethanol on responsiveness to transmitter substances thought to act there (Mancillas et al., 1984). What began as an attempt to determine the causes for apparent shifts in responsivity to afferent inputs after exposure to ethanol then led to a series of experiments to map possible transmitter interactions

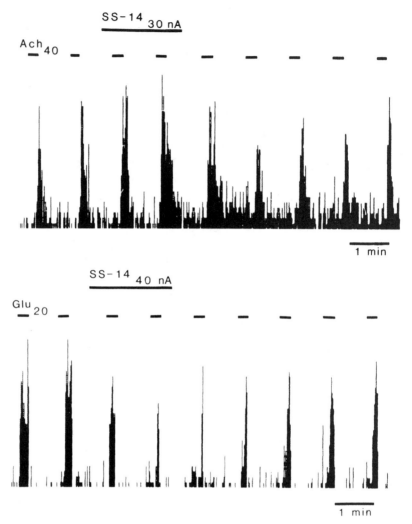

Figure 1. *Somatostatin-14 enhances excitatory responses to acetylcholine.* The activity of a single pyramidal
cell from area CA1 of the dorsal hippocampus was recorded with the center barrel of a five-
barrel pipette assembly. *Top*: Brief (15 sec) iontophoretic pulses (40 nA) of acetylcholine (ACh_{40})
delivered from one of the drug barrels caused facilitation of neuronal firing. The cell's responses
to acetylcholine were increased when somatostatin-14 ($SS-14_{30}$) was ejected concurrently with
an iontophoretic current of 30 nA from another barrel during a 2-min period. *Bottom*: Comparable
iontophoretic pulses (15 sec, 20 nA) of glutamate (Glu_{20}) also caused increased firing, which
was not enhanced by concurrent application of somatostatin-14. Rather, somatostatin-14 depressed
basal- and glutamate-induced firing. In both panels, the maximal pen excursion represents a
firing rate of 30 spikes/sec.

without the confusion of systemic ethanol. While far from complete, tests on
approximately 35 pyramidal neurons in CA1 or CA3 fields have indicated some
consistent patterns of response interactions.

In general, somatostatin produces apparently direct depressant actions on
spontaneous discharge rate. Often these effects were delayed in onset and offset
by several seconds, relative to the iontophoretic current pulses. When neurons

were tested with brief pulses of acetylcholine, which itself produces facilitation of firing, the effects of somatostatin on the acetylcholine-induced changes were dose-dependent. At doses that had little or no direct effect on spontaneous discharge rate, somatostatin only depressed the basal firing between acetylcholine pulses that produced increased firing and did not affect the magnitude of the acetylcholine-induced rate increases. This sort of effect could be regarded as "enhancing the signal-to-noise ratio" of afferent versus basal discharge rates, similar to one interpretation of noradrenergic synaptic transmission action (see Foote et al., 1983).

At higher doses of somatostatin, the most notable effect was an increased responsiveness of the test neuron to the acetylcholine pulses; under these intermediate doses of sustained somatostatin application, the cells showed more potent and somewhat longer-lasting effects of acetylcholine-induced firing (Figure 1). Interestingly, this effect of somatostatin has a more rapid onset and offset than do the "direct" depressant effects of somatostatin. Furthermore, there was no such synergistic interaction between somatostatin and the response of neurons to L-glutamate, a transmitter with classical excitatory membrane actions. In fact, somatostatin frequently depressed glutamate responses as well as basal firing.

At still higher doses of somatostatin, a combination of the lower dose interactions could be seen, depending in general on previous tests with somatostatin. Such cells could show enhancement of acetylcholine responses promptly, with more delayed mixed effects, in which both basal firing and acetylcholine responses were depressed. Depending on the degree to which other transmitter substances present in the multibarrel pipette were allowed to leak out, and depending on the test history of the neuron under investigation, the responses could appear to be chaotic. By restricting the number of possible interactions through careful monitoring of leakage, retaining, and balancing currents (see Bloom, 1974), the following interesting effects emerged: Somatostatin, even though directly inhibitory, seems capable of selectively enhancing responses to the excitatory actions of applied acetylcholine but not of glutamate. Understanding the cellular mechanisms responsible for these selective interactions will require substantial additional evidence. However, unless such forms of interaction are acknowledged and considered, the effects of somatostatin alone could be viewed as controversial or "inconsistent" when in fact they may reflect an important form of regulation of responsiveness of common target cells within the central nervous and endocrine systems. Also important will be the interactions between somatostatin and the other potentially released products of its common prohormone (for references, see Bakhit et al., 1984).

MOLECULAR GENETIC STRATEGIES FOR NEUROPEPTIDE DISCOVERY

With the very rapid emergence of recombinant DNA technologies, restriction endonucleases, and nucleotide sequencing (which make molecular genetics both powerful and rapidly progressive), a new opportunity for novel chemical messenger discovery has become available. Thus, determination of the complete sequence of the prohormone for opiocortin (Nakanishi et al., 1979) directly revealed an unanticipated biologically relevant peptide, homologous in sequence to α- and β-melanocyte-stimulating hormones. The existence of the deduced γ-melanocyte-stimulating hormone was later verified (in part) chemically and cytochemically (Bloom et al., 1980; Shibasaki et al., 1981). Subsequently, the recombinant DNA approach has been employed to obtain the prohormone structural sequences for almost every one of the previously identified neuropeptides (for references, see Bloom et al., 1985a).

These successful exploitations of molecular genetic principles indicate that better analysis of brain mRNAs might disclose the existence of additional biologically important hormones (see Bloom, 1982a,b). Such an analysis might yield not only neurotransmitters but also information important to the complete characterization of the properties of neurons and their cell assemblies.

We have used molecular cloning methods to purify randomly chosen copies (cDNAs) of rat brain mRNAs. Poly(A)$^+$ RNA was purified from the brains of adult rats, copied into double-stranded cDNA, and inserted into the plasmid pBR322 for cloning in E. coli. Clones bearing cDNA inserts that were at least 500 base pairs in length were nick-translated and evaluated for their patterns of hybridization to mRNAs isolated from brain, liver, and kidney. Those clones that hybridize to brain mRNAs, but not to mRNAs extracted from other organs, we define as being "brain-specific." The complete strategy has been reported elsewhere (Sutcliffe et al., 1983a).

This categorization has been extremely productive, since basic quantitative characterizations had not been available previously. For example, from the sizes of the mRNAs in brain, their relative abundance, and the total complexity of the brain mRNA population, it may be calculated that the rat's brain expresses about 30,000 mRNAs, of which most are brain-specific (Milner and Sutcliffe, 1983). Brain-specific mRNAs tend to be larger and rarer than the mRNAs found in other major organ systems, suggesting that genetic messages in the brain may encode more complex translation products. In addition, this phase of our research quickly yielded the wholly unanticipated finding of a cis-acting identifier or "ID" gene regulatory sequence whose presence within a gene is necessary but not sufficient for the expression of brain-specific genetic messages in particular neurons (for further details, see Sutcliffe and Milner, 1984; Sutcliffe et al., 1984a,b).

Currently, we are using the Northern blot strategy, a sensitive and rapid way of screening the very large number of brain-derived cDNAs produced from cloning whole brain mRNA (Milner and Sutcliffe, 1983; Sutcliffe et al., 1983a). This and other strategies allow us to select clones that are full-length cDNA copies of specific mRNAs. Large amounts of insert are prepared, and the nucleotide sequence is determined. Those mRNA sequences with long open reading frames are translated from the nucleotide code to deduce the amino acid sequences of the brain-specific proteins. When the sequences are obtained, they are compared to computer searches of nucleotide and peptide sequence databases so that we can focus our efforts on novel brain-specific molecules.

1B236—A BRAIN-SPECIFIC PROTEIN FOUND IN A SUBSET OF NEURONS

One of the first brain-specific mRNAs we sequenced was p1B236 (Figure 2). The strategy used to extend our characterization of 1B236 was to examine the deduced

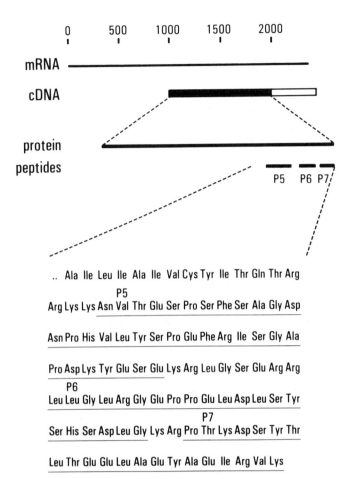

Figure 2. *Nucleotide sequence of the p1B236 cDNA insert,* showing the open reading frame (318 amino acids long), and the positions of the synthetic peptides (P5–P7) used for the immunization of rabbits and the preparation of antisera for immunocytochemistry. (From Malfroy et al., 1985.)

peptide sequence to seek out regions that might provide clues as to the function of the protein. In 1B236, we found that there were three peptides (termed by us P5, P6, and P7) clustered at the carboxyl terminus and enclosed by pairs of basic dipeptides. These peptides were synthesized and the synthetic peptides were used to raise polyclonal and monoclonal antisera. The antisera have now been used for immunocytochemistry, for Western blot analysis of immunoreactive material extractable from the brain, and for radioimmunoassays of peptidic extracts partially purified by high-pressure liquid chromatography.

In immunocytochemical mapping, antisera to each of the three nonoverlapping peptides gave virtually superimposable maps of intense immunoreactivity within a few specific neuronal systems, being most intense in the olfactory, limbic, somatosensory, and extrapyramidal motor systems (Bloom et al., 1985b). The possibility of molecular processing is still being pursued actively, but current evidence suggests that the 1B236 propeptide is processed to smaller forms that share immunoreactivity with our small synthetic peptides (Malfroy et al., 1985).

If these synthetic fragments are in fact natural processing products of the 1B236 peptide, our preliminary evidence favors their having biological activity on the cellular and behavioral levels (S. J. Henriksen, personal communication; G. F. Koob, personal communication).

Immunoreactivity was especially dense in olfactory bulb, specific preoptic and diencephalic nuclei, and also in the neostriatum, limbic, and neocortical regions. Neuropil staining was also prominent within selected thalamic and cranial nerve nuclei, as well as in the cerebellum and spinal cord. Maps constructed from the optimally reactive antisera for each of the three carboxy-terminal fragments of 1B236 gave virtually identical patterns, with some minor exceptions (Bloom et al., 1985b).

Regardless of whether 1B236 represents a transmitter or some other class of cell-specific neuronal protein whose function remains to be determined, the distribution of this marker within functional circuits of the rat brain (see Figure 3) deserves further consideration. The 1B236 protein is clearly not expressed by every neuron within any of these systems, even those that are most heavily labeled. As one traces through the circuitry of the olfactory system (Figure 4), it is clear that the primary olfactory nerves, as well as the primary output cells of the bulb—the mitral cells—are both unreactive. However, periglomerular cells, short axon cells of the internal plexiform layer, and selected large neurons within almost all regions directly innervated by the lateral olfactory tract and known to send centrifugal fibers back to the granule cells of the bulb are all strongly positive.

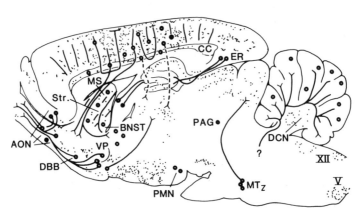

Figure 3. *Schematic overview of neuropil and perikaryonal immunoreactivity patterns.* An extensive, but virtually identical, pattern of immunoreactive fibers can be visualized throughout the normal rat central nervous system with antisera raised against P5, P6, or P7. Cell body-rich regions are represented by *circles*, neuropil-rich regions by *dots*; presumptive fiber trajectories are represented by *solid lines*, putative pathways by *dotted lines*. The source of the immunoreactive fibers ending in the granule cell layer of the cerebellum is not yet known (?); the targets of the cells seen within the periaqueductal gray and the premammillary nuclei are also unspecifiable at this time. AON, anterior olfactory nuclei; BNST, bed nucleus of the stria terminalis; CC, corpus callosum; DBB, diagonal band of Broca; DCN, deep cerebellar nuclei; ER, entorhinal cortex; MS, medial septal nucleus; MT$_z$, medial trapezoid nucleus; PAG, periaqueductal gray; PMN, premamillary nucleus; Str, striatum, V, spinal trigeminal nucleus; VP, ventral pallidal area; XII, hypoglossal nucleus.

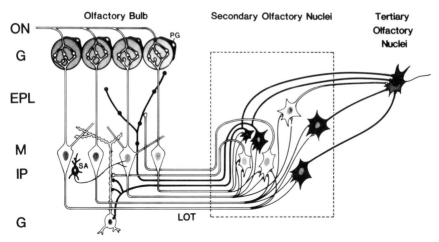

Figure 4. *Schematic representation of the pattern of 1B236 immunoreactivity for P5, P6, and P7 within the olfactory bulb.* Immunoreactive cells are represented within the bulb by the periglomerular (PG) neurons within the glomerular layer (G), and by the short axon (SA) neurons within the internal plexiform (IP) layer. Intense immunoreactivity is seen within the internal plexiform layer and in thick straight processes that occasionally course across the external plexiform layer (EPL). Centrifugal fibers are known to enter the bulb through the lateral olfactory tract (LOT), to innervate olfactory granule cells, and to arise from the secondary olfactory nuclei, where a small but significant fraction of the perikarya is immunoreactive. These regions include the accessory olfactory nuclei, the medial cortical amygdala, the diagonal band, the endopyriform nucleus, and the primary olfactory cortex. In addition, several of these immunoreactive neurons in the secondary olfactory target areas also send immunoreactive neuropil to the medial dorsal thalamic nucleus. The distribution of 1B236 peptide immunoreactivity within the olfactory system is extensive, with immunoreactive elements positioned at the interface of the hierarchical afferent links: Across the glomeruli, where immunoreactive periglomerular neurons span the synapses between nonimmunoreactive olfactory nerve fibers and nonimmunoreactive mitral (M) and tufted neurons; and at the internal plexiform layer, where the short axon cells and the centrifugal afferents may regulate the flow of information between nonimmunoreactive mitral and granule cells. One interpretation of this pattern of immunoreactive elements is that it may represent a distributed, interrupted system for the regulation of olfactory information processing.

Within the olfactory structures, immunoreactive elements alternate with non-immunoreactive elements in the multisynaptic chains of interconnected neurons that have been well studied in these functional systems. The meaning of such an alternating pattern of expression of a specific marker is not obvious. At one level, it can be directly interpreted as reflecting only that these cells contain the same protein and hence share at least one specific chemical property that may functionally relate these separated cell types.

Possibly, expression of 1B236 mRNA and its protein product reflects some primary epigenetic property shared by neurons in each of these systems as well as by cells of functionally separate systems. The common cells within each functional system may have arisen from a common progenitor cell class and during ontogenesis are further separated by cellular elements that do not express 1B236. At least for the olfactory system, the immunoreactive centrifugal connections to the olfactory bulb and the short axon and periglomerular cells within the bulb could be viewed as a distributed, interrupted system for the regulation of olfactory information processing. Cells of the different systems, and therefore the systems themselves, may also be considered to be closely related in the evolutionary sense, having descended from a common ancestral circuit of simpler dimensions. The data presently at hand favor the possibility that the 1B236 protein could function as a neurotransmitter precursor within those circuits that express it, although the evidence is far from complete (Malfroy et al., 1985).

CONCLUSIONS

If 1B236 is eventually found to meet all of the criteria of a transmitter, the catalog of other brain-specific mRNAs of this relative abundance and complexity suggests that there may be several hundred more to be found and studied. Even if 1B236 does not meet the criteria, its existence within neurons linked with specific functional systems (whose neuronal elements are far from completely characterized) suggests that our strategy may have more fundamental value. Certainly, the ability to generate synthetic fragments of an unknown gene product and to raise antisera against it offers a powerful advantage over monoclonal antibodies raised to complex mixtures of soluble or membrane-bound substances whose antigens are also unknown molecules of unknown function (Levitt, 1984).

While we are not totally ready to set aside all of our historical precedents in transmitter research, it does seem clear that the complexity and abundance of genetic messages in the brain demand that we keep an open mind concerning the kinds of factors and functions (Milner et al., 1984) that may be found if we are not to be doomed to saying that all we know now is all there can ever be. Such a view would scarcely have been compatible with the finding that somatostatin is a ubiquitous regulatory peptide within the central and peripheral nervous systems, the diffuse gastroenteric nervous system, and other endocrine tissues, nor with the fact that its actions in the brain have little or nothing to do with its actions on somatotropin secretion (Krieger, 1983). Clearly, the molecular specification of "all" regulatory factors will involve an enormous effort and considerable time. We anticipate that it will not be necessary to define every as yet undiscovered regulatory molecule before we can recognize approximately how many more categories and families of such substances there may be. Similarly, it should not be necessary to test every new factor on every possible target cell before coming to a fuller understanding of how many categories of response interactions neuronal and endocrine systems may use, and how many modes of interaction may exist for their functional control. The interactions observed thus far with peptides and amines arising from conventional discovery strategies begin to suggest that there may be a limited repertoire of response mechanisms that may be elicitable by many different substances (for a fuller discussion, see Bloom, 1984). As we and others continue to try to define these response mechanisms, important lessons will undoubtedly be learned for the advancement of endocrine and neuron science through the molecular characterization of more substances.

ACKNOWLEDGMENTS

We thank Nancy Callahan for diligent manuscript preparation, and other colleagues involved in related studies on which the present summary depended. This research was supported by grants from the National Institutes of Health (GM-32355, NS-20728) and from the McNeil Laboratories.

REFERENCES

Bakhit, C., L. Koda, R. Benoit, J. H. Morrison, and F. E. Bloom (1984) Evidence for separate compartmentalization of somatostatin 14 and somatostatin 28 (1–12) in rat hypothalamus. *J. Neurosci.* **4**:411–419.

Bloom, F. E. (1974) To spritz or not to spritz: The doubtful value of aimless iontophoresis. *Life Sci.* **14**:1819–1834.

Bloom, F. E. (1982a) Recombinant DNA strategies of neurotransmitter research. In *Advances in Pharmacology and Therapeutics II*, Vol. 2, *Neurotransmitters–Receptors*, H. Yoshida, Y. Hagihara, and S. Ebashi, eds., pp. 189–198, Pergamon, New York.

Bloom, F. E. (1982b) Prospects from retrospect. In *Molecular Genetic Neuroscience*, F. O. Schmitt, S. J. Bird, and F. E. Bloom, eds., pp. 467–475, Raven, New York.

Bloom, F. E. (1984) The functional significance of neurotransmitter diversity. *Am. J. Physiol.* **246**:C184–C194.

Bloom, F. E., E. L. F. Battenberg, T. Shibasaki, R. Benoit, N. Ling, and R. Guillemin (1980) Localization of gamma-melanocyte-stimulating hormone (γ-MSH) immunoreactivity in rat brain and pituitary. *Regul. Pept.* **1**:205–222.

Bloom, F. E., E. L. F. Battenberg, A. Ferron, J. R. Mancillas, R. J. Milner, G. R. Siggins, and J. G. Sutcliffe (1985a) Neuropeptides: Interactions and diversities. *Recent Prog. Horm. Res.* **41**:339–367.

Bloom, F. E., E. L. F. Battenberg, R. J. Milner, and J. G. Sutcliffe (1985b) Immunocytochemical mapping of 1B236, a brain-specific neuronal polypeptide deduced from the sequence of a cloned mRNA. *J. Neurosci.* **5**:1781–1802.

Dodd, J., and J. S. Kelly (1978) Is somatostatin an excitatory transmitter in the hippocampus? *Nature* **273**:674–675.

Etgen, A. M., and E. T. Browning (1983) Activators of cyclic adenosine 3′:5′-monophosphate accumulation in rat hippocampal slices: Action of vasoactive intestinal peptide (VIP). *J. Neurosci.* **3**:2487–2493.

Ferron, A., G. R. Siggins, and F. E. Bloom (1985) Vasoactive intestinal polypeptide acts synergistically with norepinephrine to depress spontaneous discharge rates in cerebral cortical neurons. *Proc. Natl. Acad. Sci. USA* **82**:8810–8812.

Foote, S. L., F. E. Bloom, and G. Aston-Jones (1983) The nucleus locus coeruleus: New evidence of anatomical and physiological specificity. *Physiol. Rev.* **63**:844–914.

Guillemin, R. (1978) Peptides in the brain: The new endocrinology of the neuron. *Science* **202**:390–402.

Klein, D. C., D. Sugden, and J. L. Weller (1983) Postsynaptic α-adrenergic receptors potentiate the β-adrenergic stimulation of pineal serotonin N-acetyltransferase. *Proc. Natl. Acad. Sci. USA* **80**:599–603.

Krieger, D. (1983) Brain peptides: What, where, and why? *Science* **222**:975–985.

Levitt, P. (1984) A monoclonal antibody to limbic system neurons. *Science* **223**:299–301.

Magistretti, P. J., and M. Schorderet (1984) VIP and noradrenaline act synergistically to increase cyclic AMP in cerebral cortex. *Nature* **308**:280–282.

Magistretti, P. J., J. H. Morrison, W. J. Shoemaker, V. Sapin, and F. E. Bloom (1981) Vasoactive intestinal polypeptide induces glycogenolysis in mouse cortical slices: A possible regulatory mechanism for the local control of energy metabolism. *Proc. Natl. Acad. Sci. USA* **78**:6535–6539.

Malfroy, B., C. Bakhit, F. E. Bloom, J. G. Sutcliffe, and R. J. Milner (1985) Brain-specific polypeptide 1B236 exists in multiple molecular forms. *Proc. Natl. Acad. Sci. USA* **82**:2009–2013.

Mancillas, J. R., G. R. Siggins, and F. E. Bloom (1984) Effects of systemic ethanol on responses of hippocampal units to iontophoretically applied neurotransmitters. *Soc. Neurosci. Abstr.* **10**:968.

Milner, R. J., and J. G. Sutcliffe (1983) Gene expression in rat brain. *Nucleic Acids Res.* **11**:5497–5520.

Milner, R. J., F. E. Bloom, C. Lai, R. A. Lerner, and J. G. Sutcliffe (1984) Brain-specific genes have identifier sequences in their introns. *Proc. Natl. Acad. Sci. USA* **81**:713–717.

Morgan, N. G., R. Charest, P. F. Blackmore, and J. H. Exton (1984) Potentiation of alpha 1 adrenergic responses in rat liver by a cAMP-dependent mechanism. *Proc. Natl. Acad. Sci. USA* **81**:4208–4212.

Morrison, J. H., and P. J. Magistretti (1983) Monoamines and peptides in cerebral cortex: Contrasting principles of cortical organization. *Trends Neurosci.* **6**:146–151.

Morrison, J. H., R. Benoit, P. J. Magistretti, N. Ling, and F. E. Bloom (1982) Immunohistochemical distribution of pro-somatostatin-related peptides in hippocampus. *Neurosci. Lett.* **34**:137–142.

Morrison, J. H., R. Benoit, P. J. Magistretti, and F. E. Bloom (1983) Immunohistochemical distribution of prosomatostatin-related peptides in cerebral cortex. *Brain Res.* **262**:344–351.

Morrison, J. H., P. J. Magistretti, R. Benoit, and F. E. Bloom (1984) The distribution and morphological characteristics of the intracortical VIP-positive cell: An immunohistochemical analysis. *Brain Res.* **292**:269–282.

Nakanishi, S., A. Inoue, T. Kita, M. Nakamura, A. C. Y. Chang, S. N. Cohen, and S. Numa (1979) Nucleotide sequence of cloned cDNA for bovine corticotropin-β-lipotropin precursor. *Nature* **278**:423–427.

Nestler, E. J., and P. Greengard (1984) *Protein Phoshorylation in the Nervous System*, Wiley, New York.

Olpe, H.-R., V. J. Balcar, H. Bittiger, H. Rink, and P. Sieber (1980) Central actions of somatostatin. *Eur. J. Pharmacol.* **63**:127–133.

Phillis, J. N., J. P. Edstrom, G. K. Kostopoulos, and J. R. Kirkpatrick (1979) Effects of adenosine and adenine nucleotides on synaptic transmission in the cerebral cortex. *Can. J. Physiol. Pharmacol.* **57**:1289–1312.

Pittman, Q. J., and G. R. Siggins (1981) Somatostatin hyperpolarizes hippocampal pyramidal cells *in vitro*. *Brain Res.* **221**:402–408.

Quik, M., P. C. Emson, J. Fahrenkrug, and L. L. Iversen (1979) Effect of kainic acid injections and other brain lesions on vasoactive intestinal polypeptide (VIP)-stimulated formation of cAMP in rat brain. *Naunyn Schmiedebergs Arch. Pharmacol.* **306**:281–286.

Shibasaki, T., N. Ling, R. Guillemin, M. Silver, and F. E. Bloom (1981) The regional distribution of γ3-melanotropin-like peptides in bovine brain is correlated with adrenocorticotropin immunoreactivity but not with β-endodorphin. *Regul. Pept.* **2**:43–52.

Siggins, G. R., and F. E. Bloom (1975) Modulation of unit activity by chemically coded neurons. In *Brain Mechanisms of Perceptual Awareness and Purposeful Behavior*, O. Pompeiano and C. A. Marsan, eds., pp. 431–448, Raven, New York.

Siggins, G. R., and E. D. French (1984) Pro-somatostatin-related peptides alter the discharge rate of rat cortical and hippocampal neurons *in vivo*: An iontophoretic study. *Soc. Neurosci. Abstr.* **10**:810.

Stone, T. W., D. A. Taylor, and F. E. Bloom (1975) Cyclic AMP and cyclic GMP may mediate opposite neuronal responses in the rat cerebral cortex. *Science* **187**:845–847.

Sutcliffe, J. G., and R. J. Milner (1984) Brain-specific gene expression. *Trends Biochem. Sci.* **9**:95–99.

Sutcliffe, J. G., R. J. Milner, T. M. Shinnick, and F. E. Bloom (1983a) Identifying the protein products of brain-specific genes using antibodies to chemically synthesized peptides. *Cell* **33**:671–682.

Sutcliffe, J. G., R. J. Milner, and F. E. Bloom (1983b) Cellular localization and function of the proteins encoded by brain-specific mRNAs. *Cold Spring Harbor Symp. Quant. Biol.* **48**:477–484.

Sutcliffe, J. G., R. J. Milner, J. M. Gottesfeld, and R. A. Lerner (1984a) ID sequences are transcribed specifically in brain. *Nature* **308**:237–241.

Sutcliffe, J. G., R. J. Milner, J. M. Gottesfeld, and W. Reynolds (1984b) Control of neuronal gene expression. *Science* **225**:1308–1314.

Section 3

Synapses in Networks

In postnatal life, the responses of networks and a major part of their historical alteration by behavior depend upon how synapses are altered. Several profound questions are prompted by a consideration of the relationship of transmitter diversity and synaptic types to the function of actual networks. In this section, important salients bearing upon this issue are considered.

Beyond the obvious needs for excitation and inhibition, one may inquire why there are multiple transmitters. Marder and her coworkers provide a possible answer to this question in reviewing their work on the stomatogastric ganglion of decapod crustaceans, a ganglion that can be studied as a model preparation for the generation of rhythmic motor activity. By application of each of the different neurotransmitters present in each of the inputs of this ganglion, a different motor pattern is elicited. Dopamine, pilocarpine, serotonin, and several neuroactive peptides were found to cause changes in frequency or in motor outputs in a ganglion preparation. Although it has not yet been shown that such dissociative effects on a single circuit are physiological, the data raise an important hypothesis: The raison d'être of multiple neurotransmitters and neuropeptides is to provide a basis for the production of many different outputs from a single "hard-wired" neuronal circuit. This intriguing concept is related to the "transmitter logic" hypothesis proposed in the last section of this book by Finkel and Edelman to account for the behavior of synapses in selective populations.

In his contribution, Sillito analyzes how the receptive field properties of cells in networks of the mammalian central visual system are influenced by the underlying synaptic organization. By applying drugs microiontophoretically, the action of specific synaptic inputs to single cells of the dorsolateral geniculate and the visual cortex could be assessed. GABAergic synapses of intrinsic thalamic and cortical neurons appeared to be a major influence in structuring receptive field selectivity; extrinsic (cholinergic and noradrenergic) inputs showed modulatory effects. Thus, upon a fixed anatomical base, a series of functional effects results from the interaction of different transmitters, each assigned to different underlying anatomy.

These findings indicate that it is the interaction between synaptic types and specific details of microcircuitry that determine functional consequences. Besides transmitter chemistry and regulation, the actual distribution of synaptic structures in a given anatomical plan is of central significance. This important issue is

discussed by Peters, who points out the consequences of the different distributions of symmetric and asymmetric synapses in the cerebral cortex. Among the
factors influencing the synaptic relationships of the neurons are: (1) the distribution
pattern of each type on different neuronal types; (2) the location and shapes of
dendritic trees; (3) the types of synapses made by intrinsic and extrinsic inputs;
and (4) the preference of these axon terminals for different postsynaptic sites.

These considerations and the selective dynamic properties reviewed in the
other chapters contained in this section indicate that a hierarchical and recursive
set of interactions ranging across anatomy, synapse type, and biochemical regulation is responsible for the various functional effects of synaptic change. One
of the impressive outcomes of this analysis is the increasing recognition of the
need for a linkage between anatomy, chemistry, and pharmacology to understand
synaptic function at any one of its levels of analysis. As discussed in the fourth
section of this book, the order in space and time of changes in such linkages in
specific evolved portions of the nervous system provides an epigenetic basis for
learning and memory.

Chapter 13

Multiple Neurotransmitters Provide a Mechanism for the Production of Multiple Outputs from a Single Neuronal Circuit

EVE E. MARDER
SCOTT L. HOOPER
JUDITH S. EISEN

ABSTRACT

The stomatogastric ganglion (STG) of decapod crustaceans is a model preparation for the study of the mechanisms underlying the generation of rhythmic motor activity. As such, it is also a useful system with which to ask questions about the function of different neurotransmitters and neurotransmitter systems within a neuronal circuit. In this chapter, we discuss how the rhythmic motor outputs of the STG are produced. The neurotransmitters present in many of the neuronal inputs to the STG are known: We show that application of each of these neurotransmitters elicits a characteristic and different motor pattern. The mechanisms underlying a shift in firing phase of one class of neurons are discussed, along with possible mechanisms that may underlie many of the modulatory actions of neurotransmitters on the output of the STG. Based on these observations, we suggest that one of the purposes of multiple neurotransmitters and neuropeptides is to provide a basis for the production of many different outputs from a single "hard-wired" neuronal circuit. The range of outputs of an array of circuits organized similarly to the STG, as may be present in vertebrate nervous systems, would be greatly increased as a result of each constituent circuit being individually capable of multiple outputs.

The ultimate aim of neuroscience is to understand how the neurons of the human nervous system interact to achieve the complex sensory, motor, and cognitive processes that make us human. Toward this end, it will certainly be necessary to understand both the basic processes of synaptic transmission and how circuits of neurons operate. Progress has been made in recent years in describing the distribution of neurotransmitter systems in the brain, and in understanding the biochemical and physiological actions of neurotransmitters and neuromodulators. However, the answers to many questions remain today almost as elusive as they were years ago.

We can still only speculate about the functions of the increasing number of neurotransmitters and neuropeptides being found in vertebrate and invertebrate nervous systems. Why so many? Why does a given neuron or set of neurons release the particular neurotransmitter or neurotransmitters that it does? Are the properties of neuronal circuits influenced by the particular neurotransmitters that are used by the neurons within them, and if so, how?

Although anatomical and immunocytochemical methods have provided a great deal of information about the organization of the circuits in the vertebrate nervous system (Kandel and Schwartz, 1981; Krieger et al., 1983), there is much that cannot be learned by anatomical methods alone. There are still relatively few neuronal circuits that provide the experimentalist with an opportunity to record from many, if not all, of their constituent units. Some invertebrate preparations do allow the investigator to record from many of the relevant neurons. Among these is the stomatogastric ganglion (STG) of decapod crustaceans.

The pyloric network of the STG is a central pattern generator responsible for the production of rhythmic contractions of the pyloric region of the stomach. Like other central pattern generators, the pyloric system neurons can continue to produce rhythmic outputs after the STG is isolated from the animal, in the complete absence of sensory feedback. In this chapter, we try to describe what is known about how this small neural network produces rhythmic outputs, and how the outputs of this ganglion are controlled. Finally, we suggest a hypothesis about the function of multiple neurotransmitters in nervous systems.

ORGANIZATION OF THE STG

The STG of decapod crustaceans contains only 30 neurons. The somata of these neurons measure 30–120 μm and encircle a central neuropil area. Most of the STG neurons are motor neurons and send axons out to the muscles of the stomach. Additionally, they make and receive numerous synaptic contacts within the neuropil of the STG. Figure 1A is a picture of the two pyloric dilator (PD) neurons from an STG of the lobster, *Panulirus interruptus*, filled with the dye carboxyfluorescein. Figure 1B is an example of a dye-filled lateral pyloric (LP) neuron. The processes of these neurons can be found throughout the whole volume of ganglionic neuropil, which is only about 0.1–0.5 mm^3. This feature of organization was well described by King (1976a,b) and is quite different from other, often larger, invertebrate ganglia in which neurons usually branch only in a portion of the ganglionic neuropil (Selverston and Remler, 1972; Kater and Nicholson, 1973; Macagno, 1980; Burrows and Siegler, 1984; Siegler and Burrows, 1984). These larger ganglia are responsible for carrying out a number of different functions, and there appears to be a spatial mapping within parts of the neuropil (Murphey et al., 1980; Liese and Mulloney, 1984). In contrast, in the STG the whole neuropil appears as if it were a single module.

WHAT DOES THE STG DO?

Unlike vertebrates, crustaceans have teeth, called the gastric mill, in their stomachs. Also unlike vertebrates, the regions of the crustacean stomach (gastric mill and pyloric region) are moved by a series of striated muscles that resemble crustacean limb muscles in many of their properties (Govind et al., 1975; Atwood et al.,

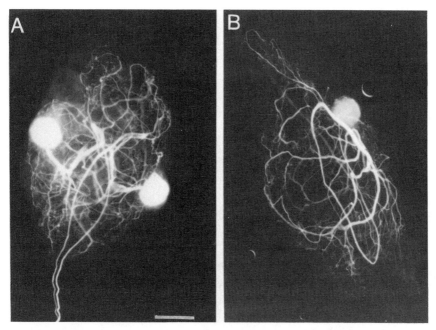

Figure 1. *Dye-filled stomatogastric (STG) neurons from the lobster,* Panulirus interruptus. Neurons were
injected with carboxyfluorescein and preparations were fixed, washed, cleared, and viewed as
whole mounts. *A:* Two pyloric dilator (PD) neurons. *B:* Lateral pyloric (LP) neuron. *Calibration
bar* = 120 μm; *bottom* of picture is posterior.

1978). More than 20 of the neurons of the STG are motor neurons that innervate
one or several of the muscles that move the stomach. The movements of the
stomach are rhythmic, not because of peristaltic muscle contractions, but because
the motor neurons that innervate the stomach muscles are rhythmically active.
The gastric mill apparatus and the pyloric region of the stomach are innervated
by different groups of STG motor neurons that produce two semiautonomous
rhythmic outputs: the gastric rhythm and the pyloric rhythm.

Figure 2 illustrates the pyloric rhythm; it shows simultaneous recordings from
STG somata, motor nerves leaving the STG, and a stomach muscle. The middle
two traces (mvn and lvn) are extracellular recordings from two of the motor
nerves leaving the ganglion, the median and lateral ventricular nerves. These
recordings reveal that the pyloric rhythm consists of alternating bursts of action
potentials in several classes of neurons, which then repeat. The bottom trace is
an intracellular recording from a muscle innervated by the LP neuron and shows
facilitating and summating excitatory junctional potentials (EJPs) associated with
each LP neuron action potential. The top three traces in Figure 2 are intracellular
recordings from three of the somata [PD, LP, and pyloric (PY)] of the neurons
that participate in the generation of the pyloric rhythm. These intracellular recordings demonstrate that the alternating bursts of action potentials seen in the
extracellular traces are associated with the periodic depolarizations of the neurons,
as they are active out of phase with each other.

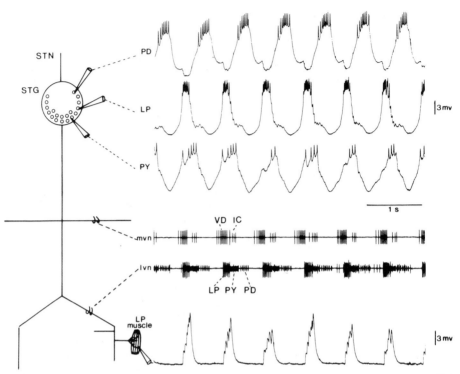

Figure 2. *STG motor patterns.* Preparation from *Panulirus interruptus.* Simultaneous intracellular recordings from somata (*top three traces*) and LP-innervated muscle (*bottom trace*) were made with potassium chloride-filled microelectrodes. Extracellular recordings from nerves were made with stainless steel pin electrodes insulated with Vaseline. Abbreviations not defined previously in text: IC, inferior cardiac; lvn, lateral ventricular nerve; mvn, median ventricular nerve; PY, pyloric; STN, stomatogastric nerve; VD, ventricular dilator.

The gastric rhythm is much slower than the pyloric rhythm, and although the two motor patterns have largely been studied independently, vigorous activity in the gastric mill (GM) motor neurons is associated with modifications of pyloric activity (Mulloney, 1977), as is illustrated in Figure 3. Additionally, the activity of pyloric neurons can influence neurons that participate in the gastric rhythm (Robertson and Moulins, 1984).

HOW DOES THE STG PRODUCE A RHYTHMIC MOTOR OUTPUT?

In most decapod species, rhythmic outputs, such as those seen in Figure 2, occur even after the STG is completely isolated from the rest of the animal by cutting the stomatogastric nerve (STN) (Maynard, 1972; Beltz et al., 1984; Marder and Hooper, 1985). In order to understand how the pyloric rhythm is generated, it is necessary to establish the pattern of synaptic connectivity among the pyloric neurons, as well as to describe the cellular properties of individual neurons that might contribute to the generation of the pattern. Both of these aims have turned out to be more difficult than was first anticipated, but the attempts to fulfill them have generated data that are more interesting than might have been predicted.

Synaptic Connectivity Among Pyloric Neurons

In addition to the classes of pyloric motor neurons shown in Figure 2, another neuron, the anterior burster (AB), is an important part of the pyloric network. The AB neuron is an interneuron, is electrically coupled to the PD neurons, and depolarizes synchronously with the PD neurons. Recordings from the AB, PD, and LP neurons are shown in Figure 4A. The electrical coupling among these neurons complicated the task of establishing the pattern of synaptic connectivity in the pyloric network (Eisen and Marder, 1982; Marder, 1984). In order to circumvent this problem, the Lucifer yellow photoinactivation technique of Miller and Selverston (1979, 1982a,b; Selverston and Miller, 1980) was used to remove selectively one or more neurons from the circuit (Figure 4B), thus permitting the study of the connections between other neurons (for details, see Eisen and Marder, 1982; Marder and Eisen, 1984a,b). The pattern of synaptic connectivity among the AB, PD, and LP neurons is shown in Figure 4C, and the complete pattern of synaptic connectivity among the pyloric neurons of *Panulirus interruptus* is shown in Figure 5.

Although the detailed firing times of the pyloric cycle neurons depend on the interplay of many synaptic and cellular properties (Figure 5), a simplified notion of the generation of the pyloric rhythm follows. The electrically coupled AB and PD neurons depolarize and together act as the pacemaker for the pyloric rhythm. As the AB and PD neurons depolarize, they inhibit all the other pyloric neurons (follower neurons), which are then constrained to fire out of phase with the PD–AB neuron group. Upon repolarization of the pacemaker group, the other neurons can start firing; the time at which each type of follower cell will fire depends on the time course of the inhibition from the AB and PD neurons, and on the inhibitory interactions among the follower neurons (for a more

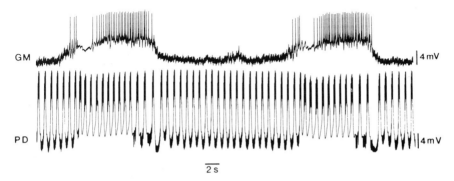

Figure 3. *Interaction between gastric mill (GM) and pyloric activity.* Simultaneous intracellular recordings from a PD neuron (*lower trace*) and a GM neuron (*upper trace*) in *Panulirus interruptus*. Bursts of action potentials in the GM neuron are associated with the disappearance of the LP-evoked inhibitory postsynaptic potentials (IPSPs) recorded in the PD neuron. Records taken in the presence of 10^{-6} M proctolin.

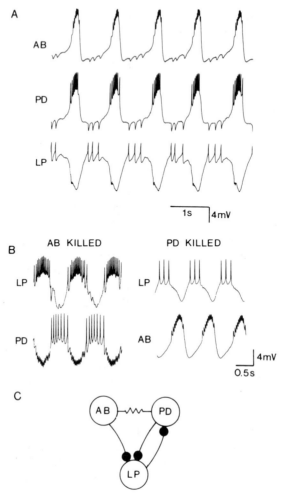

Figure 4. *Use of the Lucifer yellow photoinactivation technique to determine synaptic connectivity in the STG in* Panulirus interruptus. *A*: Simultaneous intracellular recordings from anterior burster (AB), PD, and LP neurons. LP neuron action potentials are associated with unitary IPSPs recorded in both the AB and PD neurons. When the AB and PD neurons depolarize, the LP neuron is inhibited. *B*: After the AB neuron is photoinactivated, the LP neuron action potentials continue to evoke IPSPs in the PD neuron, and the PD neuron continues to inhibit the LP neuron. After the PD neurons are photoinactivated, the LP neuron action potentials no longer evoke IPSPs in the AB neuron, but AB neuron depolarizations continue to inhibit the LP neuron. *C*: Connectivity among the AB, PD, and LP neurons. Electrical junctions are denoted by resistor symbols. *Filled circles* denote chemical inhibitory synaptic connections. (Modified from Eisen and Marder, 1982.)

complete description, see Hartline, 1979; Selverston and Miller, 1980; Miller and Selverston, 1982a,b; Selverston et al., 1983; Eisen and Marder, 1984).

Because the time at which follower neurons resume firing after depolarization of the AB and PD neurons is dependent on the time course of the inhibitory postsynaptic potentials (IPSPs) evoked by the AB and PD neurons, it is interesting that the electrically coupled AB and PD neurons release different neurotransmitters

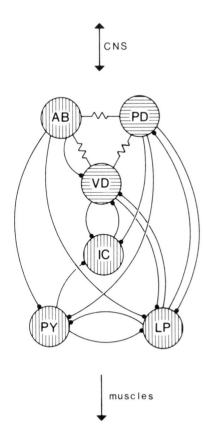

CNS

muscles

Figure 5. *Synaptic connectivity among pyloric group neurons in* Panulirus interruptus. *Resistors*: Electrical junctions. *Filled circles*: Chemical inhibitory connections. *Vertical lines*: Glutamatergic neurons. *Horizontal lines*: Cholinergic neurons. (Modified from Marder and Eisen, 1984a.)

and evoke IPSPs in follower neurons with different time courses (Figure 6) (Eisen and Marder, 1982, 1984; Marder and Eisen, 1984a). It will be seen below that this difference in time course between the IPSPs evoked by AB and PD neuron depolarization is important in understanding how the phase of PY neuron firing can be modulated by neuronal inputs from other ganglia in the crustacean nervous system.

Neurons Can Be Conditional Bursters

The rhythmic motor output of the pyloric network depends on the intrinsic ability of some of the STG neurons to generate bursting pacemaker potentials or "plateau" potentials (sharp transitions from one membrane potential to another), as well as synaptic interactions among STG neurons. Determining which of the neurons of the STG produce bursting pacemaker potentials or plateau potentials that contribute to their behavior during ongoing pyloric cycling has been difficult for two reasons. First, many of these neurons are electrically coupled. Second, some of the neurons of the STG appear to produce bursting pacemaker potentials or plateau potentials under some conditions but not under others.

Initially, it was thought that PD neurons were intrinsically bursting neurons because after the STN is cut in *Panulirus interruptus*, PD neurons routinely continue to be rhythmically active, while many of the other neurons become silent (Maynard,

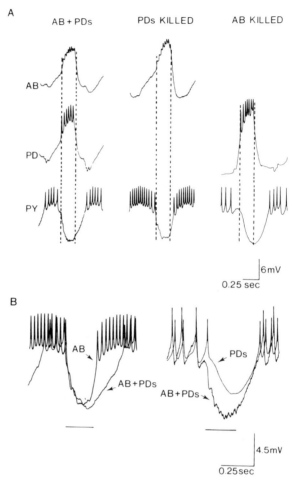

Figure 6. *Electrically coupled neurons evoke IPSPs with different time courses.* The depolarization of the AB and PD neurons evokes an IPSP in the PY neuron with an early onset and a slow recovery. After photoinactivation of the PD neurons, depolarization of the AB neuron evoked an IPSP with an early onset and a rapid recovery. After killing the AB neuron, depolarization of the PD neurons evoked an IPSP with a slow onset and a slow recovery time. *B*: Photographic superposition of the PY neuron traces before and after inactivation of the PD neurons (*left panel*) and before and after inactivation of the AB neuron (*right panel*). (Modified from Marder and Eisen, 1984a.)

1972; Maynard and Selverston, 1975). Under these conditions, PD neurons satisfy many of the criteria used to define bursting pacemakers (Selverston et al., 1976). Additionally, when PD neurons were voltage-clamped they showed membrane currents typical of bursting neurons (Gola and Selverston, 1981).

However, AB and PD neurons differ in their ability to generate bursting pacemaker potentials. Once again, by using the Lucifer yellow photoinactivation technique to remove either the AB neuron or the PD neurons from the circuit, Miller and Selverston (1982a) were able to show that the PD neurons fired tonically but did not burst after isolation from the AB neuron. The AB neuron frequently continued to burst after the PD neurons were removed from the circuit, although occasionally the AB neuron was quiescent after isolation (J. S. Eisen and E. Marder, unpublished observations; J. P. Miller and F. Nagy, personal communication). Does this mean that voltage-dependent conductances of PD and AB neuron membranes do not contribute to the generation of rhythmic bursting in the intact ganglion? As will become clear below, it is likely that *when* the pyloric system is rhythmically active, both PD and AB neurons *do* display voltage-dependent properties that contribute to bursting, although they may not always show these properties when isolated.

Many STG neurons in addition to PD and AB neurons display voltage-dependent conductances that are likely to participate in the generation of rhythmic activity only after the application of a variety of neurotransmitters or neuropeptides or after stimulation of inputs from other ganglia. Russell and Hartline (1978, 1982, 1984) first showed that inputs to the STG from the commissural ganglia (CGs) evoked plateau potentials in STG neurons. Nagy and Dickinson (1983; Dickinson and Nagy, 1983) described a neuron in the esophageal ganglion (OG) that appears to act by changing the membrane properties of many of the STG neurons. In addition, the muscarinic cholinergic agonist pilocarpine is able to cause isolated PD neurons to start bursting (Marder and Eisen, 1984b), and serotonin, pilocarpine, and dopamine can initiate bursting in isolated, quiescent AB neurons (Marder and Eisen, 1984b; Flamm and Harris-Warrick, 1986a,b). This is shown for pilo-carpine and serotonin in Figure 7.

In addition to the amines, several peptides, including proctolin and the molluscan peptide FMRFamide, can also cause quiescent STG neurons to become

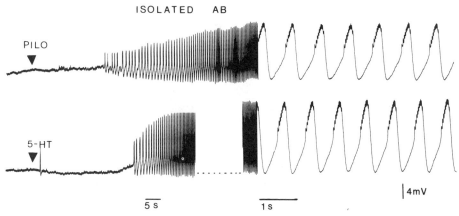

Figure 7. *Neurotransmitter induction of burst potentials in an isolated AB neuron. An AB neuron from Panulirus interruptus was isolated by photoinactivating the PD and VD neurons and cutting the STN. After these treatments, the AB neuron became quiescent. Top trace: Bath application (downward triangle) of 10^{-4} M pilocarpine to the STG resulted in bursts of action potentials in the AB neuron (expanded sweep). After washing in saline for 10 min (not shown) the bursting activity ceased. Bottom trace: Bath application (downward triangle) of 10^{-4} M serotonin (5-HT) to the ganglion resulted in bursts of action potentials (expanded sweep). At the break in the record, the amplifier saturated. Dotted line indicates the elapsed time between the records before and after the break in the record. Once again, after approximately 10 min of washing in control saline (not shown), the AB neuron ceased firing. Although not shown, dopamine (10^{-4} M) also elicited bursts in this neuron. (J. S. Eisen and E. Marder, unpublished observations.)*

rhythmically active (Hooper and Marder, 1984a,b; Marder and Hooper, 1985; Marder et al., 1986). Thus, the voltage-dependent properties of many of the neurons of the STG may be subject to modulation. Under certain conditions, some of these neurons may act as bursters, others as followers. Under other conditions, it is possible that all of the neurons within the ganglion may show voltage-dependent properties that participate in the generation of the overall rhythmic outputs of the pyloric and gastric systems.

Nonimpulse-Mediated Synaptic Transmission

The STG was one of the first preparations in which nonimpulse-mediated synaptic transmission was described (Maynard and Walton, 1975). Since then, it has become clear that a great deal of the synaptic integration in many nervous systems takes place without the intervention of action potentials (Pearson and Fourtner, 1975; Roberts and Bush, 1981; Burrows and Siegler, 1983; Reichert et al., 1983). In a series of studies, Graubard, Hartline, and Raper (Graubard, 1978; Raper, 1979; Graubard et al., 1980, 1983) have argued that although neurons in the STG do fire action potentials—and unitary synaptic potentials can be associated with these action potentials—a great deal, if not most, of the neurotransmitter released by STG neurons is released as a continuous function of membrane potential. They argue that the neurons of the STG are releasing neurotransmitter even at their most hyperpolarized level of membrane potential, as can be seen in Figure 8. In this experiment, the PY neuron was not firing action potentials

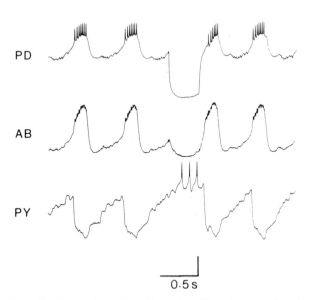

PD

AB

PY

0·5 s

Figure 8. *Nonimpulse-mediated transmitter release.* Two microelectrodes were placed in the PD neuron, and a single electrode was placed in each of the AB and PY neurons of *Panulirus interruptus*. The PD neuron was hyperpolarized, resulting in hyperpolarization of the electrically coupled AB neuron. When the PD and AB neurons were hyperpolarized by current injection, the PY neuron depolarized and fired action potentials. This indicates that even when the PD and AB neurons were at the hyperpolarizing phase of their membrane potential excursions during normal activity, they were releasing inhibitory neurotransmitter onto the PY neuron. (J. S. Eisen and E. Marder, unpublished observations.)

until the PD and AB neurons were hyperpolarized to a level below the most negative level of membrane potential reached during their typical membrane potential oscillations. Hyperpolarization of the PD and AB neurons removed this steady release of inhibitory neurotransmitter, and the PY neurons were released from inhibition and started firing.

As the neurons of the STG depolarize, they release more and more neurotransmitter. Because action potentials are rapid transients, they produce only a relatively small increment in neurotransmitter release; the slower depolarizations underlying the bursts appear to be responsible for most of the integration in the ganglion (Raper, 1979). Thus, the neuropil of the STG acts primarily as an analog device, with a digital output (action potentials) apparently important mostly for sending signals to the muscles innervated by the STG neurons.

One consequence of the analog nature of the integrative processing in the STG neuropil is that it is possible to bias the pyloric network in a graded fashion in a number of different ways. This allows the output of the circuit to be modulated in such a way that a variety of pyloric motor patterns can be produced.

MODULATION OF THE PYLORIC RHYTHM

Inputs to the STG from other ganglia influence the pyloric rhythm (Russell and Hartline, 1978, 1982; Sigvardt and Mulloney, 1982; Dickinson and Nagy, 1983; Nagy and Dickinson, 1983). In fact, merely leaving the OG and paired CGs attached to the STG produces a pyloric rhythm that is more rapid and of greater intensity than that produced by the isolated STG (Figure 9). What types of inputs to the STG are there, and how do these inputs influence neurons of the STG to change the motor patterns produced by the STG?

Characterization of Input Fibers to the STG

In order to characterize the inputs to the STG from other ganglia, biochemical, histochemical, and immunocytochemical methods are being used to identify the many different neurotransmitter substances that project into the STG (Figure 10). This approach was first used to identify several dopaminergic fibers that project from neurons in the CGs into the neuropil of the STG (Kushner and Maynard, 1977). Today we know that there are histaminergic fibers (Claiborne and Selverston, 1984), serotonergic fibers (Beltz et al., 1984), GABAergic fibers (Cazalets et al., 1985), proctolinergic fibers (Hooper and Marder, 1984; Marder et al., 1986), fibers that stain with antibodies raised against FMRFamide (Hooper and Marder, 1984; Marder et al., 1987), and fibers that stain with antibodies raised against substance P (Goldberg et al., 1986) and red pigment concentrating hormone (RPCH; Nusbaum and Marder, 1986)—all of which project into the neuropil of the STG (Figure 10).

It is interesting that many of these fibers branch throughout the neuropil of the STG and, like many of the neurons of the STG, appear to send processes into all regions of the STG neuropil (Figure 11). Figure 11A shows an acetylcholinesterase-stained STG from the crab, *Cancer irroratus*. This picture clearly shows the somata encircling the more central neuropil area. The distribution of

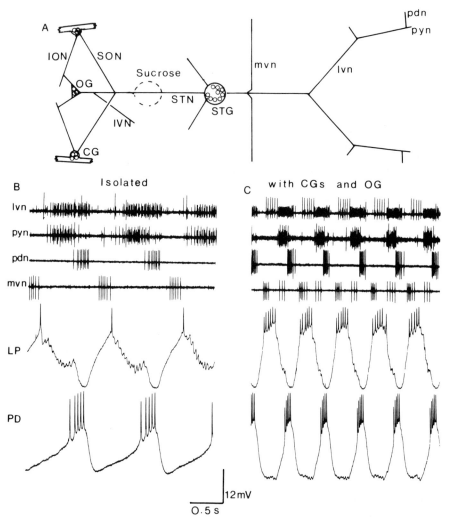

Figure 9. *Inputs from the commissural ganglia (CGs) influence the pyloric system. A*: Schematic diagram of the full stomatogastric nervous system, including the CGs, the STN, and the esophageal ganglion (OG). Nerves connecting these ganglia: IVN, inferior ventricular nerve; SON, superior esophageal nerve; ION, inferior esophageal nerve. The *dotted line* circling the STN indicates the position of a Vaseline well on the STN. When isotonic sucrose is placed in the well, all impulse traffic in the STN is blocked, thus allowing a reversible removal of inputs to the STG. *B*: Pyloric rhythm in the presence of a sucrose block to isolate the STG. *C*: Pyloric rhythm with connections from the CGs to the STG intact and functional. Note the increase in the frequency and in the amplitude of the membrane potential oscillations in both the LP and PD neurons in the presence of inputs from the CGs and OG.

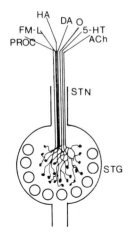

Figure 10. *The organization of neurotransmitter inputs to the STG.* A large number of different neurotransmitters are carried in input fibers to the STG. These fibers are seen to branch throughout the neuropil. ACh, acetylcholine; DA, dopamine; FM-L, FMRFamidelike peptide; HA, histamine; 5-HT, serotonin; O, octopamine; PROC, proctolin.

processes throughout the neuropil of a single PD neuron from the crab filled with carboxyfluorescein is shown in Figure 11B. Figure 11C and D shows the patterns of immunoreactivity produced with antibodies directed against serotonin and proctolin, respectively. Similar patterns were seen with antibodies against FMRFamide (Hooper and Marder, 1984; Marder and Hooper, 1985; Marder et al., 1987), substance P (Goldberg et al., 1986), and RPCH (Nusbaum and Marder, 1986).

In each case, the entire neuropil contained immunoreactive processes, but the somata of the STG were unstained. It can be seen that the terminals of the input fibers appear to blanket the entire dendritic area of the STG motor neurons. This dense intertangling of all the input fibers suggests that these fibers may release their neurotransmitters into the neuropil in a diffuse manner, and that their specificity of action may arise solely from the specificity of the receptors present on the neurons in the STG. Alternatively, the dense intertangling may mean that the distribution of synaptic contacts is highly complex but quite precise, as is the case for the synaptic contacts betwen motor neurons of the STG (King, 1976a,b).

What Do Input Neurotransmitters Do?

Two of the first input pathways to have received considerable attention were those of the inferior ventricular nerve (IVN), now known to contain histamine (Claiborne and Selverston, 1984) and possibly an additional neurotransmitter, and the dopamine-containing fibers that appear to come from somata in the CGs (Kushner and Maynard, 1977). In an analysis of the actions of these inputs on neurons of the STG, we found that the AB neurons and PD neurons responded differently to stimulation of the IVN and to dopamine applications (Marder, 1984; Marder and Eisen, 1984b). Dopamine applications inhibited the PD neurons, causing them to release less neurotransmitter. This resulted in an almost entirely AB-derived, and therefore more rapid, IPSP in the PY neurons (see Figure 6B). Consequently, the PY neurons resumed firing earlier after the AB and PD neurons repolarized (Figure 12) (Eisen and Marder, 1984). In contrast, the PD neurons

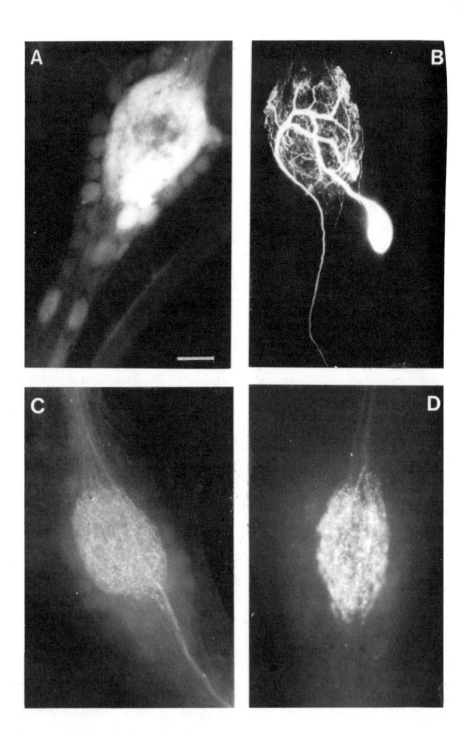

were excited by IVN stimulation, and therefore released more neurotransmitter with each burst. This prolonged the time course of the IPSP evoked in a PY neuron, since the PD neurons evoke the late, slow portion of the IPSP (see Figure 6B). This in turn caused the PY neuron to delay its resumption of firing after the depolarization of the AB and PD neurons (Figure 12) (Eisen and Marder, 1984). Thus, the difference in time course of the AB-evoked and PD-evoked IPSPs provides the basis for a mechanism to alter the time of firing of the PY neurons relative to the time of firing of the AB and PD neurons, in a way that is independent of frequency (Eisen and Marder, 1984).

Alterations in pyloric motor patterns are also produced by the other substances known to be present in input pathways to the STG (Flamm and Harris-Warrick, 1986a,b). Interestingly enough, when the substances present in input fibers to the STG are bath-applied to the STG, each elicits a characteristic and different change in the motor patterns produced by the STG (Marder and Hooper, 1985). Figure 13 shows the effects of proctolin, FMRFamide, pilocarpine, and serotonin on the pyloric rhythm produced by a single crab preparation. The preparation was extensively washed after each test application, and although the washes are not shown, the control pattern was reestablished before application of another compound. The control pyloric pattern is seen in the first panel of Figure 13. The LP neuron was firing one or two action potentials per burst, and the frequency of the pyloric cycle was about 1 Hz. The next panel shows that proctolin (10^{-6} M) produced a dramatic increase in the number of LP neuron action potentials per burst, as well as a slight increase in cycle frequency. In contrast, FMRFamide applications resulted in complete cessation of LP neuron action potentials, because of enhanced PY neuron firing that inhibited the LP neuron. Thus, these two peptides, while both being "excitatory" in that they are capable of increasing the frequency of the pyloric rhythm (Hooper and Marder, 1984; Marder et al., 1986), produce entirely different motor outputs. (In one case the muscles innervated by the LP neuron would be contracting vigorously; in the other the same muscles would be inactive.)

The effects of pilocarpine and serotonin are also shown on Figure 13. Pilocarpine greatly increased the overall frequency but produced little change in the phase relations of the firing times of the individual units. Unlike the other agents applied to the ganglion shown in Figure 13, serotonin completely disrupted the normal pattern of activity, resulting in an entirely different rhythm (Beltz et al., 1984). If these effects of serotonin applications are physiological, in terms of motor output, they might be likened to a gait change in locomotory systems (Grillner, 1981).

Figure 11. *Localization of neurons, neuropil, and input fibers.* Whole-mount pictures from the crab, *Cancer irroratus*. *A*: STG stained for acetylcholinesterase. The large central area is neuropil, and somata can be seen encircling the ganglion. *B*: Single PD neuron filled with carboxyfluorescein. Soma appears larger than it actually is because of the fluorescence. *C*: Serotoninlike immunoreactivity in STG. Ganglion was processed as a whole mount (see Beltz et al., 1984). Serotoninlike immunoreactivity was found in several fibers in the STN, in the neuropil of the STG (picture was chosen because unstained somata are faintly visible), and in several fibers exiting the ganglion in the motor nerves. *D*: Proctolinlike immunoreactivity in the neuropil of the STG (for further details, see Marder et al., 1986). Again, somata are unstained, but stained fibers fill the neuropil. In all pictures, anterior is at the top; *calibration bar* = 120 μm.

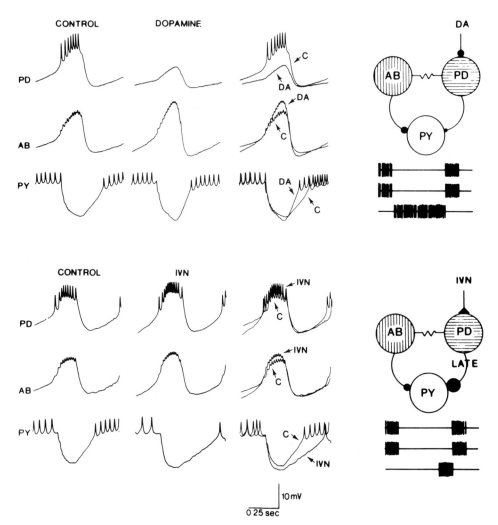

Figure 12. *Effect of inputs on the phase of PY neuron firing. Top traces*: Control, simultaneous recordings from the PD, AB, and PY neurons in control saline (*left*). Dopamine (10^{-4} M) added to the saline resulted in a hyperpolarization of the PD neuron and a smaller depolarization. At the same time, the IPSP recorded in the PY neuron is decreased in time course when compared to the control (*center*). [Photographic superposition of the control and dopamine panels is shown to facilitate comparison (*right*).] C, control; DA, dopamine. Cartoon (*top right*) shows that when the PD neuron is inhibited it releases less transmitter, thus decreasing the amplitude of the late component of the IPSP evoked by the depolarization of the PD and AB neurons. *Bottom traces*: Control as above (*left*). Stimulation of the IVN results in excitation of the PD neuron, causing it to release more transmitter, thus prolonging the IPSP recorded in the PY neuron (*center*). [Photographic superposition of the control and IVN panels is shown to facilitate comparison (*right*).] Cartoon (*bottom right*) shows that this prolonged IPSP delays the resumption of PY neuron firing. (Modified from Eisen and Marder, 1984.)

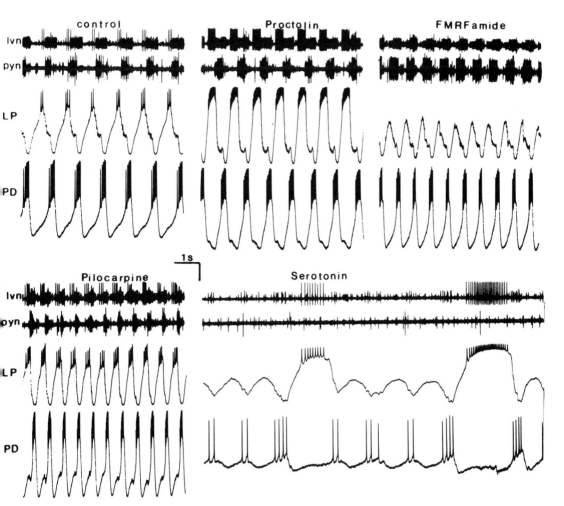

Figure 13. *Comparison of the effects of proctolin, FMRFamide, pilocarpine, and serotonin on the pyloric rhythm.* All records are from the same preparation of *Cancer irroratus*. The preparation was washed for 30 min between applications of agonists, and the motor patterns resumed control levels of activity between each application (not shown). Proctolin, 10^{-6} M; FMRFamide, 10^{-5} M; pilocarpine, 10^{-4} M; serotonin, 10^{-4} M. Each agent evoked a characteristic and different motor pattern. *Vertical calibration bar = 4 mV.*

Are the results shown in Figure 13 likely to be physiological? Since they were produced by bath application of test substances, they may or may not mimic the effects of physiological activity in the input fibers that contain, and presumably release, these or similar substances. If the fibers that release these substances make discrete, point-to-point local synapses—and the neurotransmitters released by these input fibers do not diffuse even a few microns from their site of release—then bath application of test substances may produce artifactual motor patterns from the STG. However, should many or all of the input fibers release their neurotransmitters at any distance from their targets (Jan and Jan, 1982, 1983), or should these substances be able to diffuse even several microns away from their site of release without being inactivated, then bath application may be the best way to mimic the physiological actions of these input fibers.

If it turns out that some or many of the neurotransmitters released by the input fibers do act over a relatively large distance (more than a few microns), it should be remembered that there are actually two different neuronal circuits sharing the same space in the neuropil. We have already shown that the gastric mill and pyloric systems interact (Figure 3). It is extremely likely that the strength of these interactions might be influenced by the local neurochemical environment of the ganglion. Thus, not only the output of each individual neuronal circuit but also the way in which these two circuits interact may be modulated by inputs to the STG. It should be noted that although interactions between the gastric mill rhythm and the pyloric rhythm have been described (Mulloney, 1977; Robertson and Moulins, 1984), these interactions are more pronounced in the presence of proctolin than are those routinely recorded in saline.

CONCLUSIONS

We would like to suggest that the diversity of neurotransmitters used in the control of the STG central pattern generators provides a mechanism that allows the modulation of the pyloric and gastric circuits, such that different output patterns can be produced by a single neuronal circuit. In a complex neuropil, it may not be possible to restrict neurotransmitter diffusion or receptor localization to an extremely small area. The specificity of action of a peptide- or amine-releasing fiber may then reside, not in the specific site of synaptic contact, but in the nature of the conductances and receptors affected in the target neurons (Jan and Jan, 1982, 1983). Each neurotransmitter or neurotransmitter system may then be able to elicit, from the same neuronal circuit, a characteristic and different "operational state." In this way, it would be possible to obtain a wide range of stable neuronal outputs from a single circuit. It may also be possible to obtain a wide range of interactions between semiautonomous circuits that exist in close physical proximity within a neuropil.

Much of the integration in the stomatogastric nervous system takes place in an analog fashion, in which neurotransmitter release is a continuous function of membrane potential above some release threshold. Therefore, neurons that do not reach threshold for action potential production can still reach threshold for transmitter release and thus participate in the production of rhythmic behaviors. For example, in the presence of FMRFamide (Figure 13), the LP neuron continues to show membrane potential oscillations that influence the amount of neurotransmitter that it releases onto other neurons. However, the muscle innervated by the LP neuron would receive no excitation, since the LP neuron's digital output to the muscle has been turned off.

In summary, modulation of neural output in the stomatogastric nervous system occurs in several ways. Some of the input fibers appear to act directly on voltage-dependent conductances and can stimulate or elicit bursting membrane properties. Other input fibers act by influencing the amount of neurotransmitter released by presynaptic neurons by depolarizing or hyperpolarizing them. Most likely, other mechanisms for modulating the strength of specific synaptic connections similar to those described in other preparations (Kandel and Schwartz, 1981) will be established in the future. Under some conditions, the output of the pyloric circuit includes participation from all of the pyloric neurons. At other times, although all the circuit elements may continue to participate in integration, only some of the units may reach threshold and deliver output to the next level of organization.

The variety of stable motor patterns produced by the pyloric system neurons (Figure 13) suggests the interesting possibility that the primary pacemaking function may switch among neurons in a circuit. We already know that when the pyloric rhythm is cycling slowly, the AB neuron is the pacemaker for the rhythm and appears responsible for controlling cycle frequency (Miller and Selverston, 1982a,b). In the presence of inputs from other ganglia or neurotransmitters (Russell and Hartline, 1978, 1982; Nagy and Dickinson, 1983; Dickinson and Nagy, 1983), STG neurons other than the AB neurons may exhibit plateau properties that contribute to the generation of the rhythm. It may be that when the rhythm is dramatically altered, as it is in the presence of serotonin, the timing pacemaker may no longer be the AB neuron. After the AB neuron is removed from the circuit by photoinactivation (the PD neuron fires tonically in this case), it sometimes appears that the LP neuron can act as a bursting pacemaker (J. S. Eisen and E. Marder, unpublished observations). Since the pyloric circuit is not symmetrical in its connections (e.g., the LP neuron inhibits the PD neurons but not the AB neuron; Figure 5), switching the site of the primary pacemaking function makes possible the production of quite different neuronal outputs from a single "hard-wired" circuit.

Some of what we are finding in this preparation parallels results in other preparations. Effects of amines and neuropeptides on the induction of burst potentials or pacemaker potentials have been described in a number of both invertebrate and vertebrate preparations (Levitan et al., 1979; Lingle, 1979; Dekin et al., 1984; Lent and Dickinson, 1984; Miller et al., 1984; Kuhlman et al., 1985). Work on other neural circuits is also leading toward the notion that neural circuits can produce variable neural outputs (Roberts and Roberts, 1983). The unique feature of the stomatogastric system is that the neural circuits of interest are localized to anatomically defined ganglia; this has facilitated the characterization of both the neural circuits and the transmitter pathways.

If, as we suspect, the function of multiple neurotransmitters in this preparation is to allow flexibility in neural output, how might this apply to complicated and complex vertebrate nervous systems? Many regions of vertebrate brains appear to be organized in parallel arrays of neurons, as in the retina or in the cerebellum. Small regions of these arrays may act as local circuits with many of the same properties as the STG. If so, the basic function of those regions of the brain might be "hard-wired" in the same way that the connectivity pattern of the STG is "hard-wired." Then other neuronal inputs to those regions of neuropil may also function to change the integrative functions, so that once again a given neuronal circuit might easily express a variety of states, depending on the presence or absence of one or more of many peptides and amines. Thus, there may be different kinds of "neurotransmitters": those that mediate discrete synaptic contacts, and others that act as local hormones that can change the "state" of neural circuits in specific ways. This type of organization would considerably multiply the computing power of a large neuronal circuit, as well as make possible the production of a variety of outputs from a simple neuronal circuit.

ACKNOWLEDGMENTS

We thank Mr. Michael O'Neil for help in the preparation of the figures and Ms. Carol Anderson for the acetylcholinesterase-stained preparation shown in Figure 11. We thank Drs. Brenda Claiborne and Ron Calabrese for reading earlier drafts of this manuscript. This work was supported by grant NS-17813.

REFERENCES

Atwood, H. L., C. K. Govind, and I. Kwan (1978) Nonhomogeneous excitatory synapses of a crab stomach muscle. *J. Neurobiol.* **9**:17–28.

Beltz, B., J. S. Eisen, R. Flamm, R. M. Harris-Warrick, S. L. Hooper, and E. Marder (1984) Serotonergic innervation and modulation of the stomatogastric ganglion of three decapod crustaceans (*Homarus americanus, Cancer irroratus,* and *Panulirus interruptus*). *J. Exp. Biol.* **109**:35–54.

Burrows, M., and M. V. S. Siegler (1983) Networks of local interneurons in an insect. In *Neural Origin of Rhythmic Movements,* A. Roberts and B. L. Roberts, eds., pp. 29–53, Cambridge Univ. Press, Cambridge, England.

Burrows, M., and M. V. S. Siegler (1984) The morphological diversity and receptive fields of spiking local interneurons in the locust metathoracic ganglion. *J. Comp. Neurol.* **224**:483–508.

Cazalets, J.-R., I. Cournil, and M. Moulins (1985) GABAergic inactivation of burst generating oscillations in lobster pyloric neurons. *Soc. Neurosci. Abstr.* **11**:1022.

Claiborne, B. J., and A. I. Selverston (1984) Histamine as a neurotransmitter in the stomatogastric nervous system of the spiny lobster. *J. Neurosci.* **4**:708–721.

Dekin, M. S., G. B. Richerson, and P. A. Getting (1984) Thyrotropin-releasing hormone induces spontaneous bursting in the nucleus tractus solitarius. *Soc. Neurosci. Abstr.* **10**:1116.

Dickinson, P. S., and F. Nagy (1983) Control of a central pattern generator by an identified modulatory interneurone in *Crustacea.* II. Induction and modification of plateau properties in pyloric neurones. *J. Exp. Biol.* **105**:59–82.

Eisen, J. S., and E. Marder (1982) Mechanisms underlying pattern generation in lobster stomatogastric ganglion as determined by selective inactivation of identified neurons. III. Synaptic connections of electrically coupled pyloric neurons. *J. Neurophysiol.* **48**:1392–1415.

Eisen, J. S., and E. Marder (1984) A mechanism for the production of phase shifts in a pattern generator. *J. Neurophysiol.* **51**:1374–1393.

Flamm, R. E., and R. M. Harris-Warrick (1986a) Aminergic modulation of lobster stomatogastric ganglion. I. Effects on motor patterns and activity of neurons within the pyloric circuit. *J. Neurophysiol.* **55**:847–865.

Flamm, R. E., and R. M. Harris-Warrick (1986b) Aminergic modulation of lobster stomatogastric ganglion. II. Target neurons of dopamine, octopamine, and serotonin within the pyloric circuit. *J. Neurophysiol.* **55**:866–881.

Gola, M., and A. I. Selverston (1981) Ionic requirements for bursting activity in lobster stomatogastric neurons. *J. Comp. Physiol.* **145**:191–207.

Goldberg, D., M. P. Nusbaum, and E. Marder (1986) Distribution of a substance P-like peptide in decapod stomatogastric nervous systems. *Soc. Neurosci. Abstr.* **12**:242.

Govind, C. K., H. L. Atwood, and D. M. Maynard (1975) Innervation and neuromuscular physiology of intrinsic foregut muscles in the blue crab and spiny lobster. *J. Comp. Physiol.* **96**:185–204.

Graubard, K. (1978) Synaptic transmission without action potentials: Input–output properties of a non-spiking presynaptic neuron. *J. Neurophysiol.* **41**:1014–1025.

Graubard, K., J. A. Raper, and D. K. Hartline (1980) Graded synaptic transmission between spiking neurons. *Proc. Natl. Acad. Sci. USA* **77**:3733–3735.

Graubard, K., J. A. Raper, and D. K. Hartline (1983) Graded synaptic transmission between identified spiking neurons. *J. Neurophysiol.* **50**:508–521.

Grillner, S. (1981) Control of locomotion in bipeds, tetrapods, and fish. *Handb. Physiol., The Nervous System* **3**:1179–1236.

Hartline, D. K. (1979) Pattern generation in the lobster (*Panulirus*) stomatogastric ganglion. II. Pyloric network simulation. *Biol. Cybern.* **33**:223–236.

Hooper, S. L., and E. Marder (1984) Modulation of a central pattern generator by two neuropeptides, proctolin and FMRFamide. *Brain Res.* **305**:186–191.

Jan, L. Y., and Y. N. Jan (1982) Peptidergic transmission in sympathetic ganglia of the frog. *J. Physiol. (Lond.)* **327**:219–246.

Jan, Y. N., and L. Y. Jan (1983) Electrophysiological techniques. In *Brain Peptides*, D. T. Krieger, M. J. Brownstein, and J. B. Martin, eds., pp. 547–563, Wiley, New York.

Kandel, E. R., and J. H. Schwartz (1981) *Principles of Neural Science*, Elsevier/North-Holland, New York.

Kater, S. B., and C. Nicholson, eds. (1973) *Intracellular Staining in Neurobiology*, Springer-Verlag, New York.

King, D. G. (1976a) Organization of crustacean neuropil. I. Patterns of synaptic connection in lobster stomatogastric ganglion. *J. Neurocytol.* **5**:207–237.

King, D. G. (1976b) Organization of crustacean neuropil. II. Distribution of synaptic contacts on identified motor neurons in lobster stomatogastric ganglion. *J. Neurocytol.* **5**:239–266.

Krieger, D. T., M. J. Brownstein, and J. B. Martin, eds. (1983) *Brain Peptides*, Wiley, New York.

Kuhlman, J. R., C. Li, and R. L. Calabrese (1985) FMRF-amide-like substances in the leech. II. Bioactivity on the heartbeat system. *J. Neurosci.* **5**:2310–2317.

Kushner, P. D., and E. A. Maynard (1977) Localization of monoamine fluorescence in the stomatogastric nervous system of lobsters. *Brain Res.* **129**:13–28.

Leise, E. M., and B. Mulloney (1984) Different neuropils in the adbominal ganglia of a crayfish have distinctive integrative functions. *Soc. Neurosci. Abstr.* **10**:627.

Lent, C. M., and M. H. Dickinson (1984) Serotonin integrates the feeding behavior of the medicinal leech. *J. Comp. Physiol.* **154**:457–471.

Levitan, I. B., A. J. Harmar, and W. B. Adams (1979) Synaptic and hormonal modulation of a neuronal oscillator: A search for molecular mechanisms. *J. Exp. Biol.* **81**:131–151.

Lingle, C. J. (1979) The modulatory action of dopamine on crustacean foregut neuromuscular preparations. *J. Exp. Biol.* **94**:285–299.

Macagno, E. R. (1980) Number and distribution of neurons in leech segmental ganglia. *J. Comp. Neurol.* **190**:283–302.

Marder, E. (1984) Roles for electrical coupling as revealed by selective neuronal deletions. *J. Exp. Biol.* **112**:147–167.

Marder, E., and J. S. Eisen (1984a) Transmitter identification of pyloric neurons: Electrically coupled neurons use different transmitters. *J. Neurphysiol.* **51**:1345–1361.

Marder, E., and J. S. Eisen (1984b) Electrically coupled pacemaker neurons respond differently to same physiological inputs and neurotransmitters. *J. Neurophysiol.* **51**:1362–1373.

Marder, E., and S. L. Hooper (1985) Neurotransmitter modulation of the stomatogastric ganglion of decapod crustaceans. In *Model Neural Networks and Behavior*, A. I. Selverston, ed., pp. 319–337, Plenum, New York.

Marder, E., S. L. Hooper, and K. K. Siwicki (1986) Modulatory action and distribution of the neuropeptide proctolin in the crustacean stomatogastric nervous system. *J. Comp. Neurol.* **243**:454–467.

Marder, E., R. L. Calabrese, M. P. Nusbaum, and B. Trimmer (1987) Distribution and partial characterizaton of FMRFamide-like peptides in the stomatogastric nervous systems of the rock crab, *Cancer borealis*, and the spiny lobster, *Panulirus interruptus*. *J. Comp. Neurol.* (in press).

Maynard, D. M. (1972) Simpler networks. *Ann. NY Acad. Sci.* **193**:59–72.

Maynard, D. M., and A. I. Selverston (1975) Organization of the stomatogastric ganglion of the spiny lobster. IV. The pyloric system. *J. Comp. Physiol.* **100**:161–182.

Maynard, D. M., and K. D. Walton (1975) Effects of maintained depolarization of presynaptic neuron on inhibitory transmission in lobster neuropil. *J. Comp. Physiol.* **97**:215–243.

Miller, J. P., and A. I. Selverston (1979) Rapid killing of single neurons by irradiation of intracellularly injected dye. *Science* **206**:702–704.

Miller, J. P., and A. I. Selverston (1982a) Mechanisms underlying pattern generation in lobster stomatogastric ganglion as determined by selective inactivation of identified neurons. II. Oscillatory properties of pyloric neurons. *J. Neurophysiol.* **48**:1378–1391.

Miller, J. P., and A. I. Selverston (1982b) Mechanisms underlying pattern generation in lobster stomatogastric ganglion as determined by selective inactivation of identified neurons. IV. Network properties of pyloric system. *J. Neurophysiol.* **48**:1416–1432.

Miller, M. W., J. A. Benson, and A. Berlind (1984) Excitatory effects of dopamine on the cardiac ganglia of the crabs *Portunus sanguinolentus* and *Podophthalmus vigil. J. Exp. Biol.* **108**:97–118.

Mulloney, B. (1977) Organization of the stomatogastric ganglion of the spiny lobster. V. Coordination of the gastric and pyloric systems. *J. Comp. Physiol.* **91**:1–32.

Murphey, R. K., A. Jacklet, and L. Schuster (1980) A topographic map of sensory cell terminal arborizations in the cricket CNS: Correlation with birthday and position in a sensory array. *J. Comp. Neurol.* **191**:53–64.

Nagy, F., and P. S. Dickinson (1983) Control of a central pattern generator by an identified modulatory interneurone in crustacea. I. Modulation of the pyloric motor output. *J. Exp. Biol.* **105**:33–58.

Nusbaum, M. P., and E. Marder (1986) A novel role for crustacean red pigment concentrating hormone: Neuromodulation of the pyloric CPG in the crab, *Cancer borealis. Soc. Neurosci. Abstr.* **12**:792.

Pearson, K. G., and C. R. Fourtner (1975) Nonspiking interneurons in walking system of the cockroach. *J. Neurophysiol.* **38**:33–52.

Raper, J. A. (1979) Nonimpulse-mediated synaptic transmission during the generation of a cyclic motor program. *Science* **205**:304–306.

Reichert, H., M. R. Plummer, and J. J. Wine (1983) Identified nonspiking local interneurons mediate nonrecurrent, lateral inhibition of crayfish mechanosensory interneurons. *J. Comp. Physiol.* **151**:261–276.

Roberts, A., and B. M. H. Bush (1981) *Neurones Without Impulses,* Cambridge Univ. Press, Cambridge, England.

Roberts, A., and B. L. Roberts (1983) *Neural Origin of Rhythmic Movements,* Cambridge Univ. Press, Cambridge, England.

Robertson, R. M., and M. Moulins (1984) Oscillatory command input to the motor pattern generators of the crustacean stomatogastric ganglion. The gastric rhythm. *J. Comp. Physiol.* **154**:473–491.

Russell, D. F., and D. K. Hartline (1978) Bursting neural networks: A reexamination. *Science* **200**:453–456.

Russell, D. F., and D. K. Hartline (1982) Slow active potentials and bursting motor patterns in pyloric network of the lobster, *Panulirus interruptus. J. Neurophysiol.* **48**:914–937.

Russell, D. F., and D. K. Hartline (1984) Synaptic regulation of cellular properties and burst oscillation of neuron in gastric mill system of spiny lobsters, *Panulirus interruptus. J. Neurophysiol.* **52**:54–73.

Selverston, A. I., and J. P. Miller (1980) Mechanisms underlying pattern generation in lobster stomatogastric ganglion as determined by selective inactivation of identified neurons. I. Pyloric system. *J. Neurophysiol.* **44**:1102–121.

Selverston, A. I., and M. P. Remler (1972) Neural geometry and activation of crayfish fast flexor motoneurons. *J. Neurophysiol.* **35**:797–814.

Selverston, A. I., D. G. King, D. F. Russell, and J. P. Miller (1976) The stomatogastric nervous system: Structure and function of a small neural network. *Prog. Neurobiol.* **7**:215–290.

Selverston, A. I., J. P. Miller, and M. Wadepuhl (1983) Cooperative mechanism for the production of rhythmic movements. *Soc. Exp. Biol. Symp.* **37**:55–87.

Siegler, M. V. S., and M. Burrows (1984) The morphology of two groups of spiking local interneurons in the metathoracic ganglion of the locust. *J. Comp. Neurol.* **224**:463–482.

Sigvardt, K. A., and B. Mulloney (1982) Sensory alteration of motor patterns in the stomatogastric system of the spiny lobster, *Panulirus interruptus. J. Exp. Biol.* **97**:137–152.

Chapter 14

Synaptic Processes and Neurotransmitters Operating in the Central Visual System: A Systems Approach

ADAM M. SILLITO

ABSTRACT

The receptive field properties of cells in the mammalian central visual system reflect the operation of the underlying synaptic organization. Thus, changes in the receptive field can be used as an index for assessing the effect of perturbations in the various components of this organization. Given the precision with which receptive field properties can be documented by computer-controlled stimuli, this provides a unique opportunity to study synaptic mechanisms at thalamic and neocortical levels in the intact visual system. The experimental evidence outlined here considers the effect of the use of microiontophoretic application of drugs to antagonize, or mimic, the action of specific sets of synaptic input on the receptive field properties of single cells in the dorsolateral geniculate nucleus and visual cortex.

The roles of GABAergic, cholinergic, noradrenergic, serotonergic, and peptidergic synapses are discussed in detail. The GABAergic synapses deriving from intrinsic interneurons at the thalamic and cortical levels appear to be a major influence in the structuring of receptive field selectivity. In contrast, the extrinsic nonvisual inputs mediated by acetylcholine, norepinephrine, and serotonin exert a modulatory influence, which in the case of acetylcholine in the cortex can be seen to enhance signal-to-noise levels and response selectivity. The effects of the peptides are complex and do not fall into any clearly resolved functional role. The implications of these observations for present views of the functional organization of the visual system are discussed.

Analysis of the elements of synaptic function, and the specific ionic channels influenced by given neurotransmitter agents, provides a basis for prediction and speculation about the functional significance of the various types of organization seen in particular neuronal systems. However, although superficially compelling, it is far from clear that conclusions regarding the significance of specific synaptic interactions established, for example, in the *in vitro* slice, will carry forward into the much more complex *in vivo* system, where myriad patterned interactions utilizing a range of neurotransmitters and modulators interweave in as yet undefined ways. In short, it is necessary to balance observations made in the tightly controlled *in vitro* situation with experimental verification directed to the system function *in vivo*, however complex and difficult this may turn out to be. Moreover, arguments referring to elements of the synaptic circuitry have to be formulated in terms of the operational parameters implicit to the global function of the system they subserve.

My comments in the following pages attempt to indicate the ways in which this issue can be tackled in the mammalian central visual system. There are good reasons for using the visual system as a model with which to bridge the gap between the levels of analysis referred to above. First, the level of detail in our knowledge relevant to achieving a correlation between synaptic organization, neuronal response properties, and overall system function is arguably more advanced for the visual system than for any other brain system. Second, neurons at the thalamic and cortical levels in the central visual system are precisely and reproducibly driven by particular categories of visual stimuli. These stimuli define the functional properties of the cells, collectively referred to as "receptive field organization," that can be directly related to certain aspects of visual perception and hence can be regarded as a meaningful index of overall system function. Further, it is a sine qua non that the functional properties are themselves a product of the synaptic circuitry impinging on the particular cell in question. Perturbations in the circuitry, or particular categories of synaptic input influencing a cell, will be reflected by perturbations in the visual response properties/receptive field. Hence, there is the possibility of an *in vivo* manipulation of particular categories of synaptic input, using the receptive field as an index of the consequence of this manipulation.

The technique of microiontophoresis of drugs provides one of the most direct, and from some viewpoints the only, means of providing a localized and rapidly reversible manipulation of the neurotransmitter-related events influencing neurons in the *in vivo* situation. It has been widely used to establish the likely nature of the action of putative neurotransmitters at all levels in the nervous system. Where good antagonists are available, it offers the possibility of dissecting away the influence of specific components of the synaptic circuit. The experimental data described here are based on the use of microiontophoretic techniques to apply putative neurotransmitters, their agonists, or their antagonists to the vicinity of identified cells in the dorsal lateral geniculate nucleus (dLGN) and in the visual cortex. The effects of these drugs are then assessed in terms of their action on the receptive field structure of the cell in question. The perturbations so produced provide some index of the role of the synapses utilizing a particular transmitter at a particular level in the visual system.

In this chapter, I review the relevant background information regarding the structural, neurochemical, and neurophysiological data pertinent to the central visual system and place the microiontophoretic findings in the context of this. Where possible, I attempt to establish a summary and overview of those aspects of the synaptic organization under discussion. The position adopted, however, is not intended to constitute more than a stimulus to the phrasing of further questions. One of the paradoxical features of the present state of knowledge in this field is that there is a growing realization that the synaptic organization of the visual system is considerably more complex than current theories of its operation really allow. Comprehension of the significance of particular synaptic processes is limited as much by the lack of a conceptual framework for the operational parameters of the system as it is by the lack of detailed knowledge of the ionic channels and allied events challenged by the processes. Thus, I have taken the opportunity in the discussion to indicate the ways in which the presently available data bear upon our view of the processing of the visual input.

LATERAL GENICULATE NUCLEUS

Basic Neuronal Organization

The principal elements of the neuronal circuit in the dLGN are summarized in Figure 1 and are broadly similar to those in all thalamic sensory nuclei. The presynaptic dendrites of the intrinsic inhibitory interneurons are involved in triadic synaptic arrangements in the synaptic glomeruli, where they are presynaptic to the relay cell dendrite but, together with the relay cell, are postsynaptic to the terminals of the retinal afferents (Famiglietti and Peters, 1972). It is likely, although not absolutely certain, that this arrangement is associated with the input to the dendritic spines of relay cells (Rapisardi and Miles, 1984; Wilson et al., 1984). In addition, it seems that the axonal processes of the intrinsic inhibitory interneurons make extraglomerular synaptic contacts on the dendritic shafts of the relay cells. A further inhibitory influence originates from cells in the perigeniculate nucleus (globally, reticularis thalami) and provides a recurrent collateral feedback to the relay cell (Ahlsen et al., 1982). Corticofugal fibers, in ordered retinotopic projections, make putative excitatory connections with both perigeniculate cells and relay cells. There is good evidence to support the view that both the intrinsic inhibitory interneurons and the perigeniculate cells are γ-aminobutyric acid (GABA)-ergic (O'Hara et al., 1983; Fitzpatrick et al., 1984). Furthermore, it seems likely that somatostatin (SSt) is coexistent with GABA in the perigeniculate inhibitory interneurons (Oertel et al., 1983). Extrinsic, and presumed modulatory, influences converge on the dLGN from three separate locations: a cholinergic input from the nucleus cuneiformis, a serotonergic input from the dorsal raphe nuclei, and a noradrenergic input from the locus coeruleus (Kunar et al., 1972; Hoover and Jacobowitz, 1979; Kromer and Moore, 1980).

Although the evidence is as yet inconclusive, there is a possibility that both the corticofugal pathway and the retinal input may involve excitatory amino acids (Baughman and Gilbert, 1981; Kemp and Sillito, 1981). Evidence in relation to the retinal input is somewhat confusing, because while uptake and release studies tend to exclude at least glutamate and aspartate as putative neurotransmitters at this location, the use of excitatory amino acid antagonists selective for the N-methyl-D-aspartate (NMDA) receptor block the visually driven input from X- and Y-cells without affecting the postsynaptic excitability of the relay cells (Kemp and Sillito, 1981).

GABAergic Processes

The most directly accessible facet of the dLGN neuronal organization is arguably that of the inhibitory interneurons. In most ways, the receptive fields of dLGN cells are remarkably like those of retinal ganglion cells, with X- and Y-cells subdivided into on- and off-center types, and it is only with respect to inhibitory

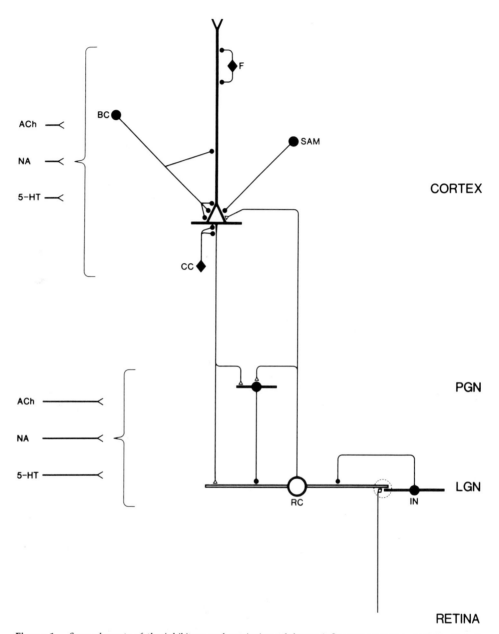

ACh
NA
5-HT

BC

F

SAM

CORTEX

CC

ACh
NA
5-HT

PGN

RC

IN

LGN

RETINA

Figure 1. *Some elements of the inhibitory and extrinsic modulatory influences operating at thalamic and cortical levels in the visual system.* Extrinsic modulatory inputs shown to the *left* of the diagram. The cortical connections are centered around a pyramidal cell. See text for further details. Abbreviations: ACh, acetylcholine; BC, basket cell; CC, chandelier cell; F, fusiform cell; 5-HT, 5-hydroxytryptamine; IN, intrinsic inhibitory interneurons; LGN, lateral geniculate nucleus; NE, norepinephrine; PGN, perigeniculate nucleus; RC, relay cell; SAM, short axon multipolar cell.

function that real distinctions can be made. The early work of Hubel and Wiesel
(1961) noted the enhanced center–surround antagonism seen in dLGN cell receptive fields with respect to those of retinal ganglion cells, a view reinforced
by intracellular data (Singer et al., 1972). Iontophoretic application of the GABA
antagonist bicuculline produces changes in the receptive field organization of
geniculate cells that are entirely commensurate with the loss of a process enhancing
center–surround antagonism (Sillito and Kemp, 1983a).

It is important to emphasize that in the dLGN, powerful postsynaptic inhibitory
inputs are elicited from both center and surround regions of the receptive field.
This is well documented by intracellular data (Singer and Creutzfeldt, 1970;
Singer et al., 1972) and can be seen as a suppression of unit firing when visual
stimuli are presented against a background discharge elicited by iontophoretic
application of an excitatory amino acid (Figure 2). This suppression of background

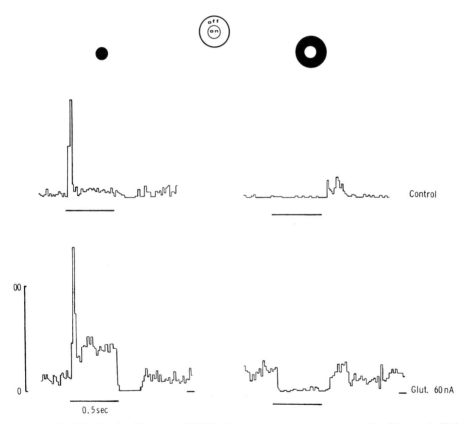

Figure 2. *Peristimulus time histograms (PSTHs) document response of an on-center X-cell to a spot of light
(0.73°) flashed over the receptive field center and an annulus (1.5–2.5°) flashed over the receptive field
surround, respectively. Region of the field stimulated is indicated by the diagrams above the
records. Upper records show the control response, lower records show the response when the
background discharge level was elevated by the iontophoretic application of glutamate. Horizontal
bars under the records indicate flash duration, 0.5 sec. Vertical calibration bar corresponds to 0–
100 counts/bin. Short horizontal bars to the right of the records indicate the level of zero count.
Bin size, 20 msecs; number of trials, 25. (From Sillito and Kemp, 1983a.)*

activity is blocked during the iontophoretic application of bicuculline (Sillito and Kemp, 1983a). Clearly, the surround-elicited inhibitory effect would be expected to be antagonistic to the center response. This is documented in Figure 3, which shows the response of an X-type on-center dLGN cell to a flashing spot of light of progressively increasing diameter. Under control conditions, the response of the cell is attenuated as the spot diameter increases and encroaches on the antagonistic surround. Conversely, during the iontophoretic application of the GABA antagonist bicuculline, the surround antagonism of the center response is markedly reduced, with the residual antagonism reflecting the level of center–surround interaction known to occur at the retinal level (Hammond, 1973).

Thus, during the blockade of GABAergic inhibition, the dLGN cells exhibit what are essentially retinal cell properties. These results apply equally to both X- and Y-group cells and their on- and off-center subgroups. Taking the simplistic view that on- and off-center cells can be regarded to detect, respectively, localized increments or decrements in the level of illumination with respect to the background (surround), the enhanced center–surround antagonism in effect serves to define more sharply the locus over which this occurs (see also discussion on responses to annuli in Sillito and Kemp, 1983a). Although, obviously, as in the control situation, there are clear distinctions in the detailed nature of the responses of

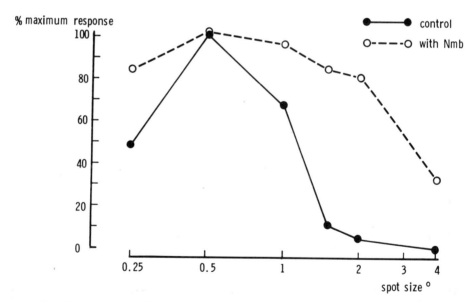

Figure 3. *Effect of inhibitory blockade on the area response curve for an on-center X-cell in the dorsal lateral geniculate nucleus (dLGN). Each point shows the average response to 25 presentations of a 0.5-sec flash of a stimulus spot, expressed as a percentage of the maximum response; abscissa shows the diameters of the test stimuli in degrees. Filled circles represent the control responses; open circles represent the responses during an inhibitory blockade elicited by iontophoretic application (60-nA ejecting current) of the γ-aminobutyric acid (GABA) antagonist N-methyl-bicuculline (Nmb). (From Sillito and Kemp, 1983a.)*

X- and Y-cells during an inhibitory blockade, the responses of both appear to be altered in a remarkably similar way with respect to the effects elicited by flashing spots and annuli. Distinctions in the apparent nature of the inhibitory contribution to the properties of X- and Y-cells do show up, however, when the fields are tested with sinusoidally modulated gratings (Berardi and Morrone, 1984). Although the contrast dependence of visual responses in both X- and Y-cells is modified, the spatial frequency selectivity of X-cells is modified at threshold and suprathreshold contrasts, while that of Y-cells is not. The X-cells show an increased sensitivity to low spatial frequencies, while neither the shape of the spatial frequency tuning curve nor the nonlinearity of the responses are affected in Y-cells.

Although ionotophoretically applied bicuculline is likely to block inhibitory effects deriving from both perigeniculate cells and intrinsic inhibitory interneurons, it seems likely that the stimulus-specific inhibitory effects seen here originate from intrinsic inhibitory interneurons. The primary reason for this view is that perigeniculate cells respond poorly to flashing spots and annuli (Dubin and Cleland, 1977; Sillito and Kemp, 1983a) and hence would not seem to be capable of generating the consistent and powerful inhibitory effects reviewed here. The perigeniculate inhibitory interneurons may exert a more generalized control over excitability levels, possibly following the suggestion of Ahlsen et al. (1982) that they serve as a variable gain control, limiting the dynamic range of the visual responses. Assuming that the intrinsic inhibitory interneurons mediate the stimulus-specific inhibitory effects, there are several factors to consider.

First, such evidence as we have suggests that they are spiking cells (Dubin and Cleland, 1977), and that they are on- or off-center X- or Y-cells with visual response properties indistinguishable from those of the relay cells. This does not, of course, imply that the properties of the cells, as determined by the action potential discharge, are of necessity predictive of the nature of the inhibitory influence exerted by the presynaptic dendrites in the glomeruli. In this situation, the "local circuit" operation may integrate information in a rather different domain. Indeed, one of the perplexing things about the triadic synaptic arrangement is that it suggests that the retinal afferents providing the excitatory drive to the relay cell initiate a short-latency inhibitory input with the same spatial and temporal properties as the excitatory input. The evidence that we have from intracellular studies (Singer et al., 1972) indicates that the latency of the inhibitory inputs elicited from both center and surround is such that it must be elicited by a center-driven (as opposed to surround-driven) visual input. This suggests that in, for example, off-center cells, the center-elicited inhibitory effect is driven by an on-center cell, and the center-antagonistic, surround-elicited inhibitory input is driven by off-center cells.

It is difficult to equate this with the superficial logic implied by the triadic arrangement. The region of visual space sampled by the inhibitory interneurons may be shifted with respect to that of the relay cells (see discussion in Sillito and Kemp, 1983a), but this hardly gets over the problem of the direct coupling of the local circuit arrangement to the cells' excitatory drive. A theoretically attractive arrangement would be to presume that the input to the presynaptic dendrites actually uncouples a tonic inhibitory input, thus producing disinhibition. The reapplication of the inhibitory input might then be very rapid following cessation of the excitatory drive, giving the impression of a short-latency, visually driven inhibitory input.

The advantage of this is that the inhibitory input would be modulated by the spatial and temporal properties of the excitatory input to produce a "mirror image" inhibitory field. This hypothesis derives some support from recent studies of the properties of dLGN off-center cells following removal of the on-center input by treatment of the retina with D,L-2-amino-4-phosphonobutyric acid (APB) (Schiller, 1982; Horton and Sherk, 1984). The loss of the on-system seems to have very little effect on off-center dLGN cell properties, with the proviso that the on-inhibition from the center may be diminished. Clearly, several factors are operating. There is good evidence for a convergence of both X- and Y-elicited, stimulus-specific inhibitory effects on individual dLGN cells (Singer and Bedworth, 1973), despite the fact that intrinsic interneurons themselves do not show such convergence (Dubin and Cleland, 1977).

On balance, this latter point is best explained by convergence of the axonal projections from X- and Y-dominated interneurons. One is tempted to speculate that the intrinsic local circuit inhibitory input to a given relay cell operates in a fashion independent of the intrinsic axonal inhibitory input. Moreover, there is indeed no reason to presume that they derive from the same cell or cells. Thus, there may be two intrinsic inhibitory processes, one representing an in-line, feed-forward disinhibitory system and the other a laterally directed, feed-forward inhibitory system. It is interesting to consider the fact that Y-cells in the dLGN appear to have a much smaller number of spines than X-cells (Wilson et al., 1984). Hence, the "process" reflecting the operation of the triadic synapses should be less prominent in Y-cells. The observations of Berardi and Morrone (1984), as discussed above, are pertinent in this respect.

The Functional Significance of the Coexistence of GABA and SSt

The possibility that GABA and the peptide SSt may coexist in perigeniculate cells (Oertel et al., 1983) raises the question of whether SSt modulates the action of GABA in a fashion similar to the modulation occurring between vasoactive intestinal polypeptide (VIP) and acetylcholine (ACh) in the control of salivary gland blood flow and secretion (Lundberg et al., 1982). We examined this possibility in the dLGN (Sillito et al., 1984) by checking the effect of both iontophoretically applied and pressure-ejected SSt on the resting discharge and visually elicited responses of dLGN cells. Furthermore, we checked for evidence of an interaction between SSt and iontophoretically applied GABA and then examined the possibility of an interaction with two other neurotransmitters influencing the dLGN circuits, norepinephrine and ACh. Although we have evidence for some small facilitatory and inhibitory effects of SSt on dLGN cell responsiveness, there is no evidence for any specific modulation of the effects of GABA, whether iontophoretically applied or associated with the GABAergic synaptic inputs mediating center–surround antagonism.

It has been reported that SSt will modulate the response of neurons in the lateral vestibular nucleus to iontophoretic pulses of GABA (Chan-Palay et al., 1982). In the dLGN, SSt does not appear to modulate the responses of cells to iontophoretic pulses of GABA, although the use of pulsed drug application and an automatic current balance control can precipitate an artefactual situation in which this appears to be the case. Similarly, it does not seem to interact with either ACh or norepinephrine. These conclusions hold for SSt-14, SSt-28, and SSt-28(1–12).

Extrinsic Modulatory Systems

While it is clear that the properties of dLGN cells are modulated *pari passu* with the level of arousal (Singer, 1977; Livingstone and Hubel, 1981), it is difficult to construct a coherent scheme attaching specific functional significance to each of the three separate subsystems thought to provide the modulatory input. One of the problems is that although the cholinergic, serotonergic, and noradrenergic inputs appear to exert distinct, and in some ways antagonistic, patterns of effect, the available evidence indicates that the activity levels in all the inputs increase in parallel with the level of arousal. ACh has for some time been associated with an input to the dLGN mediating the nonspecific effects of arousal (Deffenu et al., 1967; Phillis et al., 1967a), and Singer (1973, 1977) has postulated that the primary effect occurring in the dLGN during arousal is disinhibition. This view is indeed supported by the fact that iontophoretically applied ACh inhibits perigeniculate cells (Godfraind, 1978; Sillito et al., 1983). However, were this cholinergic input to invoke total disinhibition, it should also inhibit the intrageniculate inhibitory interneurons. By this token, iontophoretically applied ACh should inhibit the 20–25% of the dLGN cell population that represents the population of inhibitory interneurons (Sterling and Davis, 1980; Fitzpatrick et al., 1984).

In fact, iontophoretically applied ACh appears to excite all dLGN cells (Sillito et al., 1983), and during its application both stimulus-specific excitatory responses and stimulus-specific inhibitory responses can be enhanced. For example, Figure 4 shows the effects of iontophoretically applied ACh on the responses of an off-center X-cell to a flashing spot of light of progressively increasing diameter. Although the responses to stimuli within the center region are enhanced, there is no enhancement of the response to larger diameter stimuli encroaching on the surround. This lack of effect on the response to larger diameter stimuli is quite remarkable, given the potent direct excitatory effect that ACh has on dLGN cells. It contrasts sharply with the obvious "disinhibitory effect" of bicuculline in Figure 3. These observations led us to propose that the cholinergic input exerts three levels of action on the dLGN:

1. Direct facilitation of dLGN relay cells.
2. Reduction in nonspecific inhibitory influences from the perigeniculate nucleus, secondary to the direct inhibition of these cells.
3. An increase in stimulus-specific inhibitory influences acting on relay cells via a facilitatory effect on intrinsic inhibitory interneurons.

The point here is that the relative balance of the stimulus-specific inhibitory and excitatory components within the receptive field would be maintained despite an increase in the responsiveness of the cell to an optimal stimulus, such as a

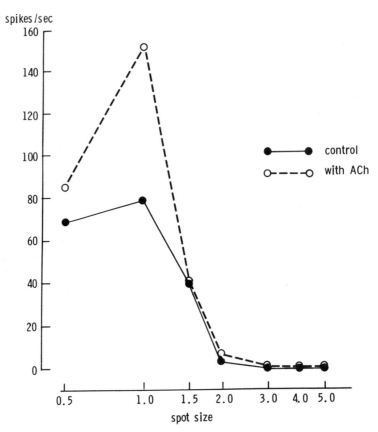

Figure 4. *Effect of acetylcholine (Ach) on the area response curve of an off-center X-cell in the dLGN. Abscissa* shows diameters of test stimuli (0.5-sec flash) in degrees; *ordinate* shows the average peak response of the cell (25 trials) in spikes/second. Iontophoretic application of ACh (45-nA ejecting current) enhances response to stimuli within the center but has no effect on response to stimuli overlapping the surround. This should be compared with the effect of bicuculline in Figure 3. It does not appear that the facilitatory effect of ACh is secondary to a disinhibition of the mechanism enhancing center–surround antagonism in the dLGN. (From Sillito et al., 1983.)

spot of light flashed within the central region of the receptive field. Were complete disinhibition at the level of intrinsic inhibitory interneurons to occur during arousal, it would suggest that the complex morphological and functional organization associated with the stimulus-specific inhibitory influences had no significant role to play in visual processing, which seems unlikely. Nonetheless, it is important to note that the data with iontophoretically applied ACh only demonstrates that stimulus-elicited inhibitory effects are present under these circumstances. It does not demonstrate that all the inhibitory effects relating to intrinsic inhibitory interneurons are present.

Thus, noting the postulate made earlier that the visual input might shunt tonic inhibition at the level of the triadic synapse, it is not inconceivable that the cholinergic input could also achieve this, leaving the intrinsic, axonally mediated inhibitory input intact. The problem here is that there are at least two distinct types of intrinsic inhibitory input, and it is not clear which aspects of the response properties are subserved by these. Interestingly, however, Livingstone and Hubel's (1981) observations on cats aroused from slow wave sleep showed shifts in the visual response of dLGN cells to flashing spots that were remarkably similar to those observed in the transition from the control state to that pertaining during iontophoretic application of ACh (Sillito et al., 1983). One of the problems associated with the data supporting the concept of disinhibition during arousal is that the shift to the aroused state was produced by electrical stimulation in the midbrain reticular formation (MRF) in otherwise anesthetized animals. It is far from evident that this situation corresponds to that occurring during natural arousal. In fact, the situation is complicated by the likelihood that MRF stimulation will affect all three modulatory systems, not just the cholinergic system, and hence the interpretation made by Singer (1977) has to take this possibility into account. As the following indicates, there is a basis for a global disinhibition, but it is not purely secondary to the cholinergic input.

The serotonergic input from the dorsal raphe nucleus is of considerable potential interest because iontophoretically applied 5-hydroxytryptamine (5-HT) has been purported to exert a presynaptic inhibitory effect on the optic nerve input to dLGN cells (Tebecis and Di Maria, 1972). This would confer a specific and unique role to this input with considerable functional implication. We have been unable to confirm this (Kemp et al., 1982); all our data point to the view that iontophoretically applied 5-HT, at all doses, exerts a direct postsynaptic inhibitory action on dLGN cells. Figure 5 illustrates that it is possible, with iontophoretically applied 5-HT, to depress excitatory effects elicited by pulses of ACh and D,L-homocysteic acid (DLH) without blocking the visual input, the converse of that which would be expected if the effect of 5-HT were primarily presynaptic.

These observations are consistent with those that Yoshida et al. (1984) obtained in the rat. They examined the effects of both iontophoretically applied 5-HT and electrical stimulation of the dorsal raphe nucleus. Their evidence favored only a postsynaptic action for both the inhibitory effects of raphe stimulation and the iontophoretic application of 5-HT. What is most interesting is that they observed that raphe stimulation inhibited relay cells, intrageniculate interneurons, and cells in the thalamic reticular nucleus. This suggests that the raphe input is capable of exerting a global disinhibitory influence, but once more this can be viewed as retaining the "balance" of the excitatory and inhibitory influences within the dLGN because, as the relay cell excitability is decreased, so is the magnitude of the attendant inhibitory mechanism.

Nonetheless, there is a clear distinction between the apparent actions of the serotonergic and cholinergic inputs. Trulson and Jacobs (1979), observing the correlation between activity in the dorsal raphe nucleus and the level of behavioral arousal, suggested that the raphe might act as a compensatory mechanism preventing hyperarousal, rather than playing a permissive role. This view would be in accord with the present evidence for the dLGN, as well as the body of literature supporting the view that 5-HT has an "inhibitory" effect on behavior.

There is good evidence for the view that activity of neurons in the locus coeruleus increases as the animal moves from the sleeping to the waking state and that, within the waking state, there are further increases during shifts from grooming type behavior to sensory-evoked, orienting responses (Aston-Jones and Bloom, 1981). Information concerning the precise nature of the action of

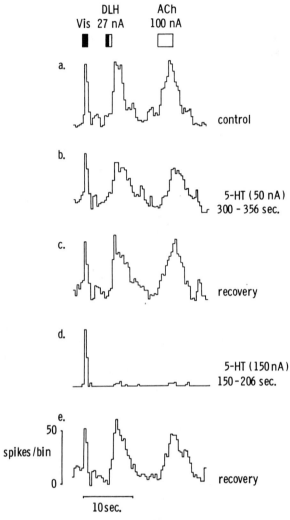

Figure 5. *The effect of 5-hydroxytryptamine (5-HT) on the responses of an on-center Y-type dLGN cell to visual stimulation (Vis) and pulsed iontophoretic application of drugs.* Visual stimulus is a spot of light flashed within the receptive field center. Durations of the flash and the drug pulses are indicated by the width of symbols above the records. Magnitudes of the drug ejection currents are indicated above the symbols. *a:* Control run with responses to visual stimulus, D,L-homocysteic acid (DLH), and ACh. *b:* Responses to the same sequence as the control but during iontophoretic application of 5-HT (50 nA) in the time period after the onset of application indicated to the *right* of the records. *c:* Recovery from 5-HT application. *d:* 5-HT application (150 nA). *e:* Recovery. These records are incompatible with the view that the primary effect of iontophoretically applied 5-HT is a presynaptic block of the optic nerve input. *Calibration bar* on the *abscissa* represents 10 sec; *calibration bar* on the *ordinate* represents the number of spikes/bin. Bin size, 400 msec; two trials. (From Kemp et al., 1982.)

340

norepinephrine in the dLGN is, however, rather contradictory. Although the original work on the cat suggested a predominance of inhibitory effects in response to iontophoretically applied norepinephrine (Curtis and Davies, 1962; Phillis et al., 1967b), several recent reports have emphasized facilitatory effects (Rogawski and Aghajanian, 1980; Kayama et al., 1982). These facilitatory effects are marked, appear to involve α-adrenoreceptors, and have been argued to be secondary to a disinhibitory mechanism (Nakai and Takaori, 1974; Jahr and Nicoll, 1982).

Kayama et al. (1982) report that both iontophoretically applied norepinephrine and locus coeruleus stimulation produce a particular pattern of effects in the dLGN that involves facilitation of perigeniculate cells and relay cells and inhibition of interneurons. This could support the possibility that the facilitatory effects of iontophoretically applied norepinephrine on relay cells are secondary to their inhibitory action on intrinsic inhibitory interneurons. We have examined this possibility by checking the effect of iontophoretically applied norepinephrine on the response of dLGN cells to a spot of light flashed within the field center and a larger spot covering both the center and the surround. From the preceding discussion, it is clear that disinhibition should invoke a relative increase in the magnitude of the response to the large spot with respect to the smaller one. This we did not see. In general, the facilitatory effects were smaller and less frequently seen (18/45 cells) than those reported by Kayama et al. (1982). An example of the facilitatory action of norepinephrine is given in Figure 6, which plots dose–response curves for the action of norepinephrine on the response to a large spot and a small spot. If anything, this suggests that the surround inhibition is enhanced rather than diminished. It must also be emphasized that in our hands the predominant effect of norepinephrine was inhibitory (25/45) at all dose ranges, and that for those cells facilitated, higher injection currents invariably produced inhibition. We also tested the effects of the α-adrenoreceptor agonists phenylephrine and methoxamine. Phenylephrine had exclusively inhibitory effects (8/8) at all dose levels, and methoxamine inhibited three cells tested and facilitated one. Our inhibitory and facilitatory effects did not correlate with any obvious physiological distinctions in terms of receptive field properties. It must be stressed, however, that the fact that norepinephrine exerts frequent inhibitory affects on dLGN cells in our experimental situation means that we cannot exclude the possibility of it inhibiting the inhibitory interneurons and producing disinhibition. The experimental point made here is that the facilitatory effects we observed secondary to the iontophoretic application of norepinephrine do not seem to be consequent upon disinhibition of those mechanisms enhancing center–surround interactions in the dLGN.

Despite certain inconsistencies in the available data, it is possible to delineate some clear distinctions in the nature of the action of the three modulatory inputs to the dLGN. The potential effects may be summarized as follows:

1. Cholinergic input: Strong excitation of relay cell activity and facilitation of intrinsic inhibitory processes relating to center–surround antagonism, but a reduction in the power of the perigeniculate inhibitory mechanisms proposed to control the dynamic range of the response.

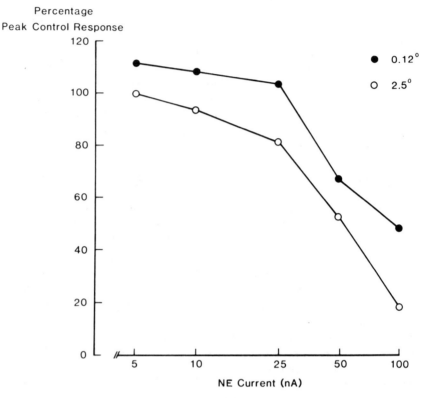

Figure 6. The effect of various doses of norepinephrine on the response of an on-center X-type dLGN cell. The *curves* plot the response to a center-located flashing spot (*filled circles*, 0.12°) and a larger spot covering the center and the surround (*open circles*, 2.5°) in the presence of increasing levels of iontophoretically applied norepinephrine; ejection current range, 5–100 nA. Each point is obtained from the average peak response to a 0.5-sec flash repeated for 25 trials, expressed as a percentage of the control response. While low doses of norepinephrine produce a slight facilitation of the response to the center spot, the response to the stimulus covering the center and the surround is unaffected at low doses and inhibited at higher doses. There is thus no evidence for a reduction in center–surround antagonism that would be commensurate with disinhibition.

2. Serotonergic input: Postsynaptic depression of relay cells and the intrinsic and perigeniculate inhibitory processes.

3. Noradrenergic input: Appears to exert strong inhibitory effects on relay cells but can also produce facilitation of responses. May enhance inhibition from perigeniculate cells and has the potential to depress the intrinsic inhibitory mechanism (although this latter effect does not seem to underlie the facilitation evoked by iontophoretically applied norepinephrine).

Even from this simplistic viewpoint, the actions of the inputs can be seen to be complementary, and a consideration of the data raises a number of important questions. Are there subtle variations in the behavioral circumstances that give rise to each input, or do they all indeed operate together, as the available data, albeit with superficial analysis, suggests? From another viewpoint, it is important to know whether there is an organization of the distribution of these terminals within the dLGN that is commensurate with a selective action in relation to cell bodies versus dendrites, proximal versus distal dendrites, or, for example, synaptic glomeruli versus other locations. These inputs may also modulate the access of the powerful corticofugal input (Wilson et al., 1984) to the dLGN relay cells. To date, studies of the influence of the corticofugal fibers have revealed surprisingly small effects, given the density of the projection. However, all the studies have been carried out in anesthetized preparations in which the output from the modulatory systems is likely to be minimal. It is not illogical to assume that arousal might correlate with an enhancement of the action of this feedback.

VISUAL CORTEX

The Neocortical Circuit

The complexity of the synaptic organization, together with the variation of detailed connectivity with cell type and lamination, makes it impossible, given the present state of knowledge, to construct any sensible circuit identifying the primary relationships underlying neocortical function. The available information enables a number of general conclusions to be drawn, however, and it is possible to identify some aspects of the functional circuitry relevant to the present account.

Visual cortical cells can be broadly subdivided into three categories: pyramidal cells, spiny stellates, and nonspiny or partially spined stellates (LeVay, 1973). The first two categories encompass the excitatory interneurons, with the spiny stellates restricted to layer IV, and the pyramidal cells occurring throughout layers II–VI. The last category encompasses the population of inhibitory inter- neurons and possibly some cells that must as yet be regarded as indeterminate in function (see below). The presumed inhibitory cells make Gray's type II synapses, which on morphological grounds are associated with inhibitory function (Gray, 1963; LeVay, 1973) and appear to be GABAergic (Iversen et al., 1971; Sillito, 1975a; Ribak, 1978; Somogyi et al., 1984). In contrast to the dLGN, inhibitory synapses, although present on dendrites, are most concentrated in the vicinity of the cell body and proximal dendrites.

A simplistic summary of the major components of the inhibitory input con- verging on a visual cortical cell is given in Figure 1. Inhibitory inputs to the cell body and proximal dendrites derive from short axon multipolar cells and basket cells (Peters and Fairén, 1978; Peters and Regidor, 1981; Martin et al., 1983, 1984). The initial segment (only in the case of pyramidal cells) receives a very specific axoaxonic input from chandelier cells (Somogyi, 1977). In addition, inputs to the distal parts of apical and basal dendrites derive from bitufted cells, basket cells, and possibly certain other cell types (Peters and Regidor, 1981; Somogyi and Cowey, 1981; Martin et al., 1983). A given basket cell may contact the soma, apical, and basal dendrites of a given pyramidal cell (Somogyi et al., 1983). Any given visual cortical cell is thus subject to a range of different GABAergic inhibitory influences deriving from neurons intrinsic to the visual cortex. Furthermore, the input from any particular type of cell derives from several such input cells, as in the case of the axoaxonic synapses, where several chandelier cells provide the input to the initial segment of a pyramidal cell. The differing patterns of dendritic and axonal arborization of the various types of inhibitory interneuron mean that they will integrate different types of input and in turn distribute it over different spatial domains. The logical consequence of this is that there is a range of distinct inhibitory circuits that must be presumed to generate different aspects of the response properties of visual cortical cells.

Not only are there several distinct sources for the inhibitory inputs converging on a visual cortical cell, but the locations contacted by these inhibitory inputs suggest that their potential influence on the cell's response properties is different. Recent evidence for both hippocampal and visual cortical pyramidal cells (Andersen et al., 1980; Alger and Nicoll, 1982a,b; Kemp, 1984) indicates that GABAergic synapses on the cell body exert a different action from those on apical dendrites. Synapses on the cell body produce the expected hyperpolarization, while those on apical dendrites cause a depolarization associated with an increased membrane conductance. Andersen et al. (1980) described the depolarizing effect as "discriminative inhibition," because by shunting currents in the vicinity of the inhibitory input it allows for a selective inhibitory influence on afferent excitatory inputs synapsing locally, while facilitating the effect of excitatory synapses at other locations in the dendritic tree. Thus, the dendritic inhibitory input must be regarded as potentially capable of gating out a specific component of the visual input.

However, the situation is rather more complex than it seems at first sight, and several additional factors should be borne in mind. The inhibitory synapses to the dendrites of visual cortical pyramidal cells may terminate on either dendritic shafts or dendritic spines (Somogyi et al., 1983). It seems likely that the significance of these two sites of termination may differ in terms of their potential influence on the excitatory input to the dendrites. A further comment is that GABA seems to exert two types of effect on dendrites: the depolarizing influence, just discussed, and a slower hyperpolarizing influence that is bicuculline-resistant and possibly mediated by $GABA_B$ receptors (Alger and Nicoll, 1982b; Nicoll and Newberry, 1984).

All this leads to the view that there may be several functionally distinct components to the inhibitory influence on dendrites, and that the concept of "discriminative inhibition" derives from data that potentially subsume all of these. An additional specific type of control is likely to derive from the chandelier cell input to the initial segment of pyramidal cells. The initial segment of the axon is considered to be the site for the initiation of the action potential (Spencer and Kandel, 1961), and hence the chandelier synapses to this zone must have the capability for a preemptive regulation of target cell activity. This in turn suggests that the chandelier control of pyramidal cells should mediate a virtually invariant facet of their visual response profile. The pyramidal cell would not respond in the stimulus circumstances precipitating a coherent chandelier cell input, and it would seem that the control would be strongly resistant to the "opposing" effects of an increase in the power of the excitatory drive (e.g., following an increase in stimulus contrast) or of overall cell excitability. Conversely, there is a clear basis for a graded interaction between excitatory and inhibitory inputs because, to give one example, visual cortical cells receive inhibitory inputs even when responding to an optimal stimulus (Creutzfeldt et al., 1974; Sillito, 1975a,b, 1979). This might be inferred to involve primarily those inhibitory inputs converging on the soma and proximal dendritic shafts. In summary, the evidence seems to favor three broad types of inhibitory influences: local discriminatory, preemptive, and graded interactive. The sources of these may be varied, as discussed in the preceding paragraph.

The inhibitory components of the neocortical circuit are an integral part of a set of interactions that includes a complex series of excitatory interconnections that feed between the different laminae of the cortex and the dLGN. These excitatory interconnections include: the projection of the dLGN to layer IV; a projection from layer IV to layers II and III; a projection from layers II and III to layer V; a projection from layer V to layer VI and to layers II and III; and a projection from layer VI to layer IV and to the dLGN (Gilbert and Wiesel, 1979, 1983; Lund et al., 1979; Martin, 1984). It is clear that each lamina is, directly or indirectly, intimately interconnected with all levels of the geniculocortical axis. The functional relevance of the patterns of connectivity is not clear despite the presence of surprisingly dense projections, as in the case of the corticogeniculate pathway. The issue is further complicated by the fact that there is an input from the A-laminae of the dLGN to the upper part of layer VI as well as to layer IV, and that the C-laminae of the dLGN project to layer I and the layer III–IV and layer IV–V border regions (LeVay and Gilbert, 1976).

Given the initial segregation of the inputs from X-, Y-, and W-cells in this projection (e.g., Ferster and LeVay, 1978; Martin and Whitteridge, 1984), it is apparent that any simple linear hierarchy is untenable. Cells in all laminae (but not all cells) seem to get a direct geniculate input (e.g., Martin and Whitteridge, 1984) and there is, for example, an apparently remarkable independence of the properties of cells in layers II, III, and part of V from the input from layer IV (Malpeli, 1983). There is obviously a potential for massive positive feedback within the system, and it seems that this must be balanced by the inhibitory components of the circuit. It needs to be emphasized that, because of the interconnectivity between the different levels of the system, the properties of each element have to be judged in terms of the overall circuit operation, with the implication that the explanation of the perturbations produced by local drug application may lie partly in terms of the changes produced in this.

There is still relatively little information available regarding the excitatory neurotransmitters operating in the visual cortex. It does seem likely that the layer VI corticogeniculate cells may utilize glutamate or aspartate, with the implication that their collaterals arborizing in layer IV will also involve one of these excitatory amino acids (Baughman and Gilbert, 1980, 1981). This view is consistent with evidence for other corticothalamic projections and for the corticostriatal projection (Kim et al., 1977; Rowlands and Roberts, 1980; Streit, 1980; Fonnum et al., 1981; Young et al., 1981; Hassler et al., 1982; Rustioni et al., 1982). There is also evidence indicating that some thalamocortical fibers may utilize glutamate or aspartate (Ottersen et al., 1983), although there are no specific observations for the visual system. Consequently, with the exception of the layer VI pyramidal cells, there is no clue as to the excitatory neurotransmitters mediating the extensive interactions that involve all other pyramidal cell types and various types of spiny stellate cells.

In contrast to the paucity of information available for pyramidal cells and spiny stellates, there is a relative abundance of data regarding the presence of peptides in the nonspiny and partially spiny cell groups. There is good evidence from immunocytochemical procedures to support the presence of VIP, SSt, cholecystokinin (CCK), and neuropeptide Y (NPY) in this cell group (McDonald et al., 1982a,b,c; Morrison et al., 1983; Hendry et al., 1984a). It should be emphasized that some of the peptides have been shown to be present in synaptosomes and released in a calcium-dependent fashion (Giachetti et al., 1977; Berelowitz et al., 1978; Iversen et al., 1978). To date, there is no reason to believe that this will not hold for all. As discussed above, the partially spined and nonspiny cell group encompasses the GABAergic inhibitory interneurons, and some of the peptides (CCK, SSt, and NPY) are colocalized with glutamic acid decarboxylase (GAD) in certain cells (Hendry et al., 1984a). However, it should be stressed that not all the GAD-positive cells contain peptides, and that in particular two morphologically distinct groups, the chandelier cells and basket cells, do not appear to contain peptides. Thus, the peptides seem to be restricted to the bipolar, bitufted, and multipolar cells, all of which except for the bipolar cells are presumed to be GABAergic. Furthermore, each peptide has a fairly distinct distribution within the population of bipolar, bitufted, and multipolar cells. Thus, for example, SSt is found in multipolar and bitufted cells that are concentrated in two bands, lying in layers II and III, and layers V and VI (McDonald et al., 1982b; Morrison et al., 1983). It seems likely that all these cells are also immunoreactive to NPY and GAD (Hendry et al., 1984a). VIP immunoreactivity is largely restricted to a population of bipolar cells influencing the laminae I–IV region (Fuxe et al., 1977; McDonald et al., 1982a; Morrison et al., 1984), and at least in the rat seems to be coexistent with ACh (Eckenstein and Baughman, 1984). These bipolar cells appear to make type I, asymmetric synapses with putative excitatory function (Peters and Kimerer, 1981). Of particular interest is evidence suggesting that VIP cells may also innervate cortical blood vessels and that, although relatively sparsely distributed, the VIP neurons are arranged in a uniform but random fashion throughout the cortex, so that on average each VIP cell can be considered to innervate a 30-μm radius column of cortex through laminae I–IV. The CCK-staining cells appear to represent a subpopulation of cells that is distinct from that of the other three peptides discussed above, in terms of both cells stained and the site of termination of the synapses (Hendry et al., 1983, 1984a,b). These are GAD-immunoreactive, bitufted, and multipolar cells in layers II and III, horizontal and multipolar cells in layer I, and small multipolar cells in layers V and VI (McDonald et al., 1982b; Peters et al., 1983; Hendry et al., 1984a,b).

There is a further small group of CCK-containing bipolar cells in laminae II–IV that may make some contacts on blood vessels, as do some VIP cells (Hendry et al., 1983). In addition, the visual cortex receives three extrinsic "nonspecific" modulatory inputs. These comprise a cholinergic input from nucleus basalis of Meynert (Henderson, 1981; Mesulam et al., 1983a,b; Price and Stern, 1983; Saper, 1984), a serotonergic input from the dorsal and median raphe nuclei (Moore et al., 1978; Lidov et al., 1980), and a noradrenergic projection from the locus coeruleus (Ungerstedt, 1971; Levitt and Moore, 1978).

GABAergic Processes

The increased complexity of the neocortical circuitry, with respect to that of the dLGN, is reflected in the much more complex stimulus requirements exhibited by visual cortical cells. As the anatomical data suggest, it does appear that inhibitory interneurons play a central role in structuring visual response properties. The intracellular data from Creutzfeldt's group has clearly demonstrated that visual stimuli, even the optimal stimulus for a given cell, generate inhibitory inputs. These appear to relate to specific visual response properties such as directional and orientation selectivity (Creutzfeldt and Ito, 1968; Creutzfeldt et al., 1974). Blockade of the GABAergic inhibitory inputs to a visual cortical cell by the iontophoretic application of bicuculline provides a demonstration of what happens to the response properties in the absence of the inhibitory control. In essence, there is an increase in response magnitude and a reduction or loss of the original receptive field selectivity (Sillito, 1974a,b, 1975a,b, 1977, 1979; Sillito et al., 1980a,b). Simple cells can lose direction selectivity, orientation selectivity, and the segregation of the receptive field into separate on and off subdivisions. Complex cells also show large changes in receptive field structure but, for example, only half the population loses orientation selectivity while the other half, although exhibiting a marked reduction in orientation tuning, retains some bias to the original optimum.

Examples of the effect of iontophoretically applied bicuculline on the orientation and directional selectivity of visual cortical cells are given in the polar tuning diagrams of Figure 7 for cells before and during drug application. These shifts in response properties are dramatic, and demonstrate clearly the importance of GABAergic processes to the generation of orientation and directional selectivity, and hence to the maintenance of the functional subdivision of the cortex into orientation columns. The significance of inhibitory mechanisms to orientation columns raises the question of whether ocular dominance columns are in any way similarly dependent. An initial consideration of the matter suggests that this is unlikely to be the case because, unlike the situation for orientation columns, there is clear evidence for a specific organization of the excitatory input to the cortex underlying the pattern of ocular dominance columns. Thus, ocular dominance columns seem to be established by the segregation of the geniculate afferents representing the two eyes in layer IV (Hubel and Wiesel, 1972; LeVay et al., 1978; Schatz and Stryker, 1978). However, during bicuculline-induced inhibitory blockade, 50% of the cells showing a preference to one eye exhibit a shift in dominance toward the other (Sillito et al., 1980a). As shown in Figure 8, this includes some cells normally dominated exclusively by one eye becoming binocularly driven, with a small but significant number equally driven by both.

Hence, although it is clear that the distribution of geniculate afferents in layer IV underlies the ocular dominance columns, a significant component of their functional integrity derives from the operation of intracortical inhibitory processes. It is, however, important to be cautious in viewing this finding. Ocular dominance per se is probably not an index of a specific functional process in the visual system, but an epiphenomenon of the neural organization underlying stereopsis. From the work of Poggio and Fischer (1977) and others, it is far from clear that the monocular testing routinely used in assessing ocular dominance will reveal the true nature of the binocular influences acting on a given cortical cell. The application of bicuculline is thus perhaps best seen as removing the influence of an inhibitory gate that provides a specific control over the conditions in which binocular interaction occurs. It relates to stereopsis, which is known to involve

Normal   With Nmb

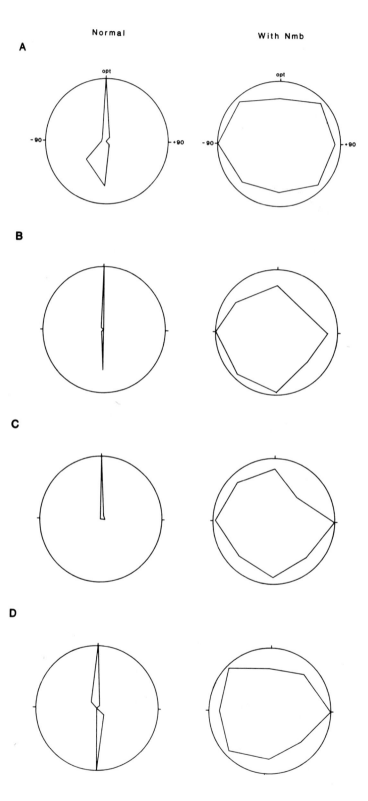

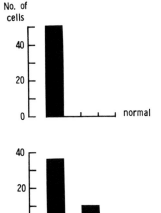

No. of
cells

Figure 8.   *Effect of an inhibitory blockade on the ocular dominance of cells normally dominated exclusively by one eye.* Cells were classified into seven ocular dominance groups after Hubel and Wiesel (1962), with group one and group seven cells being exclusively driven by either the contralateral or ipsilateral eye, respectively, and group four cells being equally driven by both. During application of the GABA antagonist N-methyl-bicuculline, a small but significant proportion of the cells develop a binocular input.

inhibitory processes, rather than to the more artificial concept of ocular dominance columns.

A detailed review of the contributions of GABAergic inhibitory processes to visual cortical organization is given elsewhere (Sillito, 1984), but I would like to emphasize several points in the present context. In any given cell, and particularly in the case of complex cells and superficial layer end-stopped cells (Sillito, 1975b, 1977, 1979; Sillito and Versiani, 1977; Sillito et al., 1980a), the various facets of receptive field structure are not equally susceptible to inhibitory blockade. Thus, ocular dominance, directional selectivity, orientation selectivity, and length preference may be affected to quite different extents. These observations stand in the face of a long period of bicuculline application and clear pharmacological block of GABA action, and suggest that for different cells the various components of the receptive field structure are dependent on different synaptic processes. It seems likely that in our experimental situation, the iontophoretically applied bicuculline should be potentially capable of reaching all the inhibitory synapses in the vicinity of the cell body and initial segment but not those, for example, on upper portions of the apical dendrites of layer V pyramidal cells. Consequently, the fact that one component of the receptive field organization is resistant to the application of bicuculline could reflect either that this component is dependent on remote inhibitory synapses, or that this property is determined by the excitatory

---

Figure 7.   *The effect of an inhibitory blockade on the orientation and directional tuning of simple cells (A, B, C) and a complex cell (D).* The polar diagrams show the normalized tuning profiles for averaged responses (assessed from peak frequency over 25 trials) to the "round the clock" range of testing orientations indicated. Response magnitude as a percentage of the maximum response for each orientation tested is represented by the distance of the points from the center. The maximum response in each situation is denoted by the point in contact with the edge of the circle. Diagrams on the *left* show the normal tuning characteristics; those on the *right* show the tuning characteristics during the iontophoretic application of the GABA antagonist Nmb. *Calibration marks* show the "normal" optimal orientation of the cell (opt), with orientation varying in a clockwise (+) and counterclockwise (−) direction to this.

input. It is relevant to note in this context that the orientation selectivity of simple cells was reduced but not eliminated by the iontophoretic application of bicuculline (Sillito, 1975b), but was eliminated by the more potent N-methyl-bicuculline (Sillito et al., 1980b), in agreement with the observations of Tsumoto et al. (1979). Given that both types of the antagonist were effective in eliminating the directional selectivity of simple cells, this raises the possibility of two components of the inhibitory process underlying simple cell orientation tuning, with one being more vulnerable than the other to inhibitory blockade.

The extent of the involvement of GABAergic inhibitory processes in the generation of orientation selectivity is a critical issue in the ongoing debate regarding the functional organization of the visual cortex. I will thus discuss this facet of the data summarized above in greater detail. The original model of visual cortical organization put forward by Hubel and Wiesel (1962) was centered around the view that simple cell orientation selectivity is established by the linear elongation of the spatial array of the receptive fields of geniculate afferents converging on single simple cells in layer IV. Once established in this way, discretely organized excitatory connections sustained the selectivity established in layer IV. These carefully formulated and elegant suggestions guided the approach to the visual cortex for the next two decades but, as is almost inevitable for any model formulated early in the development of a field, the detailed basis has been challenged by a range of observations.

First, there is the nature of the mechanisms establishing orientation selectivity at the level of the simple cell. The pharmacological data (Tsumoto et al., 1979; Sillito et al., 1980b) suggest that simple cells have access to a non-orientation-specific excitatory input, because they lose orientation selectivity during inhibitory blockade. Moreover, the extent of the response area on the peristimulus time histogram, delineated as the testing bar moves over the receptive field during inhibitory blockade, suggests that the dimensions of the excitatory discharge zone of the receptive field are similar, in directions parallel to and orthogonal to the optimal orientation (Sillito et al., 1980b). This is not compatible with the elongated field required by Hubel and Wiesel's model. The suggestion that the excitatory discharge zones of simple cell fields are more round than elongated receives support from a range of neurophysiological data, including those from intracellular studies (Creutzfeldt and Ito, 1968; Creutzfeldt et al., 1974; Schiller et al., 1976; Lee et al., 1977; Heggelund, 1981a).

The apparent elongation of center and flanks in the simple cell field can be adequately explained by overlapping but acentric, circular, inhibitory and excitatory zones, without assuming an elongated spatial array in geniculate afferent input (Heggelund, 1981a). There are thus two reasons for questioning the nature of the mechanism determining simple cell orientation selectivity: the shape of the excitatory discharge zone and the loss of orientation selectivity during inhibitory blockade. If orientation selectivity is dependent on GABAergic inhibitory processes, this in turn requires an asymmetry in either the organization of the inhibitory mechanism or the spatial relationship of the inhibitory field to the excitatory field. The partially shifted overlap seen in the inhibitory and excitatory components of simple-type cell receptive fields (Heggelund, 1981a; Albus and Wolf, 1984) certainly provides the spatial asymmetry and could constitute the basis for an orientation-tuned field (Sillito, 1984, 1985). A second-stage lateral interaction between these initial orientation filters would provide further refinement of the tuning. (These ideas are summarized in Figure 9, which is intended only as a concept diagram.)

The point at issue here is that the synaptic mechanisms required to generate orientation selectivity are well within the known complexity of the cortical circuitry and can, in essence, be regarded as variants of a simple, laterally directed, inhibitory mechanism. Furthermore, Heggelund's (1981a; Heggelund et al., 1983)

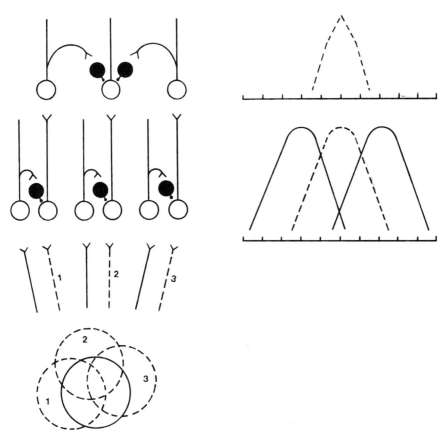

Figure 9. *Concept diagram illustrating a simple two-stage process for generating orientation selectivity from lateral inhibitory interactions.* The three facilitatory fields (*dashed circles*) overlap with a central inhibitory focus (*solid line circle*). The first crude level of orientation tuning represented by the *lower three tuning curves* derives from the interaction between the inhibitory input driven from the central focus and the respective facilitatory inputs from the three overlapping regions. The degree of spatial separation in the zones is exaggerated here for diagrammatic convenience; the overlap would actually need to be greater to generate the *curves* shown on the *right*. A second-stage lateral interaction between the broadly determined orientation channels establishes a higher level of resolution. Although this two-stage process is shown as operating in a linear sequence, the second stage could be reflected to the first to further enhance the tuning. For example, positive feedback from the second-stage central channel to its excitatory input, together with inhibitory feedback from the other two second-stage channels, would greatly improve resolution.

detailed quantitative analysis of the spatial disposition of the inhibitory and excitatory components of the simple cell receptive field reveals an organization that is compatible with that which would be theoretically required to provide the asymmetry necessary for orientation tuning and the apparent elongation of the receptive field. These points notwithstanding, it is also clear that a very small initial asymmetry in the orientation tuning of the excitatory input should, if fed into a system in which there were laterally directed interactions between adjacent cells, precipitate orientation-tuned fields. This view needs to be considered because of the data indicating that retinal ganglion cells have orientation-biased receptive fields grouped in a pattern showing a radial disposition with respect to the area centralis (Levick and Thibos, 1982). This seems to be reflected in a similar overrepresentation of radial orientations in the dLGN (Vidyasagar and Urbas, 1982) and striate cortex (Leventhal, 1983). It is important to note that the "orientation selectivity" of retinal ganglion cells is residual in comparison with that of a typical simple cell (see Figure 7A–C).

This distinction in tuning properties is further emphasized by the nature of the stimuli needed to best reveal this minimal orientation tuning of dLGN cells, for which a 15° bar seems to be necessary (e.g., Vidyasagar and Urbas, 1982). This constrasts with the fact that a 2° bar will reveal sharp orientation tuning in simple cells (e.g., Henry et al., 1974). A 2° bar reveals no significant orientation tuning in dLGN cells (B. P. Choudhury and A. M. Sillito, unpublished observations), and hence it would seem that the orientation bias established in the retina cannot be a primary determinant of simple cell orientation selectivity under these conditions. It may, however, through a relatively subtle effect that is detectable across the population of inputs, even for a 2° bar, generate the necessary asymmetry in the inhibitory circuit. Alternatively, as an early extant asymmetry in the excitatory input, it could exert an important developmental influence on the pattern of formation of the synaptic circuits delineating orientation columns in early life. Whatever applies, the suggestion is that a central component of the circuits underlying orientation selectivity involves specific patterns of inhibitory influence. Almost paradoxically, Vidyasagar (1984) has recently reported that iontophoretic application of bicuculline eliminates the orientation tuning of dLGN cells, suggesting that, even at this level, the retinal bias is in some way lost in the direct excitatory coupling of retinal input to relay cells, but translated through the inhibitory system. This is consistent with the arguments outlined above for the translation of the bias into the cortex via the inhibitory circuits.

Once orientation selectivity is established in layer IV simple cells, is it carried over to other cells in the same column by the excitatory input from the simple cells? The answer appears to be that in some cases it may occur but in other cases it does not. First, it is clear both that complex cells can receive direct geniculate input (e.g., Martin and Whitteridge, 1984), and that complex cells can be well driven by stimuli that either do not affect simple cells or even inhibit them (Hammond and Mackay, 1975). Furthermore, the work of Malpeli (1983) shows that during reversible block of the A-laminae of the dLGN, cells in layers II, III, and V can have apparently normal receptive fields at a time when cells in layer IV are unresponsive. The obvious implication of this is that the input from the C-laminae can drive cells in layers II, III, and V adequately (that is, as judged by conventional receptive field tests), and that the machinery for establishing directional and orientational selectivity is present outside layer IV. With the proviso that the excitatory and inhibitory components of the field have input from both on- and off-center mechanisms, complex cell fields can be described with the same model of overlapping but acentric zones as that used for simple cells (Heggelund, 1981b). Also as stated above, iontophoretically induced inhibitory blockade of complex cells results in half the population losing their orientation selectivity (Sillito, 1979). This indicates that they do not receive an orientation-specific excitatory input, and that their selectivity is generated by inhibitory inputs acting at the level of the cell in question. This is consistent with the data of Malpeli. On the other hand, the remainder of the complex cell population, although showing a broadening of its tuning, retains an overall bias to the original optimum during inhibitory blockade (Sillito, 1979).

This latter finding could be consistent with a broadly orientation-tuned input from layer IV, but the input could equally well derive from cells outside layer IV. A problem with the finding is that it cannot automatically be assumed that all the inhibitory synapses were blocked, since it is plausible that in these cases the synapses gating the primary excitatory drive to generate orientation selectivity were located distally on dendrites. Taken altogether, the available evidence raises the possibility that orientation selectivity could be generated *de novo* in each lamina. Alternatively, it could be established in layers III or II. The mosaic of cytochrome oxidase patches containing non-orientation-specific cells in laminae II and III of the monkey visual cortex appears to have a special relationship to the columnar structure (Horton and Hubel, 1981; Hubel and Livingston, 1981, 1982) and, given the association of cytochrome oxidase with GAD (Hendrickson et al., 1981), the patches are likely to contain a high density of inhibitory inter-neurons or terminals. Although these patches are not so well developed in the cat, their existence in the monkey does raise the possibility that synaptic processes significant to the columnar structure are established in layers II and III and not just in layer IV, as originally envisaged.

There are persuasive reasons for using an inhibitory process to maintain a common property through a column. There is a direct geniculate excitatory input to the cortex in layers I, III–IV, IVab, IVc, IV–V, and VI originating from the X-, Y-, and W-afferents. If excitatory connections formed the basis of the orientation column, these would have to be organized in a fashion that maintained the asymmetry of input established for lamina IV through all the relevant laminae. Furthermore, many pyramidal cells are in a position to sample information through a number of layers, including a mixture of direct geniculate and intracortical excitatory connections. Were the orientation bias to be established for each cell by the excitatory network, these would all have to be coherent in the orientation domain. Conversely, a common inhibitory process established, for example, in layer III and directed through the other layers could restrict the response of all the cells in a column to a common range of orientations and at the same time allow them to access a wide range of different excitatory inputs.

It is worth remembering that, even in layer IV, the vast majority of the excitatory input to spiny stellate cells derives from intracortical sources and not geniculate afferents. Presumably, the columnar structure reflects the fact that there is an advantage to be gained from maintaining one domain of coherence in the visual response properties of cells, while allowing for independent operation in other domains. The diversity of GABAergic inhibitory influences seen to reach individual cortical cells must then reflect the combined operation of processes relating to the columnar structures (e.g., orientation and ocular dominance), and other facets of receptive field properties that are independent of this. For example, moving noise analysis of the receptive fields of complex cells argues strongly for an independence of the processes underlying orientation and directional selectivity (Hammond, 1981), a view supported by a range of other findings (e.g., Sillito, 1975b, 1979; Ganz and Felder, 1984).

A final point to make is that maintaining the coherence of orientation columns by an inhibitory mechanism makes the tuning accessible to stimulus context-dependent modification. That is, it could be changed by specific patterns of intracortical interaction established by complex stimulus conditions. The flexibility postulated here is secondary to the fact that the activity of the inhibitory interneurons governing the orientation selectivity would in turn be dependent upon the integration of the stimulus-driven influences converging on them. This possibility would be less likely if orientation selectivity were a "hard-wired" phenomenon, secondary to rigid patterns of excitatory connectivity established during early development.

The Role of the Neuropeptides

Given that the available evidence suggests that the peptides in the visual cortex may be largely colocalized with GAD-immunoreactive cells (Hendry et al., 1984a), or in the case of VIP with ACh (Eckenstein and Baughman, 1984), it seems plausible that their functional significance may be seen in terms of a modulation of the action of the "conventional neurotransmitters" found in these cells, as discussed for GABA and SSt in the dLGN. It is not, however, clear that the real significance of these effects should necessarily be reflected in a direct modulation of some aspects of the "fast" processes mediating stimulus-specific responses. In the case of the VIP-containing cells, it is possible that they have a role in regulating cortical blood flow (Lee et al., 1984) and energy metabolism via the effect of VIP on cAMP (Magistretti et al., 1981). Thus, evaluation of the effects of these peptides and their "cotransmitters" on the responses of visual cortical cells needs to take account of the possibility of other modes of action.

The presently available data regarding the effects of SSt in the nervous system do not provide any clear evidence regarding its functional significance. It has been reported to have both facilitatory and inhibitory effects (Renaud et al., 1975; Ioffe et al., 1978; Dodd and Kelly, 1981; Pittman and Siggins, 1981) and to show marked tachyphylaxis with unusual dose–response curves (Delfs and Dichter, 1983). In the visual cortex, iontophoretic application of SSt-14 exerted excitatory and inhibitory effects on approximately equal numbers of cells (Salt and Sillito, 1984). In some cases, the effects were marked, as in Figure 10, where application of SSt-14 with a 40-nA current produced a dramatic enhancement of the visual response without notably affecting the background discharge level or the cell's directional selectivity. In other cases, equally pronounced inhibitory effects were seen. One immediate comment is that the effects on visual responses provide no evidence for a modulation of the effect of visually evoked GABAergic inputs, such as those underlying directional selectivity (Sillito, 1977), nor could

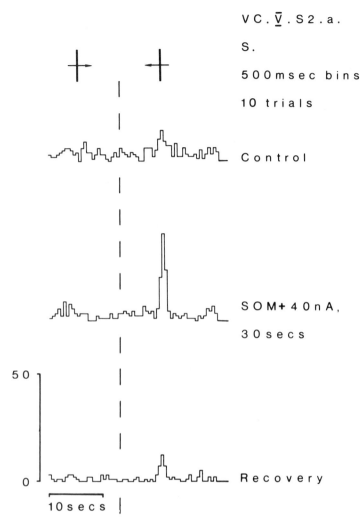

Figure 10. *Facilitatory action of somatostatin (SOM = SSt) on the responses of a single cell.* PSTHs show response of the cell to an optimally oriented bar passing forward and backward over the receptive field. Iontophoretic application of SSt causes a marked enhancement of the directionally selective response of this cell, without causing any significant increase in resting discharge level. Bin size, 500 msec; 10 trials. *Vertical calibration bar* corresponds to 0–50 counts/bin.

we obtain evidence for a modulation of the effect of iontophoretically applied GABA, other than that which would be expected to follow from a simple additive or subtractive interaction with the facilitatory and inhibitory effects elicited by SSt itself.

Following the suggestion by Bloom et al. (this volume) that SSt might influence the response to ACh, we also checked the action of SSt on the facilitatory effect of ACh on visual cortical cells but, as for GABA, we could detect no interaction beyond that which would be predicted from the direct effect of SSt. Although the facilitatory and inhibitory effects of SSt in the visual cortex did not correlate with the classification into the simple–complex groupings (Salt and Sillito, 1984), as these two groups encompass a wide range of morphologically distinct cell types it is possible that the effects of SSt may still correlate with particular morphologically (as opposed to visually) defined cell groups. Alternatively, if there are two distinct populations of SSt receptors (Delfs and Dichter, 1983; Reubi, 1984), as seems possible, the precise effects elicited may reflect the particular location of the electrode with respect to them.

The absence of any obvious modulation of GABAergic processes is puzzling. However, several additional factors have to be taken into account when interpreting this finding. First, it must be noted that it seems unlikely that the primary function of SSt would be to modulate the GABAergic processes mediated by basket cells and chandelier cells, because SSt is not contained in these cells (Hendry et al., 1984a). Second, the fact that synapses from cells in the bitufted and multipolar group contact dendrites (as well as cell bodies) raises the possibility that SSt must be judged to potentially interact with the depolarizing action exerted by GABA on dendrites. If this is the case, the excitatory "face" of SSt might reflect on action on dendrites that potentiates the depolarizing action of GABA and thus enhances the local discriminatory inhibition, while also increasing the cell's overall responsiveness to its dendritic input (Andersen et al., 1980) or even initiating a depolarization of a magnitude appropriate to a direct excitation. As discussed above, it is not yet clear which aspects of visual response properties reflect the action of GABAergic synapses on dendrites. These may exert a more subtle influence than those analyzed so far. It is tempting to speculate that the polarity of the SSt effect might reflect interaction with populations of receptors associated with SSt/GABAergic terminals either on cell bodies or dendrites, following the polarity of the action of GABA (with the caveat that precise electrode location might then determine the effect which dominates). Another possibility is that SSt modulates the action of the bicuculline-resistant hyperpolarization associated with the GABA$_B$ receptor. There is no available evidence concerning the likely role of the GABA$_B$ receptor in relation to the functional properties of visual cortical cells. Finally, recent evidence for the colocalization of NPY, SSt, and GAD (Hendry et al., 1984a) raises the possibility that the real significance of these peptides will only be seen when SSt, NPY, and GABA are applied together.

In contrast to SSt, the available evidence for CCK, which derives from studies in neocortical and hippocampal slices, suggests that it exerts only excitatory effects (Phillis and Kirkpatrick, 1980; Dodd and Kelly, 1981). The available evidence for the visual cortex shows CCK to be relatively ineffective in modifying the responses of visual cortical cells and where it is effective, as is the case for SSt, to exert either facilitatory or inhibitory effects (Grieve et al., 1985b). Once more, knowing the specific synaptic targets of the CCK-containing cells would strongly influence our interpretation of the way it might interact with GABA. It is clearly important to attempt to identify the specific patterns of distribution of SSt and CCK receptors on the dendrites and cell bodies of visual cortical cells. In the case of VIP, bipolar cells (the only cells showing immunoreactivity to VIP in the cortex) are considered to make type I synapses, and VIP is reported to exert an excitatory effect in the neocortex *in vivo* (Phillis et al., 1978; Phillis and Kirkpatrick, 1980) and in *in vitro* hippocampal slices (Dodd et al., 1979).

Recently, we have examined the effects of VIP and ACh on visual cortical cells (Grieve et al., 1985a,b). Both VIP and ACh, when iontophoretically applied to simple, complex, and special complex cells, were observed to facilitate the visual responses in a qualitatively similar fashion; this type of facilitation is discussed in detail below for ACh. Moreover, we observed summation between the actions of VIP and ACh when applied simultaneously to some cells. The available data is consistent with the view that the VIP bipolar cells may be involved in a tripartite action on cortical function via a facilitation of cell responsiveness and signal-to-noise level, an increase in cortical metabolism (Magistretti et al., 1981), and an increase in blood flow (Lee et al., 1984).

Extrinsic Modulation of Cortical Function

The cholinergic input to the visual cortex, as that to the dLGN, has been associated with mediating the effects of nonspecific arousal (Spehlman, 1971; Singer, 1979). However, most investigators have observed that only about 20% of cells in the cortex are affected by iontophoretically applied ACh (Spehlman, 1971; Spehlman et al., 1971; Wallingford et al., 1973). This contrasts with our data obtained by evaluating the effects of iontophoretically applied ACh on the visually driven responses of visual cortical cells (Sillito and Kemp, 1983b). We observed that 92% of the cells showed a modification of their response during the application of ACh. These included a group of 31% of the cells in which responses were depressed and a group of 61% of the cells in which responses were facilitated. The cells showing a depression of response were all located in the laminae III–IV region, as shown in Figure 11, raising the possibility that they may constitute a specific subgroup of visual cortical cells. Cells facilitated by ACh were found throughout all cortical layers (Figure 11).

In contrast to the effects seen in the dLGN, the facilitatory effects of ACh did not involve an obvious direct excitation of the cell with increased resting discharge, but rather an enhancement of the visually driven response. This enhancement occurred without any reduction in response selectivity and often appeared to improve it, because of the large increases in response magnitude to optimal stimuli. This is illustrated in Figure 12, which shows the response of a directionally selective simple cell to an optimally oriented bar moving over the receptive field. Iontophoretic application of ACh caused a large increase in the response to the effective direction without changing background activity. This contrasts with the effect of inhibitory blockade produced by iontophoretic application of N-methyl-bicuculline, which caused an increase in background activity and a loss of directional selectivity despite the fact that the peak response in the originally effective direction was less enhanced than it was during ACh application. The effect of ACh on the orientation and length tuning of a complex cell is documented in Figure 13. This once more emphasizes the enhancement of the response magnitude without any diminution of the tuning properties. The facilitatory effects of ACh are most parsimoniously explained by its known action on potassium channels in cortical cells (Krnjević et al., 1971; Benardo and Prince, 1982; Halliwell and Adams, 1982). It seems that it decreases the potassium conductance in relation to the voltage-dependent channel underlying the M-current and the calcium-dependent channel, the net effect being an increase in the tendency of

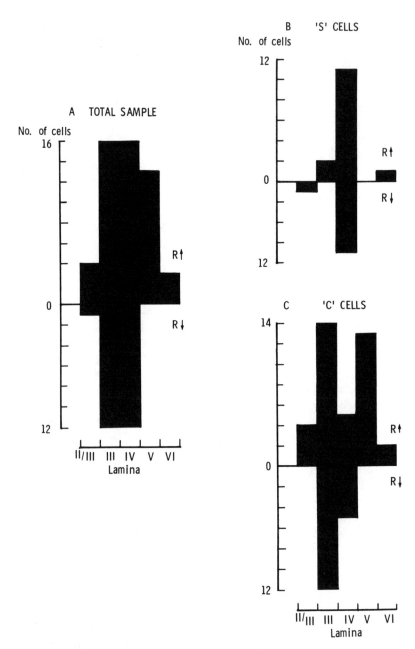

Figure 11. *Laminar distribution in the striate cortex of cells influenced by iontophoretically applied ACh.* R↑ responses were facilitated by ACh. R↓ responses were depressed by ACh. *A*: Total sample. *B*: Simple cells only. *C*: Complex cells only. (From Sillito and Kemp, 1983b.)

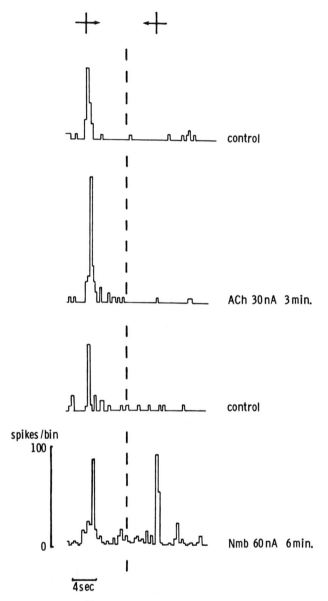

spikes/bin
100

0

4 sec

control

ACh 30 nA 3 min.

control

Nmb 60 nA 6 min.

Figure 12. *Cholinergic modulation of the response of a directionally selective simple cell.* The PSTHs show the response to motion of an optimally oriented bar of light. Shown in sequence as labeled are: A control response; the effect of ACh applied with a 30-nA ejecting current starting 3 min before the record was taken; a control for recovery; the effect of an inhibitory blockade induced by the GABA antagonist N-methyl-bicuculline, applied with a 60-nA ejecting current starting 6 min before the test. Note that the application of ACh caused a marked facilitation of the response of the cell to its preferred direction of motion and had no effect on resting discharge. An inhibitory blockade, on the other hand, results in the appearance of a response to the opposite direction of motion, a smaller enhancement of the original preferred response, and a notable increase in background activity. Bin size, 400 msec; five trials. *Vertical calibration bar* corresponds to 0–100 counts/bin. (From Sillito and Kemp, 1983b.)

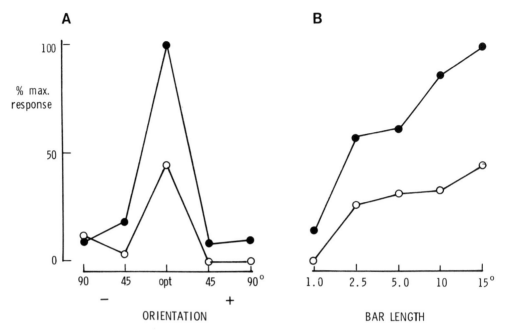

Figure 13. *Cholinergic modulation of the orientation and length tuning of a layer VI complex cell.* Responses are expressed as the percentage of maximum response, assessed from the peak frequency averaged over 10 trials. *Open circles* represent control responses; *filled circles* represent responses during the application of ACh with an 80-nA ejecting current. A: Orientation tuning; orientation shown in degrees counterclockwise (−) and clockwise (+) to the optimal. B: Length tuning assessed for response to the preferred direction of motion at optimal orientation. (From Sillito and Kemp, 1983b.)

cells to fire repetitively in response to a depolarizing input, without much direct depolarization in the absence of such an input. This is in essence exactly what we appear to have observed: an increase in responsiveness to previously effective depolarizing inputs.

It is also possible that other effects of ACh include an action on presynaptic transmitter release (Rovira et al., 1983) and even a modulation of dendritic length constants secondary to the effect on potassium conductance (Singer, 1979), but these do not seem to be necessary to explain our observations. We have no evidence to favor the view that ACh achieves an enhancement of responsiveness via a disinhibitory influence. In fact, as for the dLGN, the facilitatory effects of ACh in the cortex compare well with the observations of Livingstone and Hubel (1981) on the visual responses of cortical cells in cats passing from the sleeping to the waking state. It seems likely that the cholinergic input to the cortex could mediate some of the effects of arousal. Assuming that the stimulus selectivity of visual cortical cells has something to do with visual perception, it is appropriate that the stimulus-selective responses should be enhanced during arousal. Moreover, following evidence for the topological organization of the projection from the region of the nucleus basalis of Meynert (Lamour et al., 1982; Price and Stern, 1983; Saper, 1984), it seems that there is a potential in the cholinergic projection for activation of discrete cortical regions. This suggests that the role of the projection might also be considered in relation to selective attention. The possibility of a synergy in the actions of ACh and VIP (Lundberg et al., 1982; Grieve et al., 1985a,b) suggests that the cholinergic input could also enhance the putative effects of the VIP cells on metabolism and blood flow to match the needs of the focus of enhanced neural activity. The discrete laminar grouping of the cells inhibited by ACh suggests further that there is also a very specific cholinergic control of some facet of the cortical circuit.

While there is some distinction in the nature of the action of iontophoretically applied ACh in the cortex and dLGN, the actions of norepinephrine and 5-HT in these two locations appear rather similar. The interest in norepinephrine has been considerable, following its association with the plasticity seen in the visual cortex in early life (Kasamatsu et al., 1979), but here I refer only to its action on cell responses and activity in the adult cortex. The predominant effect of iontophoretically applied norepinephrine in the cortex is inhibitory (Krnjević and Phillis, 1963; Phillis, 1970; Stone, 1973; Reader, 1978; Videen et al., 1984; A. M. Sillito and J. A. Kemp, unpublished observations). The hyperpolarization associated with this effect appears to occur with little change in membrane resistance (Phillis, 1977). The inhibitory effect of norepinephrine has a relatively slow onset and a long duration, and is mimicked by stimulation of the locus coeruleus (Taylor and Stone, 1980). A very small proportion of cells also seem to show some facilitation (Reader, 1978; Videen et al., 1984), although Kasamatsu and Heggelund (1982) reported rather larger numbers in kittens in which the visual cortex was pretreated with 6-hydroxydopamine (6-OHDA) to deplete the natural noradrenergic input. Olpe et al. (1980) also observed a small proportion of facilitations in the rat visual cortex following locus coeruleus stimulation, although inhibitory effects predominated, and with iontophoretically applied norepinephrine they were only able to obtain inhibition. The frequency of facilitation seen with norepinephrine is certainly not as great as that seen with ACh in the visual cortex (Sillito and Kemp, 1983b, and unpublished observations). Conversely, it is interesting to note that microperfusion of norepinephrine in hippocampal slices has been reported to exert an action on calcium-dependent potassium channels, which is not readily apparent when the drug is iontophoretically applied (Haas and Konnerth, 1983). The potassium channel effect would be commensurate with an increased excitability that might only be readily apparent against the background of an ongoing excitatory input, and it is possible that the perfusion mimics the natural distribution of the transmitter evoked by locus coeruleus stimulation more effectively than iontophoresis. The objection to this argument is that stimulation of the locus coeruleus itself produces mainly inhibitory effects, although it would be useful to check the effect of this stimulation on a visually elicited input.

The other comment to make about the action of norepinephrine is that it has been considered to increase the signal-to-noise ratio in the cerebellum (Moises et al., 1981) and visual cortex (Kasamatsu and Heggelund, 1982). This interpretation has to be approached with some caution. Videen et al. (1984) point out that a slight hyperpolarization of a cell with a background discharge would automatically tend to increase the signal-to-noise ratio in relation to a strong visually evoked input. This property would be associated with any general inhibition of the cell and could be mimicked by GABA (e.g., Foote et al., 1975). Hence, the fact that norepinephrine can achieve this effect may not be particularly significant except in those cases where it causes a marked increase in response magnitude. As judged by iontophoretic experiments, ACh has a much more marked effect on the signal-to-noise level in the visual cortex (Sillito and Kemp, 1983b).

The inhibitory effect of 5-HT in the cortex is distinct from that of norepinephrine insofar as it evokes a more rapid inhibition, an effect that is matched by the response to electrical stimulation of the median raphe nuclei (Stone, 1973; Olpe, 1981). The only direct evidence available for the visual cortex suggests that 5-HT also has a predominantly inhibitory effect (Reader, 1978), although this study reports a small number of cells to have been facilitated by the drug application. A similar small percentage of facilitations in a population of cells that were predominantly inhibited by 5-HT application was seen by Olpe (1981) in the cingulate and frontal cortex. However, the cells, facilitated by the drug application, were either unaffected or inhibited by stimulation of the raphe nucleus, suggesting that the drug application was not mimicking the effect of the serotonergic input in these cases.

Given the available evidence, the predominant effects of the three extrinsic modulatory inputs would appear to be:

1. Cholinergic: Strong facilitation of stimulus-driven responses seen on cells through all laminae, but a selective depression of the responses in a subgroup of cells in the laminae III–IV region.
2. Serotonergic: Inhibition of cell activity.
3. Noradrenergic: Inhibition of cell activity and visually driven responses.

The potential significance of the cholinergic input, as discussed above, is clear and commensurate with a role in arousal and selective attention. The significance of the other two is much less so, particularly as they seem to exert broadly the same type of influence. Indeed, there would be good reason to question whether the iontophoretic data were giving a true picture of their influence were it not for the fact that similar responses were seen following stimulation of the locus coeruleus and raphe nuclei. In a positive sense, the "inhibitory" effect of these latter inputs, combined with the particular properties of the cholinergic facilitation, could be argued to maximize the signal-to-noise ratio. However, as discussed for the dLGN, it is important to delineate the precise pattern of distribution of terminals and receptor types, and to question whether a distinction can be made in the behavioral circumstances in which each input is maximally active. An additional possibility is that the proper influence of these inputs may require the concatenation of all three at the same moment in time. This should be examined, given that the available evidence militates for the view that the output of all three increases in the same behavioral conditions (see above).

COMMENT

The analysis of the functional significance of the synaptic organization of the central visual system, despite the complexity of the problem, gives intriguing insights into some of the processes underlying its operation. Virtually all avenues of investigation underline the importance of inhibitory mechanisms at the thalamic and cortical levels. There is little doubt that in the cortex, GABAergic inhibitory processes provide a major contribution to the "dynamic structuring" of receptive field properties. It is equally clear, however, that the range of different categories of effect and of morphologically distinct inhibitory interneurons indicates a subtlety of action as yet not encompassed by our models of cortical organization. In some ways, this latter comment is essential to our consideration of the role of the neuropeptides SSt and CCK in the cortex. Their apparent coexistence with GABA in a subpopulation of interneurons that may, by their synaptic contacts on dendrites, be involved in the "depolarizing discriminative inhibition" requires that we identify the functional correlate of this inhibitory mechanism in order to elucidate the role of the peptide. Likewise, the role of GABA$_B$ receptors presents a conundrum that may yet involve the neuropeptides.

It is obviously relevant to utilize the *in vitro* slice to explore the possibility of SSt–GABA and CCK–GABA interactions at the dendritic level. But as stated at the beginning of this chapter, access to the real significance of any such interactions requires their formulation in terms of the system function. The difficulty in the visual cortex at present is identifying what we would expect this type of process to achieve. One of the major limitations to our present approach is the tendency to interpret the system in terms of a linear sequence of synaptic interactions, whether in parallel lines subserving the X-, Y-, and W-systems or in a strictly hierarchical model. The morphological evidence for the organization of excitatory and inhibitory connections emphasizes the complex reciprocal interactions between the different levels of the system. They arguably define a circuit, not a linear sequence, and suggest that true appreciation of the organization may only derive from studies that attempt to model visual response properties in terms of circuit theory. This issue is already raised by the mismatch between the limited range of receptive field classes distinguished in visual cortical cells in relation to the much larger number of cells distinguished by morphology and connectivity.

When the system is considered from this viewpoint, it is apparent that the distinction between the role of inhibitory and excitatory contributions to receptive field structure may be an artificial construct derived from a poor way of looking at the system. They can be viewed as mutually dependent components of one process that cannot be strictly subdivided. In the experiments with bicuculline, lifting the inhibitory blockade in the vicinity of one cell will change the contribution that that cell, and possibly its near neighbors, make to the circuit operation; because of the extensive positive feedback between the laminae, this in turn may alter the nature of the excitatory input to the cell in question. Consequently, while this type of experiment clearly indicates the importance of the inhibitory circuit to the properties of the cell, it may not of necessity provide a reflected indication of the state of the excitatory input prior to the inhibitory blockade. These comments stand in the face of some of the arguments presented earlier in the chapter that "trail" the sequential processing view of cortical organization. I make no apology for the potential schism of viewpoint.

Even the present rudimentary evidence concerning the role of the extrinsic "neuromodulatory influences" delineates certain common features of their likely operation in relation to the enhancement of stimulus-selective responses and hence signal-to-noise levels. Moreover, there is, at least in the cortex, the implication of a level of organization commensurate with selective attention, with the possibility of a component of the circuitry operating in a synergistic fashion to regulate cortical blood flow and metabolism. It does not seem unreasonable to conclude that the evolving view of the synaptic organization of the central visual system provides great encouragement for its further use as a general model in which to evaluate the "context-dependent" operation of particular sets of synaptic processes.

ACKNOWLEDGMENTS

I am greatly indebted to a number of colleagues who have contributed to the experiments discussed here, including Dr. J. A. Kemp, Dr. P. C. Murphy, Dr. N. Berardi, Dr. K. L. Grieve, and Dr. T. E. Salt. The work would not have been possible without the financial support of the Medical Research Council and Wellcome Trust. The patient secretarial help of Miss C. S. Prout is gratefully acknowledged.

REFERENCES

Ahlsen, G., S. Lindstrom, and F. S. Lo (1982) Functional distinction of perigeniculate and thalamic reticular neurones in the cat. *Exp. Brain Res.* **46**:118–126.

Albus, K., and N. Wolf (1984) Early postnatal development of neuronal function in the kitten's visual cortex: A laminar analysis. *J. Physiol. (Lond.)* **348**:153–186.

Alger, B. E., and R. A. Nicoll (1982a) Feed-forward dendritic inhibition in rat hippocampal pyramidal cells studied *in vitro. J. Physiol. (Lond.)* **328**:105–123.

Alger, B. E., and R. A. Nicoll (1982b) Pharmacological evidence for two kinds of GABA receptor on rat hippocampal pyramidal cells studied *in vitro. J. Physiol. (Lond.)* **328**:125–141.

Andersen, P., R. Dingledine, L. Gjerstad, I. A. Langmoen, and A. M. Laursen (1980) Two different responses of hippocampal pyramidal cells to application of γ-aminobutyric acid. *J. Physiol. (Lond.)* **305**:279–296.

Aston-Jones, G., and F. E. Bloom (1981) Activity of norepinephrine-containing locus coeruleus neurons in behaving rats anticipates fluctuations in the sleep–waking cycle. *J. Neurosci.* **1**:876–886.

Baughman, R. W., and C. D. Gilbert (1980) Aspartate and glutamate as possible neurotransmitters of cells in layer 6 of the visual cortex. *Nature* **287**:848–850.

Baughman, R. W., and C. D. Gilbert (1981) Aspartate and glutamate as possible neurotransmitters in the visual cortex. *J. Neurosci.* **1**:427–439.

Berardi, N., and M. C. Morrone (1984) The role of γ-aminobutyric acid-mediated inhibition on the response properties of cat lateral geniculate nucleus neurones. *J. Physiol. (Lond.)* **357**:505–524.

Berelowitz, M., J. Mathews, B. L. Pimstone, S. Kronheim, and H. Sacks (1978) Immunoreactive somatostatin in rat cerebral cortical and hypothalamic synaptosomes. *Metabolism (Suppl.)* **27**: 1171–1173.

Benardo, L. S., and D. A. Prince (1982) Ionic mechanisms of cholinergic excitation in mammalian hippocampal pyramidal cells. *Brain Res.* **249**:333–344.

Chan-Palay, V., M. Ito, P. Tongroach, M. Sakurai, and S. Palay (1982) Inhibitory effects of motilin, somatostatin, (leu) enkephalin, (met) enkephalin, and taurine on neurons of the lateral vestibular nucleus: Interactions with gamma-amino butyric acid. *Proc. Natl. Acad. Sci. USA* **79**:3355–3359.

Creutzfeldt, O. D., and M. Ito (1968) Functional synaptic organization of primary visual cortex neurones in the cat. *Exp. Brain Res.* **6**:324–352.

Creutzfeldt, O. D., U. Kuhnt, and L. A. Benevento (1974) An intracellular analysis of visual cortical neurones to moving stimuli: Responses in a co-operative neuronal network. *Exp. Brain Res.* **21**:251–274.

Curtis, D. R., and R. Davis (1962) Pharmacological studies upon neurons of the lateral geniculate nucleus of the cat. *Br. J. Pharmacol.* **18**:217–246.

Deffenu, G., G. Bertaccini, and G. Pepeu (1967) Acetylcholine and 5-hydroxytryptamine levels of the lateral geniculate bodies and superior colliculus of cats after visual deafferentation. *Exp. Neurol.* **17**:203–209.

Delfs, J. R., and M. A. Dichter (1983) Effects of somatostatin on mammalian cortical neurons in culture; physiological actions and unusual dose–response characteristics. *J. Neurosci.* **3**:1176–1188.

Dodd, J., and J. S. Kelly (1981) The actions of cholecystokinin and related peptides on pyramidal neurones of the mammalian hippocampus. *Brain Res.* **205**:337–360.

Dodd, J., J. S. Kelly, and S. I. Said (1979) Excitation of CA1 neurones of the rat hippocampus by the octacosapeptide vasoactive intestinal polypeptide (VIP). *Br. J. Pharmacol.* **66**:125P.

Dubin, M. W., and B. G. Cleland (1977) Organization of visual inputs to interneurones of lateral geniculate nucleus of the cat. *J. Neurophysiol.* **40**:410–427.

Eckenstein, F., and R. W. Baughman (1984) Two types of cholinergic innervation in the cortex, one co-localised with vasoactive intestinal polypeptide. *Nature* **309**:153–155.

Famiglietti, E. W., and A. Peters (1972) The synaptic glomerulus and the intrinsic neuron in the dorsal lateral geniculate nucleus of the cat. *J. Comp. Neurol.* **144**:285–334.

Ferster, D., and S. LeVay (1978) The axonal arborization of lateral geniculate neurons in the striate cortex of the cat. *J. Comp. Neurol.* **182**:923–944.

Fitzpatrick, D., G. R. Penny, and D. E. Schmechel (1984) Glutamic acid decarboxylase-immunoreactive neurons and terminals in the lateral geniculate nucleus of the cat. *J. Neurosci.* **4**:1809–1829.

Fonnum, F., J. Storm-Mathisen, and I. Divas (1981) Biochemical evidence for glutamate as a neurotransmitter in corticostriatal and corticothalamic fibres in rat brain. *Neuroscience* **6**:863–873.

Foote, S. L., R. Freedman, and A. P. Oliver (1975) Effects of putative neurotransmitters on neuronal activity in monkey auditory cortex. *Brain Res.* **86**:229–242.

Fuxe, K., T. Hökfelt, S. I. Said, and V. Mutt (1977) Vasoactive intestinal polypeptide and the nervous system: Immunohistochemical evidence for localisation in central and peripheral neurons, particularly intracortical neurons of the cerebral cortex. *Neurosci. Lett.* **5**:241–246.

Ganz, L., and R. Felder (1984) Mechanism of directional selectivity in simple neurons of the cat's visual cortex analysed with stationary flash sequences. *J. Neurophysiol.* **51**:294–324.

Giachetti, A., S. I. Said, R. C. Reynolds, and F. C. Konlges (1977) Vasoactive intestinal polypeptide in brain: Localization in and release from isolated nerve terminals. *Proc. Natl. Acad. Sci. USA* **74**:3424–3428.

Gilbert, C. D., and T. N. Wiesel (1979) Morphology and intracortical projections and functionally characterised neurons in cat visual cortex. *Nature* **280**:120–125.

Gilbert, C. D., and T. N. Wiesel (1983) Clustered intrinsic connections in cat visual cortex. *J. Neurosci.* **3**:1116–1133.

Godfraind, J. M. (1978) Acetylcholine and somatically evoked inhibition on perigeniculate neurones in the cat. *Br. J. Pharmacol.* **63**:295–302.

Gray, E. G. (1963) Electron microscopy of presynaptic organelles of the spinal cord. *J. Anat.* **97**:101–106.

Grieve, K. L., P. C. Murphy, and A. M. Sillito (1985a) The actions of VIP and ACh on the visual responses of neurones in the striate cortex. *Br. J. Pharmacol. (Suppl.)* **85**:253.

Grieve, K. L., P. C. Murphy, and A. M. Sillito (1985b) An evaluation of the role of CCK and VIP in the cat visual cortex. *J. Physiol. (Lond.)* **365**:42P.

Haas, H. L., and A. Konnerth (1983) Histamine and noradrenaline decrease calcium-activated potassium conductance in hippocampal pyramidal cells. *Nature* **303**:432–434.

Halliwell, J. V., and P. R. Adams (1982) Voltage-clamp analysis of muscarinic excitation in hippocampal neurons. *Brain Res.* **250**:71–92.

Hammond, P. (1973) Contrasts in spatial organization of receptive fields at geniculate and retinal levels: Centre, surround and outer surround. *J. Physiol. (Lond.)* **228**:115–137.

Hammond, P. (1981) Simultaneous determination of directional tuning of complex cells in cat striate cortex for bar and texture motion. *Exp. Brain Res.* **41**:364–369.

Hammond, P., and D. M. Mackay (1975) Differential responses of cat visual cortex cells to textured stimuli. *Exp. Brain Res.* **22**:427–430.

Hassler, R., P. Haug, C. Nitsch, J. S. Kim, and K. Paik (1982) Effect of motor and premotor cortex ablation on concentrations of amino acids, monoamines and acetylcholine and on the ultrastructure in the cat striatum. A confirmation of glutamate as the specific corticostriatal transmitter. *J. Neurochem.* **38**:1087–1098.

Heggelund, P. (1981a) Receptive field organization of simple cells in cat striate cortex. *Exp. Brain Res.* **42**:89–98.

Heggelund, P. (1981b) Receptive field organization of complex cells in cat striate cortex. *Exp. Brain Res.* **42**:99–107.

Heggelund, P., S. Krekling, and B. C. Skotun (1983) Spatial summation in the receptive field of simple cells in the cat striate cortex. *Exp. Brain Res.* **52**:87–98.

Henderson, Z. (1981) A projection from acetylcholinesterase-containing neurones in the diagonal band to the occipital cortex of the rat. *Neuroscience* **6**:1081–1088.

Hendrickson, A. E., S. P. Hunt, and J.-Y. Wu (1981) Immunocytochemical localisation of glutamic acid decarboxylase in monkey striate cortex. *Nature* **292**:605–607.

Hendry, S. H. C., E. G. Jones, and M. C. Beinfeld (1983) CCK-immunoreactive neurons in rat and monkey cerebral cortex make symmetric synapses and have intimate associations with blood vessels. *Proc. Natl. Acad. Sci. USA* **80**:2400–2403.

Hendry, S. H. C., E. G. Jones, J. De Felipe, D. Schmechel, C. Brandon, and P. C. Emson (1984a) Neuropeptide-containing neurons of the cerebral cortex are also GABAergic. *Proc. Natl. Acad. Sci. USA* **81**:6526–6530.

Hendry, S. H. C., E. G. Jones, and P. C. Emson (1984b) Morphology, distribution and synaptic relations of somatostatin- and neuropeptide Y-immunoreactive neurons in rat and monkey neocortex. *J. Neurosci.* **4**:2497–2517.

Henry, G. H., P. O. Bishop, and B. Dreher (1974) Orientation, axis and direction as stimulus parameters for striate cells. *Vision Res.* **14**:766–778.

Hoover, D. B., and D. M. Jacobowitz (1979) Neurochemical and histochemical studies of the effect of a lesion of nucleus cuneiformis on the cholinergic innervation of discrete areas of the rat brain. *Brain Res.* **170**:113–122.

Horton, S. C., and D. H. Hubel (1981) Regular patchy distribution of cytochrome oxidase staining in primary visual cortex of macaque monkey. *Nature* **292**:762–764.

Horton, S. C., and H. Sherk (1984) Receptive field properties in the cat's lateral geniculate nucleus in the absence of on-center retinal input. *J. Neurosci.* **4**:374–380.

Hubel, D. H., and M. S. Livingston (1981) Regions of poor orientation tuning coincide with patches of cytochrome oxidase staining in monkey striate cortex. *Soc. Neurosci. Abstr.* **7**:367.

Hubel, D. H., and M. S. Livingstone (1982) Cytochrome oxidase blobs in monkey area 17. Response properties and afferent connections. *Soc. Neurosci. Abstr.* **8**:706.

Hubel, D. H., and T. N. Wiesel (1961) Integrative action in the cat's lateral geniculate body. *J. Physiol. (Lond.)* **155**:385–398.

Hubel, D. H., and T. N. Wiesel (1962) Receptive fields, binocular interaction and functional architecture in the cat's visual cortex. *J. Physiol. (Lond.)* **160**:106–154.

Hubel, D. H., and T. N. Wiesel (1972) Laminar and columnar distribution of geniculocortical fibers in the macaque monkey. *J. Comp. Neurol.* **146**:421–450.

Ioffe, S., V. Haulicek, H. Frisen, and V. Chernick (1978) Effect of somatostatin (SRIF) and L-glutamate on neurons of the sensorimotor cortex in the awake habituated rabbit. *Brain Res.* **153**:414–418.

Iversen, L. L., J. F. Mitchell, and V. Srinivasan (1971) The release of amino butyric acid during inhibition in the cat visual cortex. *J. Physiol. (Lond.)* **212**:519–534.

Iversen, L. L., S. D. Iversen, F. Bloom, C. Douglas, M. Brown, and W. Vale (1978) Calcium-dependent release of somatostatin and neurotensin from rat brain *in vitro*. *Nature* **273**:161–163.

Jahr, C. E., and R. A. Nicoll (1982) Noradrenaline modulation of dendrodendritic inhibition in the olfactory bulb. *Nature* **297**:227–229.

Kasamatsu, T., and P. Heggelund (1982) Single cell responses in cat visual cortex to visual stimulation during iontophoresis of noradrenaline. *Exp. Brain Res.* **45**:317–327.

Kasamatsu, T., J. D. Pettigrew, and M. Ary (1979) Restoration of visual cortical plasticity by local microperfusion of norepinephrine. *J. Comp. Neurol.* **185**:163–182.

Kayama, Y., T. Negi, M. Sugitani, and K. Iwama (1982) Effects of locus coeruleus stimulation on neuronal activities of dorsal lateral geniculate nucleus and perigeniculate reticular nucleus of the rat. *Neuroscience* **7**:655–666.

Kemp, J. A. (1984) Intracellular recordings from rat visual cortical cells *in vitro* and the action of GABA. *J. Physiol. (Lond.)* **349**:13P.

Kemp, J. A., and A. M. Sillito (1981) The nature of the excitatory transmitter mediating X and Y cell inputs to the cat dorsal lateral geniculate nucleus. *J. Physiol. (Lond.)* **323**:377–391.

Kemp, J. A., H. C. Roberts, and A. M. Sillito (1982) Further studies on the action of 5-hydroxytryptamine in the dorsolateral geniculate nucleus of the cat. *Brain Res.* **246**:334–337.

Kim, J. S., R. Hassler, P. Haug, and K.-S. Paik (1977) Effect of frontal cortex ablation on striatal glutamic acid levels in rat. *Brain Res.* **132**:370–374.

Krnjević, K., and J. W. Phillis (1963) Actions of certain amines on cerebral cortical neurones. *Br. J. Pharmacol.* **20**:471–490.

Krnjević, K., R. Pumain, and L. Renaud (1971) The mechanism of excitation by acetylcholine in the cerebral cortex. *J. Physiol. (Lond.)* **215**:247–268.

Kromer, L. F., and R. Y. Moore (1980) A study of the organisation of the locus coeruleus projections to the lateral geniculate nuclei in the albino rat. *Neuroscience* **5**:255–271.

Kunar, M. J., G. K. Aghajanian, and R. H. Rothe (1972) Tryptophan hydroxylase activity and synaptosomal uptake of serotonin in discrete brain regions after midbrain raphe lesions: Correlation with serotonin levels and histochemical fluorescence. *Brain Res.* **44**:165–176.

Lamour, Y., P. Dutar, and A. Jobert (1982) Spread of acetylcholine sensititivy in the neocortex following lesion of the nucleus basalis. *Brain Res.* **252**:377–381.

Lee, B. B., B. G. Cleland, and O. D. Creutzfeldt (1977) The retinal input to cells in area 17 of the cat's cortex. *Exp. Brain Res.* **30**:527–538.

Lee, T. J.-F., A. Saito, and I. Berezin (1984) Vasoactive intestinal polypeptide-like substance: The potential transmitter for cerebral vasodilation. *Science* **224**:898–901.

LeVay, S. (1973) Synaptic patterns in the visual cortex of the cat and monkey. Electron microscopy of Golgi preparation. *J. Comp. Neurol.* **150**:53–86.

LeVay, S., and C. D. Gilbert (1976) Laminar patterns of geniculo-cortical projection in the cat. *Brain Res.* **113**:1–19.

LeVay, S., M. P. Stryker, and C. J. Shatz (1978) Ocular dominance columns and their development in layer IV of the cat's visual cortex: A quantitative study. *J. Comp. Neurol.* **179**:223–244.

Leventhal, A. G. (1983) Relationship between preferred orientation and receptive field position of neurons in cat striate cortex. *J. Comp. Neurol.* **220**:476–483.

Levick, W. R., and L. N. Thibos (1982) Analysis of orientation bias in cat retina. *J. Physiol. (Lond.)* **329**:243–261.

Levitt, P., and R. Y. Moore (1978) Noradrenaline neuron innervation of the neocortex in the rat. *Brain Res.* **139**:219–231.

Lidov, H. G. W., R. Grzanna, and M. E. Molliver (1980) The serotonin innervation of the cerebral cortex in the rat—An immunocytochemical analysis. *Neuroscience* **5**:207–227.

Livingstone, M. S., and D. H. Hubel (1981) Effects of sleep and arousal on the processing of visual information in the cat. *Nature* **291**:554–561.

Lund, J. S., G. H. Henry, C. L. MacQueen, and A. R. Harvey (1979) Anatomical organization of the primary visual cortex (area 17) of the macaque monkey. *J. Comp. Neurol.* **184**:559–576.

Lundberg, J. M., A. Anggard, and J. Fahrenkrug (1982) Complementary role of vasoactive intestinal polypeptide (VIP) and acetylcholine for cat submandibular gland blood flow and secretion. III. Effects of local infusions. *Acta Physiol. Scand.* **114**:329–337.

McDonald, J. K., J. G. Parnavelas, A. N. Karamanlidis, N. Brecha, and J. I. Koenig (1982a) The morphology and distribution of peptide-containing neurons in the adult and developing visual cortex of the rat. I. Somatostatin. *J. Neurocytol.* **11**:809–824.

McDonald, J. K., J. G. Parnavelas, A. N. Karamanlidis, and N. Brecha (1982b) The morphology and distribution of peptide-containing neurons in the adult and developing visual cortex of the rat. II. Vasoactive intestinal polypeptide. *J. Neurocytol.* **11**:825–837.

McDonald, J. K., J. G. Parnavelas, A. N. Karamanlidis, and N. Brecha (1982c) The morphology and distribution of peptide-containing neurons in the adult and developing visual cortex of the rat. III. Cholecystokinin. *J. Neurocytol.* **11**:881–895.

Magistretti, P. J., J. H. Morrison, W. J. Shoemaker, U. Sapin, and F. E. Bloom (1981) Vasoactive intestinal polypeptide induces glycogenolysis in mouse cortical slices: A possible regulatory mechanism for the local control of energy metabolism. *Proc. Natl. Acad. Sci. USA* **78**:6535–6539.

Malpeli, J. G. (1983) Activity of cells in area 17 of the cat in absence of input from layer A of lateral geniculate nucleus. *J. Neurophysiol.* **49**:595–620.

Martin, K. A. S. (1984) Neuronal circuits in cat striate cortex. In *The Cerebral Cortex*, Vol. 2A, A. Peters and E. G. Jones, eds., pp. 241–284, Plenum, New York.

Martin, K. A. C., and D. Whitteridge (1984) Form, function and intracortical projections of spiny neurones in the striate visual cortex of the cat. *J. Physiol. (Lond.)* **353**:463–504.

Martin, K. A. C., P. Somogyi, and D. Whitteridge (1983) Physiological and morphological properties of identified basket cells in the cat's visual cortex. *Exp. Brain Res.* **50**:193–200.

Mesulam, M.-M., E. J. Mufson, A. I. Levey, and B. H. Wainer (1983a) Cholinergic innervation of cortex by the basal forebrain. Cytochemistry and cortical connection of the septal area, diagonal band nuclei, nucleus basalis (substantia innominata) and hypothalamus in the rhesus monkey. *J. Comp. Neurol.* **214**:170–197.

Mesulam, M.-M., E. J. Mufson, B. H. Wainer, and A. I. Levey (1983b) Central cholinergic pathways in the rat: An overview based on alternative nomenclature (Ch1–Ch6). *Neuroscience* **10**:1185–1201.

Moises, H. C., B. D. Waterhouse, and D. J. Woodward (1981) Locus coeruleus stimulation potentiates Purkinje cell responses to afferent input: The climbing fiber system. *Brain Res.* **222**:43–64.

Moore, B. Y., A. E. Halaris, and B. E. Jones (1978) Serotonin neurons of the midbrain raphe: Ascending projections. *J. Comp. Neurol.* **180**:417–438.

Morrison, J. H., R. Benoit, P. J. Magistretti, and F. E. Bloom (1983) Immunohistochemical distribution of pro-somatostatin related peptides in cerebral cortex. *Brain Res.* **262**:344–351.

Morrison, J. H., P. J. Magistretti, R. Benoit, and F. E. Bloom (1984) The distribution and morphological characteristics of the intracortical VIP-positive cell: An immunohistochemical analysis. *Brain Res.* **292**:269–282.

Nakai, Y., and S. Takaori (1974) Influence of norepinephrine-containing neurons derived from the locus coeruleus on lateral geniculate neuronal activities of cats. *Brain Res.* **71**:47–60.

Nicoll, R. A., and N. R. Newberry (1984) A possible postsynaptic inhibitory action for GABA$_B$ receptors on hippocampal pyramidal cells. *Neuropharmacology* **23**:849–850.

Oertel, W. H., A. M. Graybiel, E. Mugnaini, R. P. Elde, D. E. Schmechel, and I. J. Kopin (1983) Coexistence of glutamic acid decarboxylase- and somatostatin-like immunoreactivity in neurons of the feline nucleus reticularis thalami. *J. Neurosci.* **3**:1322–1332.

O'Hara, P. T., A. R. Lieberman, S. P. Hunt, and J.-Y. Wau (1983) Neural elements containing glutamic acid decarboxylase (GAD) in the dorsal lateral geniculate nucleus of the rat: Immunohistochemical studies by light and electron microscopy. *Neuroscience* **8**:189–212.

Olpe, H. R. (1981) The cortical projection of the dorsal raphe nucleus: Some electrophysiological and pharmacological properties. *Brain Res.* **216**:61–71.

Olpe, H. R., A. Glatt, J. Laszlo, and A. Schellenberg (1980) Some electrophysiological and pharmacological properties of the cortical noradrenergic projection of the locus coeruleus in the rat. *Brain Res.* **186**:9–19.

Ottersen, O. P., B. O. Fisher, and J. Storm-Mathisen (1983) Retrograde transport of D-[^{3}H]aspartate in thalamocortical neurones. *Neurosci. Lett.* **42**:19–24.

Peters, A., and A. Fairén (1978) Smooth and sparsely spined stellate cells in the visual cortex of the rat, a study using combined Golgi–electron microscope technique. *J. Comp. Neurol.* **181**:129–172.

Peters, A., and L. M. Kimerer (1981) Bipolar neurons in rat visual cortex: A combined Golgi–electron microscope study. *J. Neurocytol.* **10**:921–946.

Peters, A., and J. Regidor (1981) A reassessment of the forms of non-pyramidal neurons in area 17 of cat visual cortex. *J. Comp. Neurol.* **203**:685–716.

Peters, A., M. Miller, and L. M. Kimerer (1983) Cholecystokinin-like immunoreactive neurons in rat cerebral cortex. *Neuroscience* **8**:431–448.

Phillis, J. W. (1970) *The Pharmacology of Synapses*, Pergamon, Oxford.

Phillis, J. W. (1977) The role of cyclic nucleotides in the CNS. *Can. J. Neurol. Sci.* **4**:151–195.

Phillis, J. W., and J. R. Kirkpatrick (1980) The action of motilin, luteinising hormone releasing hormone, cholecystokinin, somatostatin, vasoactive intestinal peptide, and other peptides on rat cerebral cortical neurons. *Can. J. Physiol. Pharmacol.* **58**:612–623.

Phillis, J. W., A. K. Tebecis, and D. H. York (1967a) A study of cholinoceptive cells in the lateral geniculate nucleus. *J. Physiol. (Lond.)* **192**:695–713.

Phillis, J. W., A. K. Tebecis, and D. H. York (1967b) The inhibitory actions of monoamines on lateral geniculate neurones. *J. Physiol. (Lond.)* **190**:563–581.

Phillis, J. W., J. R. Kirkpatrick, and S. I. Said (1978) Vasoactive intestinal polypeptide excitation of central neurons. *Can. J. Physiol. Pharmacol.* **56**:337–340.

Pittman, Q. J., and G. R. Siggins (1981) Somatostatin hyperpolarises hippocampal pyramidal cells *in vitro*. *Brain Res.* **221**:402–408.

Poggio, G. F., and B. Fischer (1977) Binocular interaction and depth sensitivity in striate and prestriate areas of behaving rhesus monkey. *J. Neurophysiol.* **40**:1392–1405.

Price, J. L., and R. Stern (1983) Individual cells in the nucleus basalis–diagonal band complex have restricted axonal projections to the cerebral cortex in the rat. *Brain Res.* **269**:352–354.

Rapisardi, S. C., and T. P. Miles (1984) Synaptology of retinal terminals in the dorsal lateral geniculate nucleus of the cat. *J. Comp. Neurol.* **223**:515–534.

Reader, T. A. (1978) The effects of dopamine, noradrenaline and serotonin in the visual cortex of the cat. *Experientia (Basel)* **34**:1586–1588.

Renaud, L. P., J. B. Martin, and P. Brazeau (1975) Depressant action of TRH, LH-RH and somatostatin on activity of central neurones. *Nature* **255**:233–235.

Reubi, J. C. (1984) Evidence for two somatostatin-14 receptor types in rat brain cortex. *Neurosci. Lett.* **49**:259–263.

Ribak, C. E. (1978) Aspinous and sparsely-spinous stellate neurons in the visual cortex of rats contain glutamic acid decarboxylase. *J. Neurocytol.* **7**:461–478.

Rogawski, M. A., and G. K. Aghajanian (1980) Norepinephrine and serotonin: Opposite effects on the activity of lateral geniculate neurones evoked by optic pathway stimulation. *Exp. Neurol.* **69**:678–694.

Rovira, C., Y. Ben-Ari, E. Cherubini, K. Krnjević, and N. Ropert (1983) Pharmacology of the dendritic action of acetylcholine and further observations on the somatic disinhibition in the rat hippocampus *in situ*. *Neuroscience* **8**:97–106.

Rowlands, G. J., and P. J. Roberts (1980) Specific calcium-dependent release of endogenous glutamate from rat striatum is reduced by destruction of the corticostriatal tract. *Exp. Brain Res.* **39**:239–240.

Rustioni, A., R. Spreafico, S. Cheema, and M. Luenod (1982) Selective retrograde labelling of somatosensory cortical neurons after ^{3}H-D-aspartate injections in the neutrobasal complex of rats and cats. *Neuroscience (Suppl.)* **7**:5183.

Salt, T. E., and A. M. Sillito (1984) The action of somatostatin (SSt) on the response properties of cells in the cat's visual cortex. *J. Physiol. (Lond.)* **350**:28P.

Saper, C. B. (1984) Organisation of cerebral cortical afferent systems in the rat. I. Magnocellular basal nucleus. *J. Comp. Neurol.* **222**:313–342.

Schatz, C. J., and M. P. Stryker (1978) Ocular dominance in layer IV of the cat's visual cortex and the effects of monocular deprivation. *J. Physiol. (Lond.)* **281**:267–283.

Schiller, P. H. (1982) Central connections of the retinal ON and OFF pathways. *Nature* **297**:580–583.

Schiller, P. H., B. L. Finlay, and S. F. Volman (1976) Quantitative studies of single cell properties in monkey striate cortex. I. Spatiotemporal organization of receptive fields. *J. Neurophysiol.* **39**:1288–1319.

Sillito, A. M. (1974a) Modification of the receptive field properties of neurones in the visual cortex by bicuculline, a GABA antagonist. *J. Physiol. (Lond.)* **239**:36–37P.

Sillito, A. M. (1974b) Effects of iontophoretic application of bicuculline on the receptive field properties of simple cells in the visual cortex of the cat. *J. Physiol. (Lond.)* **242**:127–128P.

Sillito, A. M. (1975a) The effectiveness of bicuculline as an antagonist of GABA and visually evoked inhibition in the cat's striate cortex. *J. Physiol. (Lond.)* **250**:287–304.

Sillito, A. M. (1975b) The contribution of inhibitory mechanisms to the receptive field properties of neurones in the striate cortex of the cat. *J. Physiol. (Lond.)* **250**:305–322.

Sillito, A. M. (1977) Inhibitory processes underlying the directional specificity of simple complex and hypercomplex cells in the cat's visual cortex. *J. Physiol. (Lond.)* **271**:699–720.

Sillito, A. M. (1979) Inhibitory mechanisms influencing complex cell orientation selectivity and their modification at high resting discharge levels. *J. Physiol. (Lond.)* **289**:33–53.

Sillito, A. M. (1984) Functional considerations of the operation of GABAergic inhibitory processes in the visual cortex. In *The Cerebral Cortex*, Vol. 2A, E. G. Jones and A. Peters, eds., pp. 91–117, Plenum, New York.

Sillito, A. M. (1985) Inhibitory circuits and orientation selectivity in the visual cortex. In *Models of the Visual Cortex*, D. Rose and V. G. Dobson, eds., pp. 396–407, Wiley, New York.

Sillito, A. M., and J. A. Kemp (1983a) The influence of GABAergic inhibitory processes on the receptive field structure of X and Y cells in cat dorsal lateral geniculate nucleus (dLGN). *Brain Res.* **277**:63–77.

Sillito, A. M., and J. A. Kemp (1983b) Cholinergic modulation of the functional organization of the cat visual cortex. *Brain Res.* **289**:143–155.

Sillito, A. M., and V. Versiani (1977) The contribution of excitatory and inhibitory inputs to the length preference of hypercomplex cells in layers II and III of the cat's striate cortex. *J. Physiol. (Lond.)* **273**:775–790.

Sillito, A. M., J. A. Kemp, and H. Patel (1980a) Inhibitory interactions contributing to the ocular dominance of monocularly dominated cells in the normal cat visual cortex. *Exp. Brain Res.* **41**:1–10.

Sillito, A. M., J. A. Kemp, J. A. Milson, and N. Berardi (1980b) A reevaluation of the mechanisms underlying simple cell orientation selectivity. *Brain Res.* **194**:517–520.

Sillito, A. M., J. A. Kemp, and N. Berardi (1983) The cholinergic influence of the function of the cat dorsal lateral geniculate nucleus (dLGN). *Brain Res.* **280**:299–307.

Sillito, A. M., T. E. Salt, and J. A. Kemp (1984) GABAergic neuronal processes in the dorsolateral geniculate nucleus (dLGN) and putative interactions with somatostatin (SSt). *Neuropharmacology* **23**:875–876.

Singer, W. (1973) The effect of mesencephalic reticular stimulation on intracellular potentials of cat lateral geniculate neurons. *Brain Res.* **61**:55–68.

Singer, W. (1977) Control of thalamic transmission by corticofugal and ascending reticular pathways in the visual system. *Physiol. Rev.* **57**:386–420.

Singer, W. (1979) Central-core control of visual cortex functions. In *The Neurosciences: Fourth Study Program*, F. O. Schmidt and F. G. Worden, eds., pp. 1093–1110, MIT Press, Cambridge, Massachusetts.

Singer, W., and N. Bedworth (1973) Inhibitory interaction between X and Y units in the cat lateral geniculate nucleus. *Brain Res.* **49**:291–307.

Singer, W., and O. D. Creutzfeldt (1970) Reciprocal lateral inhibition of on- and off-center neurones in the lateral geniculate body of the cat. *Exp. Brain Res.* **10**:311–330.

Singer, W., E. Poppel, and O. D. Creutzfeldt (1972) Inhibitory interaction in the cat's lateral geniculate nucleus. *Exp. Brain Res.* **14**:201–226.

Somogyi, P. (1977) A specific "axo-axonal" interneuron in the visual cortex of the rat. *Brain Res.* **136**:345–350.

Somogyi, P., and A. Cowey (1981) Combined Golgi and electron microscopic study on the synapses formed by double bouquet cells in the visual cortex of the cat and monkey. *J. Comp. Neurol.* **195**:547–566.

Somogyi, P., Z. F. Kisvarday, K. A. C. Martin, and D. Whitteridge (1983) Synaptic connections of morphologically identified and physiologically characterised large basket cells in the striate cortex of the cat. *Neuroscience* **10**:261–294.

Somogyi, P., T. F. Freund, and Z. F. Kisvarday (1984) Different types of ^{3}H-GABA accumulating neurons in the visual cortex of the rat. Characterization by combined autoradiography and Golgi impregnation. *Exp. Brain Res.* **54**:45–56.

Spehlman, R. (1971) Acetylcholine and the synaptic transmission of non-specific impulses to the visual cortex. *Brain* **94**:139–150.

Spehlman, R., J. C. Daniel, and C. C. Smathers (1971) Acetylcholine and the synaptic transmission of specific impulses to the visual cortex. *Brain* **94**:125–138.

Spencer, W. A., and E. R. Kandel (1961) Electrophysiology of hippocampal neurons. III. Firing level and time constant. *J. Neurophysiol.* **24**:260–271.

Sterling, P., and T. L. Davis (1980) Neurons in cat lateral geniculate nucleus that concentrate exogenous [^{3}H]-γ-amino butyric acid (GABA). *J. Comp. Neurol.* **192**:737–749.

Stone, T. W. (1973) Pharmacology of pyramidal tract cells in the cerebral cortex. Noradrenergic and related substances. *Br. J. Pharmacol.* **278**:333–346.

Streit, P. (1980) Selective retrograde labelling indicating the transmitter of neuronal pathways. *J. Comp. Neurol.* **191**:429–463.

Taylor, D. A., and T. W. Stone (1980) The action of adenosine on noradrenergic neuronal inhibition induced by stimulation of the locus coeruleus. *Brain Res.* **183**:367–376.

Tebecis, A. K., and A. Di Maria (1972) A re-evaluation of the mode of action of 5-hydroxytryptamine on lateral geniculate neurones: Comparison with catecholamines and LSD. *Exp. Brain Res.* **14**:480–493.

Trulson, M. E., and B. L. Jacobs (1979) Raphe unit activity in freely moving cats: Correlation with level of behavioral arousal. *Brain Res.* **163**:135–150.

Tsumoto, T., W. Eckhart, and O. D. Creutzfeldt (1979) Modification of orientation sensitivity of cat visual cortex neurones by removal of GABA mediated inhibition. *Exp. Brain Res.* **34**:351–363.

Ungerstedt, U. (1971) Stereotaxic mapping of the monoamine pathways in the rat brain. *Acta Physiol. Scand.* (Suppl. 367) **82**:1–48.

Videen, T. O., N. W. Daw, and R. K. Radar (1984) The effect of norepinephrine on visual cortical neurons in kittens and adult cats. *J. Neurosci.* **4**:1607–1617.

Vidyasagar, T. R. (1984) Contribution of inhibitory mechanisms to the orientation sensitivity of cat dLGN neurones. *Exp. Brain Res.* **55**:192–195.

Vidyasagar, T. R., and J. V. Urbas (1982) Orientation sensitivity of cat LGN neurones with and without inputs from visual cortical areas 17 and 18. *Exp. Brain Res.* **46**:157–169.

Wallingford, E., D. Ostdahl, P. Zarzecki, P. Kaufman, and G. Somjen (1973) Optical and pharmacological stimulation of visual cortical neurones. *Nature New Biol.* **242**:210–212.

Wilson, J. R., M. J. Friedlander, and S. M. Sherman (1984) Fine structural morphology of identified X- and Y-cells in the cat's lateral geniculate nucleus. *Proc. R. Soc. Lond. (Biol.)* **221**:411–436.

Yoshida, M., M. Sasa, and S. Takaori (1984) Serotonin-mediated inhibition from dorsal raphe nucelus of neurons in dorsal lateral geniculate and thalamic reticular nuclei. *Brain Res.* **290**:95–105.

Young, A. B., M. B. Brombert, and J. R. Penney (1981) Decreased glutamate uptake in subcortical areas deafferented by sensorimotor cortex ablation in the cat. *J. Neurosci.* **1**:241–249.

Chapter 15

Synaptic Specificity in the Cerebral Cortex

ALAN PETERS

ABSTRACT

Only two morphological types of synapses—asymmetric and symmetric—seem to exist in the cerebral cortex, and all of the presynaptic elements are axons. These axons are derived from a number of sources, and although they may synapse with a variety of postsynaptic elements, all the axon terminals of a particular type of neuron form either only asymmetric or symmetric synapses. This chapter describes the morphological features of these two types of synapses and considers some of the factors that determine the synaptic interrelations of cortical neurons. One factor is that not all portions of the surfaces of each neuron are available for the formation of both types of synapses. Thus, the pyramidal cells and spiny stellate cells have only symmetric synapses on their somata, axon initial segments, and proximal dendritic lengths; most of their spines form only asymmetric synapses. In contrast, nonpyramidal cells with smooth or sparsely spinous dendrites have both symmetric and asymmetric axosomatic synapses, and their axon initial segments are usually free of synapses. What types of axon terminals are available to neurons is largely dependent on their shapes and their locations in the cortex. However, the availability of particular axon terminals does not necessarily mean that synapses are formed, because axon terminals from both extrinsic and intrinsic sources show preferences for where they synapse. Interplay between these and other factors must determine the different patterns of synaptic connections displayed by various types of cortical neurons.

Although it is generally agreed that the cerebral cortex is involved in complex information processing, morphologically the chemical synapses formed by its neurons are of only two basic types. This chapter reviews the forms of these synapses and examines some of the factors that determine the synaptic relationships of the neurons. These factors are the distribution patterns of synapses over the surfaces of different types of neurons, the locations of the neurons within the cortex and the shapes of their dendritic trees, the types of synapses formed by the terminals of axons derived from various extrinsic and intrinsic sources, and the preferences of these axon terminals for synapsing with different postsynaptic sites. All of these factors, which are probably interrelated, seem to play roles in determining the synaptic connections made by different types of neurons in the cerebral cortex.

TYPES OF CORTICAL SYNAPSES

Background

In 1959, Gray examined the visual cortex of the rat by electron microscopy, using material fixed in osmic acid. He classified the synapses into two distinct groups—type 1 and type 2. At type 1 synapses, which he encountered on dendritic spines and shafts, Gray found a large proportion of the interface between the pre- and postsynaptic elements to be involved in the formation of the synaptic junction, which was distinguished by the presence of a pronounced postsynaptic density on the cytoplasmic face of the postsynaptic membrane. At such synapses he found that the space, or synaptic cleft, between the membranes was 30-nm wide, compared to the normal intercellular distance of 20 nm, and contained a plaque of dense extracellular material, the intermediate line. Type 2 synapses, which Gray encountered on dendritic shafts and neuronal cell bodies, had a different appearance. Unlike the type 1 synapses, the junctional zone did not occupy most of the site of apposition between the pre- and postsynaptic membranes but was more confined. Also, instead of being expanded, the intercellular space at the junctions was about 20 nm, similar to that present between elements in the surrounding neuropil. Moreover, there was no intermediate line present in the synaptic cleft, and the densities associated with the cytoplasmic faces of the pre- and postsynaptic membranes were of near-equal thickness.

In Gray's (1959) material, in which osmium had been used as the primary fixative, all of the synaptic vesicles in the presynaptic axon terminals were round, but when aldehydes came to be used for primary fixation, some of the vesicles in certain of the axon terminals appeared elongated. Consequently, such terminals appeared to contain pleomorphic vesicles; that is, some were elongated, some flattened, and others round, and Valdivia (1971) among others, was able to show this to be an osmotic effect. Both the osmolarity of the buffer solutions containing the fixative and the solutions used to wash the tissue prior to osmication could affect vesicle shape, with increased osmolarity favoring increased flattening of vesicles. However, not all axon terminals were affected in this way, for in some terminals the vesicles remained round, even when the osmolarity was increased. In any event, the shapes of synaptic vesicles in aldehyde-fixed material offered another criterion for distinguishing between different types of synapses present in the cerebral cortex.

The correlation between vesicle shape and the presence or absence of a prominent postsynaptic density at cortical synapses was examined in detail by Colonnier (1968), using material fixed initially in formaldehyde. He confirmed the presence of two types of synapses in cerebral cortex using 100 micrographs of randomly selected synapses from cat visual cortex cut normal to the synaptic membranes. Colonnier showed that when these micrographs of synapses were arranged in order of decreased postsynaptic density, they fell into two groups, with an abrupt transition between those synapses with prominent postsynaptic densities and presynaptic elements containing round vesicles, and those with less obvious, more symmetrically distributed densities and presynaptic elements containing pleomorphic vesicles. Since the appearances of the synapses were somewhat different from those in Gray's (1959) osmium-fixed material, Colonnier chose to call them asymmetric and symmetric synapses, although the correspondence with Gray's type 1 and type 2 synapses is readily apparent.

Interestingly, there have been no subsequent suggestions that there are more than two morphological types of chemical synapses in the cerebral cortex, for with few possible exceptions all of the chemical synapses encountered in thin sections of cortex can be readily allocated to one of these two major categories. It should also be noted that all of the presynaptic elements in the cerebral cortex seem to be axon terminals, and there are none of the complexities that exist in the dorsal lateral geniculate nucleus, for example, where there are at least four distinct types of presynaptic processes containing pleomorphic or flattened vesicles (e.g., Guillery, 1969; Rapisardi and Lipsenthal, 1984).

Electrical synapses can also occur between cortical neurons, and when such synapses are present the plasma membranes of adjacent neurons come together to form gap junctions (see Peters et al., 1976). However, there is little evidence that electrotonic coupling is common between neurons in the mature neocortex, for the literature contains few descriptions of gap junctions between cortical neurons. Nevertheless, their presence has been recorded by Sloper (1972), and Sloper and Powell (1978), between the dendrites and somata of large nonpyramidal cells in both somatosensory and motor cortex; by Smith and Moskowitz (1979), who found them between the somata of neurons in layer IV of squirrel monkey auditory cortex; and by Peters (1980), who encountered them between dendrites and somatic spines of nonpyramidal cells in rat frontal cortex. According to Connors et al. (1983), electrical coupling is common in rat neocortex during postnatal development, as evidenced by the fact that intracellular injections of the fluorescent dye Lucifer yellow show about 70% of the neurons to be coupled between one and four days of age. But by 10–18 days of age, the percentage of coupled neurons drops to 40% and is only about 20% in the adult. Connors et al. (1983) found further that when chemical synaptic activity is blocked experimentally, there is strong evidence for neuronal coupling in the immature neocortex, but the coupling declines as chemical synapses are formed. In view of this evidence, and the infrequency with which gap junctions between neurons are encountered in the mature mammalian neocortex, it seems unlikely that electrical synapses play a prominent role in the normal synaptic activity of the cerebral cortex.

In summary then, from the viewpoint of the morphology of its synapses, the cerebral cortex appears to be one of the simpler portions of the central nervous system.

Asymmetric Synapses

Examples of asymmetric synapses in aldehyde-fixed cortical tissue are shown in Figures 1, 2, and 3; the rather wide synaptic cleft, the prominent postsynaptic density, and the round vesicles of the presynaptic axon terminal are evident. Asymmetric synapses in cerebral cortex are most commonly encountered on dendritic spines, which protrude largely from the dendrites of pyramidal cells (Figure 1) and, when such neurons are present, from the spiny stellate cells of layer IV. Usually, each dendritic spine receives only one axon terminal, and an interesting feature of these axospinous synapses is that the profiles of the head

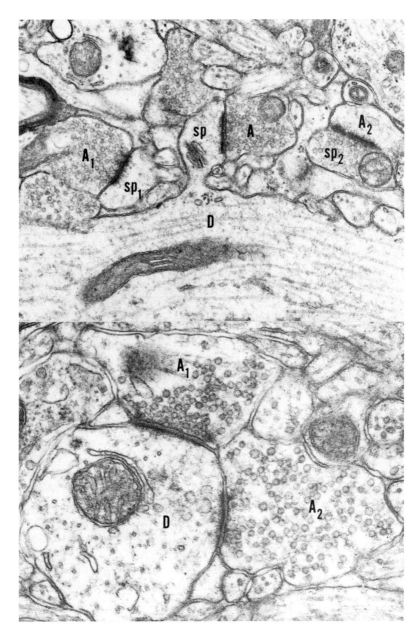

Figure 1. *Top: Electron micrograph showing the apical dendrite (D) of a pyramidal cell giving rise to a spine (sp) that forms an asymmetric synapse with an axon terminal (A).* Other asymmetric synapses between dendritic spines (sp_1 and sp_2) and axon terminals (A_1 and A_2) are present in the surrounding neuropil. Rat visual cortex. $\times$ 35,000. *Bottom: Asymmetric synapses formed betweeen two axon terminals (A_1 and A_2) and the dendrite (D) of a smooth nonpyramidal cell. Rat parietal cortex.* $\times$ 66,000.

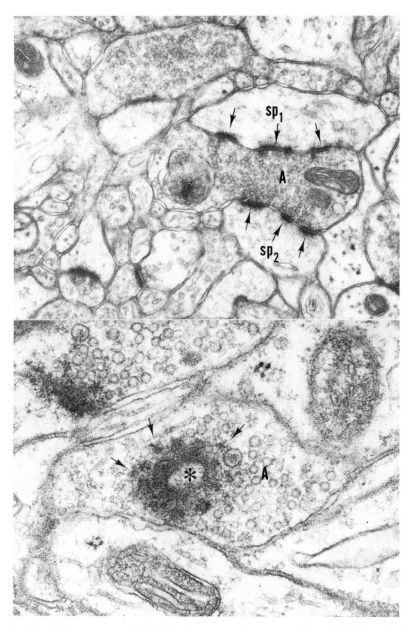

Figure 2. *Top: A large axon terminal (A) forming asymmetric synapses with two dendritic spines (sp_1 and sp_2). At the synaptic junctions, the densities (arrows) appear to be segmented. Rat parietal cortex. × 29,000. Bottom: An en face view of an asymmetrical synapse between a dendritic spine and an axon terminal (A). The synaptic junction is perforated (asterisk).* Note the small densities (*arrows*) at the periphery of the junction. These are the dense projections of the presynaptic grid. Rat visual cortex. × 62,000.

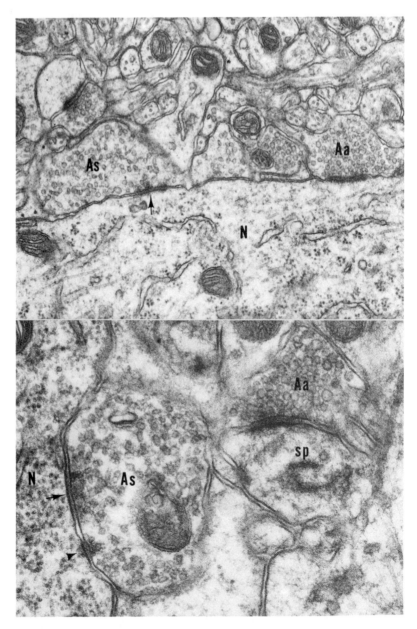

Figure 3. *Top: Synapses on the soma (N) of a nonpyramidal cell.* On the *left* is an axon terminal (As) containing pleomorphic vesicles and forming a symmetric synapse (*arrow*). The axon terminal on the *right* (Aa) has round vesicles and is forming an asymmetric synapse. Rat visual cortex. × 35,000. *Bottom:* On the *left* is an axon terminal (As) containing pleomorphic vesicles. It forms a symmetric synaptic junction (*arrow*) with the cell body (N) of a pyramidal cell. A punctum adherens (*arrowhead*) is also present between the pre- and postsynaptic membranes. On the *right* is an axon terminal (Aa) forming an asymmetric junction with a dendritic spine (sp). Monkey visual cortex. × 53,000.

of the spine and of the axon terminal often match each other in size, so that small spines seem to receive small axon terminals and large spines seem to receive large axon terminals. At these synapses, the synaptic junction tends to occupy most of the interface between the synapsing elements and, although the smaller spines show a continuous synaptic junction when sectioned normal to the plane of the synapsing membranes, synapses involving larger spines often show two or three apparently separate junctional zones (Figure 2, top).

The reason for this appearance is that the larger synaptic junctions are perforated (Peters and Kaiserman-Abramof, 1969; Cohen and Siekevitz, 1978). This can be shown either by making reconstructions of such synaptic junctions from serial thin sections, or by examining *en face* views of axospinous synapses in which the synaptic density is visible (Figure 2, bottom). Perforations tend to occur when the diameter of the synaptic junction or disk exceeds 0.5 μm, and some of the junctions that are about 1 μm in diameter can have two or three perforations. The functions of the perforations are not yet known, but Greenough et al. (1978) have found that the frequency of the occurrence of the perforations at asymmetric synapses in rat occipital cortex triples between 10 and 60 days of age, and that rats reared from weaning in complex or socially enriched environments have significantly higher proportions of synapses with perforations than do rats reared in isolation. Even when synapses with the same overall diameters are compared, the frequency of perforated synaptic junctions is greater in the socially enriched group than in the group reared in isolation. The point made by Greenough et al. (1978) is that experience and environment might produce changes in synaptic structure.

In thin sections of these asymmetric axospinous synapses, the postsynaptic density appears to contain a finely filamentous material that is continuous with the filaments of the rather flocculent matrix of the spine bulb. In preparations of isolated postsynaptic dendrites from cerebral cortex, Carlin et al. (1980) have shown that filaments 6–9 nm in diameter are attached to particles that are contained in the postsynaptic density. Presumably, these particles are the ones seen in freeze-fractured preparations when the postsynaptic membrane is exposed, and Carlin et al. (1980) suggest that the filaments may be actin. This suggestion seems to be substantiated by Matus et al. (1982), who have shown that an antibody to fish muscle actin binds to material in the dendritic spine, and by Fifková and Delay (1982), who have demonstrated the presence of actin filaments in dendritic spines of the hippocampus by decorating them with S-I myosin fragments.

In conventionally prepared material examined with the electron microscope, little is seen of the structures present on the cytoplasmic face of the presynaptic membrane, where it is known that there is a hexagonal array of dense particles attached to the presynaptic membrane. Sometimes, however, these particles can be seen in *en face* views of asymmetric synapses (see Figure 2, bottom).

Other structures that receive an abundance of axon terminals forming asymmetric synapses are the dendrites of smooth and sparsely spinous nonpyramidal cells, and most workers agree that the ratio of asymmetric to symmetric axodendritic synapses increases with distance from the cell body. Consequently, symmetric synapses are most common on the initial portions of dendrites, and the population of synapses along the more distal lengths of dendrites is almost exclusively asymmetric in form. The same distribution of asymmetric and symmetric synapses seems to occur along the shafts of pyramidal cell dendrites, but the frequency is much lower than along smooth or sparsely spinous dendrites, since pyramidal cell dendrites receive most of their synapses on spines.

Superficially at least, the appearance of the asymmetric axodendritic synapses is similar to that of the axospinous ones (Figure 1, bottom). But sometimes the postsynaptic density is less prominent and is usually continuous, only rarely showing the perforations displayed by the larger axospinous synapses.

Other locations where asymmetric synapses can occur are the cell bodies of the nonpyramidal cells. All of the cell bodies of Golgi-impregnated or HRP-filled nonpyramidal cells with smooth or sparsely spinous dendrites examined so far by electron microscopy have been found to have some asymmetric synapses on their perikarya. Usually, these synapses are formed by small axon terminals with round synaptic vesicles, and the form of the junction is similar to that of asymmetric synapses on spines and dendritic shafts (Figure 3, top). Sites from which asymmetric synapses appear to be excluded are the cell bodies of pyramidal cells and spiny stellate cells, and axon initial segments.

Symmetric Synapses

The most frequently examined symmetric synapses in the cerebral cortex are those that occur on the cell bodies of neurons, for they are the ones most easily found.

For the most part, axon terminals forming symmetric axosomatic synapses are larger than the ones forming asymmetric axosomatic synapses, and they usually contain a number of mitochondria among their pleomorphic synaptic vesicles (Figures 3–5). As mentioned above, the extent of flattening of the vesicles depends largely upon the osmolarity of the buffer in the aldehyde fixing solution, so that in some preparations elongated vesicles may not be apparent. But even when they are rounded, the vesicles at symmetric synapses are always smaller than those within axon terminals forming asymmetric synapses. Another difference from the asymmetric axosomatic synapses is that, at the symmetric synapses, the synaptic junctions lack a prominent postsynaptic density and tend to be rather short. They occupy only a fraction of the interface between the axon terminal and the cell body, and the vesicles accumulate near them, so that the junctional zones and the associated vesicles are referred to as synaptic complexes. This is emphasized because, in addition to the synaptic complexes, there are other junctional complexes that have no accumulations of associated vesicles. These latter junctions are also symmetric in form, and there is often a plate of dense material in the intercellular space. They resemble miniature zonulae adherentes, leading Peters et al. (1976) to call them puncta adherentia (Figure 3, bottom). When the forms of the junctional zones are reconstructed from serial thin sections, it becomes evident that they have the form of patches, as shown in Figure 4. As can be seen, most of these symmetric axosomatic synapses have one or two synaptic junctions and two to four puncta, although two of the junctions lack puncta. The diameters of the synaptic junctions vary between 0.4 and 0.6 μm, and the puncta adherentia are between 0.1 and 0.15 μm in diameter.

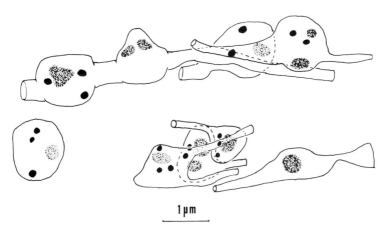

Figure 4. *Reconstructions of axonal boutons and the symmetric axosomatic synapses they form on pyramidal cell bodies in rat somatosensory cortex.* The synapses are shown *en face.* The synaptic junctions are *stippled*; the puncta adherentia are represented by *black dots.* The reconstruction is made from serial thin sections. For further explanation, see text.

Symmetric synapses are also common on the shafts of dendrites of both pyramidal (Figure 5) and nonpyramidal cells, on axon initial segments of pyramidal cells, and occasionally on dendritic spines. In some instances, particularly at symmetric synapses involving the shafts of small diameter dendrites, the synaptic junction may be more extensive than at axosomatic synapses and may occupy almost all of the interface between the pre- and postsynaptic membranes.

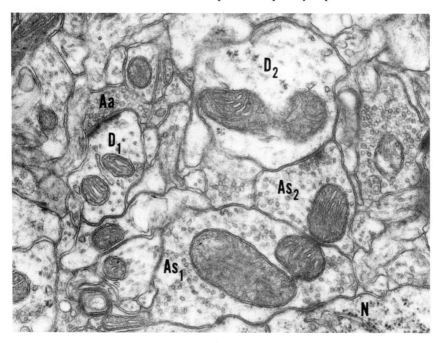

Figure 5. *Two axon terminals with pleomorphic vesicles in a neuropil.* One of the terminals (As$_1$) is forming a symmetric synapse with a cell body (N) and the other (As$_2$) with a dendrite (D$_2$). Compare these synapses with the asymmetric synapses between an axon terminal (Aa) and a dendrite (D$_1$). Rat auditory cortex. × 34,000.

SYNAPTIC PATTERNS OVER THE SURFACES OF NEURONS

In classifying neurons of the cerebral cortex on the basis of their morphology, it has become common to separate them into two broad groups, pyramidal and nonpyramidal cells (see Peters and Jones, 1984). Typically, pyramidal cells have dendrites that bear many spines and one dominant, apical dendrite that extends into layer I. Nonpyramidal cells lack this prominent dendrite and tend to have more symmetrically arranged dendritic trees. Moreover, the majority of nonpyramidal cells have dendrites that either are free of spines or have few of these protrusions, but they do not constitute a morphologically homogeneous group. They are grouped together because they lack the characteristics of pyramidal cells, rather than because they have any features in common. One type of nonpyramidal cell, the spiny stellate cell found in large numbers in layer IV of some cortices, does not fit comfortably with the other nonpyramidal cells. Like the pyramidal cells, spiny stellate cells have dendrites that bear many spines, and their synaptology is similar to that of pyramidal cells. Consequently, it is appropriate to consider the pyramidal and spiny stellate cells as members of the same neuronal group (see Lund, 1984).

Pyramidal Cells and Spiny Stellate Cells

With the possible exception of some corticotectal pyramidal cells in cat visual cortex (Kennedy, 1982), all pyramidal cells so far examined have been found to have only symmetric synapses on their perikarya (see Colonnier, 1981; Feldman, 1984), and such synapses also prevail on the neuronal processes close to the cell body. Thus, the axon initial segments of pyramidal cells have only symmetric synapses (e.g., Peters et al., 1968; Jones and Powell, 1969), and it is relatively uncommon to find other than symmetric synapses on the spine-free proximal portions of their dendrites. Asymmetric synapses seem to occur only some distance away from the cell body, and essentially their appearance coincides with that of the spines. Indeed, these protrusions are the prime receptors for axon terminals forming asymmetric synapses. However, there are some other asymmetric synapses on the shafts of the spine-bearing lengths of pyramidal cell dendrites, as well as occasional symmetric synapses, and some spines receive symmetric synapses. But in each documented example, it appears that the same spine also receives an asymmetric synapse.

Spiny stellate cells are frequent in the granule cell layers of the sensory cortices of a number of mammals, including the primary visual cortex of the cat, macaque, and tree shrew (see Lund, 1984), and the somatosensory cortex of the monkey (Jones, 1975). They also occur in layer IV of the mouse barrel field (Woolsey et al., 1975). At present, the distribution of these neurons among animal species and cortical areas is not well understood, but they are believed to be absent from some areas, so that in contrast to area 17, area 18 of monkey visual cortex lacks spiny stellate cells (Valverde, 1978; Lund et al., 1981). They also appear to be absent from area 17 of rat visual cortex, in which layer IV is largely occupied by pyramidal cells (Peters and Kara, 1984). Most likely, spiny stellate cells are a variety of pyramidal cell, because except for the absence of an apical dendrite, there is little to distinguish spiny stellate cells from pyramidal cells in Golgi preparations (see Lund, 1984), and the distribution of synapses over their surfaces is similar. An interesting observation made by Saint Marie and Peters (1984) is that among the varieties of spiny stellate cells present in layer IV of monkey area 17, the small spiny stellate cells have no synapses on their axon initial segments, whereas the medium-sized ones resemble pyramidal cells in having a number of symmetric axoaxonal synapses. The reason for this difference between the axon initial segments of these two types of spiny stellate cells is not yet known, but it may be that the medium-sized ones possess extrinsically projecting axons (Lund et al., 1975; Tigges et al., 1981), as do most pyramidal cells. If so, then the presence of symmetric synapses along the axon initial segment may be a feature of neurons with axons projecting out of the cortex. In this context, it may be noted that the smooth and sparsely spinous nonpyramidal cells, which have axons remaining in the cortex, also appear to lack axoaxonal synapses.

Smooth and Sparsely Spinous Nonpyramidal Cells

The distribution of synapses over the surfaces of the nonpyramidal cells with dendrites bearing few or no spines is quite different from that of the pyramidal and spiny stellate cells, for they have both symmetric and asymmetric axosomatic synapses. This was first noticed by Colonnier (1968) and has been borne out by subsequent studies of neurons in a variety of cortices (see Colonnier, 1981). In earlier studies, which types of nonpyramidal cells the perikarya belonged to could not be ascertained, nor whether all types of nonpyramidal cells (other than the spiny stellate cells) have both symmetric and asymmetric axosomatic synapses. However, subsequent electron microscope examination of Golgi-impregnated examples of specific types of nonpyramidal cells—such as the smooth and sparsely spinous multipolar neurons of cat (LeVay, 1973) and rat (Peters and Fairén, 1978; Peters and Proskauer, 1980) visual cortex, and the chandelier cells (Peters et al., 1983) and bipolar cells (Peters and Kimerer, 1981) of rat visual cortex—have shown that each of them has both symmetric and asymmetric axosomatic synapses. Consequently, on the basis of the available evidence, there appears to be a fundamental difference in the distribution of synapses over the cell bodies of neurons with spiny dendrites, compared to neurons with few or no spines on their dendrites.

Having a dearth of spines, the dendrites of the smoother nonpyramidal cells receive most of the synapses directly on their dendritic shafts. As with the spiny cells, symmetric synapses predominate along the proximal portions of their dendrites, the more distal lengths being occupied almost entirely by asymmetric synapses. However, even a cursory examination of the profiles of smooth and sparsely spinous dendrites reveals great differences among them in terms of the frequency with which synapses occur. For example, Davis and Sterling (1979) have shown that, in layer IV of cat visual cortex, the dendrites of neurons they designate as large type II neurons have as many as 60 synapses per 100 μm^2 of surface area, whereas their small type III neurons with varicose dendrites have only 8.1 synapses per 100 μm^2. It is not possible to equate these types of neurons with ones encountered in Golgi preparations, but White and Rock (1981) have compared the numbers of synapses along the dendrites of a bitufted and a multipolar neuron in layer IV mouse SmI cortex and found the bitufted neuron to have about twice as many synapses per unit length of dendrite as does the multipolar neuron. Symmetric synapses accounted for 26% and 20% of the total synaptic population, respectively, and examination of plots of the positions of synapses (see Figure 14 in White and Rock, 1981) clearly shows symmetric synapses to be more prevalent on the proximal than on the distal portions of the dendrites.

As mentioned earlier, those nonpyramidal cells with smooth or sparsely spinous dendrites that have so far been examined by the combined Golgi–electron microscope technique—namely, multipolar neurons (Peters and Fairén, 1978; Peters and Proskauer, 1980), chandelier cells (Peters et al., 1983), and bipolar cells (Peters and Kimerer, 1981)—have few if any synapses along their axon initial segments.

Inhibition and Excitation

As is discussed later, there is now general agreement that symmetric synapses are inhibitory in function, and that asymmetric synapses are excitatory. If this is so, then the perikarya and proximal portions of both dendrites and axons of pyramidal and spiny stellate cells form only inhibitory synapses. The excitatory synapses, most of which are formed with dendritic spines, are located away from the cell body. For smooth and sparsely spinous nonpyramidal cells, the situation is different. Most of the inhibitory synapses are still located on the cell body and proximal portions of the dendrites, but the cell bodies of these nonpyramidal cells also receive excitatory synapses, which can be expected to modify the effects of the inhibitory synapses. In addition, the smooth and sparsely spinous nonpyramidal cells, like the small spiny stellate cells, are not subject to the powerful inhibition that can be expected from the axoaxonal synapses placed along the axon initial segments of the pyramidal cells and the large spiny stellate cells.

Presumably, these different surface distribution patterns of synapses are controlled by the neurons themselves, and it would be of interest to know if the patterns are determined early in development, or if the cell bodies of spiny neurons, for example, ever form asymmetric synapses. This is difficult to ascertain, because in young animals the densities associated with the synapses are often immature in appearance, so that developing synapses cannot readily be classified as asymmetric or symmetric (see, e.g., Muller et al., 1984). However, Muller et al. (1984) concluded that in rabbit visual cortex, at least, the different synaptic patterns of pyramidal and multipolar neurons are already established by 10–14 days postnatally.

The point to be emphasized is that spiny and nonspiny neurons have different patterns of synapses over their surfaces, and that these patterns are significant in any consideration of the synaptic relationships among cortical neurons. For example, the perikarya and axon initial segments of the spiny neurons are not accessible to axon terminals that form asymmetric synapses and, for the most part, the dendritic spines of these same neurons are not available for the formation of symmetric synapses. In contrast, the smooth and sparsely spinous nonpyramidal cells exert a less rigorous "control" over where the two types of synapses are formed on their surfaces, although their cell bodies and proximal dendritic lengths are still the preferred sites for the reception of axon terminals forming symmetric synapses.

NEURONAL SHAPE

There are many different types of neurons in the cerebral cortex, and they can be classified on the basis of their appearance in Golgi preparations. How the neurons are classified, or allocated to different morphological groups, varies among different authors, but the main features used to distinguish among neuronal types are the shapes and branching patterns of their dendritic trees, the presence or absence of dendritic spines along their dendrites, the distribution patterns of their axons, and the size and locations of their cell bodies. Such classification is not intended to give an extensive account of the neuronal types that exist in the cerebral cortex, but merely to point out that the locations of their cell bodies and the shapes of their dendritic trees play an important role in determining which kinds of axon terminals can be available to them. For example, the pyramidal neurons with their long apical dendrites, which typically extend from the cell body into layer I, seem to be adapted to sampling synaptic inputs in a number of cortical laminae, although even among pyramidal cells the location of the cell body in the depth of the cortex determines what kinds of afferents the neurons can receive (Figure 6). The layer V pyramidal cells can receive callosal afferents terminating in layers V and III, as well as thalamic afferents terminating in layers IV and I. But layer IV pyramidal cells are above the callosal input to layer V, and layer III pyramidal cells can only receive the thalamic afferents terminating in layer IV on their basal dendrites, not on their apical ones.

Most of the nonpyramidal cells have much more restricted dendritic trees. The exceptions, perhaps, are the bipolar and the double bouquet cells, some of which have long and narrow dendritic trees extending vertically through a number of cortical layers (Figure 6). Most other nonpyramidal cells, like the spiny stellate cells of layer IV in some sensory cortices and the smooth, multipolar neurons, have much more localized dendritic trees. Consequently, they are only able to receive axon terminals available in the vicinities of the cell bodies.

Thus, the locations of neurons within the depth of the cortex and the shapes of their dendritic trees are significant in determining which presynaptic elements are available to synapse with them. To date, this aspect of neuronal interrelationships appears not to have been extensively investigated, for most attention has been paid to the presynaptic roles played by identified neurons, with particular emphasis on the morphological types of synapses produced by their axon terminals. As is shown later, although we know the general types of postsynaptic elements involved in the formation of synapses by certain types of neurons, in most cases it has not been possible to determine the cells of origin of the postsynaptic elements.

Another difficulty in ascertaining what neuronal populations might be available to receive synapses formed by the axons of different types of neurons has been the inability to examine much of the distribution of the axons of neurons in Golgi preparations. Some resolution of this problem has come from the recent

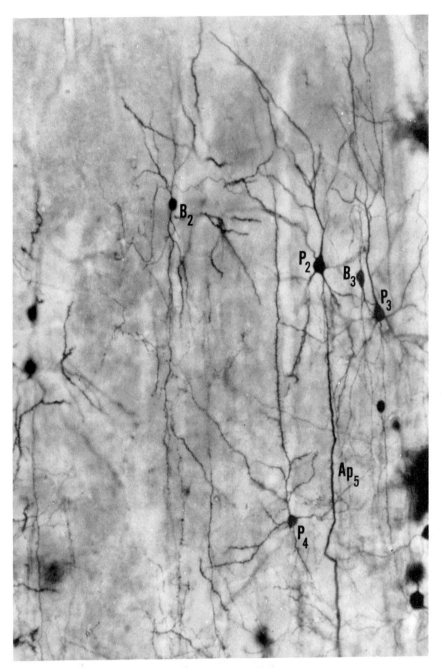

Figure 6. *Golgi-impregnated rat visual cortex.* The field contains the apical dendrite (Ap_5) of a layer V pyramidal cell, as well as pyramidal cells in layer IV (P_4), layer III (P_3), and layer II (P_2). Two bipolar cells are also present. The one in layer II (B_2) is a small cell with rather short dendrites, while the layer III bipolar cell (B_3) has descending dendrites that reach layer IV. × 275.

use of the technique of injecting neurons intracellularly with horseradish peroxidase (HRP), which fills both unmyelinated and myelinated axons. By using this technique, Gilbert and Wiesel (1981), among others, have been able to show how the axons of different types of neurons are distributed within the cortex. But until more is known about the neuronal elements with which these axon terminals synapse, we are still unable to do more than construct very simplified versions of the neuronal circuits that exist in the cerebral cortex.

It needs to be mentioned that the geographical location of a neuron within a given cortical area also determines its input. For example, within the primary visual cortex, the location of the neuron determines from which portion of the visual field the information carried by the thalamic afferents exciting it was initially derived.

Sources of Axon Terminals Synapsing in the Cerebral Cortex

As a preface to this section, it needs to be stated that the available evidence indicates that all of the axon terminals produced by a particular neuron give rise to the same morphological type of synapse. The axon terminals from a given neuron may impinge on a variety of postsynaptic elements, but all of the terminals form either asymmetric synapses only or symmetric synapses only.

Extrinsic Axons Forming Asymmetric Synapses. The sites of termination of axons projecting into the cerebral cortex have been largely examined 'either by making lesions to cause their terminals to degenerate and become electron-dense or by labeling the terminals with anterogradely transported tritiated amino acids, so that they can be recognized by autoradiography. By these methods, the sites of termination of a number of afferent inputs, including thalamocortical, commisural, and association axons, have been examined in a variety of cortical areas in a number of species (see Colonnier, 1981). Each of these afferents have been found to form asymmetric synapses.

Most of the terminals from extrinsic axons have been shown to synapse with dendritic spines, but when quantitative studies have been carried out in lesioned material, there are interesting differences between afferents with respect to what they synapse with. For example, in monkey motor cortex (Sloper and Powell, 1979) and rat auditory cortex (Cipolloni and Peters, 1983) 96–97% of the callosal terminals synapse with spines, and the remainder with the shafts of both spiny and smooth dendrites. Synapses formed by thalamic afferents in layer IV have a different distribution pattern, for only 89% of them synapse with dendritic spines in monkey motor cortex (Sloper and Powell, 1979) and only 78% in rat auditory cortex (Vaughan and Peters, 1985). In a variety of cortices, the percentage of thalamic axon terminals synapsing with spines has been given as between 70 and 90% (for tables of collected data, see Peters and Feldman, 1976; Colonnier, 1981). Thalamic afferents also synapse with dendritic shafts but, unlike the callosal afferents, some thalamic axon terminals synapse with the cell bodies of nonpyramidal cells.

It might be argued that since the callosal afferents terminate mainly in layers III and V, and since the thalamic afferents terminate in layer IV, the differences in the distribution of their synapses can be attributed to differences in the composition of the neuropil they are entering. In part this may be true, but there is evidence to indicate that some preference is exerted by the afferents themselves. This was shown in the following experiments. Vaughan and Foundas (1982) have demonstrated that if the corpus callosum is lesioned in one-month-old rats and the animals are allowed to survive for three months, thalamic afferents in auditory cortex proliferate into layer III, which ordinarily is a callosal domain. This proliferation can be demonstrated by comparing the distribution of degen- erating thalamic axon terminals in callosally lesioned animals and age-matched controls. In control animals, D. W. Vaughan (unpublished observations) found that in layer IV, 78% of thalamic afferents synapse with dendritic spines, whereas in layer III, 92% of callosal afferents in layer III synapse with dendritic spines. However, when lesions are made in the medial geniculate bodies of the callosally lesioned experimental animals and layer III is examined, 80% of the degenerating thalamic afferents that have invaded this layer now synapse with dendritic spines. In other words, synapses formed by the terminals of thalamic axons that have proliferated into layer III have a distribution pattern similar to that of the normal thalamic afferents in layer IV. To complete the picture, it needs to be stated that in the neuropil of layer III of normal rat auditory cortex, 84% of all asymmetric synapses are formed with dendritic spines. Thus, there is every indication that the relative proportions of postsynaptic elements with which thalamic and callosal afferents synapse are not solely determined by the composition of the neuropil into which they enter, but that the afferents themselves can select where to synapse.

Although the early degeneration studies were important in defining the kinds of postsynaptic elements receiving extrinsic afferent inputs, the types of neurons receiving the afferents could not be determined. This became possible only with the development of the combined Golgi–electron microscope procedure, in which Golgi-impregnated cortical neurons could first be examined with the light mi- croscope and subsequently with the electron microscope (LeVay, 1973; Fairén et al., 1977; Parnavelas et al., 1977). Use of this technique in tissue containing degenerating thalamocortical axon terminals (Peters et al., 1977), has shown that all neuronal elements contained in layer IV of cerebral cortex that are capable of forming asymmetric synapses are potential recipients of thalamocortical afferents. In rat visual cortex, this includes the spines of basal dendrites of layer III pyramidal cells, the spines of apical dendrites of layer V pyramidal cells, the dendritic spines of spiny stellate cells (Figure 7, upper left), and the perikarya and dendrites of smooth multipolar and bipolar cells (Peters et al., 1979; Peters and Kimerer, 1981).

A similar result has been obtained by White (1978), and by Hornung and Garey (1981), who have used this same technique to examine the thalamic inputs to layer IV of mouse somatosensory cortex and of cat visual cortex. It is now clear from the careful studies of White and his colleagues, who have examined the thalamic afferents to neurons in layer IV of mouse barrel field, that although these afferents can synapse with all structures capable of forming asymmetric synapses, the extent of the input to different types of neurons varies. For example, Hersch and White (1981) have demonstrated that the apical dendrites of five pyramidal cells with cell bodies in layers V and VI, and the dendrites of a spiny bitufted neuron and a nonspiny multipolar neuron with somata in layer V,

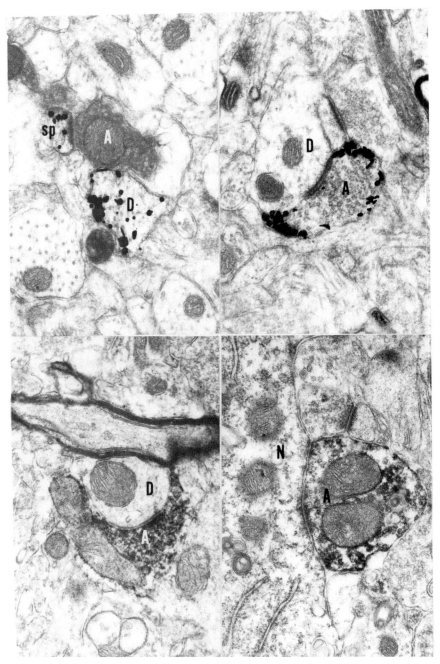

Figure 7. *Upper left: A degenerating thalamic axon terminal (A) synapsing with a spine (sp) from the dendritic shaft (D) of a sparsely spined nonpyramidal cell in layer IV of rat visual cortex.* The dendrite and its spine are from a Golgi-impregnated neuron that was gold-toned. The gold has the form of black particles. × 38,000. (From Peters et al., 1979.) *Upper right:* The gold-toned axon terminal (A) of a bipolar cell in rat visual cortex forming an asymmetric synapse with a small-diameter dendritic shaft (D). × 34,000. *Lower left:* A VIP-positive axon terminal (A) in rat visual cortex forming a symmetric synapse with a small dendrite (D). × 25,000. (From Connor and Peters, 1984.) *Lower right:* A GAD-positive axon terminal (A) forming a symmetric synapse with the cell body of a GAD-positive nonpyramidal cell (N). Rat visual cortex. × 24,000.

receive quite different proportions of their asymmetric synapses from thalamocortical afferents, again demonstrating a selectivity of where extrinsic afferent axons synapse.

Intrinsic Axons Forming Asymmetric Synapses.   At most, only 20–30% of the axon terminals forming asymmetric synapses in a particular cortical layer appear to be derived from extrinsic sources (LeVay and Gilbert, 1976; White, 1978). Consequently, most of the axon terminals producing asymmetric synapses must be intrinsic in origin, and the likely sources of most of these intrinsic axon terminals are the pyramidal cells and the spiny stellate cells. Both types of neurons have been shown to have axons forming asymmetric synapses (LeVay, 1973; Parnavelas et al., 1977; White et al., 1980; Mates and Lund, 1983; Saint Marie and Peters, 1984), and the population of pyramidal neurons is quite large, so that in rat visual cortex, for example, pyramidal cells account for as many as 69% (Winfield et al., 1980) to 85% (Peters and Kara, 1984) of all neurons present. Surprisingly though, the identified pyramidal cells so far examined by electron microscope have had axon terminals that seem to prefer to synapse with dendritic shafts rather than with dendritic spines. Thus, in their examination of 62 synapses formed by the axon collaterals of a Golgi-impregnated layer II–III pyramidal cell in monkey somatic sensory cortex, Winfield et al. (1981) found 60% of them to involve dendritic shafts and only 40% to involve dendritic spines. The same is true for the HRP-filled layer VI pyramidal cells in cat visual cortex examined by McGuire et al. (1983). The axons of these neurons terminate in layer IV, and McGuire et al. found that 71% of the terminals synapse with dendritic shafts and 29% with dendritic spines. These results are unexpected, because axospinous synapses account for about 80% of all asymmetric synapses in cortical neuropil. It is thus unclear at present what types of neurons provide the axon terminals that form axospinous synapses.

For spiny stellate cells in layer IV of monkey visual cortex, the situation is somewhat different. In an electron microscope study of the axons of Golgi-impregnated spiny stellate neurons, Saint Marie and Peters (1984) found that the axospinous synapses formed by the terminals outnumbered axodendritic ones by two to one. Many of the axon terminals seem to synapse with the spines and shafts of other spiny stellate cells, but some of the postsynaptic dendritic shafts clearly belong to smooth nonpyramidal cells.

Pyramidal neurons and spiny stellate cells are not the only neurons with axons forming asymmetric synapses, for Golgi–electron microscope studies have shown that bipolar cells of rat (Peters and Kimerer, 1981; Figure 7, upper right) and cat (Fairén et al., 1984) visual cortex, as well as some double bouquet cells of cat (Fairén et al., 1984) and monkey (Somogyi and Cowey, 1981) visual cortex, also contribute to the asymmetric synapse population. Again, the axons of these neurons have been shown to synapse with dendritic spines and shafts, and while at least some of the spines are derived from pyramidal cells (Peters and Kimerer, 1981), the identity of the other postsynaptic elements forming asymmetric synapses with these axon terminals is not yet known.

At this stage something should be added about studies employing antibodies to neurotransmitters, because bipolar cells are visualized by antibodies to a number of different putative and potential neurotransmitters. This has drawn attention to these particular neurons in the past few years, and some of the results affect the interpretation of the role of bipolar cells in the cortex. In rat visual cortex, bipolar cells are the most common type of neuron visualized by antibodies to vasoactive intestinal polypeptide (VIP) (e.g., McDonald et al., 1982a; Connor and Peters, 1984; Morrison et al., 1984), and they account for as many as 85–90% of neurons binding VIP antibody. In addition, bipolar cells in this cortex are also the most common neuronal type visualized by antibodies to acetylcholine transferase (AChE) (Houser et al., 1983a), and they also appear in preparations reacted with antibodies to cholecystokinin (CCK) (Peters et al., 1983) and avian pancreatic polypeptide (APP) (McDonald et al., 1982b). When the VIP-positive (Connor and Peters, 1984) and AChE-positive (Houser et al., 1983b) axon terminals in rat visual cortex are examined by electron microscope, they are found to form symmetric synapses that mainly involve dendritic shafts (Figure 7, lower left). The same is true for CCK-positive axon terminals present in rat and monkey cortex (Hendry et al., 1983b). In each case, the authors have commented that although the synaptic cleft is narrow, like that of a symmetric synapse, the junctional zone is long and has well-developed densities similar to those of asymmetric synapses. How to interpret this data in light of the results of the Golgi–electron microscope studies that have shown bipolar cells to have axons forming asymmetric synapses is not yet clear. A number of possibilities exist. For example, there may be two types of bipolar cells, one forming asymmetric and the other symmetric synapses, of which the former have as yet been examined only by Golgi–electron microscope procedures. Or the antibody reactions may affect the appearance of the synaptic junctions. In any case, the seeming disparity in the data has to be solved if we are to understand the role of the bipolar cells in cerebral circuitry.

Axon Terminals Forming Symmetric Synapses.   As has been shown, symmetric synapses occur on the cell bodies and dendritic shafts of all cortical neurons, and upon the axon initial segments of both pyramidal cells and large spiny stellate cells. There is no evidence that any symmetric synapses are formed by extrinsic axons entering the cortex. All of them are believed to be produced by intrinsic axons, and in recent years many of their origins have been revealed as a result of studies in which neurons have been identified by visualizing them through either Golgi impregnation or HRP intracellular filling and then determining the projections of their axons by electron microscopy. The results show that the axons of the various types of neurons giving rise to symmetric synapses differ widely in where they form their synapses (Table 1).

The axon terminals of multipolar and bitufted neurons, with local and un-myelinated axonal plexuses in rat, cat, and monkey visual cortex, form symmetric synapses with the cell bodies and dendritic shafts of both pyramidal and non-pyramidal cells, as well as with the axon initial segments of some pyramidal cells (LeVay, 1973; Peters and Fairén, 1978; Peters and Proskauer, 1980; Mates and Lund, 1983). Consequently, these neurons appear to synapse with all post-synaptic sites available for the formation of symmetric synapses. The basket cells of cat visual cortex show more specificity, for in their Golgi–electron microscope study of such neurons in the superficial layers of cortex, DeFelipe and Fairén (1982) found the basket cell axons to synapse only with the cell bodies

Table 1. Sites of Termination of Axons of Neurons Forming Symmetric Synapses[a]

Presynaptic Neuron	Pyramidal Cells				Nonpyramidal Cells		
	Somata	Dendrites	Spines	Axons	Somata	Dendrites	Axons
Smooth and sparsely spinous neurons with local plexus axons	++	++	++	+	++	++	?
Basket cells							
DeFelipe and Fairén, 1982	++	++ (proximally)			++	++ (proximally)	
Martin et al., 1983; Somogyi et al., 1983	++	++	++		+	+	
Double bouquet cells			+		+	++	
Chandelier cells				+++			

[a] +, forms synapses; ++, preferred postsynaptic element; +++, synapses exclusively.

and proximal dendrites of pyramidal and nonpyramidal cells. This is somewhat different from the intracellular HRP-filled basket cells in layers III and IV of cat visual cortex examined by Martin et al. (1983) and Somogyi et al. (1983b). About 85% of the axon terminals of these neurons synapsed with pyramidal cells: 33% with the perikarya; 20% with spines; and 20% with the apical and basal dendrites of these cells. The remaining 10% synapsed with the dendrites and somata of nonpyramidal neurons.

In contrast to this distribution of basket cell axons, the axon terminals of some double bouquet cells that form symmetric synapses in cat and monkey visual cortex prefer to synapse with dendritic shafts. This type of double bouquet cell has been examined by Somogyi and Cowey (1981, 1984) using the Golgi–electron microscope procedure. Eighty-six percent of the axon terminals of three such neurons from cat area 17 synapsed with dendritic shafts that appeared not to bear spines, 5% synapsed with dendritic spines, and 9% synapsed with the perikarya of nonpyramidal cells. For two other double bouquet cells, one in area 18 of cat visual cortex and one in area 17 of monkey, synapses on dendritic shafts were 74% and 60%, respectively. The remainder of the synapses were made with dendritic spines that also bore asymmetric synapses formed by un-impregnated axon terminals (see Somogyi and Cowey, 1984).

The other type of neuron shown to form symmetric synapses is the chandelier cell. These have been studied extensively via the Golgi–electron microscope technique, and it seems that their axons synapse exclusively with the axon initial segments of pyramidal cells (e.g., Somogyi, 1977; Fairén and Valverde, 1980; Peters et al., 1982; Somogyi et al., 1982).

Consequently, there are great differences in where the axons of the various types of neurons forming symmetric synapses terminate (see Table 1) and exert their inhibition. The evidence for considering the multipolar and bitufted cells with local plexus axons, the double bouquet cells, the basket cells, and the chandelier cells to be inhibitory neurons is that many of them have been shown to accumulate [^{3}H]GABA, and axon terminals forming symmetric synapses in cerebral cortex give a positive reaction to antibody to glutamic acid decarboxylase (GAD) (Figure 7, lower right). This has been shown in a number of studies (e.g., Ribak, 1978; Peters et al., 1982; Somogyi et al., 1983a; Hendry et al., 1983a), and there is good evidence to believe that γ-aminobutyric acid (GABA), the neurotransmitter synthesized by GAD, has an inhibitory affect in the visual cortex (e.g., Sillito, 1975).

CONCLUSIONS

It seems that there are only two distinct morphological types of chemical synapses in the neocortex, and since all of the presynaptic elements are axons, the synaptology seems to be basically simple. Despite this seeming simplicity, the neurons of the cerebral cortex are capable of carrying out complex processing and of producing well-defined responses, as seen in the physiological studies that have been carried out. This can be possible only if different types of neurons receive relatively specific inputs, and the question being asked is what determines these inputs. Within the cerebral cortex, there are two large groups of neurons, the spiny cells and the smooth or sparsely spinous cells. Not all surfaces of these neurons are equally available to all types of axon terminals, and within each group are subsets of neurons with differing dendritic arborizations. Presumably, since the dendrites are the main receptive surfaces of neurons, the forms of dendritic trees must play a significant role in determining what kinds of inputs they can receive. But even if the inputs are available in the neuropil, the various kinds of axons derived from extrinsic and intrinsic sources themselves show some preference as to where they synapse, preferring some postsynaptic elements over others. This preference, together with the postsynaptic control over where axons can synapse, must determine the neuronal connections which exist in the cerebral cortex, and while we have some knowledge of those neuronal circuits and neurotransmitters, our knowledge is still superficial. It falls far short of explaining the complex physiological responses of the neurons that have so far been recorded, and progress still has to be made toward the goal of obtaining more detailed information about the synaptic inputs of various types of neurons—and how the synapses they form interact to bring about neuronal response.

ACKNOWLEDGMENTS

The author wishes to thank Dr. M. L. Feldman for his helpful discussions about material presented in this chapter. The personal work reported herein was supported by grants NS-07016 and AG-00001 from the National Institutes of Health, United States Public Health Service.

REFERENCES

Carlin, R. K., D. J. Grab, R. S. Cohen, and P. Siekevitz (1980) Isolation and characterization of postsynaptic densities from various brain regions: Enrichment of different types of postsynaptic densities. *J. Cell Biol.* **86**:831–843.

Cipolloni, P. B., and A. Peters (1983) The termination of callosal fibers in the auditory cortex of the rat. A combined Golgi–electron microscope and degeneration study. *J. Neurocytol.* **12**:713–726.

Cohen, R. S., and P. Siekevitz (1978) Form of the postsynaptic density. A serial section study. *J. Cell Biol.* **78**:36–46.

Colonnier, M. (1968) Synaptic patterns on different cell types in the different laminae of the cat visual cortex. An electron microscope study. *Brain Res.* **9**:268–287.

Colonnier, M. (1981) The electron-microscopic analysis of the neuronal organization of the cerebral cortex. In *The Organization of the Cerebral Cortex*, F. O. Schmitt, F. G. Worden, G. Adelman, and S. G. Dennis, eds., pp. 125–152, MIT Press, Cambridge, Massachusetts.

Connor, J. R., and A. Peters (1984) Vasoactive intestinal polypeptide-immunoreactive neurons in rat visual cortex. *Neuroscience* **12**:1027–1044.

Connors, B. W., L. S. Benardo, and D. A. Prince (1983) Coupling between neurons of the developing rat neocortex. *J. Neurosci.* **3**:773–782.

Davis, T. L., and P. Sterling (1979) Microcircuitry of cat visual cortex: Classification of neurons in layer IV of area 17, and identification of the patterns of lateral geniculate input. *J. Comp. Neurol.* **188**:599–628.

DeFelipe, J., and A. Fairén (1982) A type of basket cell in superficial layers of the cat visual cortex. A Golgi–electron microscope study. *Brain Res.* **244**:9–16.

Fairén, A., and F. Valverde (1980) A specialized type of neuron in the visual cortex of cat. A Golgi and electron microscope study of chandelier cells. *J. Comp. Neurol.* **194**:761–779.

Fairén, A., A. Peters, and J. Saldanha (1977) A new procedure for examining Golgi-impregnated neurons by light and electron microscopy. *J. Neurocytol.* **6**:311–337.

Fairén, A., J. DeFelipe, and J. Regidor (1984) Non-pyramidal neurons. General account. In *Cerebral Cortex*, Vol. 1, A. Peters and E. G. Jones, eds., pp. 201–253, Plenum, New York.

Feldman, M. L. (1984) Morphology of the neocortical pyramidal neuron. In *Cerebral Cortex*, Vol. 1, A. Peters and E. G. Jones, eds., pp. 128–200, Plenum, New York.

Fifková, E., and R. J. Delay (1982) Cytoplasmic action in neuronal processes as a possible mediator of synaptic plasticity. *J. Cell Biol.* **95**:345–350.

Gilbert, C. D., and T. N. Wiesel (1981) Laminar specialization and intracortical connections in cat primary visual cortex. In *The Organization of the Cerebral Cortex*, F. O. Schmitt, F. C. Worden, G. Adelman, and S. G. Dennis, eds., pp. 167–194, MIT Press, Cambridge.

Gray, E. G. (1959) Axosomatic and axodendritic synapses of the cerebral cortex. *J. Anat.* **93**:420–433.

Greenough, W. T., R. W. West, and T.-J. DeVoogd (1978) Subsynaptic plate perforations: Changes with age and experience in the rat. *Science* **202**:1096–1098.

Guillery, R. W. (1969) The organization of synaptic interconnections in the laminae of the dorsal lateral geniculate nucleus of the cat. *Z. Zellforsch. Mikrosk. Anat.* **96**:1–38.

Hendry, S. H. C., C. R. Houser, E. G. Jones, and J. E. Vaughn (1983a) Synaptic organization of immunocytochemically identified GABA neurons in the monkey sensory-motor cortex. *J. Neurocytol.* **12**:639–660.

Hendry, S. H. C., E. G. Jones, and M. C. Beinfeld (1983b) Cholecystokinin-immunoreactive neurons in rat and monkey cerebral cortex make symmetric synapses and have intimate association with blood vessels. *Proc. Natl. Acad. Sci. USA* **80**:2400–2404.

Hersch, S. M., and E. L. White (1981) Thalamocortical synapses involving identified neurons in mouse primary somatosensory cortex: A terminal degeneration and Golgi/EM study. *J. Comp. Neurol.* **195**:253–263.

Hornung, J. P., and L. J. Garey (1981) The thalamic projection to cat visual cortex: Ultrastructure of neurons identifed by Golgi impregnation or retrograde horseradish peroxidase transport. *Neuroscience* **6**:1053–1068.

Houser, C. R., G. D. Crawford, R. P. Barber, P. M. Salvaterra, and J. E. Vaughn (1983a) Organization and morphological characteristics of cholinergic neurons: An immunocytochemical study with a monoclonal antibody to choline acetyltransferase. *Brain Res.* 266:97–119.

Houser, C. R., G. D. Crawford, P. M. Salvaterra, and J. E. Vaughn (1983b) Cholinergic neurons in rat cerebral cortex identified by immunocytochemical localization of choline acetyltransferase. *Soc. Neurosci. Abstr.* 9:80.

Jones, E. G. (1975) Varieties and distribution of non-pyramidal cells in the somatic sensory cortex of the squirrel monkey. *J. Comp. Neurol.* 160:205–268.

Jones, E. G., and T. P. S. Powell (1969) Synapses on the axon hillocks and initial segments of pyramidal cell axons in the cerebral cortex. *J. Cell Sci.* 5:495–507.

Kennedy, H. (1982) Types of synapses contacting the soma of corticotectal cells in the visual cortex of the cat. *Neuroscience* 7:2159–2164.

LeVay, S. (1973) Synaptic patterns in the visual cortex of the cat and monkey. Electron microscopy of Golgi preparations. *J. Comp. Neurol.* 150:53–86.

LeVay, S., and C. D. Gilbert (1976) Laminar patterns of geniculocortical projection in the cat. *Brain Res.* 11:1–19.

Lund, J. S. (1984) Spiny stellate cells. In *Cerebral Cortex*, Vol. 1, A. Peters and E. G. Jones, eds., pp. 255–308, Plenum, New York.

Lund, J. S., R. D. Lund, A. E. Hendrickson, A. H. Bunt, and A. F. Fuchs (1975) The origin of efferent pathways from the primary visual cortex, area 17, of the macaque monkey as shown by retrograde transport of horseradish peroxidase. *J. Comp. Neurol.* 164:287–304.

Lund, J. S., A. E. Hendrickson, M. D. Ogren, and E. A. Tobin (1981) Anatomical organization of primate visual cortex area VII. *J. Comp. Neurol.* 202:19–45.

McDonald, J. K., J. G. Parnavelas, A. N. Karamanlidis, and N. Brecha (1982a) The morphology and distribution of peptide-containing neurons in the adult and developing visual cortex of the rat. II. Vasoactive intestinal polypeptide. *J. Neurocytol.* 11:825–837.

McDonald, J. K., J. G. Parnavelas, A. N. Karamanlidis, and N. Brecha (1982b) The morphology and distribution of peptide-containing neurons in the adult and developing visual cortex of the rat. IV. Avian pancreatic polypeptide. *J. Neurocytol.* 11:985–995.

McGuire, B. A., J. P. Hornung, C. D. Gilbert, and T. N. Wiesel (1983) Layer 6 cells primarily contact smooth and sparsely spiny neurons in layer 4 of cat striate cortex. *Soc. Neurosci. Abstr.* 9:617.

Martin, K. A. C., P. Somogyi, and D. Whitteridge (1983) Physiological and morphological properties of identified basket cells in the cat's visual cortex. *Exp. Brain Res.* 50:193–200.

Mates, S. L., and J. S. Lund (1983) Neuronal composition and development in lamina 4C of monkey striate cortex. *J. Comp. Neurol.* 221:60–90.

Matus, A., M. Ackermann, G. Pehling, H. R. Byers, and K. Fujiwara (1982) High actin concentrations in brain dendritic spines and postsynaptic densities. *Proc. Natl. Acad. Sci. USA* 79:7590–7594.

Morrison, J. H., P. J. Magistretti, R. Benoit, and F. E. Bloom (1984) The distribution and morphological characteristics of the intracortical VIP-positive cells: An immunohistochemical analysis. *Brain Res.* 292:209–282.

Muller, L. J., A. Pattiselanno, B. N. Cardoza, and G. Vrensen (1984) Development of synapses on pyramidal and multipolar non-pyramidal neurons in the visual cortex of rabbits. A combined Golgi–electron microscope study. *Neuroscience* 12:1045–1069.

Parnavelas, J. G., K. Sullivan, A. R. Lieberman, and K. E. Webster (1977) Neurons and their synaptic organization in the visual cortex of the rat. Electron microscopy of Golgi preparations. *Cell Tissue Res.* 183:499–517.

Peters, A. (1980) Morphological correlates of epilepsy: Cells in the cerebral cortex. In *Antiepileptic Drugs: Mechanisms of Action*, G. H. Glaser, J. K. Penry, and D. M. Woodbury, eds., pp. 21–48, Raven, New York.

Peters, A., and A. Fairén (1978) Smooth and sparsely-spined stellate cells in the visual cortex of the rat: A study using a combined Golgi–electron microscope technique. *J. Comp. Neurol.* 181:129–172.

Peters, A., and M. L. Feldman (1976) The projection of the lateral geniculate nucleus to area 17 of the rat cerebral cortex. I. General description. *J. Neurocytol.* 5:63–84.

Peters, A., and E. G. Jones (1984) Classification of cortical neurons. In *Cerebral Cortex*, Vol. 1, A. Peters and E. G. Jones, eds., pp. 107–122, Plenum, New York

Peters, A., and I.-R. Kaiserman-Abramof (1969) The small pyramidal neuron of the rat cerebral cortex. The synapses upon dendritic spines. *Z. Zellforsch. Mikrosk. Anat.* **100**:487–506.

Peters, A., and D. Kara (1984) The neuronal composition of area 17 of rat visual cortex. I. The pyramidal cells. *J. Comp. Neurol.* **234**:218–241.

Peters, A., and L. M. Kimerer (1981) Bipolar neurons in rat visual cortex. A combined Golgi–electron microscope study. *J. Neurocytol.* **10**:921–946.

Peters, A., and C. C. Proskauer (1980) Synaptic relationships between a multipolar stellate cell and a pyramidal neuron in the rat visual cortex. A combined Golgi–electron microscope study. *J. Neurocytol.* **9**:163–183.

Peters, A., C. C. Proskauer, and I.-R. Kaiserman-Abramof (1968) The small pyramidal neuron of the rat cerebral cortex. The axon hillock and initial segment. *J. Cell Biol.* **89**:604–619.

Peters, A., S. L. Palay, and H. de F. Webster (1976) *The Fine Structure of the Nervous System: The Neurons and Supporting Cells*, W. B. Saunders, Philadelphia.

Peters, A., E. L. White, and A. Fairén (1977) Synapses between identified neuronal elements. An electron microscopic demonstration of degenerating axon terminals synapsing with Golgi-impregnated neurons. *Neurosci. Lett.* **6**:171–175.

Peters, A., C. C. Proskauer, M. L. Feldman, and L. Kimerer (1979) The projection of the lateral geniculate nucleus to area 17 of the rat cerebral cortex. V. Degenerating axon terminals synapsing with Golgi-impregnated neurons. *J. Neurocytol.* **8**:331–357.

Peters, A., C. C. Proskauer, and C. E. Ribak (1982) Chandelier cells in rat visual cortex. *J. Comp. Neurol.* **206**:397–416.

Peters, A., M. Miller, and L. M. Kimerer (1983) Cholecystokinin-like immunoreactive neurons in rat cerebral cortex. *Neuroscience* **8**:431–448.

Rapisardi, S. C., and L. Lipsenthal (1984) Asymmetric and symmetric synaptic junctions in the dorsal lateral geniculate nucleus of cat and monkey. *J. Comp. Neurol.* **224**:415–424.

Ribak, C. E. (1978) Aspinous and sparsely-spinous stellate neurons in the visual cortex of rats contain glutamic acid decarboxylase. *J. Neurocytol.* **7**:461–478.

Saint Marie, R. L., and A. Peters (1984) The morphology and synaptic connections of spiny stellate neurons in monkey visual cortex (area 17). A Golgi–electron microscopic study. *J. Comp. Neurol.* **233**:213–235.

Sillito, A. M. (1975) The contribution of inhibitory mechanisms to the receptive field properties of neurones in the striate cortex of the cat. *J. Physiol. (Lond.)* **250**:305–329.

Sloper, J. J. (1973) Gap junctions between dendrites in the primate neocortex. *Brain Res.* **44**:641–646.

Sloper, J. J., and T. P. S. Powell (1978) Gap junctions between dendrites and the somata of neurons in primate sensori-motor cortex. *Proc. R. Soc. Lond. (Biol.)* **203**:39–47.

Sloper, J. J., and T. P. S. Powell (1979) An electron microscopic study of afferent connections to the primate motor and somatic sensory cortices. *Philos. Trans. R. Soc. Lond. (Biol.)* **285**:199–226.

Smith, D. E., and N. Moskowitz (1979) Ultrastructure of layer IV of the primary auditory cortex of the squirrel monkey. *Neuroscience* **4**:349–359.

Somogyi, P. (1977) A specific "axo-axonal" interneuron in the visual cortex of the rat. *Brain Res.* **136**:345–350.

Somogyi, P., and A. Cowey (1981) Combined Golgi and electron microscopic study on the synapses formed by double bouquet cells in the visual cortex of the cat and monkey. *J. Comp. Neurol.* **195**:547–566.

Somogyi, P., and A. Cowey (1984) Double bouquet cells. In *Cerebral Cortex*, Vol. 1, A. Peters and E. G. Jones, eds., pp. 337–360, Plenum, New York.

Somogyi, P., T. F. Freund, and A. Cowey (1982) The axo-axonic interneuron in the cerebral cortex of the rat, cat and monkey. *Neuroscience* **1**:2577–2608.

Somogyi, P., T. F. Freund, J.-Y. Wu, and A. D. Smith (1983a) The section–Golgi impregnation procedure. 2. Immunocytochemical demonstration of glutamate decarboxylase in Golgi-impregnated neurons and in their afferent synaptic boutons in the visual cortex of the cat. *Neuroscience* **9**:475–490.

Somogyi, P., Z. F. Kisvarday, K. A. C. Martin, and D. Whitteridge (1983b) Synaptic connections of morphologically identified and physiologically characterized large basket cells in the striate cortex of cat. *Neuroscience* **10**:261–294.

Tigges, J., M. Tigges, S. Anschel, N. A. Cross, W. D. Ledbetter, and R. L. McBride (1981) Areal and laminar distribution of neurons interconnecting the central visual cortical areas 17, 18, 19 and MT in squirrel monkey (*Saimiri*). *J. Comp. Neurol.* **202**:539–560.

Valdivia, O. (1971) Methods of fixation and the morphology of synaptic vesicles. *J. Comp. Neurol.* **142**:257–274.

Valverde, F. (1978) The organization of area 18 in the monkey. A Golgi Study. *Anat. Embryol.* **154**:305–334.

Vaughan, D. W., and A. Peters (1985) Proliferation of thalamic afferents in cerebral-cortex altered by callosal deafferentation. *J. Neurocytol.* **14**:705–716.

Vaughan, D. W., and S. Foundas (1982) Synaptic proliferation in the auditory cortex of the young adult rat following callosal lesions. *J. Neurocytol.* **11**:29–51.

White, E. L. (1978) Identified neurons in mouse SmI cortex which are postsynaptic to thalamocortical axon terminals: A combined Golgi–electron microscopic and degeneration study. *J. Comp. Neurol.* **181**:627–662.

White, E. L., and M. P. Rock (1981) A comparison of thalamocortical and other synaptic inputs to dendrites of two non-spiny neurons in a single barrel of mouse SmI cortex. *J. Comp. Neurol.* **195**:265–277.

White, E. L., S. M. Hersch, and M. P. Rock (1980) Synaptic sequences in mouse SmI cortex involving pyramidal cells labelled by retrograde filling with horseradish peroxidase. *Neurosci. Lett.* **19**: 149–154.

Winfield, D. A., K. C. Gatter, and T. P. S. Powell (1980) An electron microscopic study of the types and proportions of neurons in the cortex of the motor and visual areas of the cat and rat. *Brain* **103**:245–258.

Winfield, D. A., R. N. L. Brook, J. J. Sloper, and T. P. S. Powell (1981) A combined Golgi–electron microscopic study of the synapses made by the proximal and recurrent collaterals of a pyramidal cell in the somatic sensory cortex of the monkey. *Neuroscience* **6**:1217–1230.

Woolsey, T. A., M. L. Dierker, and D. F. Wann (1975) Mouse SmI cortex: Qualitative and quantitative classification of Golgi-impregnated barrel neurons. *Proc. Natl. Acad. Sci. USA* **72**:2165–2169.

Section 4

Synaptic Plasticity, Memory, and Learning

The role of synapses in memory and learning is obviously a central one. The main questions concern the nature of those processes and the network properties that allow changes in synaptic efficacy to be reflected in altered behavior. In this section, the authors consider fundamental cellular and molecular processes that provide critical components related to such changes in selected regions of the brain. These range from long-term potentiation and depression, to sprouting with new synapse formation, to alterations of synapses at interneurons, to the action of proteases on postsynaptic elements, to allosteric changes of receptors.

Among the most important overall processes affecting efficacy are heterosynaptic facilitation and depression. As Andersen shows in his contribution, hippocampal synapses are superb models for such processes. While excitatory postsynaptic potentials in pyramidal cells show long- and short-term potentiation similar to those of other synapses, tetanic stimulation above a certain strength is followed by a long-lasting enhancement of synaptic transmission. Both pre- and postsynaptic mechanisms are involved, and these show particular localizations and characteristic cellular dependencies.

In contrast to potentiation events in the hippocampus, long-term depression occurs in the cerebellum. Ito discusses this phenomenon, which occurs in the synaptic transmission from parallel fibers to Purkinje cells in the cerebellar cortex. The depression follows conjunctive activation of parallel fibers and climbing fibers. Ito speculates that long-term depression may be due to desensitization of glutamate receptors. Stellate cell inhibition applied together with conditioning input from climbing fibers can abolish the potentiation, diminishing plateau potentials in Purkinje cell dendrites. This raises the possibility that increased intradendritic calcium concentration is a primary cause of long-term depression. Both Andersen's studies in the hippocampus and Ito's studies in the cerebellum bear upon the possibility that these long-term heterosynaptic effects are fundamental to memory and adaptive learning.

In his contribution, Tsukahara takes up a specific example of synaptic alteration that may also contribute to learning. Using the corticorubral synapse as a modifiable instance, and the fact that fibers to this synapse can sprout under stimulation, he shows that classical conditioning can occur by combining stimulation of corticorubral fibers as a conditioned stimulus with forelimb skin stimulation as an unconditioned stimulus. After conditioning, the change is at the corticorubral fibers. Tsukahara proposes that a tenable mechanism is that corticorubral fibers sprout onto the proximal portion of the somadendritic membrane, giving more powerful input to red nucleus neurons.

Kandel and his associates use the results of studies of the cellular and molecular mechanisms of two forms of learning in *Aplysia* to make the case for specific detailed mechanisms of synaptic change. These include modulation of ion channels at a distance by transmitter binding to other proteins, communication between them by means of an intracellular second messenger, alteration of additional substrate proteins other than the channel in the postsynaptic cell, and alteration by specific activity in the responding neuron. These processes provide a detailed picture at the molecular level of processes of potential significance to the regulation of synaptic efficacy in classical conditioning.

Siman et al. add a new and somewhat radical hypothesis to the collection of candidate mechanisms for the modifiability of synapses as it contributes to memory. They argue that transmitter release and ion fluxes are rapid and fully reversible and seem ill-suited for a role in long-term memory effects. They describe proteolytic enzymes in the brain that degrade membrane-associated proteins likely to be involved in synaptic ultrastructure. These enzymes are calcium-stimulated proteases designated calpain I and calpain II that can affect cytoskeletal proteins as substrates. The authors suggest that submembranous fodrin exerts a transmembrane control over glutamate binding sites and show that degradation of fodrin by calpain I reorganizes the cytoskeleton in such a way that previously unexposed sites become accessible to glutamate. They propose the hypothesis that membrane-associated calpain I meets many of the conditions required of an agent responsible for translating physiological events into lasting modification of synapses but are aware of the many control conditions that must be met before a believable link may be made with behavior.

Changeux and Heidemann consider the properties of a very well characterized receptor as the means by which long- and short-term changes may be introduced into activity-dependent changes in synaptic efficacy. This is the nicotinic acetylcholine receptor, for which a complete primary structure is now known. The receptor is an allosteric protein. In their chapter, the authors propose that these properties make the receptor a candidate site for short-term learning at the postsynaptic level. Data on intrinsic and extrinsic modifications of the receptor and its metabolism are then used as a basis for models of long-term learning. The explicit assumption made is that the properties of this well-studied peripheral receptor can be extended to receptors for other neurotransmitters, particularly those of central neurons.

As the reader can see, there is no dearth of candidate mechanisms at the molecular level that may be used in learning and memory. What is required to link these mechanisms? It appears that the first requirement is correlative and hierarchical—to establish how neuroanatomical arrangements and physiological activity can be correlated with synaptic change following specific biochemical mechanisms at a site shown to be involved in memory and learning. The second is related to and more directly pertinent to the global task of this volume—to show how synaptic change at different sites confers different properties on parts of neurons and populations of neurons. This is both an experimental and a theoretical task. Various experimental aspects have already been considered. The theoretical task is taken up by the accounts in the next and final section of this book.

Chapter 16

Properties of Hippocampal Synapses of Importance for Integration and Memory

PER O. ANDERSEN

ABSTRACT

Hippocampal synapses have been studied intensively over the last two decades. In pyramidal cells, excitatory postsynaptic potentials (EPSPs) have a slow onset, irrespective of dendritic location. Proximal and distal EPSPs are equally effective. Only about 100 synchronously activated synapses seem to be required to drive a cell. The EPSP shows short- and long-term potentiation, which follow the same rules and time courses as in other synapses. There is one important exception in that tetanic stimulation above a certain strength is followed by an extremely durable enhancement of synaptic transmission—long-term potentiation. This process has both pre- and postsynaptic mechanisms, both probably involving changes in membrane properties. Hippocampal cells have two types of inhibition, both mediated by γ-aminobutyric acid (GABA). Classical, chloride-dependent hyperpolarization is produced by three types of interneurons terminating upon the soma, the initial axon, and the dendrites, respectively. Depolarizing, shunting inhibition is produced by a fourth type, and is localized to dendrites only. Several systems for the powerful modulation of neuronal excitability exist, which probably control the degree of synaptic integration of the cell.

For the study of synaptic activation of cortical neurons, the hippocampal cortex offers distinct advantages. Its regular anatomy and probable involvement in emotional responses and memory have excited a large number of investigators. Studies on the hippocampus have illuminated cellular processes of importance for cortical activation—and for synaptic alterations caused by experience.

ORGANIZATION

Cortical Areas

In comparison with other cortical areas, the hippocampus, or archicortex, appears relatively simple. The hippocampus is composed of two longitudinal strips named regio inferior and regio superior by Ramón y Cajal (1893). Lorente de Nó (1934) renamed these areas CA1 and CA3–CA4, respectively. Today, the latter terms are widely used (Figure 1A). Next to the CA3–CA4 area, we find the dentate

Lamellar organization

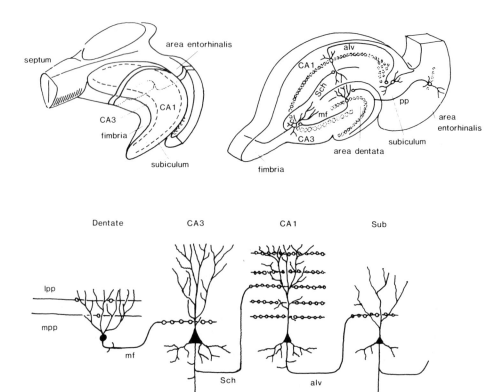

Figure 1. *Hippocampal organization.* Diagrammatic representation of the hippocampal formation showing an overview (*upper left*) and the lamellar arrangement (*upper right*). The sequence of activation of hippocampal neurons is shown from left to right (*bottom*). Two cell types give rise to the main efferent paths, pointing *downward*. Only excitatory connections are drawn. Abbreviations: alv, alveus; ang.bundle, angular bundle; fim, fimbria; lpp, lateral perforant path; mf, mossy fibers; mpp, medial perforant path; pp, perforant path; Sch, Schaffer collateral; sub, subiculum.

fascia, which forms the end of the telencephalic mantle. On the other side, CA1 borders the subiculum. In combination, the four regions make up the hippocampal formation. Further laterally, we find the parahippocampal gyrus, including the entorhinal cortex.

Main Cell Types

The CA1 cortex contains a set of relatively small pyramidal cells, whereas CA3 and CA4 have larger pyramidal cells. In the dentate fascia, the main type is the granule cell. All three areas are monolayered. In CA1 and CA3, the pyramidal cell bodies are packed together in a dense band, being about three to four cell bodies high and 80–100 μm wide (rats). All cells send their apical dendrites off in one direction. In CA1, the initial parts of these are relatively straight, giving a striped appearance in light microscope sections (stratum radiatum). The apical dendrites have particularly many branches in the outer part of CA1, the stratum moleculare. In the other direction, the basal dendrites form a dense network in a zone called stratum oriens. The dendrites of CA3 cells are similar, although the apical dendrites are not quite as long and straight as in CA1. In the dentate fascia, the granule cells are small and even more densely packed together than in the hippocampus. They have bushy dendritic trees on one side of the soma only, much like the configuration of cerebellar Purkinje cells, with axons leaving from the opposite pole. In all cell types, the dendrites are heavily covered with spines, in pyramidal cells nearly exclusively on the thinner branches (Minkwitz, 1976).

Afferent Fibers

In contrast to the situation in the neocortex, the afferent fibers run horizontally, that is, parallel to the cortical surface, and will, therefore, cross the main dendritic axis orthogonally. The fibers make synaptic contacts with boutons en passage. An afferent fiber will, therefore, activate a row of cells through synapses lying at a relatively constant distance from their somata (Figure 1C). Conversely, different parts of the dendritic tree of a given cell will be contacted by fibers coming from different sources. This arrangement allows selective activation of a population of synapses at a given distance from the soma (Lorente de Nó, 1934), or lesions of pathways synapsing on a given part of the dendritic tree. By combining histological, physiological, and chemical techniques, it has been possible to establish that excitatory synaptic connections on pyramidal cells are made by synapses of the asymmetric type making contact on dendritic spines (Andersen et al., 1966; Storm-Mathisen et al., 1983). Excitatory synapses on interneurons are distributed on the nonspinous bulbous dendrites of such neurons as well as on their somata. Interneurons probably receive less than 10% of the total number of excitatory synapses.

Interneurons

Among the interneurons, three classes of γ-aminobutyric acid (GABA)-containing cells have been identified so far. The basket cells form an axonal plexus around the somata of the pyramidal and granule cells (Ramón y Cajal, 1893) and are most likely responsible for recurrent inhibition of these neurons (Andersen et al., 1964). The chandelier cells form a dense axonal plexus around the initial axons of several hundred pyramidal cells in a given region (Somogyi et al., 1983). Both the basket and chandelier cell types and a large variety of stellate cells (Ramón y Cajal, 1893, 1911; Lorente de Nó, 1934) contain glutamic acid decarboxylase (GAD) and probably release GABA (Ribak et al., 1978; Somogyi et al., 1983). GAD-positive synapses have been found to contact shafts of middle-sized dendrites in the stratum radiatum and stratum moleculare (Storm-Mathisen et al., 1983) and are probably inhibitory in these dendritic territories (Alger and Nicoll, 1982a).

Lamella

The axons of the cells in one of the cortical strips in the hippocampal formation cross the border to the neighboring area orthogonally (Figure 1). The interconnecting axons of the main hippocampal cells lie in the same plane, nearly at right angles to the long axis of the overall structure. A thin strip of tissue with this orientation, as shown in the upper right corner in Figure 1, has been named a lamella (Andersen et al., 1971). A section along such a plane, normal to the hippocampal surface, will therefore be parallel to both the main dendritic axis of the cells and to the axons between them. This arrangement allows a thin section, the transverse hippocampal slice (Skrede and Westgaard, 1971), to be taken for *in vitro* studies. The recent interest in this preparation has greatly increased our knowledge of the properties of hippocampal cells and processes.

A final point is that the development of the hippocampal formation occurs relatively late in ontogenesis. In fact, in rats the major part of the dentate granule cells are born and develop after birth (Altman and Das, 1965; Angevine, 1965). In spite of its late development, the connections between the cells show a large degree of plasticity (Lynch et al., 1972, 1973a,b; LaVail and Wolf, 1973; Zimmer, 1973; Storm-Mathisen, 1974; Nadler et al., 1980). This appears as rearrangement and sprouting of axons after lesions, but also as an increased synaptic efficacy after short periods of intense use called long-term potentiation (LTP) (Lømo, 1966; Bliss and Gardner-Medwin, 1973; Bliss and Lømo, 1973).

PROPERTIES OF EXCITATORY HIPPOCAMPAL SYNAPSES

Excitatory Postsynaptic Potentials

When an afferent fiber bundle is stimulated, the response of a hippocampal pyramidal or granule cell consists of a depolarizing synaptic potential—an excitatory postsynaptic potential (EPSP). It shares many properties with comparable responses in other preparations. However, there are some interesting differences. The main difference is the slow rate of rise and long duration of the EPSP compared to that of other neurons, including many neocortical pyramidal cells. When stimulating fibers less than 1 mm away in order to reduce the asynchrony of the arriving fiber volley, the average rate of rise (10–90%) of the EPSP measures 3.85 msec (range, 1.8–7.6 msec). By comparison, motoneuronal EPSPs to single Ia impulses have rise times (10–90%) around 1 msec with a range from 0.2 to 2.8 msec, depending upon the cell type and synapse location (Jack et al., 1971). Another surprising feature is that the EPSP does not change greatly when synapses lying close to or far from the cell body are selectively activated (Andersen et al., 1980b). By cutting all radiatum fibers except a narrow bundle in hippocampal slices, it is possible to activate synapses at a given position along the dendritic axis selectively. With two isolated bundles placed at various distances from the soma, the shape indices for the respective EPSPs are remarkably similar (Andersen et al., 1980b). This applies to synapses lying from 50 to 450 μm away from the CA1 somata.

Recently, a more detailed analysis has shown small differences between distal versus proximal EPSPs (Andersen et al., 1986). Even in this series, however, the slight decrease in the rate of rise of the distal compared to proximal EPSPs was considerably less than expected from cable theory, assuming a unitary and passive membrane (Rall, 1962, 1967, 1970; Rall and Rinzel, 1973). In this context, a histological difference between hippocampal and neocortical pyramidal cells seems important. The neocortical pyramidal cells have relatively few and roughly equally sized apical dendritic branches from which spines emerge directly. In contrast, the hippocampal pyramidal cells have two types of apical dendritic branches. The first type starts with a main apical dendritic shaft that divides a few times in a Y-shaped fashion to form slightly thinner and relatively straight daughter dendrites with few if any spines and a moderate number of symmetric synapses on them. The branching complies with the 3/2 power law for impedance matching (Rall, 1967, 1970). The other type of apical dendritic branch is characterized by a considerably smaller diameter that branches off at right angles from the first type. After an initial naked portion, spines occur with very high density. Thus, one of the reasons for the slow rate of rise of the EPSP could be the relatively distal electrotonic location of the synapses because of high resistance in the spine neck, even for those which appear histologically close to the soma.

The amplitude of the EPSP at the spike threshold varies from cell to cell, depending upon the level of membrane potential and input resistance. However, a mean value of about 9 mV has been found (range, 6–15 mV) for CA1 pyramidal cells and 24 mV (range, 19–27 mV) for granule cells (Andersen et al., 1980b; McNaughton et al., 1981). The remarkable amplitude difference of the action potential threshold between the two cell types must be taken into account when discussing their integrative properties.

Efficacy of Excitatory Synapses

The raison d'être for excitatory synapses is, so to speak, their ability to bring the cell to discharge. Therefore, it is important to know the relative efficacy of the various excitatory synapses. There are several ways to measure this property. One is to compare the effect of stimulating different fiber bundles terminating at restricted positions of the dendritic tree. Another method is to reduce the number of afferent fibers through lesions to estimate the minimum number of synapses necessary to bring the cell to discharge. A third technique is to establish the value of single fiber EPSPs and compare this value with the minimal EPSP required to fire the cell. The latter technique requires knowledge about the degree of nonlinear summation of the EPSPs in question.

Before dealing with this question, it is useful to remember that the fibers in the hippocampal system have repeated boutons en passage that make contact with both pyramidal cells and interneurons (Figure 1). From Golgi impregnation, from reconstructions from electron micrographs, and from horseradish peroxidase (HRP) filling we know that the average distance between boutons in the perforant path fibers is about 5 μm, whereas the average distance between boutons in the radiatum fibers in CA1 is slightly less, ranging from 3 to 5 μm in various positions (P. O. Andersen, unpublished observations). Judging from field potential recordings at various positions, the efficacy of a bundle of afferent fibers in exciting cells is equal all the way along the fiber. In other words, a Schaffer collateral has an equal influence on all the CA1 cells it contacts on the way toward the subicular border. We must conclude that the action potentials are transmitted without a drop in the safety factor until the end of the fiber.

Furthermore, it would be useful to know the number of contacts a given cell has with a target cell. Let us consider a theoretical cylinder that is equivalent to the total dendritic territory of a cell and compare that with the average interbouton distance. In rat, the average transverse diameter of the soma of CA1 pyramidal cells may be taken as 20 μm. Because they are stacked about four in height in the pyramidal layer, the radius of the equivalent cylinder will be about 5 μm ($10 \ \mu m/\sqrt{4}$). Because most boutons only contact one spine, an interbouton distance of 5 μm means that a single fiber only makes two contacts with the dendrites of a particular cell. Obviously, this is a statistical number, and it does not exclude the possibility that a single fiber could have several contacts with different dendritic branches of a single cell. If so, however, the fiber would have to jump over an equivalent number of other neurons. The apical dendritic tree is found inside a tissue volume best described by a cone with its tip at the cell body. At the cone base, the transverse diameter is around 150 μm. Thus, the maximal number of contacts between a single fiber and the periphery of the dendritic tree is 30. Therefore, even in this particular case, a single fiber can only make a relatively small number of contacts with a given target cell. Although the number of theoretical contacts would rise at more distal positions of the fibers, the spatial isolation of boutons would also increase because of the dendritic branching. The situation in which a given fiber makes few contacts on a target neuron might be advantageous in that it reduces the chances for nonlinear summation and therefore the "waste" of synaptic power.

Local Stimulation of Afferent Fibers

When a microcathode activates fibers at various dendritic levels with a constant current, its effectiveness in exciting the cell is nearly the same at all levels (Figure 2A, B). This can be assessed by the amplitude of the sharp negative-going field potential, called the population spike, which is a signal of the near-synchronous discharge of many pyramidal cells. As an exception, stimulation of fibers in the molecular layer, which corresponds to the outer fifth of the apical dendritic layer, is ineffective. This could either be because the fibers in this region lack effective excitatory synapses or because of concomitant activation of fibers having an inhibitory effect that conceals the excitatory effect. This would be in accord with the high density of GAD-positive boutons on dendrites in this region. Experiments with combined stimulation and blocking of the GABA receptors might show the effectiveness of the most remote dendritic synapses.

Restriction of the Excitatory Input

Another way to assess the relative efficacy of synapses is to make a lesion that leaves only a small fraction of afferent fibers to activate the cells (Figure 2C). Such experiments have given estimates, backed by histological controls, that not

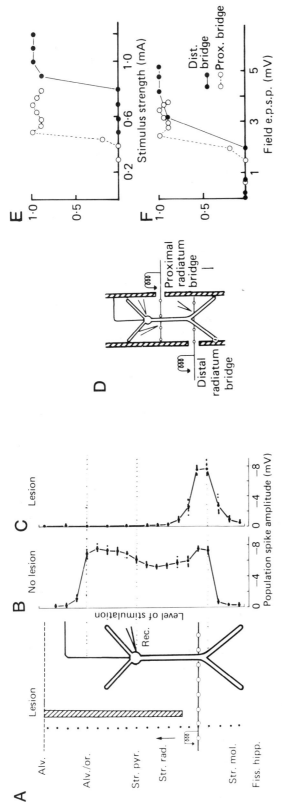

Figure 2. *Efficacy of hippocampal excitatory synapses. A:* Diagram showing the position of the stimulating cathode (*dots*) and lesion (*hatched*), leaving only distally located fibers (*line* with *open circles*) to influence the cells. *B:* Graph with the amplitude of population spike as a function of the level of afferent fibers stimulated with a constant current pulse. *C:* As in *B*, but after the lesion shown in *A. D:* Diagram indicating two double lesions to form two restricted synaptic inputs to a group of CA1 neurons. *E:* The probability of firing of a single pyramidal cell in response to increasing the two inputs is shown. *F:* The same data, plotted against the size of the corresponding field excitatory postsynaptic potential (EPSP) to give an index of the number of synapses activated. The two inputs are equally effective. (From Andersen et al., 1980b.)

409

more than 3–5% of the total number of dendritic synapses are needed to activate virtually all neurons in a sample population in CA1 (Andersen et al., 1980b). This figure is an upper estimate, since many of the fibers near the border of the lesion were also probably damaged by mechanical disturbance or edema. Therefore, only 100–400 synapses seem to be needed for synchronous activation to drive a CA1 pyramidal cell. Experiments of this nature have not been performed in CA3 or in the dentate area.

A third way to establish the efficacy of excitatory synapses is to measure the size of single fiber EPSPs and compare that with the EPSP at spike threshold. Because of the small diameter and unmyelinated nature of most hippocampal fibers, this is a difficult technique. Therefore, it has only been undertaken for the lowest threshold fibers of the perforant path–granule cell synapse (McNaughton et al., 1981). Three methods were used. First, by gently increasing the stimulus strength, small steps in the averaged response were looked for. Second, the coefficient of variation of the amplitude of a large number of small amplitude EPSPs were calculated to estimate the quantal content. Third, the amplitude histogram of a series of small EPSPs was subjected to Fourier transformation. The occurrence of frequencies with statistically more power than a control series without stimulation was taken as index of a minimal amplitude contribution, probably single fiber EPSPs. All three methods indicated that the perforant path–dentate granule cell synapse had single fiber EPSPs of around 0.1 mV. This is similar to the value given for single Ia fiber EPSPs on motoneurons (Kuno and Miyahara, 1969; Jack et al., 1971; Edwards et al., 1976). Assuming that fibers with higher thresholds have the same EPSP, taking 24 mV as the threshold amplitude for spike discharge, and correcting for nonlinear summation by the EPSP versus fiber volley amplitude relation, McNaughton et al. (1981) came up with 400 synapses as the necessary minimum for synchronous activation to drive a dentate granule cell. Without correction for nonlinear summation, the number would be 240 synapses. Remembering that dentate granule cells have between 10,000 and 50,000 synapses on their dendritic trees (West and Andersen, 1980), this appears to be a remarkably low percentage.

Assuming that the single fiber EPSPs for radiatum fibers to CA1 neurons also measure 0.1 mV, and that the EPSP at spike threshold is 6–10 mV, the number of excitatory synapses needed to be activated synchronously to drive a CA1 cell would only be 60–100. This represents about 1% of the total population, assuming that there are 10,000 synapses on a pyramidal cell (Wenzel et al., 1981). This finding is in accord with experiments with stimulation of a restricted input. Stimulation of various fiber groups indicated that thin but equally wide fiber bundles were able to discharge the cell with high probability (Figure 2D–F).

In conclusion, the results from stimulation and lesion experiments suggest a remarkable equipotentiality of excitatory synapses, irrespective of their position on the dendritic tree. The exception is the outer fifth of the apical dendrites where the situation is unclear, perhaps because of the large amount of GABA synapses. Furthermore, a surprisingly small number of excitatory synapses seems necessary to drive a cell. Under physiological circumstances, however, such numbers may have relatively little meaning. We do not know how often a cell is at what we take to be a normal resting potential and is activated by a reflexlike synchronous impulse volley in a number of fibers. It is perhaps more likely that the cells receive a more or less asynchronous synaptic bombardment, moving the membrane potential closer to the firing level so that the number of activated synapses required to drive a cell may be considerably lower. Furthermore, modulation by various neurotransmitters or neuromodulators may also assist the cell in discharging, making the required number for activating synapses even smaller. At the lowest limit, only one additional excitatory synapse is required to drive the cell, provided that other fibers have set up the necessary background depolarization.

Types of Synaptic Summation

When several synapses are activated simultaneously, the resulting depolarization depends in part upon the type of summation. Because of the reduction of the driving electromotive force, taken as the difference between the membrane potential and the equilibrium potential for the EPSP, the latter of two EPSPs is diminished if it is elicited during the voltage change of the first EPSP. Obviously, this effect increases in importance the closer the synapses are spaced. The greatest interference is found within a single synapse between different quanta released at a given active site.

As a first estimate, Langmoen and Andersen (1983) produced two 50- or 100-μm-thick fiber bundles and measured the summation of the EPSPs elicited by stimulation of these bundles (Figure 3). With small EPSPs (0.5–1.5 mV), there was a perfectly linear summation, although the separation of the two fiber bundles along the apical dendritic axis was only 75 μm. With stronger stimulation, there appeared to be a nonlinear summation in most cells. However, this was probably due to the addition of a recurrent inhibitory postsynaptic potential (IPSP), because linear summation was again obtained when the cell was polarized to the equilibrium potential for the IPSP, or when the IPSPs were blocked by penicillin or picrotoxin. Thus, EPSPs produced in neighboring dendritic territories (75 μm apart) summate linearly. Because of the occlusion of the fiber volley, it has not been possible so far to test the situation with more closely spaced synapses. It is possible that synapses lying on the same thin secondary dendritic branch sum nonlinearly. However, the electrical isolation provided by the high resistance in the spine neck on CA1 secondary dendrites makes nonlinear summation less likely than in cells in which the spines are short and located directly on a large shaft, as in many neocortical pyramidal cells (Koch and Poggio, 1983).

In dentate granule cells, McNaughton et al. (1981) tried to estimate the degree of linear summation by comparing the amplitude of the EPSP with the size of the presynaptic afferent fiber volley. The amplitude of the fiber volley was assumed to be linearly related to the number of activated fibers and synapses. The growth of the EPSP amplitude with increasing presynaptic volleys was nonlinear. The degree of nonlinear summation was calculated to increase gradually until it gave about a 40% reduction of the EPSP close to the threshold for spike discharge. The larger degree of nonlinear summation in the dentate, compared to CA1, is in accord with the shorter length of the dendrites and the smaller degree of branching, but perhaps is particularly due to the fact that the spines do not sit on a particular category of thin dendrites but on the ordinary dendritic

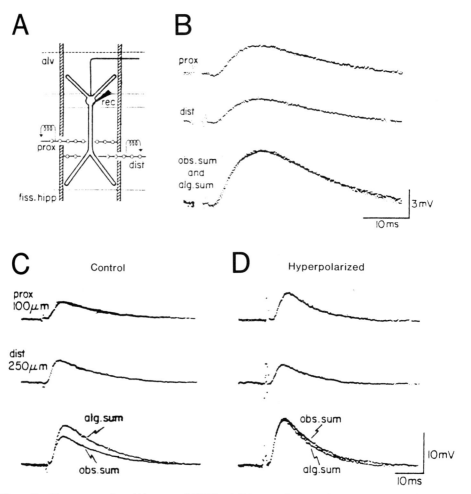

Figure 3. *Linear summation of hippocampal EPSPs. A:* Diagram showing the experimental arrangement. *B:* Averaged EPSPs (*n* = 30) in response to the proximal input (*top*), the distal input (*middle*), and the superimposition of the response to combined stimulation (obs.sum); the algebraic sum of the two records above (alg.sum) is also shown (*bottom*). *C:* A similar sequence with a different input from another cell. *D:* As in C, but after the cell has been hyperpolarized to the equilibrium potential for the inhibitory postsynaptic potential (IPSP). Abbreviations: fiss. hipp., hippocampal fissure; rec, recording electrode.

branches having diameters of 2–3 μm (Laatsch and Cowan, 1966; Matthews et al., 1976).

Excitatory Transmitters

The most likely transmitter candidates for excitatory synapses in the hippocampal formation are glutamate and aspartate (Storm-Mathisen, 1974, 1979; Nadler et al., 1976, 1977; Storm-Mathisen et al., 1983). The evidence for glutamate is based upon the presence of the compound, the excitation of pyramidal and granule cells when it is applied locally (Biscoe and Straughan, 1966; Dudar, 1974; White et al., 1977), fast depolarization that occurs when glutamate is added to particular hot spots corresponding to dendritic synapse territories (Schwartzkroin and Andersen, 1975), the release of glutamate by depolarizing agents in the presence of calcium (Nadler et al., 1976), the presence of a high-affinity, sodium-dependent uptake mechanism (Storm-Mathisen, 1975), and the observation of immunoreactive glutamate attached to vesicles in asymmetric spine synapses (Storm-Mathisen et al., 1983).

Aspartate is also released from synaptosome fractions from dentate and CA1 preparations (Nadler et al., 1976), is taken up by the same high-affinity uptake system, and will drive cells when applied iontophoretically. The detailed localization of hot spots has not been determined for aspartate.

Receptors

The synaptic transmission of various radiatum fibers onto CA1 is blocked by glutamic diethylester (GDEE), suggesting that the glutamate receptor in action belongs to the quisqualic acid type (Cotman and Nadler, 1981; Watkins, 1981; Collinridge et al., 1983). In the dentate region, the synapses of the middle perforant path fibers are blocked by GDEE, whereas the lateral perforant path fibers seem to be blocked better by 2-amino-5-phosphonobutyric acid (APB) (Cotman and Nadler, 1981). There is evidence that the synapses for the lateral perforant path and the commissural input to the dentate fascia may release aspartate.

In addition to the quisqualic receptor, there is evidence for the presence of an N-methyl-D-aspartate (NMDA) receptor for glutamate (Cotman and Nadler, 1981; Collinridge et al., 1983). This is based upon the effectiveness of NMDA applied iontophoretically in territories where excitatory synapses are known to exist. However, the best blockers for NMDA receptors do not change the synaptic activation of CA1 cells by radiatum fibers (Cotman and Nadler, 1981; Collinridge et al., 1983). The NMDA receptor is, therefore, probably not engaged in the synaptic activation of excitatory synapses in CA1. It is, however, more likely that this receptor is engaged in the LTP process that is discussed below. Both glutamate and aspartate are taken up by the same high-affinity uptake mechanism (Davies and Johnston, 1976). Recently, Storm-Mathisen et al. (1983) have demonstrated that antibodies to aldehyde-linked glutamate bind to vesicles in asymmetric dendritic synapse configurations both in CA1 and the dentate fascia. Detailed information on the location of aspartate is not yet available.

Local iontophoresis of glutamate to areas very close to excitatory synapses produces discharges of CA1 pyramidal and dentate cells (Biscoe and Straughan, 1966; Dudar, 1974) and depolarization of cells (Schwartzkroin and Andersen, 1975). The sensitive area is found within the envelope of the dendritic tree of the impaled cell. A penetrating iontophoretic electrode produces short-latency depolarization only at specific points, called hot spots. The dimension of a hot spot is of the order of 7–10 μm, probably corresponding to a thin dendritic branch with its associated spines and excitatory boutons. Local application of glutamate at a hot spot causes a relatively short-latency (around 10 msec) depolarization. This occurs even if the spot is two thirds of the distance between the cell body and the dendritic tip. However, glutamate is only efficient inside a volume best described as a double cone with its tips at the cell body corresponding to the overall distribution of the dendritic tree of the impaled cell (Dudar, 1974). Glutamate causes a dose-dependent depolarization that ends in a plateau. There is an initial resistance increase that turns into a decrease after some seconds, depending upon the dose. After cessation of the iontophoretic ejection, the membrane potential returns to its precontrol level within 1–2 sec. In contrast to the findings of Cotman and Nadler (1981), application at hot spots in CA1 caused remarkably little desensitization of the intracellular record in response to repeated applications with relatively short interejection intervals (3–5 sec) (Ø. C. Hvalby and P. Andersen, unpublished observations).

Strong evidence for glutamate as an excitatory transmitter was provided by Hablitz and Langmoen (1982), who recorded with cesium-filled electrodes and found that glutamate depolarization has the same equilibrium potential as or- thodromically activated EPSPs, both being close to zero.

The response to NMDA application is strikingly different from the glutamate response. First, the dose necessary to drive CA1 cells is very much lower than for glutamate application. The latency of the NMDA effect is relatively long. However, even with small doses of NMDA, there is a gradually increasing depolarization that leads to a burst discharge of the impaled cells. With continued application, the sodium channels inactivate, as judged by the increased width and reduced amplitude of the spikes, coupled with a slow reduction of the depolarizing plateau. This declining response may be seen for several seconds after the ejection current is terminated. Following the plateau of depolarization, there is a slow recovery, compared with the situation after glutamate ejection. Characteristically, after NMDA application, the membrane potential becomes more negative than the preejection level and stays at a more negative level for a longer time (minutes) than after glutamate ejection (5–20 sec). Initially, the period in which the membrane is hyperpolarized after NMDA ejection is associated with a reduced membrane resistance. However, in the last part of the recovery period the membrane resistance appears normal. NMDA application does not seem to affect the size or shape of orthodromically activated synaptic potentials. However, the drug greatly influences the size of the LTP following a tetanic activation of the same synapses (Cotman and Nadler, 1981; Collinridge et al., 1983). Conversely, GDEE effectively blocks the orthodromic activation of radiatum fiber EPSPs in CA1 cells but is without any effect on the LTP potential of the same synapses unless large doses are used to block synaptic transmission com- pletely.

PROPERTIES OF INHIBITORY SYNAPSES

Interneurons

There are a number of interneurons in the hippocampal cortex, some of which have been identified as inhibitory interneurons (Figure 4). The candidates are the basket cells, which terminate with synapses on the soma of pyramidal and dentate granule cells, the chandelier cells, which terminate on the initial axon segment in the CA1 region, and a large number of stellate cells, which are found

Transmitters and modulators

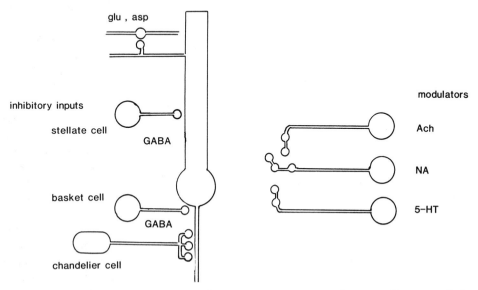

Figure 4. *Hippocampal transmitters and modulators.* Diagram indicating the types of synapses, their approximate position, and the associated transmitters for hippocampal pyramidal cells. To the *right* are some of the modulating neurons and their transmitters.

in the apical and basal dendritic territories in CA3 and CA1, in the hilus, and, to a smaller extent, in the molecular layer of the dentate fascia. By combining evidence from immunohistochemical studies of GAD distribution and the appearance of symmetric synapses with pleomorphic vesicles, the majority of the stellate cells seem to terminate on the shafts of middle-sized and small dendrites. However, they do not seem to be common on the thinner spine-bearing dendrites. In the dentate region, stellate cells are seen to terminate on the dendrites and only occasionally on spine heads (Gottlieb and Cowan, 1972).

Transmitters

All these classes of interneurons contain the enzyme GAD and therefore probably release GABA. The best-known instance is that of the basket cells (Ramón y Cajal, 1893; Lorente de Nó, 1934), which by immunocytochemical methods have been shown to contain GAD both in their somata and in their terminals on pyramidal and granule cell somata. By physiological techniques, Andersen et al. (1964) concluded that basket cells were inhibitory to CA1. The equivalent cells in the dentate region cause hyperpolarizing inhibitory responses in dentate granule cells, also by synapses located on their somata. Kandel et al. (1961)

found that the hyperpolarization was chloride-sensitive. The inhibitory chloride current is most likely driven down a gradient produced by an outward chloride pump (Allen et al., 1977), because the hyperpolarization is influenced by changes in the chloride concentration both inside and outside the cell. In slices, somatic application of GABA causes a chloride-dependent hyperpolarization of both pyramidal and granule cells associated with inhibition, most likely conveyed by the basket cell pathway. However, dendritic application as far as 300 μm from the cell body depolarizes the same cells (Andersen et al., 1980a; Alger and Nicoll, 1982a). The local dendritic depolarization by GABA application produces a conductance increase locally, shunting neighboring excitatory synaptic currents to give a local inhibition. The effect is direct, since it persists in low-calcium media. The equilibrium potentials for the hyperpolarizing GABA response and the recurrent IPSP are similar and lie at about −75 mV. The equilibrium potential for the dendritic application is less easily determined, because the cells are often lost during application of large depolarizing currents. However, by extrapolation, the equilibrium potential appears to be near −40 mV. The effect is partly dependent upon the external chloride concentration. Alger and Nicoll (1982b) could selectively block either the somatic or the dendritic GABA effect by local application of bicuculline, picrotoxin, penicillin, or pentylene tetrazol. In view of the relatively negative level of the equilibrium potential, the ion responsible for the depolarizing effect of dendritic GABA application does not seem to be chloride only. The conductance is perhaps due to the opening of a nonspecific channel where sodium ions are also involved. Such sites could be located extrasynaptically, although only indirect evidence exists on this point. If only chloride ions are involved, an efficient inward chloride pump is required in the dendritic tree. Coupled to the outward chloride pump at the soma, this interpretation presupposes a chloride circle with a resting inward pump at the soma and an outward pump in the dendrites, an energetically expensive solution. Furthermore, Alger and Nicoll (1982a) observed that hyperpolarizing dendritic IPSPs did not reverse their polarity even when released on top of a depolarizing GABA-mediated response.

The importance of the dendritic GABA effect lies in its ability to shunt the membrane resistance locally. This leads to an efficient decoupling of local synapses of both the depolarizing and hyperpolarizing variety. In addition to a reduction of local synaptic efficacy, dendritic GABA application could, because of its synaptic depolarizing effect, assist other excitatory synapses lying sufficiently far away to escape the shunting effect.

The histological substrate of the GABA dendritic effect has not been determined with certainty. However, both Ramón y Cajal (1893, 1911) and Lorente de Nó (1934) noted the large amount of interneurons in the layer of apical and basal dendrites of both pyramidal and granule cells. Later electron microscope work has shown an appreciable number of symmetrical synapses located on large and middle-sized dendrites. Immunocytochemical data indicate that these boutons may contain GAD and thus release GABA (Ribak et al., 1978; Storm-Mathisen et al., 1983). Thus, symmetric synapses on smooth, middle-sized dendrites remain candidates for GABA-releasing boutons in the hippocampal formation. The majority probably come from the variety of short axon cells, which may collectively be called stellate cells. Alger and Nicoll (1982a) have presented evidence that a feed-forward pathway operates dendritic depolarizing synapses, probably activating stellate cells by collaterals of afferent fibers.

Recently, a third cell type with a relatively short but profusely branching axon and containing GAD has been described (Somogyi et al., 1983). This type of cell—the chandelier cell—is found in or near the pyramidal layer in CA1 and has a greatly ramifying axonal tree terminating in an open plexus of axonal branches that twine themselves around the initial axon segments of many neighboring pyramidal cells. Its synapses are symmetric and are particularly concentrated next to the initial myelin segment. Although no physiological investigation has been undertaken, it is likely that these cells may have a GABA-mediated hyperpolarizing effect on the initial axons of CA1 and CA3 cells and thereby inhibit their axonal discharge. Thus, hyperpolarizing inhibition may be a feature of the initial axon segment, the soma, and the middle-sized dendrites of the pyramidal cell. So far, the depolarizing effect of GABA has been established only in the dendritic territory.

SYNAPTIC POTENTIATION

Types of Potentiation

A particular feature of the hippocampal synapses is their ability to change their efficacy during particular types of operations. In particular, the frequency of activation seems of paramount importance. The types of change seen are facilitation, depression, augmentation, posttetanic potentiation, and LTP.

Short-term facilitation is produced by a single impulse, as indicated by an increased response to a second stimulus following within 100 msec after the first (Figure 5). In addition, following a short tetanic stimulation, augmentation and posttetanic potentiation are present. Facilitation, depression, augmentation, and posttetanic potentiation follow the same rules as do corresponding reactions in other synapses (del Castillo and Katz, 1954; Kuno, 1964; Martin and Pilar, 1964; Magleby, 1973; Magleby and Zengel, 1976), particularly in situations in which the quantal content is low. However, in addition to the three types of facilitatory processes, the hippocampal synapses show one particular type of considerable interest, LTP (Figures 5, 6). In 1966, Lømo discovered that a short tetanic stimulation of the perforant path caused a very long lasting enhancement (hours) of the synaptic transmission between perforant path fibers and granule cells. Bliss and Lømo (1973) showed further that the effect follows both a relatively small number of stimuli delivered at physiological frequencies (Ranck, 1973) and a shorter, high-frequency tetanic stimulation.

Furthermore, the effect was seen as synaptic because it was not produced by antidromic activation of the target cells. Bliss and Gardner-Medwin (1973) showed that LTP not only occurred in awake animals, but that the process lasted for days and even weeks after a single tetanic activation. Further work has shown that the process exists in all hippocampal synapses studied so far. In addition, a similar process has been seen in the rostral colliculus, the medial geniculate body, the goldfish optic tectum and, in the activation of the visual cortex (Lee, 1982; Swanson et al., 1982). LTP is also present in hippocampal slices (Schwartzkroin

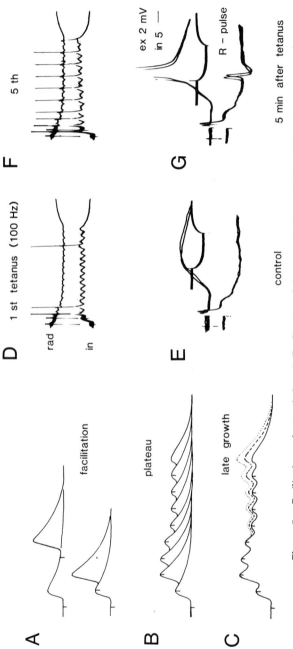

Figure 5. *Facilitation and potentiation. A:* Facilitation of the second of two EPSPs, delivered up to 30 sec apart. *B:* Plateau produced by summed EPSPs, with large variations in the individual amplitude with time. *C:* With repeated tetani, a late cumulative depolarization occurs. *D:* Responses of a CA1 pyramid to a short tetanic stimulation or to radiatum fibers (in) and to stimulation from the layer of the activated synapses (rad). *E:* A control EPSP (*top*), a resistance pulse (*middle*), and an extracellular response from the input level (*bottom*). *F:* The responses to the fifth tetanus, delivered with 5 sec between each stimulation. *G:* Test response 5 min after the five tetani; compare with *E.*

418

and Wester, 1975). Using two independent afferent bundles, one for tetanization and the other as a control, LTP was shown to be a homosynaptic phenomenon (Andersen et al., 1977, 1980c). Lynch et al. (1977) confirmed these results by local stimulation without lesions.

Cooperativity

McNaughton et al. (1978) showed that LTP requires stimulation above a certain strength for its development. They termed this effect the cooperativity phenomenon and postulated that the number of activated fibers or postsynaptic structures somehow issue a controlling signal to neighboring elements. Thus, LTP was seen as the result of a certain mass of afferent fibers and/or the postsynaptic cells activated by these fibers. As an alternative explanation, Hvalby and Andersen (1983) have suggested that the pairing of local dendritic depolarization and synaptic activation may act as the essential condition for LTP development. During tetanic activation, summated EPSPs produce a depolarization plateau that shows cumulative growth when repeated (Figure 5B–F). A certain enhancement of this plateau is required for LTP to develop. A sufficient degree of dendritic depolarization would normally occur only when the number of activated fibers surpass a certain value. However, in other circumstances, when depolarization is caused by other means (modulators, local synaptic barrage, environmental ionic changes) one could envisage that a sufficient depolarization could exist locally to produce a change of the described nature in the receiving cells, affecting a small proportion of synapses, all the way down to a single bouton. A test of these two proposals awaits the development of a preparation with single fiber activation of hippocampal synapses.

Locus of Enhancement

LTP may be due to changes in the presynaptic bouton of its release of transmitter, to a change in the local postsynaptic environment of the cell, or to both (Figure 6). The possibility that the potentiation is due to a general change in the excitability of the postsynaptic cell has been ruled out (Andersen et al., 1980c), since neither the membrane potential nor the membrane input resistance changes during LTP.

Presynaptic Changes

As evidence for a presynaptic site for the facilitation, Hamberger et al. (1978) reported a stimulus-evoked increase of glutamate synthesis. Skrede and Malthe-Sørenssen (1981) further reported that LTP was associated with an increased release of D-aspartate in hippocampal slices. In view of the reported correlation between glutamate and aspartate release (Davies and Johnston, 1976), these data are suggestive. Dolphin et al. (1982) applied radioactive glutamine to hippocampal slices; this was taken up by terminals in the slices and converted to glutamate. Following repetitive activation, slices showing LTP development also showed an increased release of "hot" glutamate. Because the soma membrane potential and membrane input resistance do not change during LTP (Andersen et al., 1980c), augmented transmitter release may best explain the increased EPSP seen

LTP,   possible presynaptic and

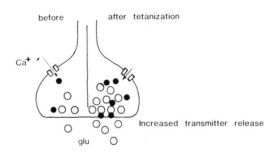

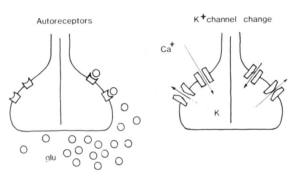

Figure 6.   *Long-term potentiation (LTP) changes.* Diagram illustrating possible pre- and postsynaptic changes responsible for LTP. In all drawings with a *vertical midline*, the *left side* shows the control and the *right side* shows the changed situation. *Open circles* represent glutamate or aspartate, and *filled circles* represent calcium ions. Presynaptic changes may involve increased transmitter release because of enhanced calcium influx (*top left*). Autoreceptors may alter the reaction over time, and long-lasting changes could be due to biochemical changes activated by calcium. Alteration of potassium channels by phosphorylation seems a realistic candidate mechanism (*bottom left*). Postsynaptic changes could involve the unmasking of receptors, an N-methy-D-aspartate (NMDA) receptor-induced alteration of the spine membrane, or morphological changes of the spine (*top right*). An NMDA mechanism could be operated either by glutamate at higher release sites, or by a specific aspartate mechanism (*bottom right*).

during intracellular recording (Deadwyler et al., 1976; Andersen et al., 1977, 1980c; Lynch et al., 1977).

A possible explanation may be that tetanic activation produces an enhanced influx of calcium ions in the activated fibers associated with a long-lasting increase of transmitter release (Figure 6). Another possibility is that an increased calcium influx is caused by a special agent released by the activated fibers. Finally, the existence of autoreceptors for glutamate has been reported in hippocampal synapses (Collins et al., 1983), so that an enhanced release of glutamate because of repeated activation could lead to a depolarization of the fibers. The result could be increased transmitter release, either because of the depolarization per se or because of an increased calcium influx caused by the depolarization.

postsynaptic mechanisms

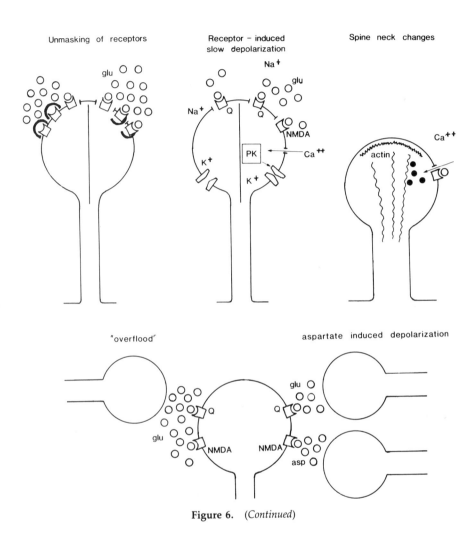

Figure 6. *(Continued)*

There is a discrepancy between the relatively modest or nonexistent increase of the EPSP intracellularly and the very clear increase of the extracellular field potential corresponding to this EPSP. Therefore, it appears as if the local inward current might be due to a double phenomenon, partly an inward synaptic current and partly another current, which is not seen by the intrasomatic electrode.

Postsynaptic Changes

When input–output curves are constructed for an LTP effect, the efficacy of a given number of input fibers in discharging the cells is larger than can be explained by the EPSP increase. Therefore, the idea that a local postsynaptic process is also involved was put forward (Andersen, 1983), supporting earlier suggestions by Bliss and Lømo (1973) and Lynch et al. (1977). To look for a postsynaptic change associated with LTP, intracellular recordings have been made in parallel with extracellular dendritic recordings from the layer of the activated synapses (Hvalby and Andersen, 1983). Tetanic stimulation is associated with a plateau of dendritic depolarization produced by a summation of a series of EPSPs (Figure 5). Provided that this depolarization is above a certain critical level, subsequent testing shows that LTP occurs. This minimal depolarizing level of dendrites may be the correlate of the cooperativity phenomenon described by McNaughton et al. (1978).

In order to test the theory that local dendritic depolarization is essential for subsequent LTP production, Ø. C. Hvalby and P. O. Andersen (unpublished observations) have subjected CA1 pyramidal cells to three different types of conjunctive depolarization and synaptic activation. Depolarization by current injection through the intrasomatic electrode, coupled with low-frequency synaptic activation, did not change the efficacy of the latter, however. Furthermore, the passage of a longitudinal current through the dendritic tree to produce local dendritic depolarization was also without any effect. However, local spine depolarization caused by iontophoretic glutamate ejection, coupled with low-frequency synaptic activation, resulted in an enhanced synaptic transmission for 10–40 min in about half of the cells. The glutamate depolarization was given as 800 msec pulses, coupled with a single shock of orthodromic activation just before the end of the pulse. The conjunction was repeated 10–20 times at a frequency of 0.5 Hz. When the glutamate dose was above a certain level, the associated conductance change was so large that the coupling lost its facilitatory effect. In essence, the situation is similar to the conjunctive stimulation of parallel and climbing fibers on Purkinje cells in the cerebellum. In the latter case, the climbing fiber produces a long-standing dendritic depolarization, which when coupled to parallel fiber activation causes a long-lasting change in the efficacy of the parallel fiber–Purkinje cell synapses, in this case a depression, however.

Involvement of NMDA Receptor

Since the NMDA receptor blocker 2-5-APV (Watkins, 1981) was reported to prevent the development of LTP but not synaptic transmission in CA1 (Cotman and Nadler, 1981; Collinridge et al., 1983), we repeated these experiments. We applied NMDA locally to a dendritic region of CA1 apical dendrites. Small doses of NMDA caused a gradual depolarization of the cells associated with high-voltage extracellular potentials because of the highly synchronous discharge of a number of pyramidal cells. In spite of continued application, the effect subsided, probably because of a conductance shunt. Following an NMDA application of less than 1 sec, there was a long-lasting (30 min) enhancement of synaptic transmission, even without any conjunctive stimulation of the afferent pathways. Thus, dendritic NMDA application produces a change in synaptic transmission that has many features in common with the LTP.

Since NMDA probably activates a receptor that may normally be activated by aspartate, this raises the possibility that aspartate fibers may produce the local dendritic depolarization needed for the creation of LTP. One might say that aspartate fibers may act as "teachers" instructing the glutamate-containing synapses to change their efficacy.

An alternative scenario might be as follows: During normal, low-frequency synaptic activation, glutamate may be released in small amounts sufficient to diffuse to nearby quisqualic acid-type glutamate receptors and cause an ordinary synaptic activation. However, following a short burst of impulses at high frequency, the amount of glutamate released may be considerably higher than normal, sufficient to activate more distantly placed receptors, including the NMDA variety. This could cause a prominent depolarization, possibly through a nonspecific conductance increase, most likely for both sodium and potassium (Nowak et al., 1984). This may be possible, since glutamate is a flexible molecule that can activate both the quisqualic and the NMDA receptor and thus may have a dual role, depending upon the availability of different receptor sites or the glutamate concentration.

A third possibility is raised by the recent finding of interference with NMDA by magnesium (Ault et al., 1980). The effect of NMDA at membrane potentials above -40 mV depends upon the local concentration of magnesium ions (Nowak et al., 1984). With normal magnesium concentrations (around 1 mM), NMDA application causes a regenerative inward current carried mostly by sodium ions. By removing magnesium ions from the fluid, the membrane behaves in a more linear fashion, without the negative slope conductance at hyperpolarized levels. (Mayer et al., 1984; Nowak et al., 1984). Thus, by reducing the extracellular magnesium concentration, NMDA may increase its effectiveness in depolarizing cells. To what extent physiological circumstances may change the extracellular magnesium concentration in brain tissue is unknown.

The types of lasting changes induced postsynaptically are also unknown. Interesting candidates (Figure 6) are morphological changes of the spines (Lee et al., 1980; Fifková and Anderson, 1981) or a loosening of the cytoskeleton that unmasks glutamate receptors. The increased calcium that enters during tetanic stimulation could stimulate the enzyme calpain to change the structural protein fodrin (Lynch and Baudry, 1984).

MEMBRANE CONDUCTANCE CHANGES

Control of Slow Conductances

Until recently, the efficacy of synaptic transmission has been discussed in the context of a constant resting membrane potential. However, recent evidence indicates that the excitability of the membrane is dramatically dependent upon the previous condition of the membrane potential. In order to mimic a continuous asynchronous bombardment, Lanthorn et al. (1984) passed small, long-lasting currents through CA1 pyramidal cells. At stronger depolarizations, the cell behaved as described earlier by Gustafsson and Wigström (1981) and by Schwartzkroin (1978). However, at currents just above the threshold for discharge, it appeared that the initial latency was particularly long, and that the cell was able to sustain a low-frequency discharge (around 0.5–1 Hz). Similar discharges were seen in the adapted stage with stronger currents. In these circumstances, each spike was preceded by a slowly depolarizing potential, called a slow prepotential. Further analysis (J. Storm, personal communication) has shown that this pre-potential depends upon the level of the membrane potential before the depolarizing test pulse. Prehyperpolarization produces an increase in the slow depolarizing ramp potential, while predepolarization acts conversely. Neither 4-aminopyridine nor tetraethylammonium gives clear changes of the slow ramp potential. However, calcium and manganese cause a partial but very slow reduction, suggesting that a slow inward calcium current could be involved. A full understanding must await further analysis, however. Alternative explanations involve changes in potassium channels. Hippocampal pyramidal cells have I_A channels (Gustafsson et al., 1982) that give rise to a transient outward current lasting about a second in response to depolarization. They also have an I_M current in response to depolarization from -60 mV (Halliwell and Adams, 1982) that is reduced by muscarinic agonists. Prominent modulation follows the application of acetylcholine to hippocampal cells (Dodd et al., 1981; Benardo and Prince, 1982a,b) because of a resistance increase, no doubt resulting from the closure of I_M channels. The resulting depolarization and enhancement of EPSPs cause an effective facilitation of synaptic transmission.

Following predepolarization, the slow ramp potential (lasting from 1 to 15 sec) is abolished, but each spike is still preceded by a prepotential, this time with a duration of only about 100 msec. This intermediate prepotential is tetro-dotoxin-sensitive and is not changed by applications of cadmium, manganese, or cobalt. It is probably because of an inward sodium current, possibly a slow activation of the fast sodium current.

Other modulators, like norepinephrine, have many actions on the membrane. An important aspect is the reduction of adaptation to steady depolarization, notably by blocking the calcium-stimulated potassium channel I_C (Madison and Nicoll, 1982). Monoamines are also involved in the state-dependent control of transmission through the hippocampal circuit (Winson and Abzug, 1978).

Active Dendritic Membrane

A final point in discussing the efficacy of dendritic synapses during normal and tetanic situations is the assumption of a passive dendritic membrane that often is made in modeling. Electrical coupling between pyramidal cells has been dem-onstrated (MacVicar and Dudek, 1980). Evidence from LTP experiments shows a greatly enhanced occurrence of small (3–8 mV) all-or-nothing spikes. These events may be interpreted as dendritic spikes that are blocked before reaching the soma. When LTP develops further, the small spikes are seen to trigger full spikes that appear at various positions on the EPSP, including its declining part, suggesting their initiation in the dendritic tree. Schwartzkroin and Slawsky (1977) demonstrated slow calcium spikes in CA1 cells. Benardo et al. (1982) were able to record regenerative spikes from dendrites in a preparation in which the somata of CA1 cells were surgically separated from the dendritic region. The large dendritic spikes (around 50 mV) were probably due to calcium currents, since the sodium channels had been blocked by tetrodotoxin. With regenerative properties in patches of the dendritic membrane, the integrative property of the cell would be quite different from that hitherto supposed. Clearly, this point is of paramount interest and should be the focus of attention for investigators in this field for years to come.

REFERENCES

Alger, B. E., and R. A. Nicoll (1982a) Feed-forward dendritic inhibition in rat hippocampal pyramidal cells studied *in vitro*. *J. Physiol. (Lond.)* **328**:105–123.

Alger, B. E., and R. A. Nicoll (1982b) Pharmacological evidence for two kinds of GABA receptor on rat hippocampal cells studied *in vitro*. *J. Physiol. (Lond.)* **328**:125–141.

Allen, G. I., J. C. Eccles, R. A. Nicoll, T. Oshima, and F. J. Rubia (1977) The ionic mechanisms concerned in generating the i.p.s.p.s of hippocampal pyramidal cells. *Proc. R. Soc. Lond. (Biol.)* **198**:363–384.

Altman, J., and G. D. Das (1965) Autoradiographic and histological studies of postnatal neurogenesis. I. A longitudinal investigation of the kinetics, migration and transformation of cells incorporating tritiated thymidine in neonate rats, with special reference to postnatal neurogenesis in some brain regions. *J. Comp. Neurol.* **126**:337–390.

Andersen, P. (1983) Possible cellular basis for prolonged changes of synaptic efficiency—A simple case of learning. *Prog. Brain Res.* **58**:419–426.

Andersen, P., J. C. Eccles, and Y. Løyning (1964) Location of postsynaptic inhibitory synapses of hippocampal pyramids. *J. Neurophysiol.* **27**:592–607.

Andersen, P., T. W. Blackstad, and T. Lømo (1966) Location and identification of excitatory synapses on hippocampal pyramidal cells. *Exp. Brain Res.* **1**:236–248.

Andersen, P., T. V. P. Bliss, and K. K. Skrede (1971) Lamellar organization of hippocampal excitatory pathways. *Exp. Brain Res.* **13**:222–238.

Andersen, P., S. H. Sundberg, O. Sveen, and H. Wigström (1977) Specific long-lasting potentiation of synaptic transmission in hippocampal slices. *Nature* **266**:736–737.

Andersen, P., R. Dingledine, L. Gjerstad, I. A. Langmoen, and A. Mosfeldt Laursen (1980a) Two different responses of hippocampal pyramidal cells to application of gamma amino butyric acid. *J. Physiol. (Lond.)* **305**:279–296.

Andersen, P., H. Silfvenius, S. H. Sundberg, and O. Sveen (1980b) A comparison of distal and proximal dendritic synapses on CA1 pyramids in hippocampal slices *in vitro*. *J. Physiol. (Lond.)* **307**:273–299.

Andersen, P., S. H. Sundberg, J. N. Swann, and H. Wigström (1980c) Possible mechanisms for long-lasting potentiation of synaptic transmission in hippocampal slices from guinea pigs. *J. Physiol. (Lond.)* **302**:463–482.

Andersen, P., J. Storm, and H. V. Wheal (1986) Thresholds of action potentials evoked by synapses on the dendrites of pyramidal cells in the rat hippocampus *in vitro*. *J. Physiol. (Lond.)* (in press).

Angevine, J. B., Jr. (1965) Time of neuron origin in the hippocampal region: An autoradiographic study in the mouse. *Exp. Neurol. (Suppl.)* **2**:1–70.

Ault, B., R. H. Evans, A. A. Francis, D. J. Oakes, and J. C. Watkins (1980) Selective depression of excitatory amino acid induced depolarizations by magnesium ions in isolated spinal cord preparations. *J. Physiol. (Lond.)* **307**:413–428.

Benardo, L. S., and D. A. Prince (1982a) Cholinergic excitation of mammalian hippocampal pyramidal cells. *Brain Res.* **249**:315–331.

Benardo, L. S., and D. A. Prince (1982b) Ionic mechanisms of cholinergic excitation in mammalian hippocampal pyramidal cells. *Brain Res.* **249**:333–344.

Benardo, L. S., L. M. Masukawa, and D. A. Prince (1982) Electrophysiology of isolated hippocampal pyramidal dendrites. *J. Neurosci.* **2**:1614–1622.

Biscoe, T. J., and D. W. Straughan (1966) Micro-electrophoretic studies of neurones in the cat hippocampus. *J. Physiol. (Lond.)* **183**:341–359.

Bliss, T. V. P., and A. R. Gardner-Medwin (1973) Long-lasting potentiation of synaptic transmission in the dentate area of the unanaesthetized rabbit following stimulation of the perforant path. *J. Physiol. (Lond.)* **232**:357–374.

Bliss, T. V. P., and T. Lømo (1973) Long-lasting potentiation of synaptic transmission in the dentate area of the anaesthetized rabbit following stimulation of the perforant path. *J. Physiol. (Lond.)* **232**:331–356.

Collinridge, G. L., S. J. Kehl, and H. McLennan (1983) Excitatory amino acids in synaptic transmission in the Schaffer collateral commissural pathway of the rat hippocampus. *J. Physiol. (Lond.)* **334**: 33–46.

Collins, G. G. S., J. Anson, and L. Surtees (1983) Presynaptic kainate and N-methyl-D-aspartate receptors regulate excitatory amino acid release in the olfactory cortex. *Brain Res.* **265**:157–159.

Cotman, C. W., and J. V. Nadler (1981) Glutamate and aspartate as hippocampal transmitters: Biochemical and pharmacological evidence. In *Glutamate: Transmitter in the Central Nervous System*, P. J. Roberts, J. Storm-Mathisen, and G. A. R. Johnston, eds., pp. 117–154, Wiley, New York.

Davies, L. P., and G. A. R. Johnston (1976) Uptake and release of D- and L-aspartate by rat brain slices. *J. Neurochem.* **26**:1007–1014.

Deadwyler, S. A., V. Gribkoff, C. W. Cotman, and G. Lynch (1976) Long-lasting changes in the spontaneous activity of hippocampal neurons following stimulation of the entorhinal cortex. *Brain Res. Bull.* **1**:1–7.

del Castillo, J., and B. Katz (1954) Statistical factors involved in neuromuscular facilitation and depression. *J. Physiol. (Lond.)* **124**:574–585.

Dodd, J., R. Dingledine, and J. S. Kelly (1981) The excitatory action of acetylcholine on hippocampal neurones of the guinea pig and rat maintained *in vitro. Brain Res.* **207**:109–127.

Dolphin, A. C., M. L. Errington, and T. V. P. Bliss (1982) Long-term potentiation of the perforant path *in vivo* is associated with increased glutamate release. *Nature* **297**:496–498.

Dudar, J. D. (1974) *In vitro* excitation of hippocampal pyramidal cell dendrites by glutamic acid. *Neuropharmacology* **13**:1083–1089.

Edwards, F. R., S. J. Redman, and B. Walmsley (1976) Statistical fluctuations in charge transfer at Ia synapses on spinal motoneurones. *J. Physiol. (Lond.)* **259**:665–688.

Fifková, E., and C. L. Anderson (1981) Stimulation-induced changes in dimensions of stalks of dendritic spines in the dentate molecular layer. *Exp. Neurol.* **74**:621–627.

Gottlieb, D. I., and W. M. Cowan (1972) On the distribution of axonal terminals containing spheroidal and flattened vesicles in the hippocampus and dentate gyrus of the rat and cat. *Z. Zellforsch. Mikrosk. Anat.* **129**:413–429.

Gustafsson, B., and H. Wigström (1981) Shape of frequency–current curves in CA1 cells in the hippocampus. *Brain Res.* **223**:417–421.

Gustafsson, B., M. Galvan, P. Grafe, and H. Wigström (1982) A transient outward current in a mammalian central neurone blocked by 4-aminopyridine. *Nature* **299**:252–254.

Hablitz, J. J., and I. A. Langmoen (1982) Excitation of hippocampal pyramidal cells by glutamate in the guinea-pig and rat. *J. Physiol. (Lond.)* **325**:317–331.

Halliwell, J. V., and P. R. Adams (1982) Voltage-clamp analysis of muscarinic excitation in hippocampal neurons. *Brain Res.* **250**:71–92.

Hamberger, A., G. Chiang, E. S. Nylén, S. W. Scheff, and C. W. Cotman (1978) Stimulus-evoked increase in the biosynthesis of the putative neurotransmitter glutamate in the hippocampus. *Brain Res.* **143**:549–555.

Hvalby, Ø. C., and P. Andersen (1983) Evidence for both pre- and postsynaptic changes during long-term potentiation of CA1 hippocampal synapses. *Acta Physiol. Scand.* **118**:29A.

Jack, J. J. B., S. Miller, R. Porter, and S. J. Redman (1971) The time course of minimal excitatory post-synaptic potentials evoked in spinal motoneurones by group Ia afferent fibres. *J. Physiol. (Lond.)* **215**:353–380.

Kandel, E. R., W. A. Spencer, and F. J. Brinley (1961) Electrophysiology of hippocampal neurons. I. Sequential invasion and synaptic organization. *J. Neurophysiol.* **24**:225–242.

Koch, C., and T. Poggio (1983) A theoretical analysis of electrical properties of spines. *Proc. R. Soc. Lond. (Biol.)* **218**:455–477.

Kuno, M. (1964) Mechanism of facilitation and depression of the excitatory synaptic potential in spinal motoneurones. *J. Physiol. (Lond.)* **175**:100–112.

Kuno, M., and J. T. Miyahara (1969) Non-linear summation of unit synaptic potentials in spinal motoneurones of the cat. *J. Physiol. (Lond.)* **201**:465–477.

Laatsch, R. H., and W. M. Cowan (1966) Electron microscopic studies of the dentate gyrus of the rat. I. Normal structure with special reference to synaptic organization. *J. Comp. Neurol.* **128**:359–396.

Langmoen, I. A., and P. Andersen (1983) Summation of excitatory postsynaptic potentials in hippocampal pyramidal cells. *J. Neurophysiol.* **50**:1320–1329.

Lanthorn, T., J. Storm, and P. Andersen (1984) Current-to-frequency transduction in CA1 hippocampal pyramidal cells: Slow prepotentials dominate the primary range firing. *Exp. Brain Res.* **53**:431–443.

LaVail, J. H., and M. K. Wolf (1973) Postnatal development of the mouse dentate gyrus in organotypic cultures of the hippocampal formation. *Am. J. Anat.* **137**:47–66.

Lee, K. S. (1982) Sustained enhancement of evoked potentials following brief, high-frequency stimulation of the cerebral cortex *in vitro. Brain Res.* **239**:617–623.

Lee, K. S., F. Schottler, M. Oliver, and G. Lynch (1980) Brief bursts of high-frequency stimulation produce two types of structural change in rat hippocampus. *J. Neurophysiol.* **44**:247–258.

Lømo, T. (1966) Frequency potentiation of excitatory synaptic activity in the dentate area of the hippocampal formation. *Acta Physiol. Scand. (Suppl.)* **68**:128.

Lorente de Nó, R. (1934) Studies on the structure of the cerebral cortex. II. Continuation of the study of the ammonic system. *J. Psychol. Neurol. (Lpz.)* **46**:113–117.

Lynch, G. S., and M. Baudry (1984) The biochemistry of memory: A new and specific hypothesis. *Science* **224**:1057–1063.

Lynch, G. S., D. A. Matthews, S. Mosko, T. Parks, and C. Cotman (1972) Induced acetylcholinesterase-rich layer in rat dentate gyrus following entorhinal lesions. *Brain Res.* **42**:311–318.

Lynch, G. S., S. Deadwyler, and C. Cotman (1973a) Postlesion axonal growth produces permanent functional connections. *Science* **180**:1364–1366.

Lynch, G. S., S. Mosko, T. Parks, and C. W. Cotman (1973b) Relocation and hyperdevelopment of the dentate gyrus commissural system after entorhinal lesions in immature rats. *Brain Res.* **50**:174–178.

Lynch, G. S., T. Dunwiddie, and V. Gribkoff (1977) Heterosynaptic depression: A postsynaptic correlate of long-term potentiation. *Nature* **266**:737–739.

McNaughton, B. L., R. M. Douglas, and G. V. Goddard (1978) Synaptic enhancement in fascia dentata: Cooperativity among coactive afferents. *Brain Res.* **157**:277–293.

McNaughton, B. L., C. A. Barnes, and P. Andersen (1981) Synaptic efficacy and EPSP summation in granule cells of rat fascia dentata studies *in vitro. J. Neurophysiol.* **46**:952–966.

MacVicar, B. A., and F. E. Dudek (1980) Dye-coupling between CA3 pyramidal cells in slices of rat hippocampus. *Brain Res.* **196**:494–497.

Madison, D. V., and R. A. Nicoll (1982) Noradrenaline blocks accommodation of pyramidal cell discharge in the hippocampus. *Nature* **299**:636–638.

Magleby, K. L. (1973) The effect of tetanic and post-tetanic potentiation on facilitation of transmitter release at the frog neuromuscular junction. *J. Physiol. (Lond.)* **234**:353–371.

Magleby, K. L., and J. Zengel (1976) Augmentation: A process that acts to increase transmitter release at the frog neuromuscular junction. *J. Physiol. (Lond.)* **257**:449–470.

Martin, A. R., and G. Pilar (1964) Presynaptic and post-synaptic events during post-tetanic potentiation and facilitation in the avian ciliary ganglion. *J. Physiol. (Lond.)* **175**:17–30.

Matthews, D. A., C. Cotman, and G. Lynch (1976) An electron microscopic study of lesion-induced synaptogenesis in the dentate gyrus of the adult rat. I. Magnitude and time courses of degeneration. *Brain Res.* **115**:1–21.

Mayer, M. L., G. L. Westbrook, and P. B. Guthrie (1984) Voltage-dependent block by Mg^{2+} of NMDA responses in spinal cord neurones. *Nature* 309:261–263.

Minkwitz, H. G. (1976) Zur Entwicklung der Neuronenstruktur des Hippocampus während der prä- und postnatalen Ontogenese der Albinoratte. I. Mitteilung: Neurohistologische Darstellung der Entwicklung langaxoniger Neurone aus den Regionen CA3 und CA4. *J. Hirnforsch.* 17:213–231.

Nadler, J. V., K. W. Vaca, W. F. White, G. S. Lynch, and C. W. Cotman (1976) Aspartate and glutamate as possible transmitters of excitatory hippocampal afferents. *Nature* 260:538–540.

Nadler, J. V., W. F. White, K. W. Vaca, D. A. Redburn, and C. W. Cotman (1977) Characterization of putative amino acid transmitter release from slices of rat dentate gyrus. *J. Neurochem.* 29: 279–290.

Nadler, J. V., B. W. Perry, C. Gentry, and C. W. Cotman (1980) Loss and reacquisition of hippocampal synapses after selective destruction of CA3–CA4 afferents with kainic acid. *Brain Res.* 191: 387–403.

Nowak, L., P. Bregestovski, P. Ascher, A. Herbert, and A. Prochiantz (1984) Magnesium gates glutamate-activated channels in mouse central neurones. *Nature* 307:462–465.

Rall, W. (1962) Electrophysiology of a dendritic neuron model. *Biophys. J.* 2:145–167.

Rall, W. (1967) Distinguishing theoretical synaptic potentials computed for different somadendritic distributions of synaptic input. *J. Neurophysiol.* 30:1138–1168.

Rall, W. (1970) Cable properties of dendrites and effects of synaptic location. In *Excitatory Synaptic Mechanisms*, P. Andersen and J. K. S. Jansen, eds., pp. 175–187, Universitetsforlaget, Oslo.

Rall, W., and J. Rinzel (1973) Branch input resistance and steady attenuation for input to one branch of a dendritic neuron model. *Biophys. J.* 13:648–688.

Ramón y Cajal, S. (1893) Beiträge zur feineren Anatomie des grossen Hirns. I. Uber die feinere Struktur des Ammonshornes. *Z. Wiss. Zool.* 56:615–663.

Ramón y Cajal, S. (1911) *Histologie du Système Nerveux de l'Homme et des Vertébrés*, Vol. 2, Maloine, Paris (trans. by S. Azoulay).

Ranck, J. B., Jr. (1973) Studies on single neurons in dorsal hippocampal formation and septum in unrestrained rats. Part I. Behavioral correlates and firing repertoires. *Exp. Neurol.* 41:461–531.

Ribak, C. E., J. E. Vaughn, and K. Saito (1978) Immunocytochemical localization of glutamic acid decarboxylase in neuronal somata following colchicine inhibition of axonal transport. *Brain Res.* 140:315–332.

Schwartzkroin, P. A. (1978) Secondary range rhythmic spiking in hippocampal neurons. *Brain Res.* 149:247–250.

Schwartzkroin, P. A., and P. Andersen (1975) Glutamic acid sensitivity of dendrites in hippocampal slices *in vitro*. *Adv. Neurol.* 12:45–51.

Schwartzkroin, P. A., and M. Slawsky (1977) Probable calcium spikes in hippocampal neurons. *Brain Res.* 135:157–161.

Schwartzkroin, P. A., and K. Wester (1975) Long-lasting facilitation of a synaptic potential following tetanization in the *in vitro* hippocampal slice. *Brain Res.* 89:107–119.

Skrede, K. K., and D. Malthe-Sørenssen (1981) Increased resting and evoked release of transmitter following repetitive electrical tetanization in hippocampus: A biochemical correlate to long-lasting synaptic potentiation. *Brain Res.* 208:436–441.

Skrede, K. K., and R. H. Westgaard (1971) The transverse hippocampal slice: A well-defined cortical structure maintained *in vitro*. *Brain Res.* 35:589–593.

Somogyi, P., M. G. Nunzi, A. Gorio, and D. A. Smith (1983) A new type of specific interneuron in the monkey hippocampus forming synapses exclusively with the axon initial segments of pyramidal cells. *Brain Res.* 259:137–142.

Storm-Mathisen, J. (1974) Choline acetyltransferase and acetylcholinesterase in fascia dentata following lesion of the entorhinal afferents. *Brain Res.* 80:181–197.

Storm-Mathisen, J. (1975) High-affinity uptake of GABA in presumed GABA-ergic nerve endings in rat brain. *Brain Res.* 84:409–427.

Storm-Mathisen, J. (1979) Tentative localization of glutamergic and aspartergic nerve endings in brain. *J. Physiol. (Paris)* 75:677–684.

Storm-Mathisen, J., A. K. Leknes, A. T. Bore, J. Line Vaaland, P. Edminson, F.-M. S. Haug, and O. P. Ottersen (1973) First visualization of glutamate and GABA in neurones by immunocytochemistry. *Nature* **301**:517–520.

Swanson, L. W., T. J. Teyler, and R. F. Thompson (1982) Hippocampal long-term potentiation: Mechanisms and implications for memory. *Neurosci. Res. Program Bull.* **20**:611–769.

Watkins, J. C. (1981) Pharmacology of excitatory amino acid receptors. In *Glutamate: Transmitter in the Nervous System*, P. J. Roberts, J. Storm-Mathisen, and G. A. R. Johnston, eds., pp. 1–24, Wiley, New York.

Wenzel, J., G. Stender, and G. Duwe (1981) Zur Entwicklung der Neuronenstruktur der Fascia Dentata bei der Ratte. Neurohistologisch–morphometrische, ultrastrukturelle und experimentelle Untersuchungen. *J. Hirnforsch.* **22**:629–683.

West, M. J., and A. H. Andersen (1980) An allometric study of the area dentata in the rat and mouse. *Brain Res. Rev.* **2**:317–348.

White, W. F., J. V. Nadler, A. Hamberger, C. W. Cotman, and J. T. Cummins (1977) Glutamate as transmitter of the hippocampal perforant path. *Nature* **270**:356–357.

Winson, J., and C. Abzug (1978) Neuronal transmission through hippocampal pathways dependent on behavior. *J. Neurophysiol.* **41**:716–732.

Zimmer, J. (1973) Extended commissural and ipsilateral projections in postnatally deentorhinated hippocampus and fascia dentata demonstrated in rats by silver impregnation. *Brain Res.* **64**:293–311.

Chapter 17

Long-Term Depression as Memory Process in the Cerebellum

MASAO ITO

ABSTRACT

The long-term depression (LTD) induced in synaptic transmission from parallel fibers to Purkinje cells in the cerebellar cortex appears to be the physiological counterpart of memory in the cerebellum. LTD is induced after conjunctive activation of parallel fibers and climbing fibers by a variety of experimental arrangements. The timing of the conjunctive activation is allowed a rather wide range, suggesting that LTD depends on some variable factors, such as enhancement of the correlation between the firing of parallel fibers and that of climbing fibers. The sensitivity of Purkinje cell dendrites to glutamate, a putative neurotransmitter of parallel fibers, undergoes an LTD when glutamate is applied iontophoretically in conjunction with the activation of climbing fibers. LTD may therefore be due to desensitization of glutamate receptors, but the possibility remains that it is caused by constriction of the neck of dendritic spines, which would reduce glutamate-induced postsynaptic currents. LTD is abolished by conditioning the climbing fiber activation with stellate cell inhibition, which diminishes plateau potentials induced in Purkinje cell dendrites by climbing fiber impulses. Since the plateau potentials represent a voltage-dependent increase of calcium permeability, it is suggested that an increased intradendritic calcium concentration is the primary cause of LTD. Purkinje cells in the cerebellar flocculus that innervate relay cells of the vestibuloocular reflex (VOR) alter their simple spike responsiveness to head rotation during adaptive changes of VOR in a manner consistent with the hypothesis that LTD acts as a memory device in the adaptive and learning control functions of the cerebellum.

Synaptic plasticity implies a wide range of long-term changes of synaptic transmission efficacy, either increases or decreases, that occur under certain functional conditions of synapses. The type of plasticity in which a long-term change is triggered by relatively short-term stimulation, in a manner somewhat comparable to opening or closing a switch, would serve as a memory device in neuronal networks of the central nervous system. Typical examples of this sort have been found in the hippocampal cortex of vertebrate brains (see Andersen et al., 1982) and also in the ganglia of *Aplysia* (see Klein and Kandel, 1980). Long-term depression (LTD) is another example of presumably memory-related plasticity, which is displayed by synapses on Purkinje cells in the cerebellar cortex and which may play a central role in the learning processes of the cerebellum. Plasticity

431

of parallel fiber–Purkinje cell synapses had been suggested theoretically a decade ago (Marr, 1969; Albus, 1971), but LTD has been discovered only recently (Ito et al., 1982).

Theoretical arguments concerning the plasticity of these synapses originated from considerations of the functional meaning of the characteristic dual innervation of cerebellar Purkinje cells with parallel fibers and climbing fibers. Parallel fibers are axons of granule cells in the cerebeller cortex. These axons initially ascend from the granular layer to the molecular layer through the Purkinje cell layer and then bifurcate to form bundles of parallel fibers that run over a distance of a few millimeters. Parallel fibers supply numerous spine synapses on the dendrites of Purkinje cells, and each spine synapse exerts weak excitatory action on the dendrite. Climbing fibers are axons of inferior olive neurons in the medulla oblongata, and dendrites of each Purkinje cell receive powerful excitatory synapses from one climbing fiber. Stimulation of the parallel fibers elicits *simple* spikes and that of climbing fibers *complex* spikes in Purkinje cells.

Referring to Hebb's (1949) idea that correlated presynaptic and postsynaptic activity would induce plastic changes of synaptic efficacy, Brindley (1964) suggested that convergent inputs from parallel fibers and climbing fibers would produce such correlated activities and consequently a plastic change at parallel fiber–Purkinje cell synapses. Grossberg (1969) also suggested a similar process in analogy to the associative memory processes postulated for classical conditioning. Based on such assumptions of plasticity, theories of the cerebellar neuronal network incorporating learning capabilities were developed by Marr (1969) and Albus (1971). Marr (1969) assumed an enhancement of transmission efficacy at parallel fiber–Purkinje cell synapses, whereas Albus (1971) postulated the opposite, that is, a depression. These two assumptions have similar theoretical implications, but there are certain differences in their practical implications.

Direct evidence in support of the assumption of plasticity for the cerebellar neuronal circuitry has now been obtained with a variety of testing methods (Figure 1) and has consistently revealed the occurrence of a long-term change in transmission efficacy subsequent to conjunctive stimulation of the parallel fibers and climbing fibers. The change observed has been LTD, in conformity with Albus's (1971) assumption. At present, no evidence has been obtained for facilitation. This chapter describes properties of LTD and discusses its possible mechanism. The possibility that LTD is the physiological counterpart of memory processes in the cerebellum is examined on the basis of experimental data about the cerebellar control of eye movements.

PROPERTIES OF LTD

LTD has been induced in *in vivo* preparations with the following four experimental paradigms (Figure 1).

The first of these is indirect stimulation of parallel fibers via mossy fiber afferents in conjunction with stimulation of climbing fibers, and recording from individual Purkinje cells with an extracellular microelectrode. Ito et al. (1982) tested the responsiveness of floccular Purkinje cells by applying single pulse stimuli to a vestibular nerve that projects to the cerebellar flocculus as mossy

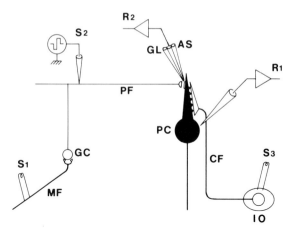

Figure 1. *Experimental arrangement for testing long-term depression (LTD).* Abbreviations: AS, aspartate; CF, climbing fiber afferent; GL, glutamate; IO, inferior olive; MF, mossy fiber afferent; PC, Purkinje cell; PF, parallel fiber afferent; R_1, single glass microelectrode; R_2, recording barrel in a multibarreled pipette; S_1, S_2, S_3, stimulating electrodes.

fiber afferents. These stimuli excited Purkinje cells with a latency of 3–6 msec, presumably via granule cells and parallel fibers. The firing index for the excitation of Purkinje cells was calculated from the number of spikes initiated above the spontaneous firing level, during 100 sweeps repeated at the rate of 2 pulses/sec (Figure 2). Conjunctive stimulation of climbing fibers and mossy fibers was performed by applying 4-Hz stimuli to the inferior olive and 20-Hz stimuli to a vestibular nerve simultaneously for a period of 25 sec. Thus, 100 climbing fiber impulses and 500 vestibular mossy fiber impulses were given to the flocculus. A stimulation of 4 Hz was chosen, as it is about the maximum climbing fiber discharge observed in alert rabbits; 20 Hz is a moderate frequency for discharge evoked in vestibular nerve fibers by head rotation.

These parameters reveal that conjunctive stimulation effectively depresses the vestibular mossy fiber responsiveness of flocculus Purkinje cells (Figure 2). Although the depression diminishes in about 10 min, there is usually a slow phase of weak depression that lasts for more than one hour. This effect was specific to the vestibular nerve involved in the conjunctive stimulation; no depression occurred in the responsiveness to inputs from the opposite vestibular nerve. Therefore, the effect of a conjunctive stimulation is not due to general depression in Purkinje cells, but is specific to a site or sites in the mossy fiber–granule cell–Purkinje cell pathway involved in the conjunctive stimulation.

Conjunctive stimulation of climbing fibers and mossy fibers did not affect the responsiveness of basket cells to mossy fiber inputs. Field potentials recorded in the granular layer and white matter of the flocculus were not affected. These responses represent impulse transmission in the mossy fibers and the cortical network, exclusive of the parallel fiber–Purkinje cell synapses. Therefore, it can be concluded that signal transmission at parallel fiber–Purkinje cell synapses undergoes an LTD after conjunctive activation of the climbing fiber impinging on the same Purkinje cell.

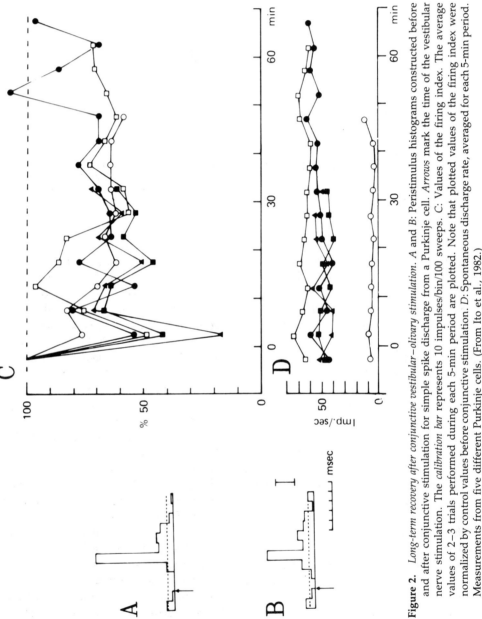

Figure 2. *Long-term recovery after conjunctive vestibular–olivary stimulation. A* and *B*: Peristimulus histograms constructed before and after conjunctive stimulation for simple spike discharge from a Purkinje cell. *Arrows* mark the time of the vestibular nerve stimulation. The *calibration bar* represents 10 impulses/bin/100 sweeps. *C*: Values of the firing index. The average values of 2–3 trials performed during each 5-min period are plotted. Note that plotted values of the firing index were normalized by control values before conjunctive stimulation. *D*: Spontaneous discharge rate, averaged for each 5-min period. Measurements from five different Purkinje cells. (From Ito et al., 1982.)

434

A similar long-term depression can be demonstrated by repetitive impulses applied to a vestibular nerve at a frequency of 20 Hz (Ito, 1982b). Such constant rate stimulation may mimic vestibular inputs occurring during a linear head acceleration. When the number of impulses evoked during the 20-Hz stimulation for 2.5 sec above the spontaneous firing level was measured as an index of the responsiveness of the Purkinje cell to vestibular mossy fiber inputs, an LTD could be demonstrated to occur, as with single pulse testing (Figure 3).

A second paradigm involves conjunctive stimulation of parallel fibers and climbing fibers, and recording of mass field potentials from the molecular layer of the cerebellar cortex. In an experiment by Ito and Kano (1982), parallel fibers were stimulated directly through a glass microelectrode placed in the molecular layer. Application of brief impulses (0.2 msec duration) of 20–60 µA excites a narrow beam of parallel fibers, along which double-peaked negative field potentials are recorded with another microelectrode. The first peak (n_1) represents volleys conducted along parallel fibers, and the second peak (n_2) represents the post-synaptic excitation thereby evoked in dendrites of Purkinje and other cortical cells. When the parallel fiber stimuli were paired with stimuli to the inferior

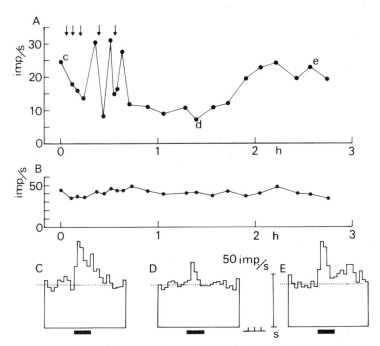

Figure 3. *Depression of mossy fiber responsiveness of a flocculus Purkinje cell after conjunctive stimulation of mossy fibers and climbing fibers, tested with repetitive mossy fiber stimulation. A:* The average increase of simple spike discharges from the Purkinje cell during 20-Hz stimulation of the vestibular nerve is plotted as a function of time. *Arrows* mark the moments of conjunctive stimulation of the vestibular nerve at 20 impulses/sec and the contralateral inferior olive at 4 impulses/sec for 25 sec at a time. *c–e* are plotting points obtained from the histograms of *C–E,* respectively. *B:* plot of spontaneous discharge rate. *C–E:* Peristimulus histograms constructed during five sweeps. *Black bars* indicate the period of stimulation of the ipsilateral vestibular nerve at 20 Hz. *Dotted lines* indicate the levels of spontaneous firing. (From Ito, 1982b.)

olive with a time delay of 6–2 msec, and repeated at a rate of 4 pulses/sec for one or two minutes, the n_2 wave often exhibited a small but significant depression that lasted for more than one hour.

The depression detected in the n_2 wave of the field potentials in the molecular layer is usually small (10–20%) and is often difficult to detect, in contrast to the frequent occurrence of a prominent depression in unit spike responses of Purkinje cells, as described in what follows. This discrepancy may be explained by the heterogeneous origin of the n_2 wave from Purkinje, basket, stellate, and Golgi cells. There may also be a nonlinear relationship between the excitatory synaptic currents and the resultant membrane excitation. The possibility also remains that the conjunctive activation of parallel fibers and climbing fibers depresses not only the synaptic transmission mechanisms but also the excitability of the local postsynaptic membrane, as postulated for the prolonged potentiation of synaptic transmission in hippocampal neurons (Andersen et al., 1982). If this were so, changes in postsynaptic potentials would be smaller than those to be expected from changes in the firing index, which reflects both the postsynaptic potentials and the postsynaptic membrane excitability.

In the third paradigm, parallel fibers and climbing fibers are conjunctively stimulated, and recordings from individual Purkinje cells are taken. When the recording microelectrode is placed in the Purkinje cell layer, activation of single Purkinje cells by parallel fiber volleys can be observed (Ekerot and Kano, 1983). Conjunctive stimulation of a parallel fiber beam and the inferior olive at 1–4 Hz regularly produced a prominent depression in the responsiveness of Purkinje cells to parallel fiber stimulation (Figure 4). The depression usually developed in two steps: an early phase lasting for about 10 min, and a late phase lasting for a succeeding period of more than one hour. Some Purkinje cells could be excited through two separate parallel fiber beams. When one of the two beams was stimulated in conjunction with the inferior olive, the responsiveness of the Purkinje cell to that parallel fiber beam was specifically depressed; the responsiveness to the other beam remained unchanged. This specificity supports earlier observations made by stimulating vestibular nerves (see above).

The timing of effective conjunctions of parallel fiber and climbing fiber stimulation has been studied by C.-F. Ekerot and M. Kano (personal communication) and found to be allowed an unexpectedly wide latitude, in contrast to the critical timing postulated by Marr (1969). Parallel fiber impulses falling during the period between 20 msec prior to and 150 msec subsequent to the stimulation of climbing fibers are nearly equally potent in inducing LTD. Even those occurring at 250 msec after a climbing fiber impulse induce LTD, though with less predictability. Therefore, the conjunction stimulation of parallel fibers and climbing fibers does not need to be critically timed; rather, LTD may depend on some more variable factors, such as enhancement of the correlation between the firing of parallel fibers and that of climbing fibers, as recently postulated in Fujita's (1982a) adaptive filter model of the cerebellum. The need for critical timing is also unrealistic in view of the characteristically irregular pattern of climbing fiber discharge under natural stimulating conditions.

The fourth and final paradigm involves the application of glutamate, the putative neurotransmitter for parallel fibers, in conjunction with climbing fiber stimulation. Ito et al. (1982) replaced parallel fiber stimulation with the iontophoretic

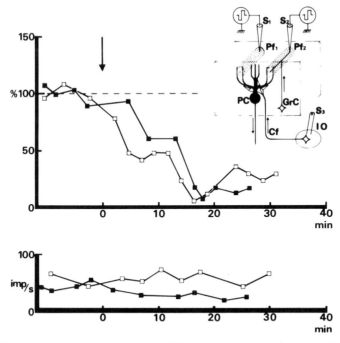

Figure 4. *Effect of conjunctive activation of parallel fibers and climbing fibers on the parallel fiber–Purkinje cell transmission. Inset* shows the experimental arrangements for stimulating two beams of parallel fibers in the molecular layer and climbing fibers in the inferior olive, and for recording extracellularly from a Purkinje cell. Abbreviations: Cf, climbing fiber; GrC, granule cell; IO, inferior olive; PC, Purkinje cell; Pf₁, Pf₂, parallel fibers; S₁, S₂, stimulating microelectrodes; S₃, stimulating metal electrode. *Upper graph* plots the firing index at the peaks of the peristimulus histogram. *Arrow* indicates the moment of conjunctive stimulation of Pf₁ and IO. *Lower graph* plots the spontaneous firing level. (Courtesy of Drs. C. F. Ekerot and M. Kano.)

application of glutamate, which is a putative neurotransmitter of parallel fibers. The application of glutamate and aspartate through a multibarreled pipette normally excited Purkinje cells. The application of glutamate in conjunction with 4-Hz stimulation of the inferior olive effectively depressed the glutamate sensitivity of Purkinje cells; aspartate sensitivity, tested as control, was depressed to a much lesser degree (Figure 5). The depression diminished in about 10 min and was followed by a slow depression lasting for one hour. The depression of glutamate sensitivity was obtained only when there was an initially high glutamate sensitivity, higher than control aspartate sensitivity, suggesting that the electrode was close to parallel fiber–Purkinje cell junctions. When the electrode tip was placed in the molecular layer, such high glutamate sensitivity was obtained in about one-third of the trials, whereas in the other two-thirds the glutamate sensitivity was relatively low, even lower than the control aspartate sensitivity. In these two-thirds, LTD of glutamate sensitivity could not be induced by conjunctive application of glutamate with climbing fiber stimulation. This suggests that Purkinje cell dendrites may have potent extrajunctional glutamate receptors that do not behave as the junctional receptors under the conjunctive application of glutamate with climbing fiber stimulation.

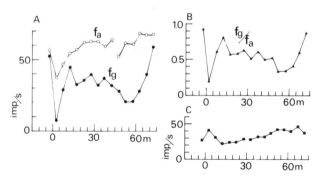

Figure 5. *Long-term recovery after glutamate–olivary conjunction.* A: f_g is the increased simple spike discharge resulting from the application of glutamate with a 9-nA current; f_a is that resulting from the application of aspartate with a 69-nA current. Each point represents the average value of 2–3 tests during each 5-min period. B: The f_g/f_a ratio. C: Plot of the spontaneous discharge rate. (From Ito et al., 1982.)

The causal relationship assumed between the effect demonstrated in parallel fiber–Purkinje cell transmission and that seen in the glutamate sensitivity of Purkinje cells has been examined by Kano and Kato (1985). When glutamate is applied to a dendritic region of a Purkinje cell in conjunction with the stimulation of climbing fibers, the responsiveness of the Purkinje cell to stimulation of a parallel fiber bundle that passes the dendritic site of glutamate application undergoes LTD, just like LTD obtained with conjunctive stimulation of parallel fibers and climbing fibers. Therefore, both the third and the fourth paradigms appear to test the same LTD.

Thus, LTD apparently represents the physiological counterpart of the synaptic plasticity postulated theoretically as the memory device of the cerebellar neuronal network. The entire duration of LTD is still uncertain because of the limitations of present recording techniques for *in vivo* preparations. Even though LTD was observed to continue for three to four hours in a limited number of cases, it is urgently desirable to determine the whole time course of LTD and its dependence on stimulus parameters.

It may be questioned whether only LTD accounts for the entire process of learning in the cerebellar cortex. Is there no need for a positive facilitation in addition to the depression? Fujita (1982a) assumed that, around a certain resting level, a decreased incidence of simultaneous activation of a climbing fiber and a parallel fiber will lead to a facilitation opposite to the depression that takes place under an increased incidence of simultaneous activation. If so, there will be a facilitation because of the withdrawal of LTD. It is desirable to verify this assumption experimentally.

MECHANISMS OF LTD

The Hebbian type of plasticity, which suggests that the coincidence of presynaptic and postsynaptic impulses plays a key role in the modification of synaptic efficacy, does not apply to LTD for several reasons: (1) Parallel fiber volleys that excite Purkinje cells are not sufficient to produce a plastic change in parallel fiber–Purkinje cell synapses; (2) iontophoretic application of glutamate, which excites Purkinje cells, does not modify the glutamate sensitivity of Purkinje cells; and (3) climbing fiber impulses are effective at a low rate of 1–4 Hz, implying that postsynaptic impulses evoked by climbing fiber stimulation may not play a major role in producing LTD.

The second possibility, originally suggested by Marr (1969), is that climbing fiber terminals liberate a "change" substance which induces LTD. The change substance might be something like thyrotropin-releasing hormone (TRH), which selectively depresses glutamate sensitivity in cerebral cortical cells (Renaud et al., 1979). TRH is present in the cerebellum, especially in the vestibulocerebellum (Pachero et al., 1981). However, TRH induces only a short-lasting depression of the glutamate sensitivity of Purkinje cells (M. Ito and M. Kano, unpublished observations) so that TRH by itself cannot account for LTD. Furthermore, the following observations by Ekerot and Kano (1985) eliminate the possibility of a change substance and suggest a third possible mechanism of LTD.

Stellate cells, which innervate a Purkinje cell under examination in a conjunctive stimulation paradigm, can be activated transsynaptically by stimulating a parallel fiber bundle passing near the Purkinje cell. Conditioning of the climbing fiber stimulation with stellate cell activation abolishes LTD. Since such stellate cell conditioning removes the climbing fiber-induced plateau potentials in Purkinje cell dendrites that represent a voltage-dependent increase of the calcium permeability of the dendritic membrane (Llinás and Sugimori, 1980), it is possible that an increased intradendritic calcium concentration affects subsynaptic glutamate receptors of Purkinje cell dendrites in the manner suggested for desensitization phenomena in neuromuscular junctions (Miledi, 1980; Ekerot and Oscarsson, 1981), or that it causes a change in the shape of dendritic spines, which are the sites of parallel fiber–Purkinje cell synapses (Figure 6). These spines are 1.5–2.0 μm long, with a head diameter of 0.4–0.5 mm. If the neck of a spine undergoes a constriction, there will be an increase in the electrical resistance through the shaft of the spine. This could, under certain conditions, effectively reduce the synaptic current flowing into the dendritic shaft. This possibility is analogous, though the direction is opposite, to what has been assumed for plastic enhancement

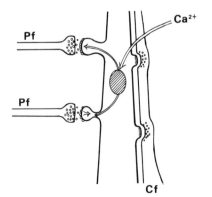

Figure 6. *Possible mechanisms of modification of parallel fiber–Purkinje cell transmission following conjunctive activation of parallel fibers and climbing fibers.*

of synaptic efficacy; if the shaft of a spine shortens, there will be an increased efficacy of the postsynaptic currents in influencing the membrane potential in the dendritic shaft and cell soma (Crick, 1982; Koch and Poggio, 1983; Kawato et al., 1984). Thus, the mechanism of LTD should be investigated further with these various possibilities in mind.

ROLES OF LTD

The possibility that LTD plays a key role in cerebellar functions has been substantiated by studies of the flocculo-vestibuloocular system. The flocculus is a phylogenetically old part of the cerebellum and projects Purkinje cell axons to relay cells of the vestibuloocular reflex (VOR). These Purkinje cells receive vestibular signals as a mossy fiber input and visual signals as a climbing fiber input (Figure 7). It seems that the visual climbing fiber afferents convey "instruction" signals to the flocculus as to the effectiveness of VOR eye movements compensating for head movements. If these climbing fiber signals act to modify the signal transfer characteristics of the vestibular mossy fiber–granule cell–Purkinje cell pathway in the flocculus in the manner predicted by the plasticity assumption, modification will then occur in VOR dynamics toward improved visual stability. This "flocculus hypothesis of VOR control," proposed a decade ago (Ito, 1970, 1972, 1974, 1982a), has been tested and supported by examining the effects of lesioning the flocculus (Ito et al., 1974; Robinson, 1976; Ito et al., 1982; Nagao, 1983), by recording Purkinje cell responses (Ghelarducci et al., 1975; Ito, 1977; Dufossé et al., 1978; Watanabe, 1984), and also by a computer simulation study (Fujita, 1982a,b).

VOR can be modified by imposing visual–vestibular interacting conditions. The wearing of dove prism goggles, which reverse the right–left polarity of the visual field, acts to reduce VOR gain, and even to reverse the polarity of VOR (Gonshor and Melvill Jones, 1976), while 2× telescopic lenses increase VOR gain

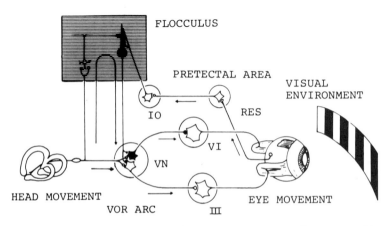

Figure 7. *Connections of the flocculus with the horizontal vestibuloocular reflex (VOR).* Abbreviations: IO, inferior olive; RES, retinal error signals; VN, vestibular nuclei.

(Miles and Fuller, 1974; Gauthier and Robinson, 1975). Combined rotation of the visual field with the whole-body rotation of an animal causes similar effects. The out-phase combination, in which the visual field rotates 180° out of phase with the animal, causes an enhancement of VOR gain, whereas the in-phase combination, in which the visual field rotates together with the animal, causes a decrease of VOR gain. The initial changes of VOR gain are rapid, so that a combined rotation for a few hours produces a substantial gain change of about 0.2. Lesions of the flocculus abolished the VOR adaptation (Ito et al., 1974; Robinson, 1976; Ito et al., 1982; Nagao, 1983). Interruption of the visual climbing fiber pathway produced similar effects (Ito and Miyashita, 1975; Demer and Robinson, 1982). Administration of Harmaline, which produces abnormal rhythmic activity in climbing fibers, also impaired the lens-induced VOR adaptation (Gauthier et al., 1983). These observations are in accordance with the flocculus hypothesis.

Events in the flocculus have been investigated during sinusoidal head rotation on the horizontal plane in rabbits and monkeys. When Purkinje cells were selected from the floccular area (H-zone) in which local electrical stimulation with the recording microelectrodes induced abduction of the ipsilateral eye, indicating involvement of the Purkinje cells in the horizontal VOR (Dufossé et al., 1978; Watanabe, 1984), the major observations were the following:

1. Floccular Purkinje cells modulate discharge of simple spikes in various phase relationships with head velocity. As discharges in primary vestibular afferents are modulated in phase with head velocity (Fernandez and Goldberg, 1971), simple spike modulation in phase with head velocity will have the effect of depressing VOR as it cancels excitatory vestibular inputs to VOR relay cells. In contrast, simple spike modulation out of phase with head velocity will have the effect of enhancing VOR, as the inhibitory Purkinje cell signals that modulate out of phase wax and wane opposite to the excitatory vestibular signals. The flocculus can therefore either depress VOR through Purkinje cells that modulate in phase or enhance it through Purkinje cells that modulate out of phase (Figure 8).

2. Complex spike discharges are also modulated by optokinetic stimuli involved in the combined visual–vestibular stimulation. Complex spikes are facilitated by temporonasal, and depressed by nasotemporal, movement of visual stimuli. Thus, when the visual field moves in phase with the head, complex spikes are modulated out of phase, while the out-phase-moving visual field modulates complex spikes in phase with the head velocity (Figure 9F, G).

3. During combined visual–vestibular stimulation, the simple spike modulation alters in parallel with adaptive changes of VOR gain. During the out-phase combination, which adaptively increases VOR gain, the simple spike modulation became less in phase, more out of phase, or was even converted from the in-phase to the out-phase type (Figure 9C, D). During the in-phase combination, which adaptively decreases VOR gain, the simple spike modulation became less out of phase, more in phase, or even converted from out of phase to in phase. It is a corollary observation that complex spike modulation causes a reciprocal change in simple spike modulation: in-phase complex spike modulation leads to more out-phase simple spike modulation, whereas out-phase complex spike modulation leads to more in-phase simple spike modulation.

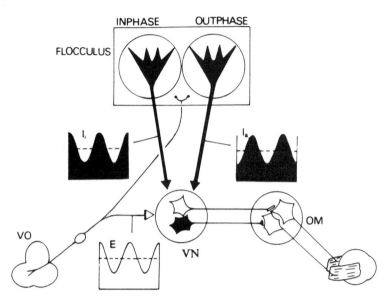

Figure 8. *Modification of the vestibuloocular reflex by in-phase and out-phase responses of flocculus Purkinje cells. E is a spike density histogram for the primary vestibular afferent impulses; I_i and I_a are those for Purkinje cell discharges. Note that when superposed on second-order vestibular neurons (VN), I_i cancels E, whereas I_a reinforces E. OM, oculomotor neurons; VO, vestibular organ. (From Ito, 1976.)*

The reciprocal relationship between the complex spike modulation and the shift of simple spike modulation can be explained on the basis of LTD at parallel fiber–Purkinje cell synapses (Ito, 1977). Imagine that simple spike modulation in Purkinje cells is due to summation of parallel fiber activities that are modulated by various phase relationships with head velocity. During combined stimulation, complex spikes would act to depress the synaptic effects of parallel fibers whose impulses collide with the complex spikes on Purkinje cells. Only those parallel fibers modulating reciprocally with the complex spikes will escape LTD, and their synaptic action will become more predominant in determining the simple spike responsiveness of Purkinje cells.

The various phase relationships between the modulation in mossy fibers and that in parallel fibers may be created by several factors. First, primary mossy fiber signals generated from the two vestibular organs are 180° out of phase with each other. Second, signals in secondary vestibular mossy fibers relayed by vestibular nuclei would have a shift of phase from those of primary vestibular fibers. Third, according to Fujita's (1982a) adaptive filter model of the cerebellum, the mossy fiber–granule cell relay attached to Golgi cell recurrent inhibition creates subsets of signals with varied phase relationships. LTD would act to remove the effect of those parallel fibers modulating in parallel with, and intensify the relative effects of those modulating reciprocally to, complex spikes. Fujita's (1982b) adaptive filter model, constructed along this idea and incorporated in the model of the oculomotor system, reproduces the adaptive behavior of VOR with fidelity (Fujita, 1982b).

The same applies to the observations of Gilbert and Thach (1977), who recorded from Purkinje cells in the intermediate cortex of the monkey's lobules III–V and demonstrated that after the load to a moving arm was suddenly changed, there was an increase in the occurrence of complex spikes just after the load change (at 50–150 msec). This increase persisted for many trials before returning to the base line. There was a concurrent change in simple spike occurrence after the load change; it gradually decreased over time and remained decreased after the complex spike firing frequency had returned to its prior level. The changes in complex and simple spike discharges were over a time course similar to that of the improvement in motor performance. These observations are consistent with the view that, as in VOR adaptation, motor learning takes place in the cerebellum through a decrease (LTD) in the strength of transmission of parallel fiber synapses on Purkinje cells caused by the climbing fiber inputs.

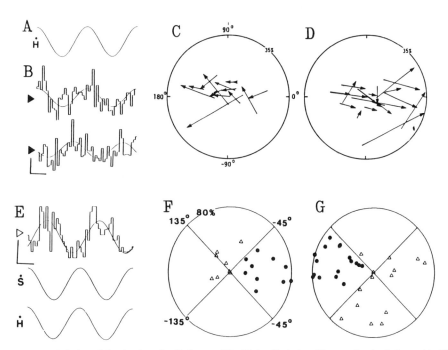

Figure 9. *Modulation of the simple spike discharge of Purkinje cells induced by rotation in darkness (A–D) and that of complex spikes induced during combined rotation (E–G). A: The time course of head velocity (H) change (0.3 Hz by 500 peak to peak). B: Simple spike density histograms taken from the same Purkinje cell in response to head rotation in darkness. Upper trace, before, and lower trace, after, horizontal VOR gain decreased adaptively. Horizontal calibration bar represents 1 sec; vertical calibration bar represents 10 impulses/sec. Filled triangles mark a spike frequency of 60 impulses/sec. C and D: Arrows represent changes in the modulation pattern of each H-zone Purkinje cell before and after horizontal VOR adaptation on polar diagrams. C, out-phase combination; D, in-phase combination. E: Upper trace is a density histogram for complex spikes in H-zone Purkinje cells. Middle and lower traces indicate screen velocity (S) and head velocity (H), respectively. Open triangle marks a spike frequency of 1 impulse/sec. F and G: Modulation patterns of complex spikes observed during out-phase and in-phase combination, respectively. Filled circles represent cells in the H-zone and open triangles those in other zones. (From Watanabe, 1984.)*

COMMENTS

It now seems evident that LTD represents a memory device in the cerebellar neuronal circuitry and plays a key role in the adaptive control of the vestibuloocular reflex. Possibilities that LTD plays key roles in various adaptive and learning control functions of the cerebellum in general are discussed in a recent monograph by this author (Ito, 1984). Experimental examination of these possibilities will fruitfully lead to a more complete understanding of the mechanisms and the implications of synaptic plasticity in central nervous system function.

REFERENCES

Albus, J. S. (1971) A theory of cerebellar function. *Math. Biosci.* **10**:25–61.

Andersen, P., S. H. Sundberg, O. Sveen, J. W. Swan, and H. Wingstrom (1982) Possible mechanism for long-lasting potentiation of synaptic transmission in hippocampal slice from guinea-pigs. *J. Physiol. (Lond.)* **302**:463–482.

Brindley, G. S. (1964) The use made by the cerebellum of the information that it receives from sense organs. *IBRO Bull.* **3**:80.

Crick, F. (1982) Do dendritic spines twitch? *Trends Neurosci.* **5**:44–46.

Demer, J. L., and D. A. Robinson (1982) Effects of reversible lesions and stimulation of olivocerebellar system on vestibulo-ocular reflex plasticity. *J. Neurophysiol.* **47**:1084–1107.

Dufossé, M., M. Ito, P. J. Jastreboff, and Y. Miyashita (1978) A neuronal correlate in rabbit's cerebellum to adaptive modification of the vestibuloocular reflex. *Brain Res.* **150**:511–616.

Ekerot, C.-F., and M. Kano (1983) Climbing fibre-induced depression of Purkinje cell responses to parallel fibre stimulation. *Proc. IUPS (Sydney)* **15**:393.

Ekerot, C.-F., and M. Kano (1985) Long-term depression of parallel fibre synapses following stimulation of climbing fibres. *Brain Res.* **342**:357–360.

Ekerot, C.-F., and O. Oscarsson (1981) Prolonged depolarization elicited in Purkinje cell dendrites by climbing fibre impulses in the cat. *J. Physiol. (Lond).* **318**:207–221.

Fernandez, C., and J. M. Goldberg (1971) Physiology of peripheral neurons in innervating semicircular canals of the squirrel monkey. II. Response to sinusoidal stimulation and dynamics of peripheral vestibular system. *J. Neurophysiol.* **34**:661–675.

Fujita, M. (1982a) Adaptive filter model of the cerebellum. *Biol. Cybern.* **45**:195–206.

Fujita, M. (1982b) Simulation of adaptive modification of the vestibuloocular reflex with an adaptive filter model of the cerebellum. *Biol. Cybern.* **45**:207–214.

Gauthier, G. M., and D. A. Robinson (1975) Adaptation of the human vestibuloocular reflex to magnifying lenses. *Brain Res.* **92**:331–335.

Gauthier, G. M., E. Marchetti, and J. Pellet (1983) Cerebellar control of vestibuloocular reflex (VOR) studied with injection of Harmaline in the trained baboon. *Arch. Ital. Biol.* **121**:9–36.

Ghelarducci, B., M. Ito, and N. Yagi (1975) Impulse discharge from flocculus Purkinje cells of alert rabbits during visual stimulation combined with horizontal head rotation. *Brain Res.* **8**:66–72.

Gilbert, P. F. C., and W. T. Thach (1977) Purkinje cell activity during motor learning. *Brain Res.* **128**:309–328.

Gonshor, A., and G. Melville Jones (1976) Extreme vestibulo-ocular adaptation induced by prolonged optical reversal of vision. *J. Physiol. (Lond.)* **256**:381–414.

Grossberg, S. (1969) On learning of spatiotemporal patterns by networks with ordered sensory and motor components. I. Excitatory connections of the cerebellum. *Studies Appl. Math.* **48**:105–132.

Hebb, O. (1949) *The Organization of Behavior: A Neurophysiological Theory*, Wiley, New York.

Ito, M. (1970) Neurophysiological aspects of the cerebellar motor control system. *Int. J. Neurol.* **7**:162–176.

Ito, M. (1972) Neural design of the cerebellar motor control system. *Brain Res.* **40**:81–84.

Ito, M. (1974) The control mechanisms of cerebellar motor system. In *The Neurosciences: Third Study Program*, F. O. Schmitt and F. G. Worden, eds., pp. 293–303, MIT Press, Cambridge, Massachusetts.

Ito, M. (1976) Cerebellar learning control of vestibulo-ocular mechanisms. In *Mechanisms in Transmission of Signals for Conscious Behavior*, T. Desiraju, ed., pp. 1–22, Elsevier, Amsterdam.

Ito, M. (1977) Neuronal events in the cerebellar flocculus associated with an adaptive modification of the vestibulo-ocular reflex of the rabbit. In *Control of Gaze by Brain Stem Neurons*, R. Baker and A. Berthoz, eds., pp. 391–398, Elsevier, Amsterdam.

Ito, M. (1982a) Cerebellar control of the vestibuloocular reflex–around the flocculus hypothesis. *Annu. Rev. Neurosci.* **5**:275–296.

Ito, M. (1982b) Experimental verification of Marr–Albus plasticity assumption for the cerebellum. *Acta Biol. Acad. Sci. Hung.* **33**:189–199.

Ito, M. (1984) *The Cerebellum and Neural Control*, Raven, New York.

Ito, M., T. Shiida, N. Yagi, and M. Yamamoto (1974) The cerebellar modification of rabbit's horizontal vestibulo-ocular reflex induced by sustained head rotation combined with visual stimulation. *Proc. Jpn. Acad.* **50**:85–89.

Ito, M., and Y. Miyashita (1975) The effects of chronic destruction of the inferior olive upon visual modification of the horizontal vestibulo-ocular reflex of rabbits. *Proc. Jpn. Acad.* **51**:716–720.

Ito, M., and M. Kano (1982) Long-lasting depression of parallel fiber–Purkinje cell transmission by conjunctive stimulation of parallel fibers and climbing fibers in the cerebellar cortex. *Neurosci. Lett.* **33**:253–258.

Ito, M., P. J. Jastreboff, and Y. Miyashita (1982) Specific effects of unilateral lesions in the flocculus upon eye movements of rabbits. *Exp. Brain Res.* **45**:233–242.

Ito, M., M. Sakurai, and P. Tongroach (1982) Climbing fiber-induced depression of both mossy fiber responsiveness and glutamate sensitivity of cerebellar Purkinje cells. *J. Physiol. (Lond.)* **324**: 113–134.

Kano, M., and M. Kato (1985) Long-term depression of parallel fiber–Purkinje cell transmission induced by conjunctive local glutamate application with climbing fiber stimulation in the cerebellar cortex of the rabbit. *Neurosci. Res. (Suppl.)* **1**:S126.

Kawato, M., T. Kamaguchi, F. Murakami, and N. Tsukahara (1984) Quantitative analysis of electrical properties of dendritic spines. *Biol. Cybern.* **50**:447–454.

Klein, M., and E. R. Kandel (1980) Mechanism of calcium current modulation underlying presynaptic facilitation and behavior sensitization in *Aplysia*. *Proc. Natl. Acad. Sci. USA* **77**:6912–6916.

Koch, C., and T. Poggio (1983) A theoretical analysis of electrical properties of spines. *Proc. R. Soc. Lond. (Biol.)* **218**:445–447.

Llinás, R., and M. Sugimori (1980) Electrophysiological properties of *in vitro* Purkinje cell dendrites in mammalian cerebellar slices. *J. Physiol. (Lond.)* **305**:197–213.

Marr, D. (1969) A theory of cerebellar cortex. *J. Physiol. (Lond.)* **202**:437–470.

Miledi, R. (1980) Intracellular calcium and desensitization of acetylcholine receptors. *Proc. R. Soc. Lond. (Biol.)* **209**:447–452.

Miles, F. A., and J. H. Fuller (1974) Adaptive plasticity in the vestibulo-ocular responses of the rhesus monkey. *Brain Res.* **80**:512–516.

Nagao, S. (1983) Effects of vestibulocerebellar lesions upon dynamic characteristics and adaptation of vestibulo-ocular and optokinetic responses in pigmented rabbits. *Exp. Brain Res.* **53**:36–46.

Pachero, M. F., J. F. McKelvy, D. J. Woodward, C. Loudes, P. Joseph-Bravo, L. Krulich, and W. S. T. Griffin (1981) TRH in the rat cerebellum. I. Distribution and concentration. *Peptides* **2**:277–282.

Renaud, L. P., H. W. Blume, Q. J. Pittman, Y. Lamour, and A. T. Tan (1979) Thyrotropin releasing hormone selectively depressed glutamate excitation of cerebral cortical neurons. *Science* **205**: 1275–1277.

Robinson, D. A. (1976) Adaptive gain control of vestibulo-ocular reflex by the cerebellum. *J. Neurophysiol.* **39**:954–969.

Watanabe, E. (1984) Neuronal events correlated with long-term adaptation of horizontal vestibulo-ocular reflex in the primate flocculus. *Brain Res.* **297**:169–174.

Chapter 18

Cellular Basis of Classical Conditioning Mediated by the Red Nucleus in the Cat

NAKAAKIRA TSUKAHARA

ABSTRACT

Evidence accumulated over the past decade indicates that sprouting occurs in adult central neurons in various loci of the central nervous system. In the cat's red nucleus (RN), for example, corticorubral fibers that initially terminate on the distal dendrites of RN neurons can sprout under various circumstances and form new functional connections onto the proximal portion of the somatodendritic membrane of RN cells. Of particular interest is the fact that sprouting can take place in normal central neurons without any lesions to their synaptic input, which previously had been the most common method used to induce sprouting. We have focused our attention on the question of whether sprouting may be a neuronal basis of learning. Such a question can best be addressed by using the corticorubral synapse as a modifiable element and then demonstrating that classical conditioning can be synthesized by combining corticorubral fiber stimulation (the conditioned stimulus) with forelimb skin stimulation (the unconditioned stimulus). Our experiments indicate that classical conditioning can indeed be reproduced in this way and that the sites of the conditioned change are the corticorubral synapses. One possible mechanism for which we have some evidence is that corticorubral fibers sprout onto the proximal portion of the somatodendritic membrane, thus giving more powerful synaptic input to RN neurons. The possibility of other mechanisms is also considered.

The neuronal mechanisms of learning and memory in the mammalian brain represent a fascinating problem for neurobiologists, but clarifying this problem has proved to be a frustrating task. Consequently, some neurobiologists have turned to studying this problem in relatively simple animals and have succeeded in identifying some aspects of memory mechanisms (see Kandel, 1978). Two of the problems in mammalian learning studies are to identify the neuronal circuit involved in any form of complex learning behavior and to pinpoint the site at which modification takes place during learning. One approach is to analyze a modifiable element of the system first, and then to reconstruct the modification of behavior produced by a pathway that contains the modifiable element.

As an example of such an approach, we first analyzed the plasticity of the red nucleus (RN) in cat brain and found that corticorubral synapses from the cerebral cortex onto the red nucleus have remarkable plasticity; that is, sprouting and the formation of new functional synapses occur under several circumstances.

Then we tried to use this sprouting synapse as a modifiable element and attempted to reconstruct classical conditioning. We could reproduce classical conditioning by using corticorubral fiber stimulation as a conditioned stimulus (CS) and forelimb electric shock as an unconditioned stimulus (US). By training the cat with CS–US pairing, it was possible to induce classical conditioning in these monosynaptic corticorubral synapses. In this situation, we can analyze the primary site at which the conditional change takes place, since it is both monosynaptic and modifiable. Indeed, it turned out that the primary site was the corticorubral synapse.

SPROUTING OF CORTICORUBRAL SYNAPSES

Lesion-Induced Sprouting of Excitatory Corticorubral Synapses

It was already known in the 1950s that collateral sprouting of intact motor nerve fibers in the peripheral nervous system results in the reinnervation of muscles after partial transection of the motor nerve. The experimental evidence for sprouting in the brain is mostly of recent origin. Raisman (1969) has shown, using electron microscopy, that new synapses are formed by sprouting of fibers in the rat brain. Now there is a growing list of investigations dealing with the formation of new synapses by sprouting of fibers, and it is clear that the phenomenon is widespread (Cotman et al., 1981; Tsukahara, 1981).

The large size and ease of identification, together with the unique synaptic organization of the RN, make it a particularly favorable target for the electro-physiological investigation of synaptic plasticity. Of particular importance is the discrete segregation of the two major synaptic inputs: those from the nucleus interpositus (IP) of the cerebellum that terminate on the somatic portions of the cell membranes, and those from the cerebral cortex that form synapses on the distal dendrites.

Stimulation of the two excitatory inputs to an RN neuron produces monosynaptic excitatory postsynaptic potentials (EPSPs) of a different time course, as shown in Figure 1A. Stimulation of the IP produces fast-rising EPSPs, whereas stimulation of the efferent fibers of cerebral cortical neurons at the level of the cerebral peduncle (CP) produces slow-rising EPSPs. Also, it has been shown that the EPSPs induced from the CP are less sensitive to membrane potential displacement than are those induced from the IP (not illustrated). These phenomena have been interpreted as supporting a qualitative difference between synaptic sites on the somatic and dendritic membranes of RN cells, a view that is supported by electron microscope evidence (Nakamura et al., 1974; Murakami et al., 1982).

Our question is whether the corticorubral fibers sprout when one of the inputs—IP, for example—is destroyed. If sprouting takes place onto the proximal portion of the somatodendritic membrane, then we can expect that the time course of the corticorubral EPSPs might change as a result of the smaller electrotonic distance. In this case, one would expect a fast-rising EPSP superimposed on the preexisting slow-rising corticorubral EPSPs. This is indeed the case (see Figure 1). The data shown in the figure were taken to indicate that new, functionally active synapses are formed at the proximal portion of the somatodendritic membrane of the RN cells. It should be noted that a change in the cable properties

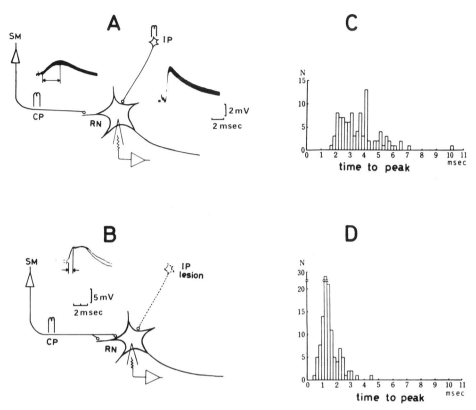

Figure 1. *Lesion-induced sprouting in the adult feline red nucleus (RN). A:* Synaptic organization of the normal RN. Monosynaptic excitatory input from the ipsilateral sensorimotor cortex (SM) through the cerebral peduncle (CP) impinges on the distal dendrites and that from the contralateral nucleus interpositus (IP) of the cerebellum on the soma. Stimulation of CP produces a slow-rising excitatory postsynaptic potential (EPSP) in an RN cell and stimulation of IP produces a fast-rising EPSP, as shown in the *insets. B:* After IP lesion, a fast-rising component appears superimposed on the slow-rising CP EPSPs, as shown in the *inset. C:* Frequency distribution histogram of the time-to-peak values of the CP EPSPs of normal cats, measured as in the *inset* in *A. D:* Frequency distribution histogram of the time-to-peak values of CP EPSPs of cats with chronic IP lesions, measured as in the *inset* in *B.* Note that the time-to-peak values are shorter in *D* than they are in *C.* (Modified from Tsukahara et al., 1975b.)

of RN neurons after IP lesions accounts for less than 5% of the observed time-to-peak change in corticorubral EPSPs.

Rall's (1964) theoretical analysis of the shape of EPSPs predicts that the EPSPs produced by proximal synapses are larger in amplitude and shorter in rise time than those of distal ones. Are the newly appeared corticorubral EPSPs consistent with this prediction? We analyzed the unitary EPSPs and found that the relation of the time to peak and the amplitude of the corticorubral unitary EPSPs before and after chronic lesions of IP can be fitted to the theoretical calculation derived from Rall's compartment model (Figure 2B). The time course of the theoretical EPSPs generated at each of five compartments is illustrated in Figure 2D. The theoretical relation between time to peak and amplitude is shown by the dotted

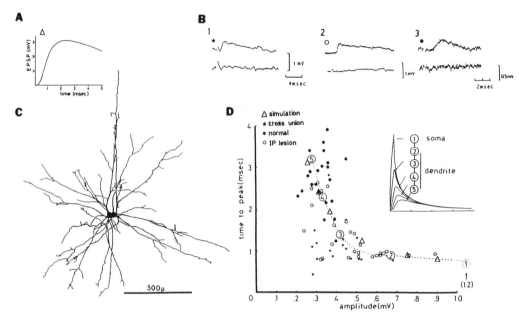

Figure 2. *Corticorubral unitary EPSPs and theoretical EPSPs based on a neuronal model. A: A theoretical EPSP calculated with the Butz and Cowan theorem, based on the morphology shown in C. Ordinate, amplitude in millivolts; abscissa, time in milliseconds. B1: Intracellular EPSP evoked by stimulation of CP in an RN cell of a cross-innervated cat. B2: Intracellular EPSP evoked by stimulation of the SM in a cat with a lesion of the IP 27 days before acute experiment. B3: Same as B1, but in a normal cat. B1–B3: Upper traces, intracellular potentials; lower traces, extracellular field potential corresponding to the upper traces. C: Three-dimensional reconstruction of a horse-radish peroxidase (HRP)-filled RN neuron. D: Relation between the time to peak and amplitude of unitary EPSPs. Open circles, unitary EPSPs of IP-lesioned cats; asterisks, those of cross-innervated cats more than two months before recording; closed circles, those of normal cats; circled numbers, time to peak and amplitude of theoretical EPSPs derived from Rall's compartment model, initiated at each compartment of a five-compartment chain. The time course of the theoretical EPSPs generated in the compartments is shown in the inset of the figure. Triangles represent theoretical EPSPs partly shown in A, calculated by using the Butz and Cowan theorem and the morphological parameters of the RN neuron shown in C.*

curve. The experimental data are well fitted to this curve and the points derived from normal cats are concentrated in the distal compartment, whereas those from cats with lesions of the IP are scattered in all compartments. It is likely that new synapses are formed at the proximal compartments.

Recently, Kawato et al. (1984) extended this analysis by using measured parameters obtained from the three-dimensional reconstruction of the geometry of horseradish peroxidase (HRP)-filled RN cells. Electrical parameters were also obtained by electrophysiological measurements. First, HRP was injected into electrophysiologically identified RN neurons of adult cats, as has been described by Murakami et al. (1982). After processing, the three-dimensional morphology of an RN cell was reconstructed by using serial sections (Figure 2C). After determining the overall branching structure, the diameter of each dendritic segment was determined and the dendritic tree was approximated by a series of cylindrical segments (179 cylinders for cell A and 79 cylinders for cell B). Each segment whose diameter did not change by more than 20% was described as an equivalent cylinder of length l and an average diameter of d. The soma of the RN cells was described as a spheroid. In a previous report on RN cells, the average input resistance and membrane time constant were 2.5 MΩ and 5.6 msec (Tsukahara et al., 1975a), respectively. We used the electrical parameters of specific membrane resistance, $R_M = 2800\ \Omega\text{cm}^2$ and $C_M = 2\ \mu\text{F/cm}^2$, and of specific axoplasmic resistance, $R_I = 50\ \Omega\text{cm}$, so that after numerical calculation, the input resistance and membrane time constant calculated by a series of cylinders, each based on the morphology, matched the electrophysiological data.

Butz and Cowan (1974) developed a graphical calculus that can be used to generate analytical solutions to the Laplace transform of functions representing the voltage transient at any point along the dendritic tree of neurons. It can be applied for arbitrary dendritic geometries responding to current inputs at any point. By using the fast inversion of the Laplace transform (FILT) algorithm (Hosono, 1981) for numerical inversion of the Laplace transform to obtain the voltage transient as a function of time, and by devising another algorithm that numerically calculates the solution of the Butz and Cowan theorem by a recurrence formula, we could calculate the theoretical EPSPs (Figure 2D). Kawato et al. (1984) calculated the unitary EPSP produced by a synapse situated directly on the soma of cell A. The α-function, $g(t) = c\alpha^2(t/\tau_m)\exp(-\alpha t/\tau_m)$, was chosen as a time-varying synaptic conductance. The amplitude and the duration of the synaptic conductance can be adjusted by varying c and α and can be determined experimentally by observing the corticorubral unitary EPSP. The maximal values of the synaptic conductance and peak time were estimated as 43 nS and 0.3 msec, respectively, and it was at these values that the observed amplitude (0.9 mV) and the time to peak (0.9 msec) were reproduced best.

The triangles in Figure 2D show the calculated unitary EPSPs that were produced by the conductances estimated above at different locations directly on the dendritic shafts. As can be seen, the electrophysiological data and the simulated results are in good agreement for an overall range of amplitudes and time to peak of the EPSPs, although we used the same synaptic conductance. This fact validates the use of this estimated synaptic conductance for all corticorubral synapses without regard to their location on the somadendritic membrane.

How fast does sprouting occur? This is an important question, because in order to correlate the sprouting phenomenon with learning behavior, it is necessary to have some idea of the time course of the development of sprouting. The time course of development of the newly formed corticorubral synapses, as investigated in the time to peak changes of CP EPSPs, is illustrated in Figure 3. Here, the relationship between the average time to peak of the corticorubral EPSPs and the number of days after lesions of the IP for each experimental animal are shown. Four days after lesion of the IP, there is already a significant shortening of the time to peak. After 10 days, the shortening reaches its maximum.

Are there any morphological correlates for these physiological findings? Electron microscope studies (Nakamura et al., 1974; Murakami et al., 1982) provide evidence in support of the physiological outcome of sprouting. Previous electron microscope studies of the RN were not able to survey the whole neuronal surface because of the extended nature of the dendritic trees of these neurons. However, intra-

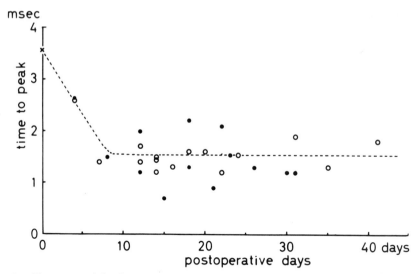

Figure 3.   *Time course of the change in the rise time of the CP EPSPs after IP lesion. Ordinate,* time to
peak of the CP EPSPs; *abscissa,* days after IP lesion; *open circles,* the mean time to peak of the
CP EPSPs of more than six RN cells; *filled circles,* the mean time to peak of the CP EPSPs of
two to five RN cells. Each point represents data from one cat. The "x" indicates the mean time
to peak of the CP EPSPs of 100 RN cells in normal cats. (From Tsukahara et al., 1975b.)

cellular HRP injection with microelectrodes has now made it possible to survey
entire labeled neurons with the electron microscope. This technique, which
involves degeneration of the presynaptic terminals, has enabled us to locate the
sites of termination of the two major inputs to the RN: those from the cerebral
cortex and those from the IP of the cerebellum.

Quantitative measurement of the dendritic tree by a computer-assisted image-
processing system developed in our laboratory revealed that the diameters of
dendritic branches decrease monotonically. Therefore, it is possible to estimate
the position of synapses on RN cell dendrites by measuring the minor diameter
of cross sections of dendritic branches in electron micrographs of HRP-filled
RN cells. Furthermore, corticorubral synapses can be distinguished by the degeneration of their terminals after lesions of the cerebral sensorimotor cortex
(Figure 4A, B).

Degenerating terminal boutons resulting from the destruction of the sensorimotor cortex were found mainly on dendritic branches with small diameters,
that is, 1–4 μm. Figure 4C and D shows the frequency distribution of the cross
section when the shape of the cross section was not round. These histological
findings support the results of the electrophysiological studies discussed above.
They show that cerebral inputs terminate on the distal dendrites of RN neurons,
whereas inputs from the IP terminate on the soma.

Murakami et al. (1982) studied the location of degenerating terminals of corticorubral fibers on the dendritic surfaces of RN cells that were stained by intracellular injection of HRP. These terminals end on dendrites with diameters
of 1–4 μm (Figure 4A, C). Degenerated corticorubral terminals were also studied

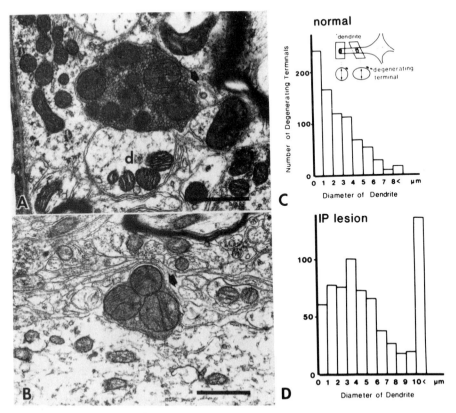

Figure 4.   *Degenerating corticorubral terminals. A:* Normal cat; an electron-dense degenerating terminal
(*arrow*) making synaptic contact with a dendrite (d) of small cross section. Synaptic vesicles are
recognizable. *B:* Cat with IP lesion; a degenerating terminal (*arrow*) in synaptic contact with a
large dendritic profile. *C* and *D:* Frequency distribution of the dendritic diameters in which
degenerating terminals of corticorubral synapses were found. *C:* Normal cat. *D:* Cats with
chronic destruction of the IP. *Ordinate,* number of degenerating presynaptic terminals; *abscissa,*
minor diameters of dendrites on which the corticorubral degenerating terminals were found.
Calibration bars in *A* and *B* = 1 μm. (Modified from Murakami et al., 1982.)

in cats in which the IP had been destroyed about three months previously. In
these animals, in accordance with the physiological findings, the cerebral synapses
were found to terminate not only on the distal dendrites but also on the proximal
dendrites and on the somatic portion of the RN cells (Figure 4B, D).

Lesion-Induced Sprouting of Inhibitory Synapses

RN neurons are disynaptically inhibited by collaterals of fast-conducting pyramidal
tract fibers (Tsukahara et al., 1968), in addition to being excited monosynaptically
by slow-conducting pyramidal tract and corticorubral fibers. The transmitter
mediating the inhibition seems to be γ-aminobutyric acid (GABA). GABA hyperpolarizes the RN cell membrane and is associated with a conductance increase
when tested in an *in vitro* slice preparation (Sakaguchi et al., 1984). GABA release

from such a preparation has been demonstrated (Kubota et al., 1983). The existence of glutamic acid decarboxylase (GAD) in the RN region also has been shown (Nieoullon and Dusticier, 1981), and Murakami et al. (1983) demonstrated GABAergic synapses on RN cells by using immunohistochemistry of GAD combined with intracellular injection of HRP. GAD-immunoreactive axon terminals outline the somata and large dendrites of RN cells. Furthermore, Katsumaru et al. (1984) have shown that small GAD-immunoreactive neurons with a major

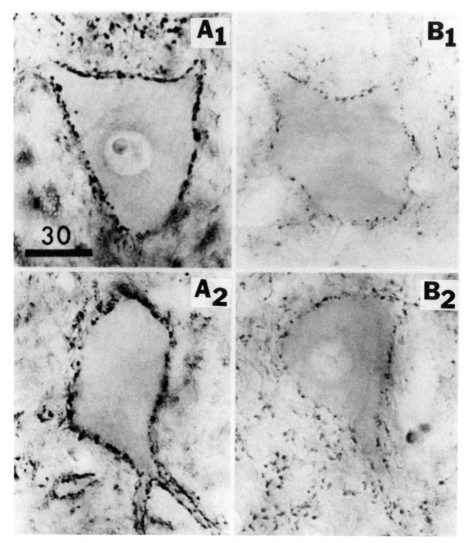

Figure 5.   *Photomicrographs of RN neurons surrounded by GAD-immunoreactive puncta in 100-μm-thick sections obtained from one animal. A_1 and A_2:* Experimental side (contralateral to the IP lesion side). *B_1 and B_2:* Control side. RN neurons on the experimental side are surrounded by intensely stained puncta or by strings of puncta that are laid one upon another. *Calibration bar = 30* μm. (From Katsumaru et al., 1985.)

diameter of 16 μm were observed under both light and electron microscopy to be uniformly distributed throughout the RN. They were considered to be inhibitory interneurons, since they receive afferent fibers from the cerebral sensorimotor cortex. The existence of such interneurons was expected from the presence of disynaptic inhibition on RN cells, preceded by the activation of fast-conducting pyramidal tract fibers.

Whether the GABAergic inhibitory axon terminals also undergo modification after lesions of the IP can be answered by observing the number of GAD-positive terminals on RN neurons. A possible change in the GAD-positive terminals was tested in kitten RN after lesions of the IP, and the results show a marked increase (100%) in GAD-positive terminals on the somata of the RN neurons (Figure 5). This suggests that sprouting of the inhibitory synapses also takes place, although the possibility that an increase in GAD production did take place without any morphological change cannot be completely excluded.

SPROUTING OF NORMAL CENTRAL NEURONS

Although much evidence has been provided to show that sprouting can and does take place after denervation in the mammalian central nervous system, we still have little idea of what triggers this process. For example, does the presence of degenerating fibers initiate sprouting? In this context, we might ask to what extent sprouting occurs in circumstances other than denervation.

Published attempts to use controlled cross-innervation of peripheral nerves to investigate central reorganization are quite old. Sperry (1947) investigated the functional compensation of movement disorders that followed cross-innervation of nerves innervating flexor and extensor muscles in various species of mammals. He found that motor relearning occurs in monkeys, and that the reversed action is inhibited while new, correct, and smoothly coordinated movements are learned. Eccles et al. (1962) investigated possible changes in the synaptic connections of spinal motoneurons after cross-innervation of the flexor and extensor nerves of the hindlimbs in the cat. Although they found evidence that new synapses formed on motoneurons after cross-innervation, it was restricted to the groups of motoneurons whose axons had been severed. Thus the extent of the reorganization was very limited. Subsequently, motivated by these experiments, we performed cross-innervation experiments in cats to determine whether synaptic reorganization occurred at the supraspinal level. The corticorubrospinal system is one of the major motor outflows from the cerebrum to the spinal cord. Therefore, if synaptic reorganization at the supraspinal level should occur, the corticorubrospinal system might well be affected. If so, it should be possible to detect the changes by using techniques similar to those described previously.

For cross-innervation of the forelimb nerves, the musculocutaneous, median, radial, and ulnar nerves were cut at the axillary region, and the central stumps of the radial nerves were united with the peripheral stumps of the musculocutaneous, median, and ulnar nerves by suturing the nerve sheaths. A similar procedure was applied to the peripheral stumps of the radial nerve; those stumps were united with the central stumps of the musculocutaneous, median, and ulnar nerves.

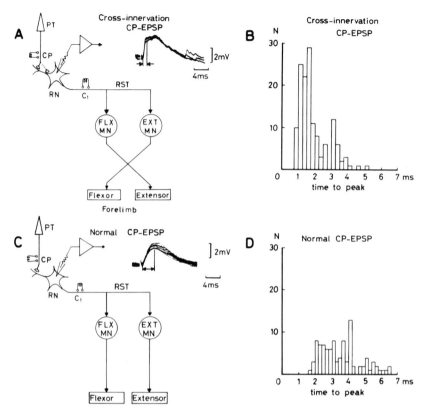

Figure 6. *Corticorubral EPSPs in cross-innervated cats.* A: Traces show intracellular responses of an
RN neuron from a cross-innervated cat 176 days before acute experiment. C: Traces show
intracellular responses of an RN cell in a normal cat. The diagrams in *A* and *C* illustrate the
experimental arrangements. C_1, spinal segment; EXT MN, extensor motoneuron; FLX MN,
flexor motoneuron; PT, pyramidal tract cell; RST, rubrospinal tract. B: The frequency distribution
of the time to peak of CP EPSPs in cross-innervated cats. The number of cells employed is
shown on the *ordinate*; the time to peak of CP EPSPs in milliseconds is shown on the *abscissa*.
D: Same as B, but of CP EPSPs in normal cats.

These studies (Fujito et al., 1982; Tsukahara et al., 1982) showed that two to
six months after cross-innervation, the rising time of the corticorubral EPSPs
induced by stimulating the CP became shorter than those in normal cats. A
typical slow EPSP evoked by stimulating the CP in a normal cat is illustrated in
Figure 6C. In contrast, the EPSPs shown in Figure 6A are from a cat with cross-
innervation of the forelimb nerves. Recordings are from cells innervating the
upper spinal segments (C cells). The EPSPs had a much faster rising time course
than those in normal cats. In these experiments, C cells were identified by the
antidromic excitation produced by stimulating the C_1 spinal segment. The frequency
distribution of the time to peak of the CP EPSPs in cross-innervated cats is
shown in Figure 6B. The mean time to peak of CP EPSPs of C cells in cats cross-
innervated more than two months previously (1.9 + 0.9 msec; n = 160) was
significantly shorter than that of the normal cats (3.6 + 1.4 msec; n = 100). The
slower time to peak in C cells was also found when recordings were performed

less than two months after cross-innervation. Therefore, the data indicate that the EPSPs of RN cells in the normal cat had a much slower rise time than those of C cells in cross-innervated cats (Figure 6D).

A fast-rising component appeared in the corticorubral unitary EPSPs of the cross-innervated cats. This was not accompanied by an appreciable change in the dendritic cable properties of the RN neurons, and there was no change in the number of synapses of the interpositorubral terminals, as estimated physiologically (Fujito et al., 1982). By analogy with the previous experiments, these findings all suggest that new synapses had been formed on the proximal portions of the somatodendritic membrane of the RN cells by corticorubral fibers that

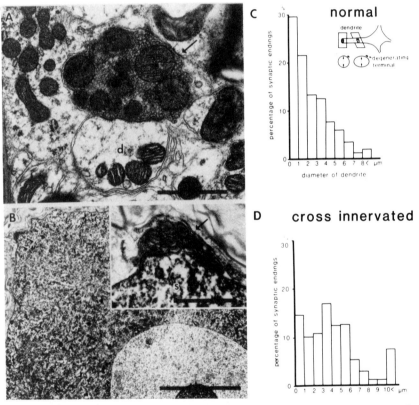

Figure 7. *Morphological evidence of sprouting of corticorubral synapses in cats with cross-innervation of the peripheral flexor and extensor nerves. A and B*: Corticorubral axon terminals synapsing upon a dendrite (*A*) and a soma (*B*) of an HRP-filled RN neuron in a normal animal (*A*) and in a cat with cross-innervation of the peripheral flexor and extensor nerves (*B*). Degenerating terminals are indicated by *arrows*. d, dendrite; s, soma. *Calibration bars* = 1 μm. *C and D*: Histograms illustrating the relation between the number of degenerating corticorubral terminals and the diameter of dendrites. *C*: The distribution of degenerating terminals in normal cats. *Ordinate*, the number of degenerating synaptic endings, as expressed by the percentage of terminals; *abscissa*, the minor diameter of dendrites contacted by the degenerating terminals; the measurements were taken from electron micrographs. *D*: Similar distribution of degenerating terminals found in cats with cross-innervation. (From Murakami et al., 1984.)

normally terminate on the distal dendrites. It appears, therefore, that sprouting can occur in central neurons without direct lesions of synaptic inputs.

In order to correlate these physiological findings with electron microscope data, we developed a computer system that enabled us to measure dendritic diameters along the center line of a dendritic tree as a function of distance from the somatic center. It was found that in both normal and cross-innervated cats, dendritic diameters of RN cells decrease monotonically as the distance from the somatic center increases. Based on this measurement, it is possible to estimate the location of synapses on dendrites of an RN cell by measuring the smallest diameter of the dendritic cross section in electron micrographs of HRP-filled RN cells. Additional corticorubral synapses can be identified by the presence of degenerating terminals after lesions of the sensorimotor cortex.

Degenerating terminals in normal cats are found mainly on dendrites with small diameters (Figure 7A, C). On the other hand, degenerating terminals in cats with cross-innervation are found on the distal dendrites, the proximal dendrites, and the soma (Figure 7B, D) (Murakami et al., 1984). This is consistent with physiological findings and supports the formation of new synapses on the proximal portion of the RN cell membrane. There is no damage of the direct synaptic input to RN cells after cross-innervation, so this result represents one of a few examples of sprouting of intact central neurons.

LONG-TERM POTENTIATION OF THE CORTICORUBRAL SYNAPSES

In addition to the sprouting phenomenon, the corticorubral input is characterized by another aspect of synaptic plasticity, long-term potentiation. It has been reported that the corticorubral input is characterized by short-term plasticity of its synaptic transmission, such as paired pulse potentiation (Tsukahara and Kosaka, 1968) and posttetanic potentiation (Murakami et al., 1977). Recently, we tested long-term effects in corticorubral synaptic transmission.

Figure 8 illustrates an example of *in vivo* experiments. In order to facilitate the recording of field potentials resulting from corticorubral synaptic activation, corticorubral sprouting was induced by lesions of the IP of the cerebellum in the kitten. The amplitude of the field potentials that represent the corticorubral synaptic currents was measured before and after tetanic stimulation of the CP. It was noted that after tetanic stimulation of the CP with 100 Hz for 3 min, there was an increase of the amplitude of the field potentials lasting for an hour or so. This increase of corticorubral synaptic transmission could also be noted in the corticorubral EPSPs (Figure 8). However, with lower tetanic frequencies, the potentiation tended to be much smaller or even absent. It is likely that corticorubral synaptic transmission is characterized by long-term potentiation.

FROM SYNAPTIC PLASTICITY TO LEARNING BEHAVIOR

A large body of studies has dealt with the neuronal correlates of classical conditioning. In the mammalian central nervous system, it is not easy to distinguish local neuronal changes at the site of the recording from those occurring at distant

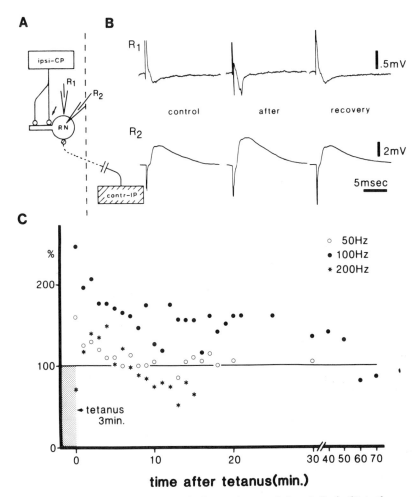

Figure 8. *Long-term potentiation of corticorubral synaptic transmission. A*: To facilitate the recording of field potentials resulting from corticorubral synaptic transmission, corticorubral sprouting was induced by lesion of the IP. contr-IP, contralateral nucleus interpositus; ipsi-CP, ipsilateral cerebral peduncle. *B*: Specimen records of field potentials and intracellular corticorubral EPSPs before, just after tetanic stimulation, and 50 min after tetanic stimulation. R_1, extracellular microelectrode; R_2, intracellular microelectrode. *C*: Amplitude of the field potentials (*ordinate*) is plotted against time after tetanic stimulation for 3 min (*abscissa*). *Filled circles*, data after tetanic stimulation at 100 Hz. *Open circles*, data after tetanic stimulation of 50 Hz. *Asterisks*, data after tetanic stimulation at 200 Hz. (Modified from Kosar et al., 1985.)

sites. One strategy for isolating the primary site of change is to simplify afferent pathways for the conditioned responses. Hitherto, the mammalian RN has been used to investigate neuronal plasticity such as sprouting. In an extension of these studies, an attempt was made to use the plasticity of corticorubral synapses as a modifiable element in the reconstruction of a simplified learning paradigm. There are experiments indicating that midbrain structures play an important role in the conditioned avoidance response. Smith (1970) has reported that rubral lesions abolished the conditioned forelimb flexion responses paired by tone as CS and forelimb electric shock as US.

A classical conditioning paradigm was therefore used in our study. Our question was whether known synaptic plasticity such as sprouting constitutes a neuronal basis for classical conditioning. In order to facilitate the identification of the primary site of conditioning, the CS was delivered to the left CP as an electric shock. Furthermore, the cortical outflow was restricted mainly to the corticorubral fibers by lesions of corticofugal fibers below the level of the RN. This procedure eliminates the contribution of the pyramidal tract, as well as the corticoponto-cerebellar fibers and some other corticobulbar fibers in this reflex. The CS was the electric pulse train to the CP, and forelimb electric shock was used as the US (Figure 9A). It was found that after pairing the CS–US in close temporal association, initially ineffective stimulus intensities of CS gave rise to flexion of the contralateral forelimb (Figure 9B).

Cats were mounted on a frame using bags with holes from which their heads and right forelimbs protruded. The shoulder was fixed to the frame to maintain the forelimb at the predetermined resting position. The movement of the elbow joint was measured by a potentiometer attached to the joint. Electromyograms of the biceps brachi muscle and the triceps brachi muscle were recorded.

A series of stimuli was given daily during the training session. The CS was a train of five pulses with 2-msec intervals. The US was an electric shock and was preceded by the CS by 60–200 msec, but most frequently by 100 msec. CS–US pairing of 120 trials with an interval of 30 sec constituted the training of the day. Once every five trials only the CS was given. The ratio of positive responses of 24 such trials without the US gives the score of performance for the day. The extinction procedure was CS alone, or reversing the sequence of stimulus to US–CS. At the end of the training session, the flexion responses were tested by changing the stimulus intensities for CS, and the relation between the score of performance and the applied current was determined.

After training, the score of performance gradually increased, and after about one week the score attained a plateau. Figure 9B shows the mechanogram of elbow flexion on the first and seventh days of training. CS (S_1) is the stimulus to the CP and US (S_2) is the stimulus to the forearm. On the first day, the CS alone produced no response. After the seventh day, the CS produced elbow flexion.

Figure 9C shows the time course of the acquisition and extinction of conditioned responses. The performance score increased gradually, attaining a plateau after about one week. In parallel to the increase in the performance score, the minimum current intensity necessary for producing 100% performance (100% performance current) decreased. After establishing the conditioned responses by CS–US pairing, backward pairing was used to extinguish the conditioned responses, as shown in Figure 9C. Random control experiments were also performed in two cats, and the results are illustrated in Figure 10. The CS presented at regular intervals of 30 sec was followed by the US presented randomly, as determined by the microcomputer-controlled stimulating system. With this mode of stimulation, neither the score of performance nor the 100% performance current changed appreciably with training. In a third cat, the US was presented by itself for 10 days. In this case, the 100% performance current did not show any appreciable

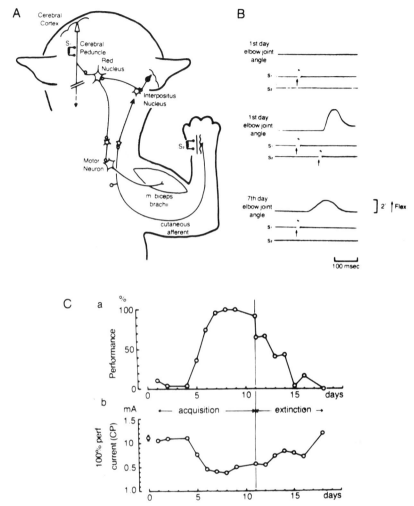

Figure 9. *Associative learning mediated by the RN. A*: Arrangement of the experimental setup. S₁, conditioned stimulus (CS); S₂, unconditioned stimulus (US). *B*: Specimen record of elbow flexion on the first day (*top traces*) and seven days (*bottom trace*) after conditioning. *Arrows* indicate the onset of the stimulus. *C*: The change in performance (*a*) and change in minimum current necessary for eliciting 100% performance (100% performance current) during forward and backward pairing (*b; ordinates*). *Abscissae*, days after the onset of training; CS–US interval of 100 msec. After the 11th day, the stimulus sequence was reversed to US–CS, with an interval of 900 msec. (Modified from Tsukahara et al., 1981.)

change. Therefore, it seems likely that the behavioral modification can be considered an example of classical conditioning.

The pathway mediating the conditioned response in this experimental paradigm is considered to be relatively simple in view of the fact that corticofugal fibers are surgically eliminated just caudal to the RN and also because the CS electrodes were implanted within the CP, which contains corticorubral fibers that are presynaptic to the cells in the RN.

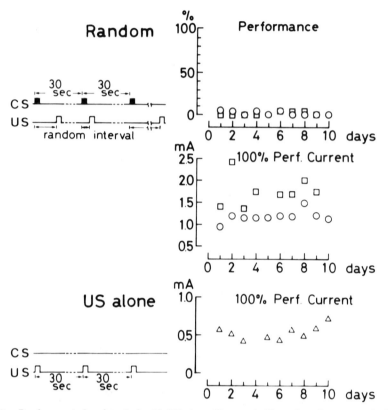

Figure 10. *Random control and control with US alone. Top graph*: Plot of random control. *Ordinate,* performance scores from random control experiments with two cats, using the stimulus parameters shown at the *top left; abscissa,* days after CS–US pairing with random intervals. *Open circles* and *open squares* represent each animal's performance. *Middle graph*: Plot of random control. *Ordinate,* 100% performance current in the same cats as in the *upper graph* (symbols as before); *abscissa,* days after CS–US pairing with random intervals. *Bottom graph*: Plot of conditioning US alone. *Ordinate,* 100% performance current; *abscissa,* days after onset of conditioning with US alone.

The latency of electrical activity elicited in the biceps muscle in response to the CS also supports this view; the shortest latency recorded in the electromyograms from the biceps brachi muscle was 8 msec, which is in accord with the shortest time required for the transmission of impulses along the corticorubrospinal pathway to the muscle. Therefore, it is likely that the conditioned responses are mediated by the corticorubrospinal system.

The primary site of the neuronal change in this pathway was tested. The RN cells receive another excitatory input from the IP of the cerebellum. Therefore, if the primary sites of the neuronal change are below the RN, we should be able to see an increase in the score of performance by stimulating the IP or a decrease in current intensity to maintain the same score of performance. This possibility was tested, and the results are summarized in Figure 11. There is no appreciable decrease in current intensities for eliciting the same score of performance by stimulating the IP, although the conditioned responses were already established by the stimulation of the CP. This result indicates that the site of neuronal change is not situated below the RN. It is also unlikely that the general excitability of RN neurons has been changed by conditioning. Therefore, the most likely site is the corticorubral synapses, which as we already know, are characterized by prominent plasticity.

ANALYSIS OF MODIFICATION OF THE CORTICORUBRAL SYNAPSES FOLLOWING CONDITIONING

The next question is whether transmission through the corticorubral synapses was indeed facilitated after conditioning. We tested this by counting the extracellular unitary spikes of RN cells in awake conditioned cats. Figure 12 shows a comparison of the firing probability of RN neurons to the same CS before and after establishment of the conditioned reflex. The firing probability, as measured by the number of spikes fired in response to the stimuli applied to the CP, increased in some RN neurons after conditioning (Oda et al., 1981). This result is consistent with the interpretation suggested by the behavioral experiment mentioned earlier that transmission through the corticorubral pathway increases after conditioning.

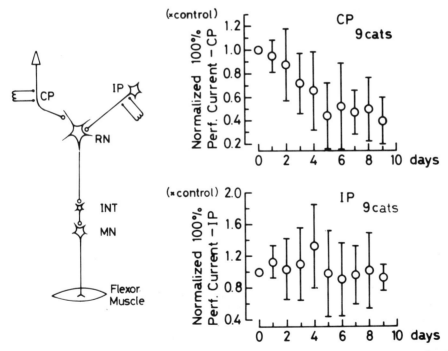

Figure 11. *Diagram of the primary site of conditioned changes (left).* INT, interneurons interpolated in the rubrospinal system; MN, flexor motoneurons. *Top graph:* Current intensity producing 100% performance to CS. *Bottom graph:* Current intensity producing 100% performance by stimulating IP with the same train of impulses in the same cats used for the experiments illustrated by the *top graph. Ordinates,* 100% performance current; *abscissae,* days after the onset of presentation of CS to the CP, and of US to the skin of the forelimb. Mean data from nine animals ± SDM.

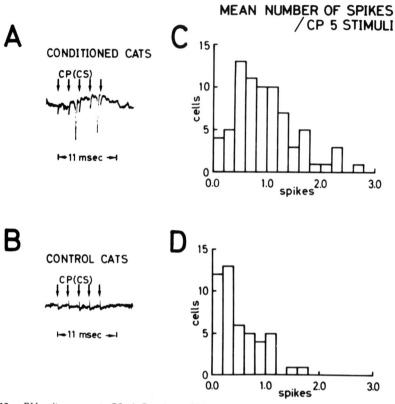

Figure 12. *RN unit response to CS. A:* Specimen RN unit responses in a conditioned cat on the ninth
day after conditioning. CS consisting of five impulses (marked by *arrows*) was delivered to the
CP. *B:* No spike response in a control cat, in which the conditioned response was extinguished
by presenting the CS alone for six days. *C and D:* Histograms of the number of spikes induced
in each RN unit by CS in a conditioned and a control cat, respectively. *C: Abscissa,* mean number
of spikes induced in each RN unit by CS. *D: Abscissa,* mean number of spikes during the initial
11 msec after onset of the CS in each unit. *Ordinates,* number of RN cells. (From Oda et al.,
1981.)

There still remains a question of whether the sprouting of corticorubral fibers
is the anatomical basis for observed conditioned responses. If the sprouting is
really the cause, then one would expect to see changes in corticorubral EPSPs
after the establishment of the conditioned reflex that are similar to changes
observed after lesions of the IP, or after cross-innervation. We tested this by
intracellular recording from RN neurons in conditioned as well as in control
cats. It was found that after the establishment of the conditioned reflex, a new
fast-rising component appears in the corticorubral dendritic EPSPs (Tsukahara
and Oda, 1981).

The training procedures used in our experiments were the same as before.
Control cats had corticofugal lesions like the conditioned animals, but were not
subjected to any training regime. As shown in Figure 13A, in conditioned animals,
a fast-rising component is superimposed on the slow-rising dendritic CP EPSPs.
A similar fast-rising component is also evident in EPSPs induced by stimulating

the sensorimotor cortex, as shown in Figure 13B. In contrast, the CP EPSP shown in Figure 13C from a nonstimulated control cat shows only a slow-rising time course, as is seen in normal unlesioned cats (Figure 13D). The time to peak of the CP EPSPs was measured in both conditioned and control cats, and the frequency distributions of the time to peak are illustrated in Figure 13E and F. Data are from anesthetized animals. If dual peaks occurred, the first peak was measured to determine the time to peak of the EPSPs. The time to peak of CP EPSPs in conditioned cats appears shorter than that of control, nonstimulated cats, which according to our test was significant statistically ($p = 0.01$). In Figure 13G, the frequency distribution of the CP EPSPs in normal unlesioned cats from our previous experiments (Tsukahara et al., 1975b) is illustrated. It should be noted that in some nonstimulated, peduncular-lesioned cats, the time to peak of the CP EPSPs is faster than that in the unlesioned control cats.

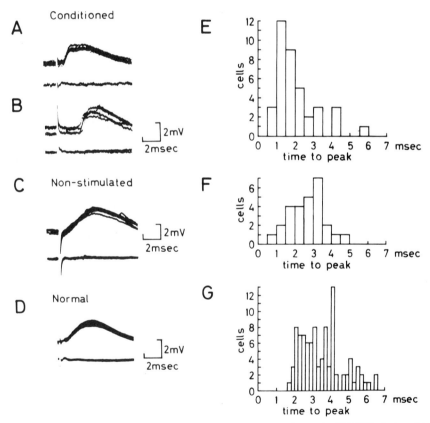

Figure 13. *Corticorubral EPSPs from conditioned and nonconditioned cats. A*: CP EPSPs induced in RN cell after the eighth day of conditioning, when conditioning is fully established. *B*: Same cell, but an EPSP induced by stimulating the SM. *C*: CP EPSPs induced in an RN cell in a nonconditioned control cat. *D*: CP EPSPs induced in an RN cell in a normal cat. *Upper traces,* intracellular potentials; *lower traces,* extracellular records corresponding to the *upper traces*. Time and voltage calibration of *B–D* also applies to *A. E* and *F*: Frequency distribution of the time to peak of CP EPSPs in conditioned (*E*) and nonconditioned (*F*) cats. *G*: The same histogram, but of the CP EPSPs of normal cats. The number of cells is shown on the *ordinates* and the time to peak of CP EPSPs, recorded in milliseconds, on the *abscissae*. (From Tsukahara and Oda, 1981.)

The most likely interpretation of these results seems to be that, by analogy with the previous experiments using IP lesions or cross-innervation, the corticorubral fibers sprout after conditioning to form new functional synapses on the proximal portion of the somatodendritic membrane of RN cells. However, another possibility exists. For example, shortening of the spine where corticorubral terminals are located could be possible, since this might result in shortening of the electrotonic length of transmission of corticorubral synaptic currents, as recorded from the RN cell soma. We calculated the effect of morphological changes in spines on the postsynaptic potential by using the Butz and Cowan theorem in the following way. At the beginning of this chapter, we described the calculation of theoretical EPSPs based on the three-dimensional reconstruction of HRP-filled RN cells. Kawato et al. (1984) calculated the EPSPs caused by the activity of a single synapse on a dendritic spine in cell A, for which we have a detailed knowledge of branching patterns and electric properties. Each spine was modeled as a narrow thin cylinder, called a spine stalk, with a spine head of a fixed surface area of $1 \ \mu m^2$. Three spine stalks of different lengths (ls) and different diameters (ds) were chosen: (1) $ls = 0.5 \ \mu m$ and $ds = 0.2 \ \mu m$; (2) $ls = 1 \ \mu m$ and $ds = 0.1 \ \mu m$; and (3) $ls = 2 \ \mu m$ and $ds = 0.05 \ \mu m$.

Figure 14A and B shows the theoretical EPSPs recorded at the soma by this spine synapse. Morphological changes in the spine were simulated by "spines" 3, 2, and 1. The spine was assumed to change its shape from spine 3 to spine 1, and finally to the shaft synapse, where the synapse attaches directly to the dendritic shaft. Although the amplitudes of the EPSPs were increased by this morphological change, the time to peak of these theoretical EPSPs remained more or less the same. The difference in the amplitudes and the time to peak values is accounted for by the fact that the amplitude of the synaptic current was reduced because of the nonlinearity introduced by the reversal potential, while the cable properties of the spines essentially remained unaffected, as we have theoretically shown (Kawato and Tsukahara, 1983, 1984). Based on the calculations shown in Figure 14, it is clear that even if a morphological change in the spine does take place, this cannot account for the changing time course of corticorubral EPSPs after the establishment of conditioning.

A possible explanation for the increased transmission of corticorubral synapses that takes place after the establishment of conditioning is increases in postsynaptic potentials because of prolonged increases in synaptic transmission such as long-term potentiation. The presence of long-term potentiation in corticorubral synaptic transmission invites speculation on its role in the initial phase of conditioning. Recent studies by McNaughton et al. (1978) and Levy and Steward (1979) suggest that it is indeed possible to demonstrate heterosynaptic enhancement of one input by conjunctive stimulation of two inputs, similar to associative learning. Moreover, a recent study by Parnas et al. (1984) on the lobster neuromuscular junction indicates that several days before sprouting produced by lesion of neighboring axons, enhancement of synaptic transmission takes place. It seems likely that sprouting and the enhancement of synaptic transmission are coupled in some way. Therefore, it is not unreasonable to speculate that long-term potentiation plays a significant role at an early stage of conditioning. It would be an interesting future task to test this hypothesis.

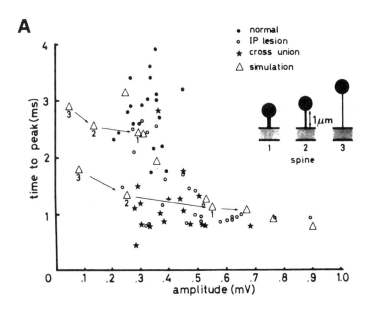

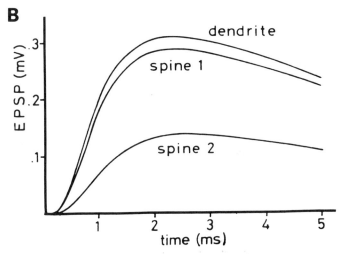

Figure 14. *The relation between the time-to-peak values and the amplitude of corticorubral unitary EPSPs. Filled circles, unitary EPSPs of normal cats; open circles, those of IP-lesioned cats; stars, those of cross-innervated cats more than two months before recording; triangles, time-to-peak values and amplitudes of the theoretical EPSPs calculated from the morphology of cell A (see text). Triangles with index numerals below them represent the time-to-peak values and amplitudes of the theoretical EPSPs that are produced by the activation of the synapse on a spine; the spine's changing shape and size is correspondingly numbered and represented in the inset of the figure by "spines" 1, 2, and 3. B: Time courses of the theoretical EPSPs produced by the activation of the synapse on spines 1 and 2 (shown in A), and that produced by the activation of a synapse on a dendritic shaft (dendrite). Note that the amplitudes of the theoretical EPSPs increase with the morphological changes in the spine that are simulated by spine 3, spine 2, spine 1, and dendrite, but the time-to-peak values of the theoretical EPSPs do not change appreciably (for further explanation, see text). (Modified from Kawato et al., 1984.)*

467

As for the nature of the change in CP EPSPs associated with classical conditioning, I believe that sprouting of corticorubral synapses constitutes at least one of the neuronal mechanisms for the following reasons: (1) The site of conditional changes is the corticorubral synapses, where sprouting was found; (2) sprouting of corticorubral synapses occurs without lesions of the input, adding considerable strength to this view; (3) the change in corticorubral EPSPs that one would expect from sprouting of the corticorubral synapses at the proximal portion of the somatodendritic membrane of RN cells was observed after establishment of conditioning; and (4) the time course of the acquisition and extinction of conditioning is a slow process, requiring one week or so, and is similar to the time course of sprouting, which takes about one week. Further experimental efforts are required to substantiate this hypothesis.

REFERENCES

Butz, E. G., and J. D. Cowan (1974) Transient potentials in dendritic system of arbitrary geometry. *Biophys. J.* **14**:661–689.

Cotman, C. W., M. Nieto-Sampedro, and E. W. Harris (1981) Synapse replacement in the nervous system of vertebrates. *Physiol. Rev.* **61**:684–784.

Eccles, J. C., R. M. Eccles, C. N. Shealey, and W. D. Willis (1962) Experiments utilizing monosynaptic excitatory action on motoneurons for testing hypothesis relating to specificity of neuronal connection. *J. Neurophysiol.* **25**:559–579.

Fujito, N., N. Tsukahara, Y. Oda, and M. Yoshida (1982) Formation of functional synapses in the adult cat red nucleus from the cerebrum following cross-innervation of forelimb flexor and extensor nerves. II. Analysis of newly-appeared synaptic potentials. *Exp. Brain Res.* **45**:13–18.

Hosono, T. (1981) Numerical inversion of Laplace transform and some applications to wave optics. *Radio Sci.* **16**:1015–1019.

Kandel, E. R. (1978) *A Cell-Biological Approach to Learning*, Society for Neuroscience, Bethesda, Maryland.

Katsumaru, H., F. Murakami, J.-Y. Wu, and N. Tsukahara (1984) GABAergic intrinsic interneurons in the red nucleus of the cat demonstrated with combined immunocytochemistry and anterograde degeneration methods. *Neurosci. Res.* **1**:35–44.

Kawato, M., and N. Tsukahara (1983) Theoretical study on electrical properties of dendritic spines. *J. Theor. Biol.* **103**:507–522.

Kawato, M., T. Hamaguchi, F. Murakami, and N. Tsukahara (1984) Quantitative analysis of electrical properties of dendritic spines. *Biol. Cybern.* **50**:447–454.

Kosar, E., Y. Fujito, F. Murakami, and N. Tsukahara (1985) Morphological and electrophysiological study of sprouting of corticorubral fibers after lesions of the contralateral cerebrum in kitten. *Brain Res.* **347**:217–224.

Kubota, M., H. Sakaguchi, and N. Tsukahara (1983) Release of endogenous GABA from the cat red nucleus slices. *Brain Res.* **270**:190–192.

Levy, W. B., and O. Steward (1979) Synapses as associative memory elements in the hippocampal formation. *Brain Res.* **175**:233–245.

McNaughton, B. L., R. M. Douglas, and G. V. Goddard (1978) Synaptic replacement in fascia dentata: Cooperativity among coactive afferents. *Brain Res.* **157**:227–293.

Murakami, F., N. Tsukahara, and Y. Fujito (1977) Analysis of unitary EPSPs mediated by the newly-formed corticorubral synapses after lesion of the interpositus nucleus. *Exp. Brain Res.* **30**:233–243.

Murakami, F., H. Katsumaru, K. Saito, and N. Tsukahara (1982) A quantitative study of synaptic reorganization in red nucleus neurons after lesion of the nucleus interpositus of the cat: An electron microscopic study involving intracellular injection of horseradish peroxidase. *Brain Res.* **242**:41–53.

Murakami, F., H. Katsumaru, J.-Y. Wu, T. Matsuda, and N. Tsukahara (1983) Immunocytochemical demonstration of GABAergic synapses on identified rubrospinal neurons. *Brain Res.* **267**:357–360.

Murakami, F., H. Katsumaru, J. Maeda, and N. Tsukahara (1984) Reorganization of corticorubral synapses following cross-innervation of flexor and extensor nerves of adult cat: A quantitative electron microscopic study. *Brain Res.* **306**:299–306.

Nakamura, Y., N. Mizuno, A. Konishi, and M. Sato (1974) Synaptic reorganization of the red nucleus after chronic deafferentation from cerebellorubral fibers; an electron microscope study in the cat. *Brain Res.* **82**:298–301.

Nieoullon, A., and N. Dusticier (1981) Glutamate decarboxylase distribution in discrete motor nuclei in the cat brain. *J. Neurochem.* **37**:202–209.

Oda, Y., K. Kuwa, S. Miyasaka, and N. Tsukahara (1981) Modification of rubral unit activities during classical conditioning in the cat. *Proc. Jpn. Acad. (Phys. Biol. Sci.)* **57**:402–405.

Parnas, I., J. Dudel, I. Cohen, and C. Frank (1984) Strengthening of synaptic contacts of an excitatory axon on elimination of a second excitatory axon innervating the same target. *J. Neurosci.* **4**:1912–1923.

Raisman, G. (1969) Neuronal plasticity in the septal nuclei of the adult rat. *Brain Res.* **14**:25–48.

Rall, W. (1964) Theoretical significance of dendritic trees for neuronal input–output relations. In *Neural Theory and Modeling*, R. F. Reiss, ed., pp. 73–87, Stanford Univ. Press, Stanford, California.

Sakaguchi, H., K. Kubota, M. Nakamura, and N. Tsukahara (1984) Effects of amino acids on cat red nucleus neurons *in vitro*. *Exp. Brain Res.* **54**:150–156.

Smith, A. M. (1970) The effects of rubral lesions and stimulation on conditioned forelimb flexion responses in the cat. *Physiol. Behav.* **5**:1121–1126.

Sperry, R. W. (1947) Effect of crossing nerves to antagonistic limb muscles in the monkey. *Arch. Neurol. Psychiatry* **58**:452–473.

Tsukahara, N. (1981) Synaptic plasticity in the mammalian central nervous system. *Annu. Rev. Neurosci.* **4**:351–379.

Tsukahara, N., and K. Kosaka (1968) The mode of cerebral excitation of red nucleus neurons. *Exp. Brain Res.* **5**:102–117.

Tsukahara, N., and Y. Oda (1981) Appearance of new synaptic potentials at corticorubral synapses after the establishment of classical conditioning. *Proc. Jpn. Acad. (Phys. Biol. Sci.)* **57**:398–401.

Tsukahara, N., D. R. G. Fuller, and V. B. Brooks (1968) Collateral pyramidal influences on the corticorubrospinal system. *J. Neurophysiol.* **31**:467–484.

Tsukahara, N., H. Hultborn, and F. Murakami (1975a) Electrical constants of neurons of the red nucleus. *Exp. Brain Res.* **23**:49–64.

Tsukahara, N., H. Hultborn, F. Murakami, and Y. Fujito (1975b) Electrophysiological study of formation of new synapses and collateral sprouting in red nucleus neurons after partial denervation. *J. Neurophysiol.* **38**:1359–1372.

Tsukahara, N., Y. Oda, and T. Notsu (1981) Classical conditioning mediated by the red nucleus in the cat. *J. Neurosci.* **1**:72–79.

Tsukahara, N., Y. Fujito, Y. Oda, and J. Maeda (1982) Formation of functional synapses in adult cat red nucleus from the cerebrum following cross-innervation of forelimb flexor and extensor nerves. I. Appearance of new synaptic potentials. *Exp. Brain Res.* **45**:1–12.

Tsukahara, N., Y. Fujito, and M. Kubota (1983) Specificity of the newly-formed corticorubral synapses in the kitten red nucleus. *Exp. Brain Res.* **51**:45–56.

Chapter 19

Synaptic Modulation and Learning: New Insights into Synaptic Transmission from the Study of Behavior

ERIC R. KANDEL
MARC KLEIN
BINYAMIN HOCHNER
MICHAEL SHUSTER
STEVEN A. SIEGELBAUM
ROBERT D. HAWKINS
DAVID L. GLANZMAN
VINCENT F. CASTELLUCCI
THOMAS W. ABRAMS

ABSTRACT

Studies of the cellular and molecular mechanisms of two forms of learning in Aplysia (sensitization and classical conditioning) have led to a broader understanding of synaptic transmission and its regulation by modulatory neurotransmitters and neuronal activity. Specifically, the study of learning has contributed to the analysis of eight new features of chemical synaptic action: (1) Transmitters can operate to close ion channels that are open at the resting potential. (2) The receptor for the transmitter and the ion channel controlled by it need not be part of the same protein, but can be separate proteins located some distance from one another. (3) When the receptor and ion channels are separate proteins, communication between them can be achieved by a diffusible intracellular second messenger. (4) The channel regulated by the transmitter can contribute to the currents of the action potential. (5) The receptor and the channel it controls are not necessarily restricted in location to the cell body and dendrites (where they control the excitability of the cell), but can also be located on the presynaptic terminal (where they can regulate the release of transmitter). (6) Transmitters, acting through a second messenger, can affect additional substrate proteins other than the channel within the postsynaptic cell. (7) The action of the transmitter on this molecular cascade can be enhanced by spike activity in the responding neuron. (8) A number of different transmitters can converge upon a common molecular cascade.

Since 1894, when Ramón y Cajal and Sigmund Freud independently suggested that learning could lead to alterations in the strength of synaptic connections, the study of learning and the study of synaptic transmission have been joined conceptually. In the last few years, it has also become possible to link them experimentally. This linkage has been instructive in two ways. First, it has given us initial insights into the mechanisms of several forms of learning and has shown how they are interrelated. Second, and perhaps more surprising, it has revealed new aspects of synaptic function.

In this chapter, we examine the novel aspects of synaptic transmission that have emerged over the last decade from the study of learning. A historical perspective reveals that, as with other central concepts in biology—such as species, gene, and antibody—our understanding of synaptic transmission is still evolving. We now have a fairly good understanding of the rapid *mediating synaptic actions* that directly control the probability of discharging the target cell. By contrast, we know much less about the slower *modulating synaptic actions* that act to regulate the strength of the mediating synaptic actions. Studies of learning have been particularly useful in uncovering and analyzing the mechanisms of synaptic modulation.

In a larger sense, a historical perspective also illustrates that the distinction between *slow modulatory actions* and *fast mediating actions* is only the most recent of several mechanistic distinctions to emerge, as intracellular recordings and subsequent methodological advances made it possible to study synaptic transmission directly, first at neuromuscular synapses, and later at a variety of central synapses.

THE MODERN ANALYSIS OF SYNAPTIC TRANSMISSION

As recently as 1950, many scientists believed that there was only one mode of synaptic transmission in the brain, and controversy raged over whether that mode was electrical or chemical (Figure 1). Fifteen years earlier, biochemically oriented physiologists had already shown that acetylcholine (ACh) is released at the heart, the adrenal medulla, and the sympathetic ganglion, and that ACh accounts for the slow muscarinic synaptic actions at these synapses (see, for example, Loewi, 1921; Loewi and Navratil, 1926; Feldberg and Gaddum, 1934; Dale et al., 1936). Feldberg, Dale, and their colleagues then went on to find that ACh can even account for the fast nicotinic synaptic actions at the neuromuscular junction. As a result, the almost unanimous opinion of these physiologists was that transmission at central synapses was likely to be chemical. But some biophysically oriented physiologists, including Erlanger, Forbes, Gasser, Lapique, Lorente de Nó, Eccles, and Grundfest argued that fast synaptic transmission between nerve and muscle and between central nerve cells was electrical (see Eccles, 1936, 1949; Erlanger, 1939; Gasser, 1939; Lorente de Nó, 1939).

As the debate continued, Bernard Katz evaluated the evidence in 1939 in his usual meticulous way:

> The work of Dale and his colleagues . . . has established that the motor nerve impulse releases a chemical substance, acetylcholine, after its arrival at the junctional region, and that the same substance, if applied by intra-arterial injection, causes a short tetanic contraction. Quantitatively the amounts, liberated and injected, are of entirely different orders of magnitude; but this is only to be expected. . . . Furthermore, a single nerve impulse can be made to cause repetitive firing of the

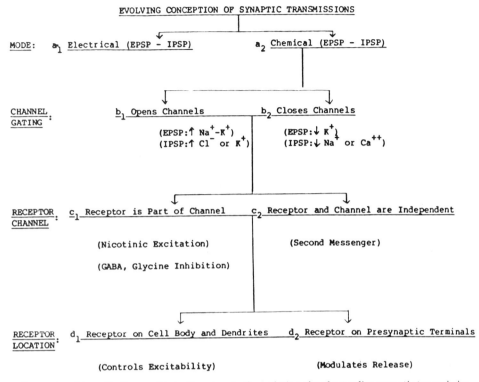

Figure 1. *Schematic diagram illustrating steps in the evolution of understanding synaptic transmission.*

muscle if the liberated amount of acetylcholine is preserved against the destruction by a specific enzyme (Brown et al., 1936) normally accumulated around the junctional region (Marnay and Nachmansohn, 1937).

. . . In spite of the recent date of these discoveries, it is almost generally agreed by now that acetylcholine plays an important part in the transmission process.

. . . As a whole, the idea of electric transmission from nerve to muscle might still be regarded as a "working hypothesis," but all the evidence for it is indirect and controversial, and obviously weighs very little when comparing it with the amount of evidence which has been added recently to the theory of electric propagation in nerve by Hodgkin's (1937) observations.

Given the nature of the evidence available in 1939, it is amazing, in retrospect, that the dispute continued until 1950, and for some participants, beyond. Even after Eccles accepted chemical transmission in 1951, Chandler Brooks, Harry Grundfest, and a few others held out. In a general review published in 1952, Grundfest, one of the most astute modern investigators of synaptic transmission, argued that: "Following through the consequences of the assumption that the synaptic response acts in the nature of an amplifier . . . makes unnecessary the successive surrender by Eccles of an electrical transmission mechanism at the myoneural junctions and at the central nervous synapses." Not until 1954, in his lecture at the Macy Conference on the Nerve Impulse, did Grundfest accept chemical mechanisms. In that lecture, he also explained the intellectual basis of the physiologists' earlier intransigence: "Eccles (1953) has recently adopted the position that this transmission is chemically mediated. Some of us have opposed this view, but much of our thinking has been influenced by data obtained with electrical stimulation of nerve cells. We may have been in error. If the neuron has a dual excitable mechanism dispersed in its membrane, the existence of only chemically activated synaptic transmission would not be disclosed by tests with electrical excitation."

The controversy was resolved experimentally only in the early 1950s, as the development of intracellular recordings made it possible to analyze synaptic transmission more directly at the nerve–muscle synapse and in the large motor cells of the spinal cord. Using intracellular recordings, first Fatt and Katz (1951), then Eccles (1953), and finally Grundfest (1956, 1957; see also Altamirano et al., 1955) found that synaptic transmission is in fact not electrical at the neuromuscular junction in frogs and crabs, at the synapses between the Ia afferent fibers and motor neurons in cats, or between motor neurons and electroplax in electric fish. At all of these synapses, then, the evidence indicated that transmission occurred through a chemical mediator. This dramatic set of findings caused Eccles and Grundfest not only to change their views but even to argue that *all* synaptic transmission is chemical! (See, for example, Eccles, 1957; Grundfest, 1959.)

However, not all participants in this debate were committed to a single mode of transmission. Remarkable for his foresight was Katz's colleague, Paul Fatt. In a classic review published in 1954 entitled "Biophysics of Junctional Transmission," Fatt clearly spelled out the alternative hypotheses:

> Although there is every indication that chemical transmission occurs across those junctions which have been discussed in this review and which are most familar to the physiologist, it is probable that electrical transmission occurs at certain other junctions. The geometry of the junction is decidedly unfavorable for electrical transmission at the junctions which have been mentioned. The pre-junctional structure, which according to the electrical hypothesis would generate the electric current for transmission, is usually much smaller than the post-junctional structure, which would have its excitatory state altered by those currents. Conditions are much more favorable for transmission in the reverse direction, and, in fact, the excitation of pre-junctional motor nerve fibers by the action currents of post-junctional muscle fibers has been observed to occur in mammalian muscle. This argument does not hold when one considers the synapses between giant nerve fibers where the pre- and post-junctional structures have usually about the same dimensions. In this case some electrical interaction will be expected, its intensity depending on how closely the fibers approach each other. One possible arrangement, which may be envisaged to give a high degree of interaction, is for the two fibers to be actually touching and for the membrane in contact to have a low electric resistance compared with that in neighboring parts of the fibers. The synapse would then serve to direct current between the interior of the two fibers, while active membrane changes would occur in neighboring regions. The ultimate development of such a system would be the elimination of the contacting membrane to secure greatest efficiency of transmission, should other factors permit this. This view of electrical transmission has been taken because it is possible to observe in certain giant fiber preparations

a protoplasmic continuity existing between, what in an earlier stage of phylogenetic development, must have been independent, synapsing nerve cells. The available evidence, however, does not indicate that a single mechanism of transmission operates at all giant fiber synapses.

In 1957, shortly after this review appeared, Edwin Furshpan and David Potter, then postdoctoral fellows at University College London, discovered in the giant fiber system of crayfish the first example of electrical transmission. Soon thereafter, Michael Bennett (1960) described a family of additional examples (for a review, see Bennett, 1979). We now accept with equanimity that there are two major modes of synaptic transmission, electrical and chemical, each of which can give rise to inhibitory and excitatory synaptic actions. Moreover, our insights into the mechanisms of both modes of transmission has greatly deepened since Furshpan and Potter's groundbreaking paper. Here, however, we are concerned only with the evolution of our understanding of chemical transmission.

Between 1950 and 1970, several chemical synaptic actions were analyzed. All of them were found to be of one type. In each case, the chemical transmitter was shown to bind to a receptor that directly regulated the opening (or gating) of an ion channel. This gating results in a flow of either inward or outward ionic current that modifies the excitability of the neuron, increasing or decreasing the probability that the target cell will generate an action potential (for reviews, see Eccles, 1964; Katz, 1966). Nicotinic excitation at the neuromuscular junction of vertebrates is the prototype for this class of synaptic action. Here the recognition site to which ACh binds, and the channel through which ions flow, are simply two different domains of a single multimeric protein (Karlin et al., 1983; Numa et al., 1983). A similar principle is thought to govern synaptic excitation in the spinal cord, where the transmitters, still unknown, open a channel for sodium and potassium, as well as synaptic inhibition, where GABA or glycine opens channels for chloride.

These rapid-mediating synaptic actions lasting milliseconds, the first to be studied, remain the best understood. Recently, however, studies of central neurons in a variety of contexts have revealed an additional subclass of chemical synaptic actions that are of much longer duration (minutes) and that typically serve to modulate fast synaptic actions. Several features of this subclass were first encountered in studies of learning. In turn, the discovery of this subclass of slow modulatory chemical synaptic actions has broadened our understanding of synaptic transmission in several ways. Specifically, the study of synaptic modulation has uncovered eight new features of chemical synaptic action. These are:

1. Transmitters can operate to *close* ion channels that are open at the resting potential.
2. The receptor for a given transmitter and the ion channel controlled by it need not be part of the same protein, but can be *separate* proteins located some distance from one another.
3. When the receptor and the ion channels are separate proteins, communication between them can be achieved by an *intracellular second messenger*.
4. The channel regulated by the transmitter can sometimes also be regulated by membrane voltage. As a result, synaptically activated channels can be

multiply gated and can therefore contribute to the currents of the action potential.

5. The receptor and the channel are not necessarily restricted in location to the cell body and dendrites, where they control the excitability of the cell, but can also be located on the *presynaptic terminal*, where they can regulate the release of transmitter.

6. Transmitters, acting through a second messenger, can affect other substrate proteins within the postsynaptic cell besides the channel, and therefore activate a *coordinated molecular response*.

7. The action of the transmitter on a molecular cascade can be enhanced by *spike activity* in the responding neuron.

8. A number of different transmitters can act together by converging on a common molecular cascade.

These eight features have broadened our view of synaptic transmission by emphasizing that the synaptic action mediated by a given synapse can be *modulated* by other transmitters that act on the synapses either presynaptically or post-synaptically. Here we examine these eight features by focusing on a particular modulatory synaptic connection, that from facilitating neurons to the mechano-sensory neurons in the marine snail, *Aplysia*. This synaptic connection produces a slow synaptic action that modulates transmitter release from the sensory neurons to their central target cells, the interneurons and motor neurons of the gill and siphon withdrawal reflexes. This slow synaptic action is of particular interest for two reasons. One, it is important for two types of learning in *Aplysia*: sensitization and classical conditioning. Two, it provides a particularly instructive case for analyzing the relationship between a mediating and a modulating synaptic pathway.

Before considering these eight features, we briefly review some basic features of the gill and siphon reflex system, and the learning process that modifies their expression.

A SIMPLE REFLEX IN *APLYSIA* CAN BE MODIFIED BY BOTH ASSOCIATIVE AND NONASSOCIATIVE LEARNING

The defensive reflex withdrawal of the gill and siphon can be elicited by weak stimuli applied either to the mantle skin or to its caudal extension, a fleshy spout called the siphon (Figure 2). As with other defensive reflexes, the gill and siphon withdrawal reflex is readily modified by three forms of learning: habituation, sensitization, and classical conditioning. Here we focus on sensitization—specifically short-term sensitization—and on classical conditioning.

Sensitization is a nonassociative form of learning produced by applying a noxious stimulus to some part of the body surface. We have primarily used the tail (or neck). In nonassociative learning, an animal acquires information about a single stimulus. Thus, following a shock to the tail (or neck), an *Aplysia* learns about the presence of a dangerous stimulus and enhances its defensive responses for a period ranging from minutes to hours (Carew et al., 1971). In addition to

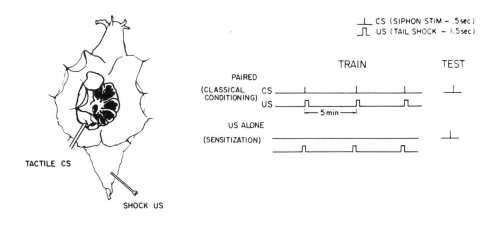

A

TACTILE CS

SHOCK US

B

⊥ CS (SIPHON STIM – .5sec)
Л US (TAIL SHOCK – 1.5sec)

TRAIN   TEST

PAIRED
(CLASSICAL   CS
CONDITIONING)   US
      ⟵ 5 min ⟶

US ALONE
(SENSITIZATION)

C

MEAN SIPHON WITHDRAWAL (sec)

60
50
40
30
20
10

●——● PAIRED (N=8)
△——△ US ALONE (N=8)

PRE ↑   1   2   3   4   5

TRAINING   RETENTION (DAYS)

Figure 2. *Comparison of classical conditioning and sensitization.* A: Dorsal view of *Aplysia* with the parapodia and mantle shelf retracted to reveal the gill. The conditioned stimulus (CS) was a weak tactile stimulus to the siphon, delivered either by a nylon bristle or by electrodes implanted in the siphon skin. The unconditioned stimulus (US) was a strong electrical shock to the tail, delivered either by hand-held spanning electrodes or by implanted electrodes. B: Diagrammatic representation of classical conditioning and sensitization. The US-alone group received pure sensitization training. After training in each case, learning was measured in the test period as the response to the CS alone. A pretest with the CS alone was given before training to match groups and to permit statistical comparisons within each group. C: Amplitude and time course of retention of the conditioned and sensitized response. After testing (PRE), the two groups were given 30 trials of paired or US-alone training (*arrow*) and then were tested with the CS alone every 24 hours. Within-group comparisons showed significant retention of the learned response in the paired group up to and including day three. The US-alone group, while significantly lower in retention than the paired group ($p < 0.01$), showed significant sensitization up to and including day two. Data in this and all other figures are expressed as means ± SEM. (From Carew et al., 1981.)

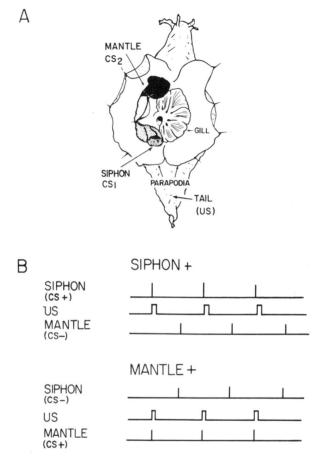

Figure 3. *Differential conditioning of the defensive withdrawal reflex.* A: Dorsal view of *Aplysia* illustrating
the two sites used to deliver conditioned stimuli: the siphon and the mantle shelf. The US was
an electric shock delivered to the tail. For illustrative purposes, the parapodia are shown intact
and retracted. However, the behavioral studies were all carried out in freely moving animals
whose parapodia had been surgically removed. B: Paradigm for differential conditioning: one
group (Siphon+) received the siphon CS (CS+) paired with the US and the mantle CS (CS−)
specifically unpaired with the US; the other group (Mantle+) received the mantle stimulus as
CS+ and the siphon stimulus as CS−. The intertrial interval was 5 min.

showing short-term memory following a single sensitizing stimulus, an *Aplysia*
shows long-term memory for the consequence of the stimulus if the sensitization
trials are repeated (Pinsker et al., 1973). Thus, when four stimuli a day are given
for four days, the defensive behavior is enhanced for over a week.

The gill and siphon withdrawal reflex can also be modified by classical conditioning, an associative form of learning (Carew et al., 1981). In associative
learning, animals learn about the predictive relationship between two stimuli
(Rescorla, 1968; Kamin, 1969). The animal learns that the conditioned stimulus
(CS) predicts the occurrence of the unconditioned stimulus (US).

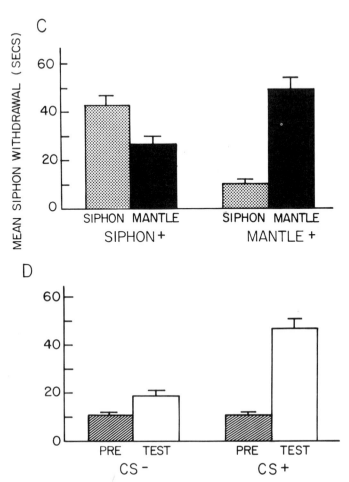

Figure 3. *(continued)* C: Results of an experiment using the paradigm of B. Testing was carried out 30 min after 15 training trials. The Siphon+ group ($n = 12$) showed significantly greater responses ($p < .05$) to the siphon CS than to the mantle CS, whereas the Mantle+ group ($n = 12$) showed significantly greater responses ($p < .01$) to the mantle CS than to the siphon CS. D: Pooled data from C. Test scores from the unpaired (CS−) and paired (CS+) pathways are compared to their respective pretest scores. The CS+ test scores are significantly greater than the CS− test scores ($p < .005$), demonstrating that differential conditioning has occurred. (From Carew et al., 1983.)

When a very weak stimulus to the siphon or the mantle shelf (which produces a weak gill and siphon withdrawal reflex) is repeatedly paired with a tail shock (which produces a powerful withdrawal reflex), the paired sensory pathway will produce a significantly enhanced reflex response, compared to another pathway that is stimulated in an unpaired manner or exposed to the US alone (sensitized). Classical conditioning here differs from sensitization in three ways: (1) It produces reflex enhancement of greater amplitude (Figure 2); (2) the enhancement is specific to the paired pathway (Figure 3); and (3) it requires a precise temporal pairing of the two inputs—the conditioning will work only when the CS precedes the US by 500 msec to 1 sec (Figure 4).

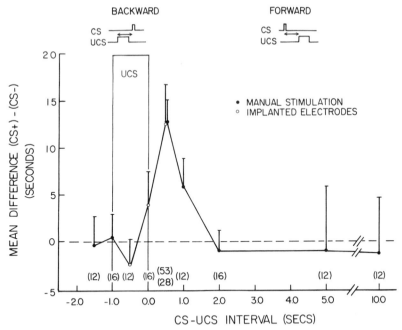

Figure 4. *The time window for classical conditioning.* The effect of various interstimulus intervals was examined by varying the time between presentation of the CS and the US in different groups of animals (at least 12 animals per group), stimulated either manually or through implanted electrodes. Significant differential conditioning was obtained when the onset of the CS+ preceded the onset of the US by 0.5 sec. Marginal conditioning resulted when the interstimulus interval was prolonged for 1 sec. No significant learning occurred when the onset of the US preceded that of the CS (backward conditioning), when the onsets of the two stimuli were simultaneous, or when the US followed the CS by 2 or more sec. In each animal, the particular interstimulus interval examined for a given input (CS+) was compared with a specifically unpaired input (CS−), and the difference between the two was used as a measure of learning. Note that scores for forward conditioning begin at time zero on the *abscissa*. (From Hawkins et al., 1983b.)

ANALYSIS OF SENSITIZATION AND CLASSICAL CONDITIONING

The mantle shelf and the siphon are each innervated by a separate cluster of about 24 sensory cells, one located on the left side (the siphon or LE sensory neurons) and the other on the right side of the abdominal ganglion (the mantle or the RE sensory neurons) (Byrne et al., 1974). The sensory neurons from each cluster make excitatory monosynaptic connections with interneurons and motor neurons that produce the withdrawal reflex. We focus here only on changes in the monosynaptic component (for a discussion of interneurons, see Frost and Kandel, 1984). The monosynaptic portion of the reflex circuit, consisting of the sensory neuron–motor neuron connection, is illustrated in Figure 5. A sensitizing stimulus applied to the tail activates facilitating neurons that produce a slow modulatory excitatory synaptic potential in both clusters of sensory neurons, those for the siphon as well as those for the mantle shelf (Klein and Kandel, 1978, 1980). This slow synaptic action has the time course of short-term sensitization

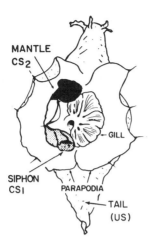

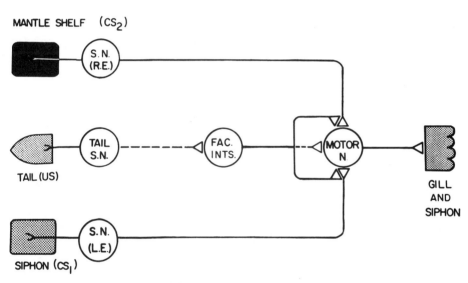

Figure 5. *Gill and siphon withdrawal reflex: Anatomy and neural circuit. A*: Dorsal view of *Aplysia* illustrates the respiratory cavity containing the gill. *B*: Schematic representation of the neural circuit for the gill and siphon withdrawal reflex. Stimulation of the mantle or the siphon excites the sensory neurons that innervate these regions, whose cell bodies are located in the RE and LE clusters in the abdominal ganglion. These sensory neurons make direct excitatory synaptic connections with motoneurons that project to the gill and siphon. During sensitization and classical conditioning training, noxious stimuli applied to the tail excite a population of facilitator interneurons. These interneurons in turn produce a slow modulatory synaptic action on the mantle and siphon sensory neurons, which results in enhanced synaptic transmission between the sensory neurons and motoneurons.

and leads to a process we have called *presynaptic facilitation*, the enhancement of transmitter release from the presynaptic terminals of the sensory neurons (Castellucci and Kandel, 1976).

How does classical conditioning differ from sensitization? We have so far only examined this question in the monosynaptic component of the reflex—the connection between sensory neurons and their cellular target cells. Our studies suggest that pairing siphon and tail stimuli, as in classical conditioning, causes sensory neurons of the siphon to be active—to fire action potentials—just before the facilitatory neurons are activated by the unconditioned stimulus. We have found that when the sensory neurons are active just before they are acted upon by the facilitating transmitter, the effectiveness of the facilitating transmitter is enhanced, producing greater presynaptic facilitation (Hawkins et al., 1983a). Thus, the effectiveness of the action of the facilitatory neuron on the sensory neuron can be amplified by preceding activity in the sensory neuron. We have therefore called this mechanism of classical conditioning *activity-dependent amplification of presynaptic facilitation*. The temporal requirements of activity-dependent enhancement are similar to those of classical conditioning (Clark, 1984).

We do not as yet understand the facilitating system in cellular detail because we have not yet identified all of the neurons in it. We have so far identified two groups of cells and have reason to believe there is a third. Based on immunocytochemical studies (Kistler et al., 1983, 1985), and on their ability to simulate the natural action of tail stimuli, we think that each of these three groups uses a different transmitter (Brunelli et al., 1976; Abrams et al., 1984b); serotonin, two closely related peptides (SCP_A and SCP_B), and a third, as yet unidentified transmitter released by the L29 cells. As we discuss later, each of the other transmitters produces actions similar to those produced by serotonin (5-HT). We have therefore used 5-HT as a model for analyzing the slow excitatory synaptic actions produced by the facilitating system, and we use it here to illustrate the eight new features of synaptic actions revealed in studies of learning (Figure 6B).

CHEMICAL TRANSMITTERS CAN CLOSE ION CHANNELS THAT ARE OPEN AT THE RESTING LEVEL OF MEMBRANE POTENTIAL

In addition to opening ion channels that are closed at rest, transmitter actions have been discovered that close ion channels that are open at rest. The membrane potential normally is leaky to potassium and to a lesser degree to sodium. Closure

Figure 6. *Synaptic facilitation at the synapse between mechanoreceptor neurons and motor neurons. A_1:* Ventral aspect of the abdominal ganglion of *Aplysia*, illustrating simultaneous recording from gill motor neuron L7 and a mechanoreceptor sensory neuron. A_2: Depression and subsequent facilitation of a monosynaptic excitatory postsynaptic potential (EPSP) after a strong electrical stimulus to the left connective. *Arrows* indicate the last EPSP before the facilitating stimulus and the first EPSP after the stimulus. M.N., motor neuron; S.N., sensory neuron. (From Castellucci and Kandel, 1976.) B: Slow EPSP elicited in sensory neuron (S.N.) by nerve stimulation (*upper trace*) and serotonin (*lower trace*). The *vertical lines* are hyperpolarizing pulses that were injected into the cell at a constant frequency to measure membrane resistance. Resistance increased by 40% in response to connective stimulation (CONNECTIVE) and by 48% in response to serotonin application (5-HT). (From Klein and Kandel, 1978.)

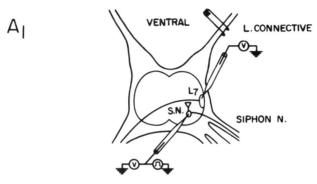

A_1

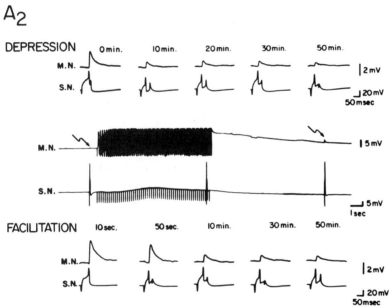

A_2

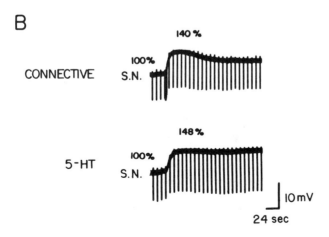

of either of these two channels moves the membrane potential toward the equilibrium potential of the other ion, the ion whose channel is still open. Thus, in addition to excitation occurring by the opening of a channel permeable to both sodium and potassium, as it does at nicotinic synapses, excitation has been found to occur in a variety of neurons by closing of a potassium channel.

Synaptic excitation produced by closure of a potassium channel was first encountered by Weight and Votava (1970) in sympathetic neurons and has now been analyzed in detail in a variety of other central and peripheral synapses of vertebrate and invertebrate animals (Carew and Kandel, 1976; Brown and Adams, 1980; Klein and Kandel, 1980; Paupardin-Tritsch et al., 1981; Jan and Jan, 1982). In each of these cases, closure of potassium channels produces a slow-modulating synaptic action that is characteristically different from the more conventional fast-mediating synaptic actions produced by opening ion channels.

A particularly interesting form of modulatory synaptic action was encountered in the study of sensitization of the gill and siphon withdrawal reflex (Klein and Kandel, 1980). When the tail of an *Aplysia* is stimulated so as to produce sensitization, a slow modulatory synaptic action is produced in the sensory neurons by the facilitating neurons (Figure 6). This slow synaptic action parallels the time course of presynaptic facilitation (and short-term sensitization). Measurements of the input conductance of the sensory neurons with constant current pulses reveal that during the slow EPSP the ionic conductance of the membrane decreases, presumably because of reduction of a resting potassium current. To test this idea directly, Klein and Kandel (1980) voltage-clamped the sensory neuron and found that the net outward potassium current was indeed depressed during the slow excitatory postsynaptic potential (EPSP).

Klein et al. (1982) next attempted to determine which, if any, of the several common potassium currents present in the sensory neurons is modulated by 5-HT: (1) the delayed voltage-dependent potassium current; (2) the early potassium current; and (3) the calcium-activated potassium current. In fact, none of these currents was affected by 5-HT. Rather, 5-HT was found to modulate a novel potassium current that Klein et al. named the "S-current" because it is sensitive to serotonin. As we illustrate later, this current is also modulated by the other putative facilitating transmitters.

THE RECOGNITION SITE (THE RECEPTOR) FOR THE TRANSMITTER AND THE IONIC CHANNEL CAN BE SEPARATE PROTEIN MOLECULES

Using the patch clamp technique that allowed them to study the properties of individual ion channels (see Neher and Sakmann, 1976), Siegelbaum et al. (1982) searched for and found a new class of potassium channels that had properties consistent with the macroscopic S-current. They called this channel the serotonin-sensitive (S)-potassium channel, because this S-channel is closed by serotonin. In addition, the S-channel has another interesting feature: The channel is structurally independent of the receptor. The channel protein does not seem to contain the recognition site for the modulatory transmitter. When 5-HT is applied to the cell membrane *outside* the area of the patch electrode, the ion channels

A

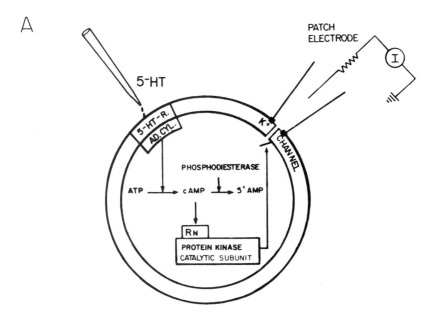

Figure 7. *Modulation of the serotonin-sensitive (S)-potassium channel by serotonin.* A: Diagram of a siphon
sensory neuron illustrating the experimental design and the components of the cAMP cascade.
Single S-channel currents were recorded by pressing a fire-polished glass patch electrode against
the cell body of a sensory neuron. With the application of gentle suction, a high-resistance seal
forms between the electrode glass and the cell membrane. Seal resistance is generally about
$10-100 \, G\Omega$; this seal forms an effective diffusion barrier between the bath and the membrane
under the patch electrode. Following the establishment of the gigaseal and the recording of
control S-channel currents, serotonin (5-HT) is added to the bath. 5-HT binds to a receptor (5-
HT-R) coupled to the enzyme adenylate cyclase (AD. CYL.), which catalyzes the conversion of
ATP to cyclic AMP (cAMP). cAMP binds to the regulatory subunits of cAMP-dependent protein
kinase (Rn) and causes them to dissociate from the catalytic subunits. Free catalytic subunit is
then available to phosphorylate a number of substrate proteins, one or more of which act to
modulate the S-channel. The cAMP cascade is terminated by the enzyme phosphodiesterase,
which hydrolyzes cAMP to 5′ AMP. Because bath-applied 5-HT is unable to diffuse directly to
the area of membrane under the patch electrode, this experiment can test the idea that 5-HT
is separate from the potassium channel and acts on it via an intracellular second messenger.
(*Figure continued on p. 486.*)

within the patch electrode are closed, even though they are not directly accessible
to the 5-HT. This experiment provided the first direct evidence in nerve cells
that a channel can be structurally independent of the receptor that regulates it
(Figures 7, 8).

THE RECEPTOR IS LINKED TO THE CHANNEL BY MEANS
OF A SECOND MESSENGER

How do these two spatially separate membrane proteins interact? How does the
activation of the receptor lead to the closure of the channel? Bernier et al. (1982)
found that the binding of the facilitating transmitter to its receptor in the sensory

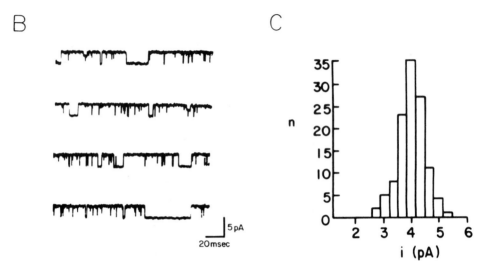

Figure 7. *(continued) B*: The S-channel is tonically active in the absence of 5-HT. Representative sweeps show single S-channel currents recorded from a siphon sensory neuron in the absence of bath-applied 5-HT. The channel undergoes rapid conformational changes between the conducting and nonconducting states, a process referred to as channel gating. Open channel contributes outward current, shown as upward deflection of the current trace. Open periods are characterized by brief closures (flickers) and are punctuated by longer closed periods. Potential across the patch is 0 mV. *C*: S-channel currents are a discrete size. Frequency histogram plots the number of observations (*n*) against the single channel current amplitude for S-channel currents measured at +11 mV. The amplitudes cluster around a single peak at 4 pA, indicating that S-channel currents are homogeneous in size at a given membrane potential and represent current flow through a single class of channels.

neuron leads to activation of adenylate cyclase and a rise in intracellular cAMP. The cAMP then activates cAMP-dependent protein kinase, resulting in the phosphorylation of various substrate proteins (for a general review of the cyclase system, see Schramm and Selinger, 1984; for a review of protein phosphorylation, see Nestler and Greengard, 1984).

Consistent with this finding, Siegelbaum et al. (1982) found that the channel can also be closed by direct injection of cAMP into sensory neurons (Figure 9). This decrease in potassium conductance produced by cAMP results from the activation of the cAMP-dependent protein kinase and the subsequent phosphorylation of some as yet unknown substrate protein (Castellucci et al., 1980, 1982; Shuster et al., 1985).

These findings raised the following question: Is the critical substrate protein, which is acted on by the protein kinase, cytoplasmic or membrane-associated? To address this point, Shuster et al. (1985) applied the purified catalytic subunit of cAMP-dependent protein kinase to cell-free, inside-out patches of membrane and found that protein kinase is capable of closing S-channels (Figure 10). These experiments suggest that the critical substrate protein is membrane-linked; it might be either the channel itself or a regulatory protein closely linked to the channel in the membrane.

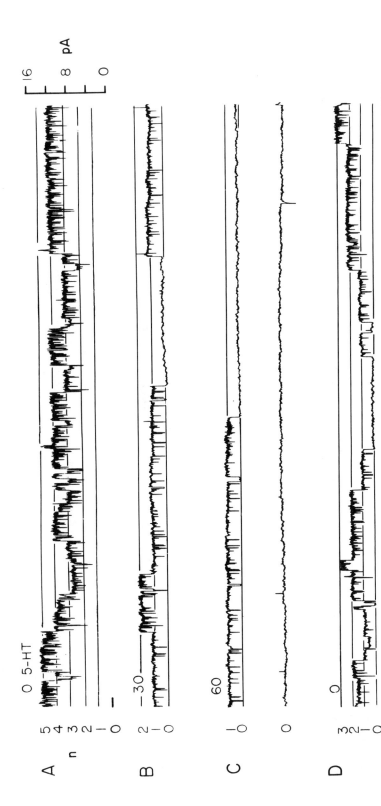

Figure 8. *5-HT acts to reduce the number of functional S-channels. A:* Control record showing an S-channel current in the absence of 5-HT. Current flows across a patch of membrane containing five active S-channels. *Ordinate* at *left* shows the level of current associated with zero through five (*n*) simultaneously open S-channels. *B* and C: Following the addition of 30 μM 5-HT and 60 μM 5-HT, 30 μM 5-HT (*B*) caused three of the five active channels to close. Following the dropout of three channels, current level fluctuated between zero and two open channels. After 5-HT concentration is elevated to 60 μM (C) the remaining two channels drop out, and no current flows across the patch. *D:* Following washout of 5-HT from the bath, the S-channels begin to recover. (From Siegelbaum et al., 1982.)

487

488

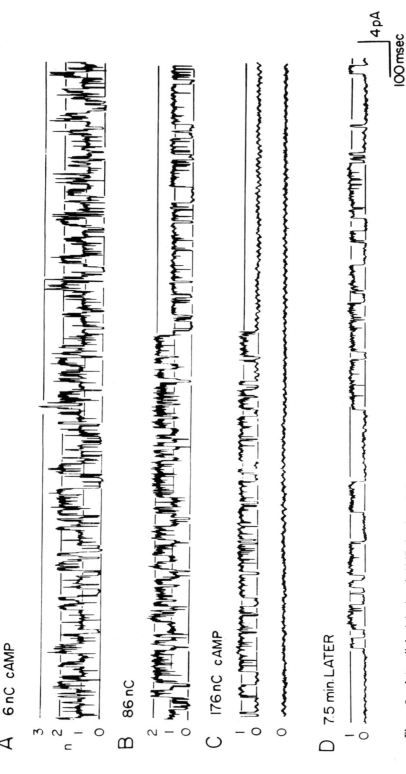

Figure 9. *Intracellular injection of cAMP also closes S-channels. A–C: S-channel currents recorded from a cell impaled with a cAMP-filled microelectrode. Patch initially contained three active S-channels. Following injection of 86 nC of cAMP, one of the three channels closes (B). After 176 nC of cAMP has been injected, the remaining two channels drop out (C). This result provides further evidence that 5-HT is acting through the cAMP second messenger system. D: Partial recovery of S-channel current flow, after removal of cAMP electrode from cell. One of three channels reopens 7.5 min after removal of the cAMP electrode. (From Siegelbaum et al., 1982.)*

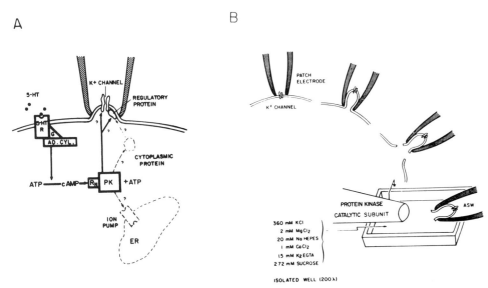

Figure 10. *Cell-free patch provides a means of identifying the location of the phosphoproteins required for S-channel modulation. A:* Diagram of the adenylate cyclase system and the location of possible substrates for cAMP-dependent protein kinase. Occupation of 5-HT receptor (5-HT R) by 5-HT activates adenylate cyclase (AD. CYL.) and results in the conversion of ATP to cAMP and the subsequent activation of the catalytic subunit of the cAMP-dependent protein kinase. Active catalytic subunit then phosphorylates a family of substrate proteins, one or more of which produce the all-or-none closure of the S-channel. In principle, this action of 5-HT could be mediated by the phosphorylation of a cytoplasmic regulatory protein, a membrane-associated regulatory protein, or perhaps by direct phosphorylation of the channel itself. *B:* Ripped-off patch provides a means of asking if the critical substrate for the protein kinase is membrane-associated or cytoplasmic. The patch electrode is placed against the soma of the LE cell. Gentle suction is applied to form a high-resistance gigaseal between the patch electrode and the cell membrane. In addition to allowing the high-resolution recording of single S-channel currents, the gigaseal is mechanically stable. The electrode can be pulled away from the cell surface, forming an isolated patch of membrane containing the S-channel protein and other membrane-associated proteins. The cytoplasmic surface of the membrane faces the bath (inside-out patch configuration). Following isolation of the inside-out patch, the electrode is moved to a small isolation well filled with a high-potassium, low-calcium intracellularlike medium. Control currents are recorded, and catalytic subunit of cAMP-dependent protein kinase is added to the isolation well, along with Mg-ATP to determine whether channels can be modulated in the absence of cytoplasmic proteins. (*Figure 10 continues on p. 490.*)

We then asked: How does protein phosphorylation alter channel gating? How is the potassium current that flows through the S-channel reduced by cAMP-dependent protein phosphorylation? In principle, potassium current could be reduced in one of four ways: (1) by decreasing the conductance of the channel; (2) by decreasing the probability of channel opening; (3) by increasing the probability of closing; or (4) by reducing the number of channels that are open in the membrane. Siegelbaum et al. (1982) and Shuster et al. (1985) examined this question in both cell-attached and cell-free patches and found that 5-HT, cAMP, and the cAMP-dependent protein kinase all act in a common manner; they reduce the number of channels that are open in an all-or-none fashion.

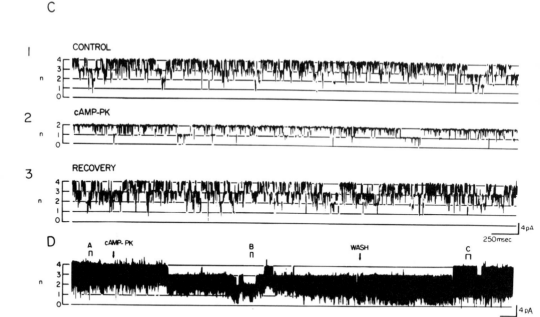

Figure 10. (*continued*) *C*: cAMP-dependent protein kinase closes S-channels in inside-out membrane patches. Expanded record of channel currents before, during, and after application of cAMP-dependent protein kinase catalytic subunit, respectively. 1 mM Mg-ATP was present initially. *Ordinate* shows the number of open channels (*n*). C_1: Before the addition of kinase, the patch contained four active channels open for a large fraction of the time. The current record fluctuates from one to four channels open simultaneously because of the rapid random opening and closing of individual channels. The patch contained a fifth channel that opened occasionally throughout the experiment (seen as brief upward spikes in *D*) and was not analyzed further. C_2: 3 min after the addition of cAMP-dependent protein kinase catalytic subunit (0.1 μM final concentration) plus 1 mM Mg-ATP (2.0 mM final concentration), the current level fluctuates from zero to two channels open, but the amplitude and probability of opening of the remaining active channels are unchanged from those of the control. C_3: After recovery, the channels again fluctuate between four levels. *D*: Closure and reopening of the same channels shown in *A*–*C*, but on a slower time sweep. Channel currents were recorded for over 8 min before the addition of the cAMP-dependent protein kinase catalytic subunit, during which time there were no closures longer than 10 sec. At the *arrow*, enzyme and Mg-ATP were added to the bath. After a latency of 3 min, one channel closed (downward step in maximal current level), and after a further 4 min, a second channel closed. The two closed channels then reopened (upward step changes in maximal current level in *C*), followed by a final prolonged channel closure. On washout of the enzyme, the remaining closed channel reopened after 5 min. The mean duration of the enzyme-produced closures in this experiment was 3 min. The expanded records were taken from the regions indicated by brackets labeled A, B, and C in *D*. (From Shuster et al., 1985.)

TRANSMITTERS CAN MODULATE ION CHANNELS THAT CONTRIBUTE TO THE ACTION POTENTIAL

What does closure of the channel accomplish? What is its physiological function? The actions of the nicotinic ACh receptor channel and other transmitter-activated channels that were initially studied were found to be independent of voltage, unlike the sodium, potassium, and calcium channels that contribute to the action potential. Indeed, this distinction seemed so fundamental that Grundfest and others suggested that ion channels fall into two mutually exclusive categories: voltage-gated channels that are electrically excitable and chemically gated channels that are electrically inexcitable. However, the S-potassium channel (as well as other potassium and certain calcium channels that are modulated by transmitters) has been shown to be both modestly voltage-sensitive as well as chemically gated (Klein et al., 1982). As a result, the channel can directly affect the cell's mechanisms for generating action potentials.

Because it can be modified by either voltage or a chemical transmitter, closure of the S-channel has two novel functions:

1. Closure of the potassium channel by 5-HT increases the excitability of the cell by removing an inhibitor brake, the shunt produced by the background potassium conductance; 5-HT reduces an outward potassium current that opposes the initiation of the action potential by the inward sodium current (Klein et al., 1986). This can best be illustrated by injecting a depolarizing current in the cell. Under normal circumstances, adaptation of the firing occurs after the first one or two action potentials. Following activation of the facilitatory neurons by nerve stimulation, or the application of 5-HT, the same current pulse now elicits a nonadapting train of action potentials (Figure 11). Normally, the presence of the S-current contributes to adaptation by providing a braking action in the generation of action potentials. The depression of the S-current by the 5-HT removes this braking action. This feature is shared by other modulating synaptic actions that close potassium channels, such as the muscarinic or peptidergic modulation of the M-channel or the noradrenergic modulation of the calcium-activated potassium channel, as first shown by Roger Nicoll (1982) and Paul Adams (Adams et al., 1982; Pennefather et al., 1985).

2. In addition, 5-HT increases the duration of each individual action potential (Klein and Kandel, 1978; Klein et al., 1980). The S-channel controls an important component of the outward current that repolarizes the action potential. Closure of the S-channels by 5-HT (or by other facilitating transmitters) slows the repolarization and broadens the spike (Figure 12).

RECEPTORS FOR TRANSMITTER CAN ALSO BE LOCATED ON PRESYNAPTIC TERMINALS OF NEURONS

Until 1960, the accepted view of synaptic action was that put forward by Ramón y Cajal at the turn of the century. According to Ramón y Cajal, synaptic contacts between neurons were located only on the cell body and dendrites of the post-synaptic neurons. Since the discovery of presynaptic inhibition (Frank and Fuortes, 1957; Dudel and Kuffler, 1961) and presynaptic facilitation (Kandel and Tauc, 1965a,b; Castellucci and Kandel, 1976), it has become clear that there also are synapses on the presynaptic terminals. These differences in location are now known to be important functionally. When a transmitter binds to receptors on the cell body and dendrites, it influences the excitability of the neuron, its probability of firing an action potential. But when the transmitter binds to receptors

492

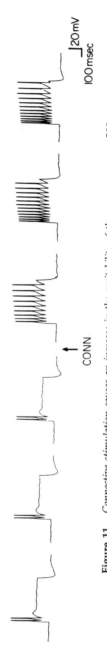

Figure 11. *Connective stimulation causes an increase in the excitability of the sensory neuron.* 500-msec depolarizing current steps were imposed at 30-sec intervals in order to elicit action potentials. Prior to connective stimulation, the action potentials accommodate to long, depolarizing pulse input because of the shunting action of the S-current. After connective stimulation (CONN), this accommodation was greatly reduced as the shunt produced by S-current was reduced. (Spikes are truncated as a result of the slow-frequency response of the pen recorder.) (From Klein et al., 1986.)

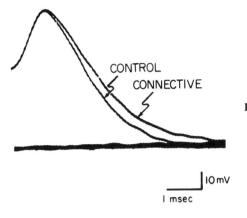

CONTROL
CONNECTIVE

Figure 12. *Spike broadening induced by connective stimulation.* Action potentials recorded in normal seawater solution broaden by 10–15% after stimulation of the left connective. (From Klein et al., 1980.)

10 mV

1 msec

on or near the presynaptic terminals, it can also alter the currents underlying the action potential and can thereby regulate the transmitter release caused by a single action potential.

The slow modulatory synaptic actions in *Aplysia* that contribute to sensitization and classical conditioning are exerted not only on the cell body, but also on the presynaptic terminals where the broadening of the action potential can increase calcium influx, which in turn can enhance transmitter release (Figures 6, 13). Until recently (Belardetti et al., 1986), it has not been possible to record directly from the synaptic terminals. Therefore, we have used the membrane cell body as a model for changes in the presynaptic terminals (for rationale, see Klein and Kandel, 1978; Klein et al., 1980). Thus, Brunelli et al. (1976), Klein and Kandel (1978), and Castellucci et al. (1980) found that injection of cAMP or of the cAMP-dependent protein kinase into the sensory neurons produces not only broadening of the action potential in the cell body but also enhancement of transmitter release (Figure 13).

Most nerve cells quite likely have several different kinases. Are other kinases also activated by 5-HT? Do they contribute to the broadening of the action potential and to the enhancement of transmitter release? To determine to what degree the action of the cAMP-dependent protein kinase is specific for naturally occurring facilitation, Castellucci et al. (1982) injected the Walsh inhibitor, a specific protein inhibitor of the cAMP-dependent protein kinase, into the sensory neuron. They found that the inhibitor blocked the broadening of the action potential and the facilitation of transmitter release (Figure 14). A similar blockage was obtained after injection of GDP$_\beta$-S, a blocker of adenylate cyclase (Castellucci et al., 1983; Schwartz et al., 1983).

Based on these experiments, Klein and Kandel (1980; see also Klein et al., 1980) proposed a working molecular model of this slow synaptic action and its modulation of transmitter release (Figure 15). They proposed that the facilitating transmitters act through cAMP-dependent protein phosphorylation to close a special class of potassium channels. The closure of these channels enhances excitability and broadens the action potential. Broadening the action potential

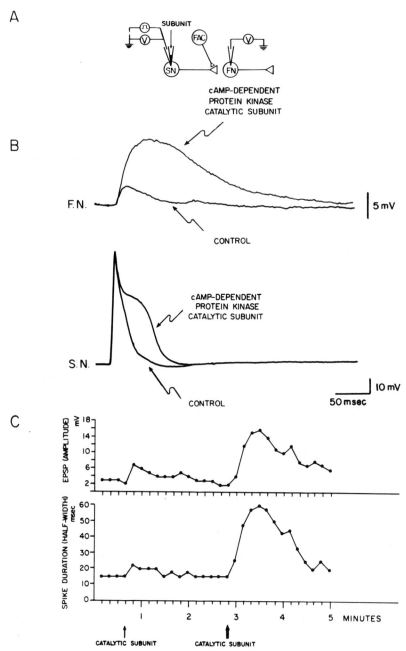

Figure 13. *Injection of the catalytic subunit enhances transmitter release.* A: Diagram of the simplified neuronal circuit of the gill withdrawal reflex, illustrating the experimental procedure involving injection of the catalytic subunit in the sensory neuron (SN) and recording from a follower neuron (FN). B: Superimposed recordings of the action potentials in the sensory cell and the monosynaptic EPSPs in the follower neuron before and after injection of the catalytic subunit. After intracellular injection of the enzyme into the sensory cell, the duration of both the sensory cell action potential and its transmitter release were increased. C: Quantification of the effect of intracellular injection of the catalytic subunit on spike duration and EPSP amplitude. Action potential duration and transmitter release from a single sensory neuron were monitored at 10-sec intervals. After a small injection (*thin arrow*), the action potential duration and transmitter release (size of the monosynaptic EPSP) increased in a parallel fashion. After a larger injection (*thick arrow*), both physiological effects were much larger. (From Castellucci et al., 1980.)

494

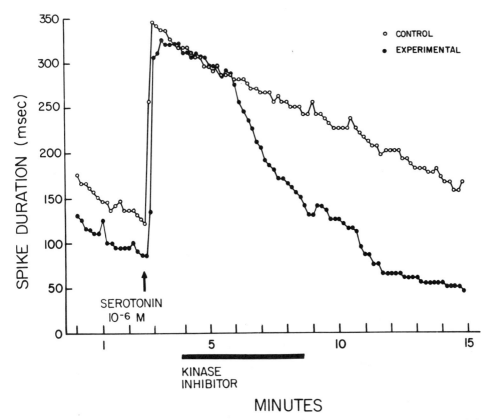

Figure 14. *Injection of the kinase inhibitor reverses the action of 5-HT.* Action potentials were recorded simultaneously every 10 sec from a pair of sensory neurons and allowed to respond to 5-HT. One cell was injected with the inhibitor; injection is indicated by the *bar*. Note that the spike-broadening response decayed more rapidly in the injected cell. (From Castellucci et al., 1982.)

in turn increases calcium influx and enhances transmitter release. This model gives rise to two predictions: (1) broadening of action potential should simulate facilitation; and (2) because the action potential is broader, the facilitated EPSP should have a slower time to peak.

Hochner et al. (1986a,b; see also Klein et al., 1980) have tested these two predictions. They applied brief depolarizing pulses to the sensory neuron under voltage clamp conditions, so as to substitute these for action potentials. They found that even slight broadening of the action potential causes substantial increases in transmitter release. Thus, a 20% increase in pulse duration, from a duration of 2.0 to 2.5 msec, can cause a twofold increase in transmitter release (Figure 16). Since the normal action potentials are 2.0–3.0 msec in duration, transmitter release seems to be highly sensitive to changes in the duration of the action potentials. Moreover, broadening of the action potential affects the shape of the EPSP, increasing the time it takes to reach its peak amplitude. Comparable slowing in the time to peak is seen with naturally occurring presynaptic facilitation produced by tail nerve stimulation or 5-HT.

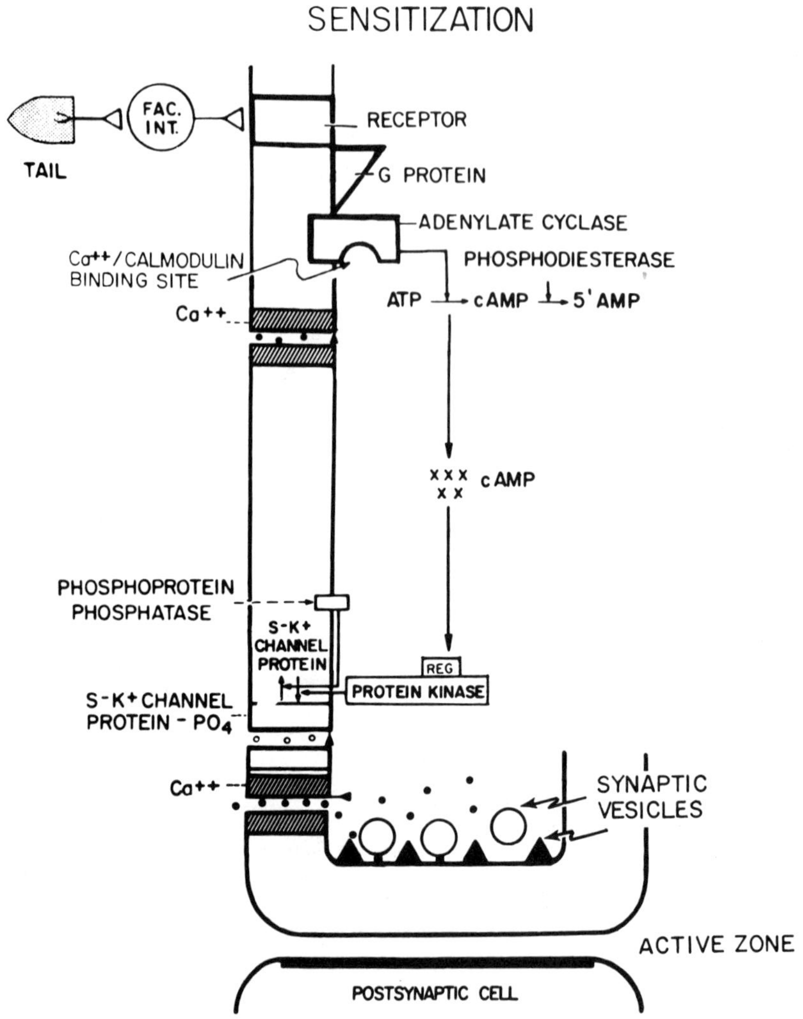

SENSITIZATION

Figure 15. *Diagram summarizing the intracellular mechanism thought to be involved in short-term sensitization of the defensive withdrawal reflex.* Noxious stimuli to the tail excite facilitator interneurons that stimulate adenylate cyclase in the siphon sensory neurons, increasing the synthesis of cAMP (XXX). The catalytic subunit of the cyclase is shown coupled to the receptor for the facilitatory transmitter via the regulatory G protein. cAMP binds to the regulatory unit of the protein kinase, which then releases from the catalytic unit of the kinase, activating it. Phosphorylation of either the S-potassium channel protein or another membrane-associated protein results in the closing of this potassium channel. Subsequent to this S-channel closure, action potentials in the sensory neurons are prolonged, resulting in more time for calcium influx through the voltage-dependent calcium channel (shown adjacent to the active zone, the release site for synaptic vesicles). (From Kandel et al., 1983.)

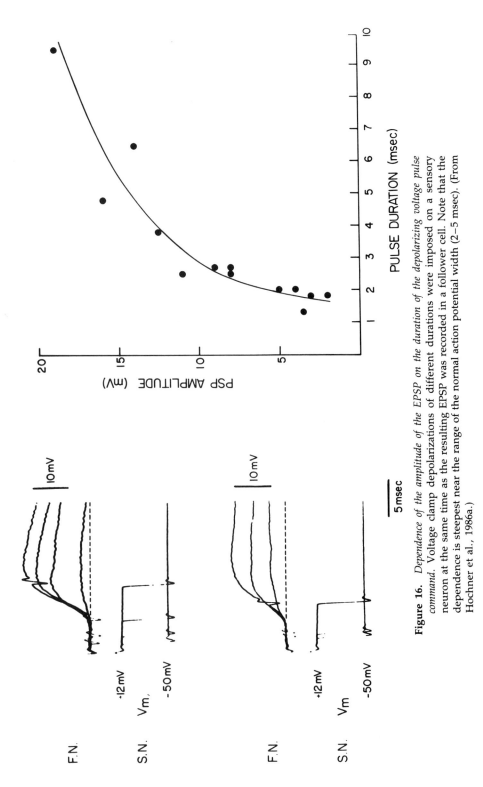

Figure 16. *Dependence of the amplitude of the EPSP on the duration of the depolarizing voltage pulse command.* Voltage clamp depolarizations of different durations were imposed on a sensory neuron at the same time as the resulting EPSP was recorded in a follower cell. Note that the dependence is steepest near the range of the normal action potential width (2–5 msec). (From Hochner et al., 1986a.)

THE TRANSMITTER ENGAGES A FAMILY OF REGULATORY
PATHWAYS WITHIN THE CELL

The finding that broadening of the action potential because of closure of potassium channels by cAMP-dependent protein phosphorylation can contribute to presynaptic facilitation does not imply, however, that the kinase produces only one effect in the sensory neuron and that presynaptic facilitation is fully accounted for by closure of the potassium channel. The possibility that cAMP has additional actions within the cell arises from several independent lines of evidence.

First, Schwartz and his colleagues have found that the kinase phosphorylates at least 10 substrate proteins in the sensory neuron. It would thus appear that the closure of the potassium channel is only one member of the cell's family of responses to the modulatory transmitters. The transmitters produce other changes in the activity of molecules within the cell that are not immediately apparent in either the resting or the action potential. A clue that additional intracellular events are initiated by the facilitating transmitters came from the experiments of Boyle et al. (1984). They measured intracellular free calcium transients in the sensory neuron cell bodies, using the calcium-sensitive dye arsenazo III. As might be predicted from this discussion, they found that increases in the duration of the depolarizing command under voltage clamp conditions increased the free calcium transient (by increasing calcium influx). But they also found that at any given duration, 5-HT increased the free calcium transients further by 75%. This increase in the free calcium transients is not merely secondary to the changes in the potassium current, since it can be observed under voltage clamp conditions when the duration of the command is held constant (Figure 17).

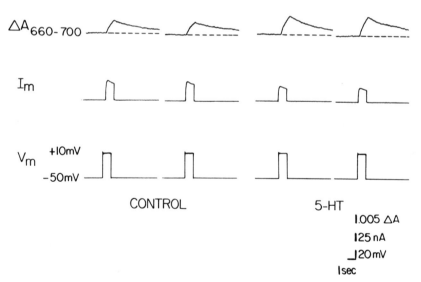

Figure 17.   *Increase by 5-HT in the depolarization-induced calcium transient.* An arsenazo-filled sensory neuron was depolarized for 1 sec at 1-min intervals. When 5-HT was added, the differential light absorbance signals ($A_{660-700}$) increased, indicating an increase in the calcium transients, while membrane currents became less outward (I_m, *middle traces*). *Bottom traces* show membrane voltage (V_m). (From Boyle et al., 1984.)

SENSITIZATION

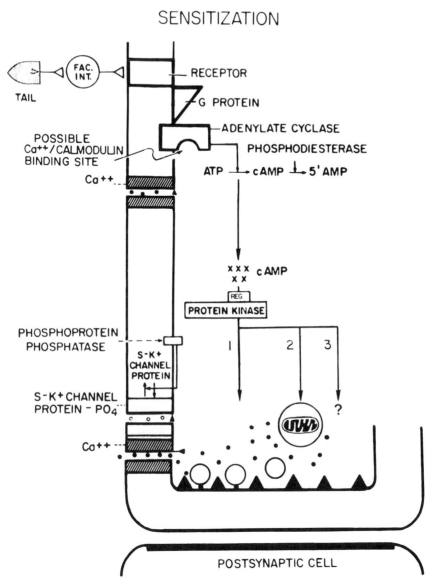

Figure 18. *cAMP-dependent protein phosphorylation has diverse effects within the siphon sensory neurons.* In addition to causing closure of the S-potassium channel, cAMP seems to modulate intracellular handling of calcium ions and may also produce other actions.

Recent experiments by Hochner et al. (1986b) suggest that this increase in free calcium transients reflects not an increase in calcium influx, but a change in calcium handling by the cell: either a reduction in intracellular calcium sequestration or a release of calcium from intracellular stores. Preliminary experiments indicate that this alteration in calcium handling may also be dependent on cAMP (Figure 18).

We think it likely that the enhancement of calcium accumulation and the reduction in potassium current act synergistically in producing short-term presynaptic facilitation. Perhaps the calcium accumulation is important in the mobilization of the synaptic vesicles to the release sites (see also Gingrich and Byrne, 1985; Hochner et al., 1986b). Mobilization of this sort may be more important when transmitter release is sustained or, as in habituation, when transmitter release has previously been depressed. In addition, since calcium also is an important second messenger within the cell, the modulation of calcium handling by 5-HT might contribute to other processes that depend on calcium, such as long-term sensitization or classical conditioning.

THE RESPONSE OF THE ADENYLATE CYCLASE SYSTEM TO A GIVEN TRANSMITTER CAN BE AMPLIFIED BY IMPULSE ACTIVITY WITHIN THE CELL

During classical conditioning, the response of a sensory neuron to facilitatory input is enhanced because the sensory neuron of the CS pathway has recently fired action potentials (Figure 19). How does this come about? Abrams, Bernier, and their colleagues (1984a) have examined this question and found that 5-HT produces a greater increase in cAMP when the sensory neurons are active prior to the application of 5-HT, compared to cells that were not active (see also Ocorr et al., 1985). These experiments indicate that the response of the adenylate cyclase complex to a given amount of transmitter can be regulated and amplified by recent action potentials within the cell itself.

What aspect of the action potential provides the signal that regulates the cyclase? Is it the sodium influx, the calcium influx, the potassium efflux, or the change in membrane potential? Abrams et al. (1983) have found the activity-dependent enhancement of the facilitation response requires the calcium influx that occurs with the action potential. The enhancement disappears with elimination of calcium influx either by reducing extracellular calcium or by intracellular injection of the calcium chelator EGTA (Figure 20). The discovery that the molecular signal for the US is the release of the facilitating transmitters, and that at least part of the signal for the CS is the influx of calcium produced by activity of the sensory neurons, has allowed us to examine where the two signals interact within the sensory neurons. Stated another way: Where does the actual association

---

Figure 19. *Activity-dependent facilitation of monosynaptic EPSPs in the neuronal circuit for the withdrawal reflex.* A: Circuit for pathway-specific enhancement of presynaptic facilitation during conditioning. Both sensory pathways receive facilitatory input in response to the tail stimulus (US), but those sensory neurons that have been activated by a CS just before the US occurs experience enhanced presynaptic facilitation. B: Protocol for the cellular experiments. One siphon sensory neuron (S.N.) was caused to fire a 0.5-sec train of action potentials immediately prior to the tail stimulus (US). The control (unpaired) siphon sensory neuron was similarly caused to fire a train of action potentials, but 2.5 min after the US. In other experiments, the control sensory neuron was not stimulated during training and served as a US-alone, or sensitization, control. C: Comparison of cellular data showing differential facilitation of EPSPs and behavioral data showing sensitization and differential conditioning of the withdrawal reflex. Behavioral data are from experiments on the conditioning of the withdrawal reflex, with the same experimental protocol and parameters as physiological data. (From Hawkins et al., 1983a.)

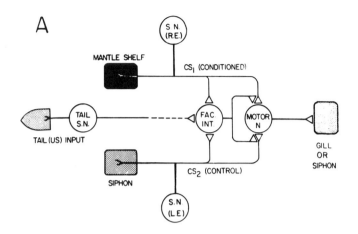

A

S.N. (R.E.)

MANTLE SHELF

CS₁ (CONDITIONED)

TAIL S.N.

TAIL (US) INPUT

FAC. INT.

MOTOR N

GILL OR SIPHON

SIPHON

CS₂ (CONTROL)

S.N. (L.E.)

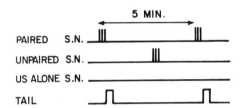

B

5 MIN.

PAIRED S.N.

UNPAIRED S.N.

US ALONE S.N.

TAIL

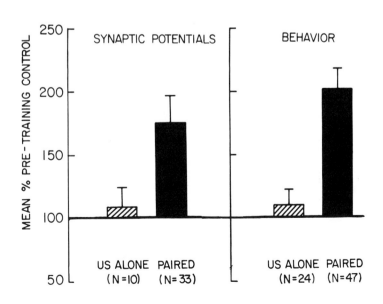

C

RETENTION

SYNAPTIC POTENTIALS

BEHAVIOR

MEAN % PRE-TRAINING CONTROL

250

200

150

100

50

US ALONE (N=10) PAIRED (N=33)

US ALONE (N=24) PAIRED (N=47)

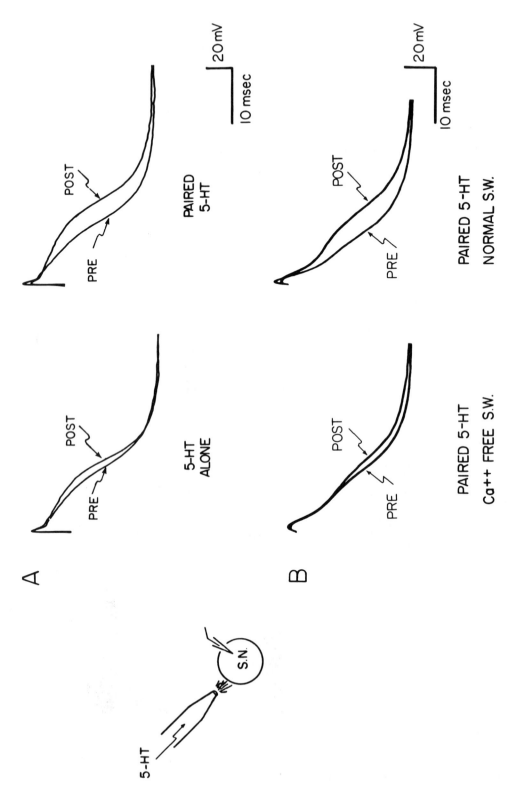

502

Figure 20. *Activity-dependent enhancement of siphon sensory neuron responses to brief applications of 5-HT.* Brief (1 sec) puffs of 5-HT were pressure ejected from an extracellular micropipette onto the soma of a single sensory neuron (shown at *left*). *A*: Influence of paired spike activity on the 5-HT response, measured as the increase in action potential duration. In alternate trials, the 5-HT puff was delivered alone or immediately following a 0.5-sec, 10-Hz train of action potentials. The effect on the action potential duration was then measured 60 sec after the puff. Sufficient time was allowed between trials for the spike broadening response to decay completely. A differential spike broadening from one typical experiment is shown. Action potentials before (PRE) and after (POST) the puff alone and the paired puff are superimposed. Recordings were made in normal saline (without TEA). To allow more accurate measurement of the change in the action potential during pre- and post-tests, the neuron was fired repetitively at 20 Hz for 2.5 sec, and the action potentials were measured at the end of the train. Because two other potassium currents (I_A and I_K) are inactivated during repetitive firing, the contribution of the S-potassium current in repolarizing the action potential is increased; thus the action potential at the end of these spike trains is particularly sensitive to any changes in the S-current. Note that although the duration of the action potential increased only slightly after the 5-HT puff alone, there was substantially more spike broadening after the paired 5-HT puff. *B*: The role of calcium influx in activity-dependent enhancement of the 5-HT response. In single sensory neurons, 0.5-sec, 10-Hz trains of action potentials were paired with brief 5-HT puffs alternately in calcium-free (10^{-7} M calcium) saline and in normal (10^{-2} M calcium) saline (S.W.). Action potential duration was measured in normal saline both before and 90 sec after pairing in each solution. In calcium-free saline trials, the bath was rapidly switched from normal calcium to low calcium for the paired 5-HT puff and back to normal saline for the post-test 90 sec after the puff. An example of pre- and post-puff action potentials from one experiment is shown. Note that after action potentials were paired with 5-HT in normal saline, the increase in action potential duration was substantially greater than after pairing in the absence of calcium influx. Pre- and post-tests were conducted, using 2.5 sec of high-frequency repetitive firing as in *A*. (Calcium was included with 5-HT in the puff solution to control for any calcium requirement of the receptor. Thus, in the calcium-free saline trials, calcium was present during the pre- and post-tests and during the puff, and was absent only during the paired spike train.) (From Abrams et al., 1983.)

that underlies classical conditioning occur? At what molecular steps do the CS and US converge?

We do not as yet know the answer to these questions. But as an initial approach we asked: How does calcium influx lead to the increase in cAMP? Does it cause a depression in the activity of the degradative enzyme cAMP phosphodiesterase, or does it cause a stimulation of adenylate cyclase? Abrams and Kandel (1985) explored these questions in a particulate membrane preparation from *Aplysia* central nervous system enriched in sensory neurons and found that calcium did not depress phosphodiesterase, and at higher concentrations actually stimulated it. By contrast, calcium did stimulate the activity of adenylate cyclase in the particulate membrane preparation. As a result, we think that one likely point for the convergence is adenylate cyclase (Figure 21; see also Ocorr et al., 1983). Transmitter-sensitive cyclases are complex enzymes, consisting of a transmitter receptor, one of several GTP-binding regulatory subunits, and one

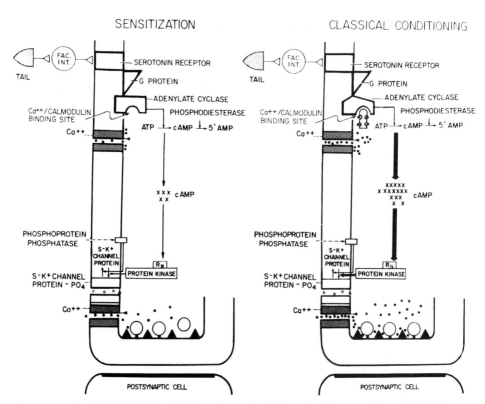

Figure 21. *A model of classical conditioning illustrating the hypothesis that preceding activity leads to an influx of calcium in the sensory neurons of the CS pathway.* Calcium/calmodulin binds to adenylate cyclase, leading to a conformational change in this enzyme. This change promotes the synthesis of a greater amount of cAMP than would occur in the absence of calcium binding, resulting in the closure of more S-potassium channels. During subsequent action potentials (as indicated at the *bottom* of the diagrams), more calcium will enter the terminals of the sensory neurons with the larger cAMP response. (Modified from Abrams et al., 1983, 1984a.)

of two types of catalytic subunits. When the transmitter binds to the receptor, the receptor activates a stimulating GTP-binding regulatory subunit (called G_s). The G_s protein interacts with and activates the catalytic subunit, so that the enzyme converts ATP to cAMP. Recent studies indicate that the catalytic subunit exists in two isozymic forms (Brostrom et al., 1978). There is a universal catalytic subunit, thought to be present in all cells, that does not require calcium for activity. In addition, there is a second catalytic subunit, first identified in brain cells, that is activated by calcium/calmodulin.

Thus, it seems possible that calcium may interact with 5-HT by modulating the calcium/calmodulin-dependent adenylate cyclase response to 5-HT (Figure 21). In testing this idea further, Abrams and Kandel (1985) found that the ability of 5-HT to stimulate adenylate cyclase in this particulate membrane preparation is substantially reduced if the endogenous calmodulin in the membrane is removed or inhibited (Figure 22). The addition of mammalian calmodulin restores the sensitivity to both calcium and to 5-HT.

This particulate preparation has one further advantage. It may give us an approach through which to explore the temporal specificity of classical conditioning on the molecular level. Does the interaction between the calcium and the adenylate cyclase account for the temporal specificity of classical conditioning? The two critical features of classical conditioning are: (1) that the CS must precede the US by only a narrow time interval (1000 msec or less); and (2) that the two stimuli are noncommutable—the CS must precede the US (Hawkins et al., 1983b). These features are mirrored on the cellular level. Enhanced presynaptic facilitation does not result if the stimuli are paired but the US precedes the CS (Clark, 1984).

What determines the narrow time window of classical conditioning (Figure 4)? Why must the CS precede the US by only 500–1000 msec? Why can the interval not be longer? Why can't the US precede the CS? Preliminary experiments with transient pulses of calcium suggest that, just as in classical conditioning, the calcium pulse must temporally overlap the exposure to 5-HT to enhance cyclase stimulation (Figure 23). If the calcium pulse precedes the 5-HT by several seconds, it has no effect on the response of the cyclase to 5-HT (Abrams and Kandel, 1985).

It is attractive to think that these features might be explained by the characteristic features of impulse activity and the calcium/calmodulin-dependent) form of the cyclase (Figure 23). First, the critical duration of the CS–US interval might be determined *by the time during which the intracellular free calcium level is elevated in the sensory neurons by impulse activity, so as to prime the calcium/calmodulin-dependent cyclase.* This short time window may reflect the speed with which calcium is taken up by buffering organelles. A corollary to this finding is that the increase in free calcium produced by 5-HT might serve to enhance even further the calcium action on the cyclase after the first pairing trial. Second, the noncommutable feature of classical conditioning cannot be explained in this manner and must involve another mechanism. Perhaps the cyclase will not bind calcium/calmodulin once it has been activated by the facilitatory transmitter (Figure 23). We are currently testing these ideas.

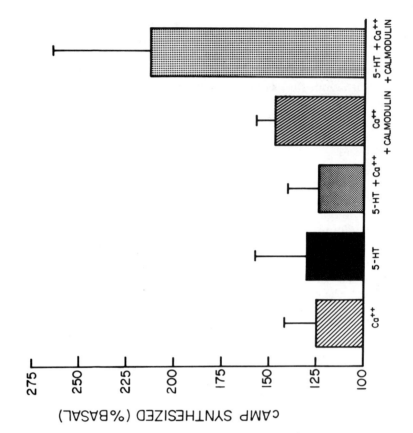

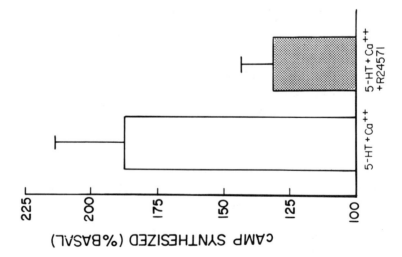

506

Figure 22. *Calcium/calmodulin potentiates the activation of serotonin-sensitive adenylate cyclase. Left:* Effect of a calmodulin inhibitor, R24571, on adenylate cyclase stimulation. *Aplysia* pleural ganglia, which contain all the tail sensory neurons in the animal, were desheathed, homogenized, and centrifuged to prepare a membrane pellet, which was then resuspended in a low-calcium EGTA buffer with 5 mM magnesium. Basal synthesis of cAMP was assayed with 10 μM GTP and 50 μM ATP. Assays were also carried out with 10^{-4} M 5-HT and with 1 μM free calcium, with or without the addition of 5×10^{-6} M R24571. cAMP synthesis is expressed as percentage of basal. Data are averaged from five experiments with three replicates each. Note that the calmodulin inhibitor substantially reduced stimulation by 5-HT and calcium. *Right:* Adenylate cyclase activity in particulate membrane preparation that has been stripped of calmodulin. After homogenization, membrane from pleural ganglia was stripped of endogenous calmodulin by sequential washing with trifluoperazine (which binds calmodulin in the presence of calcium) and then with EGTA. After stripping, only slight stimulation occurred with either calcium or 5-HT. However, after addition of calmodulin from mammalian brain, both 5-HT and calcium sensitivity were restored.

507

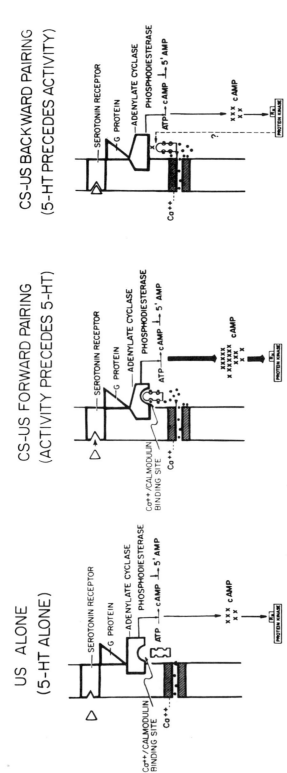

Figure 23. *Hypothetical model suggesting how allosteric properties of the calcium/calmodulin-dependent adenylate cyclase may account for the association mechanisms of classical conditioning in Aplysia.* Left: US alone. In the absence of spike activity and calcium influx in the sensory neuron, the facilitating transmitter released by the US is shown producing a modest activation of the cyclase, stimulating a small amount of cAMP synthesis. The calcium channel is shown closed, and calmodulin is shown without calcium bound. *Middle:* Forward pairing; CS precedes US. The CS has caused spike activity in the sensory neuron, thereby transiently opening calcium channels and allowing calcium influx. Calcium/calmodulin is shown binding to adenylate cyclase. If the US occurs during this period of calmodulin activation, stimulation of the cyclase is shown to be potentiated, causing a greater synthesis of cAMP. *Right:* Backward pairing; US precedes CS. Some mechanism must prevent the enhancement of facilitation by the spike activity that follows the US. We speculate that the initial small activation of the cyclase by facilitatory transmitter may block subsequent modulation of the cyclase by calcium/calmodulin, possibly through an action of the cAMP-dependent protein kinase. Thus, with backward pairing, only a modest activation of the cyclase may occur, as with the US alone. (Modified from Abrams et al., 1983, 1984a; Abrams and Kandel, 1985.)

508

DIFFERENT TRANSMITTERS CAN CONVERGE
ON A COMMON cAMP CASCADE

At least three transmitters besides 5-HT seem able to bind to different receptors that converge on adenylate cyclase to increase cAMP levels and stimulate protein kinase, thereby closing a common potassium channel. The evidence is most complete for two neuropeptides endogenous to *Aplysia*, the small cardioactive peptides SCP$_A$ and SCP$_B$. Bioassays of HPLC fractions of abdominal ganglion extracts indicate that both SCPs (and 5-HT) are present in the ganglion in large quantities (Abrams et al., 1984b). Immunocytochemical studies indicate that their processes come in close contact with the siphon sensory neurons (Kistler et al., 1983, 1985; Lloyd et al., 1985). Like 5-HT, the two peptides are capable of both producing facilitation of synaptic transmission from siphon mechanosensory neurons and enhancing the defensive withdrawal reflex which these sensory neurons mediate. Moreover, single channel recording has revealed that these peptides close the same S-channel that is modulated by 5-HT and cAMP. Finally,

CONVERGENCE

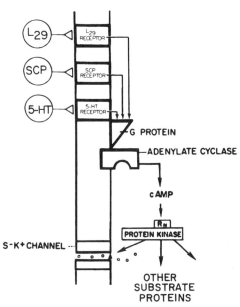

Figure 24. *Convergence of several facilitatory transmitters on the adenylate cyclase of the sensory neurons.* The neuropeptides SCP$_A$ and SCP$_B$ are thought to activate the cyclase via one receptor (because of cross-desensitization), whereas 5-HT seems to stimulate the cyclase via a second receptor. Although the mechanism of action of the L29 transmitter has not yet been determined, L29 neurons produce a broadening of the action potential similar to that produced by the SCPs and 5-HT. Therefore, we suggest in this diagram that the L29 effect on the sensory neurons may also be mediated via adenylate cyclase. The cAMP-dependent protein kinase is shown phosphorylating a number of substrate proteins, in addition to the protein responsible for the closure of the S-potassium channel. Thus, there is convergence at the beginning of the cAMP cascade and divergence at the end, with the phosphorylation of a family of substrate proteins. (Based on Abrams et al., 1984b; Glanzman et al., 1984.)

like 5-HT, the peptides produce their action by increasing cAMP levels in these sensory neurons (Abrams et al., 1984b). Thus, both small conventional transmitters such as 5-HT, and peptides such as SCP_A and SCP_B, can act through a common cAMP cascade to close the S-potassium channel. A similar convergence of ACh and luteinizing hormone releasing hormone (LHRH) for another potassium channel, the M-channel of vertebrates, was noted earlier by Adams and Brown (1980).

It appears likely that a third class of transmitters can also converge on the cyclase. Kistler et al. (1983, 1985), and Lloyd et al. (1985) have found that one group of identified facilitatory interneurons, the L29 cells, does not contain either the SCPs or 5-HT. These cells seem to use yet another facilitatory transmitter (Glanzman et al., 1984).

Thus, several transmitters can converge to produce presynaptic facilitation in the sensory neurons of the defensive withdrawal reflex. The three transmitters studied so far, the SCPs and 5-HT, all appear to act via the identical molecular cascade: cAMP-dependent closure of the S-potassium channel, broadening of the presynaptic action potential, increased calcium accumulation, and facilitation of transmitter release. Preliminary exploration of the action of L29 suggests that it may also engage this cascade, but more detailed comparisons will require identification of the L29 transmitter (Figure 24; see Glanzman et al., 1984).

AN OVERALL VIEW

Perspectives on Mediating and Modulating Synaptic Actions

The modern analysis of chemical transmission dates to the beginning of the twentieth century and to the work of John Langley (1906) and Henry Dale (1914). Langley appreciated that drugs do not act diffusely on target cells but bind to specific membrane sites. He called these sites *receptors* (see also Ehrlich, 1913). Thus, Langley found that nicotine produced its actions on muscle by acting on receptors localized to the end-plate region.

In the course of studying the esters and ethers of choline, Dale discovered ACh as a natural constituent of the brain. He then found that ACh simulated the actions of nicotine on muscle cells and those of muscarine on gland cells and smooth muscle. Dale therefore postulated that ACh produced two kinds of actions—nicotinic and muscarinic—by acting on two different receptors. The nicotinic receptor produced fast actions; the muscarinic receptor, slow actions.

Three quarters of a century later, we realize that in making this distinction, Dale (in his usual prescient manner) had in fact delineated the two prototype actions we now call fast *mediating* (nicotinic) and slow *modulating* (muscarinic). Indeed, nicotinic actions at the neuromuscular junction involve a receptor in which the recognition site for the ligand and the channel for ion translocation represent separate loci on a common macromolecule. By contrast, as Adams and his colleagues (Adams et al., 1982; Pennefather et al., 1985) and R. A. Nicoll and his colleagues (unpublished observations) have now shown, muscarinic receptors work in a manner analogous to the action of 5-HT on the S-channel—the muscarinic receptor activates a second messenger to close a potassium channel. Presumably here, as with the S-channel, the recognition site and the channel are different molecular entities.

Similar Modulatory Actions Have Now Been Encountered in Several Instances of Learning

Two instances of sensitization (gill and tail withdrawal reflexes in *Aplysia*), and four instances of classical conditioning (gill and tail withdrawal in *Aplysia*, leg lift in locust, and phototaxis in *Hermissenda*), have now been partially analyzed on the cellular level. All of these involve (at least in part) closure of a potassium channel. In *Hermissenda*, second messengers and protein phosphorylation are also thought to be involved much as they are in *Aplysia*. Although the specific potassium channel and the specific second messengers vary, closure of a potassium channel by second messenger-mediated protein phosphorylation is emerging as an important mechanism whereby learning alters both neuronal excitability and synaptic strength. Moreover, in each case the learning is selective rather than instructive. Learning does not involve the *de novo* formation of new synaptic contacts but a modulation in the strength of preexisting synaptic connections (for discussions of selective mechanisms, see Jerne, 1967; Edelman, 1979; Changeux et al., 1984).

These modulatory actions may also be important for controlling the behavior of vertebrates. Nicoll (1982, and unpublished observations) and Adams (Adams et al., 1982; Pennefather et al., 1985) have found that slow modulatory actions mediated by ACh, norepinephrine, and by certain peptides involving closure of a potassium channel by a second messenger, are important in regulating the excitability of neurons in the hippocampus and cerebral cortex. It will therefore be interesting to see to what degree simple forms of sensitization and classical conditioning in vertebrates also utilize these modulatory mechanisms.

Studies of Learning Have Also Given Us Insights into the Functions of the cAMP Cascade

Studies of modulatory action involved in learning have revealed new features not only about synaptic actions but also about the functioning of the cAMP cascade in nerve cells. We consider three of these features here: (1) sites of regulation within the cascade; (2) the generality of the cascade for learning; and (3) the importance of isozymes and other forms of molecular microheterogeneity in a universal molecular cascade.

There are Separate Points Within the cAMP Cascade that Mediate the Readout of Learning and the Timekeeping Step for Memory. The finding that the S-potassium channel is separate from the recognition site for 5-HT (the 5-HT receptor) illustrates one specific function of the cAMP cascade: to couple the information flow between the receptor and the channel. The cAMP cascade, in turn, has at least two major points of regulation: the *kinase* and the *cyclase*. We can now ask: What are their respective functions? Which, if any, of these is concerned with the time course of the memory? Studies by Castellucci et al. (1982, 1983), using selective inhibitors of the cyclase and the kinase, reveal that the kinase is concerned with the readout of the short-term memory, the closure of the potassium channel, and the regulation of transmitter release from the presynaptic nerve terminal. But this enzyme does not, as far as we can tell, determine the full time course of short-term memory. The time course is determined in part by the persistent activation of adenylate cyclase (Castellucci et al., 1983; Schwartz et al., 1983). Thus, by having the cyclase, the kinase, and the channel within a presynaptic terminal, a modulatory synaptic action can activate a complete *memory module* in which persistent activation of the cyclase by the modulating transmitter leads to a prolonged enhancement of transmitter release.

Thus, studies of learning illustrate how even in a simple memory process the key enzyme in a molecular cascade can have separate functions. Perhaps more surprising, however, is the suggestion that classical conditioning achieves amplification by the activation, through calcium influx, of calmodulin-sensitive adenylate cyclase. The existence of two species of cyclase has repeatedly raised the question: What is their distinctive physiological function? Our studies suggest that calcium/calmodulin cyclase serves as a molecular convergence point for an associative mechanism, a convergence that might depend upon allosteric properties of calmodulin-sensitive cyclase (for a discussion of allostery, see Changeux and Heidmann, this volume).

Different Sites of the cAMP Cascade Are Disrupted by Single Gene Learning Mutant in **Drosophila.**   One would expect that the most general features of a particular class of learning would emerge not only on the cellular but even more on the molecular level. This is indeed what appears to be happening. Evidence for the involvement of the cAMP cascade in learning is also emerging from the application of a genetic approach to the fruit fly, *Drosophila*. Seymour Benzer and his colleagues first used *Drosphila* to explore how single genes control behavior. Subsequently, Quinn et al. (1974) found that the fruit fly can be conditioned. Using genetic selection procedures, Dudai et al. (1976) and Quinn and his colleagues have isolated single gene mutants that fail to learn (for a review, see Quinn, 1984). Four of these learning mutants have now been studied in detail and have two interesting features. First, some of the mutants that are unable to learn by conditioning also cannot learn by sensitization. This finding suggests that in *Drosophila*, as in *Aplysia*, sensitization and classical conditioning share common molecular components. Second, all of the four learning mutants so far isolated have a defect in one or another step in the cAMP cascade. One lacks cAMP phosphodiesterase, the enzyme that degrades cAMP. As a result, the fly has abnormally high levels of cAMP that are thought to be out of the range of normal activation of the cAMP-dependent protein kinase. Other learning mutants have defects in the 5-HT receptor, biogenic amine transmitters, or calcium/calmodulin-dependent adenylate cyclase (Dudai and Zvi, 1984; Livingstone et al., 1984; Quinn, 1984). Thus, both cell biology approaches in *Aplysia* and genetic approaches in *Drosophila* indicate that the cAMP cascade is important in elementary forms of learning and memory storage.

The cAMP Cascade Has Both General and Particular Features.   The studies in *Drosophila* and in *Aplysia* also address an even broader question: How can a universal set of mechanisms such as cAMP-dependent protein phosphorylation be used for a highly specialized task such as learning? Every cell in the body has the machinery of the cAMP cascade. How then do some cells achieve the specificity necessary for learning? The results in *Aplysia* and in *Drosophila* indicate that although cAMP has a ubiquitous role in the organism, there are both circuit and molecular features that are more specific to learning than they are for other physiological processes (for earlier discussions of this point, see Schwartz et al., 1983; Livingstone et al., 1984).

First, learning derives a major part of its specificity from the precision of the neural connections, the wiring of the brain. Given that the developmental program establishes the basic circuit of a behavior, the underlying mechanism for learning may, at least in certain instances, be reduced to the strengthening (or weakening) of preexisting synaptic connections. Thus, the so-called biological constraints on learning—which have often been used as arguments against general mechanisms of learning—may simply represent biological constraints in the wiring. Learning cannot result from pairing any arbitrary CS and US, because only certain stimuli will be able to converge such that the US can facilitate the CS.

Second, only certain target cells and not others will have an adenylate cyclase coupled to the appropriate receptor for a given modulatory transmitter that is released by the facilitating neuron that ends on the target cell.

Third, of the very large family of *substrate proteins* of the cAMP-dependent protein kinase, only some will be present in *any particular cell*. Consider, for example, only the S-channel modulated by 5-HT and the substrate proteins responsible for the modulation of calcium handling by the cell in response to 5-HT. These proteins are present in the sensory neurons but seem, in functional tests, to be absent from many other nerve cells of the body. Other substrate proteins that are likely to be present in some, but not in other, cells include various channels, receptors, structural proteins, and even other kinases such as calcium/calmodulin kinase and protein kinase C.

Finally, and in some ways most interestingly, the proteins in the cAMP cascade—the cyclase, kinase, phosphodiesterase, and phosphatase—exist in multiple (isozymic) forms (Eppler et al., 1982). As a result, in any cell each of the isozymic forms may have slightly different functions, and different cells may preferentially utilize some of these isozymic forms but not others. Thus, whereas all cells have a calcium-independent cyclase, only some have a calcium-dependent one. Perhaps only these latter cells can be engaged in classical conditioning and other contingency-dependent processes.

In a broader sense, the heterogeneity provided by isozymic forms allows for parallel processing of information on the molecular level. As pointed out by Livingstone et al. (1984), the importance of parallel processing on the molecular level is particularly clear from studies of the *Drosophila* mutants, *dunce* and *rutabaga*. These have gross biochemical defects in cAMP metabolism, yet are behaviorally almost normal except when examined for learning. One might rather have expected that flies with major defects in an important enzyme, such as phosphodiesterase or adenylate cyclase, would not be viable. In both *dunce* and *rutabaga*, however, even though one enzyme seems to be missing, at least one other form of the same enzyme exists and is functional. Perhaps the existing forms of the enzyme fulfill the basic functions necessary for survival, whereas the missing form is generally the more dispensable form of the enzyme—the form that is primarily concerned with behavioral plasticity. Thus, there may be isoenzymes within the cAMP cascade that are more specifically related to the machinery for memory and less related to other more routine physiological functions. The finding by Schwartz and his colleagues (Eppler et al., 1982) that there are several types of regulatory subunits of cAMP-dependent protein kinase supports this possibility.

In the context of the universality of cellular mechanisms revealed by modern molecular biology, learning may be seen as a regulatory process that emerged in evolution by using preexisting molecular machinery, such as the cAMP cascade (and other second messenger systems), that already existed in cells for the coordination of other cellular processes.

A Major Question Persists: How Are Long-Term Changes in Synaptic Transmission Initiated and Maintained?

The modulatory actions we have considered last from minutes to hours and are only responsible for the short-term memory resulting from sensitization and classical conditioning. A task now facing those who study learning in *Aplysia* is to examine the modulation that underlies long-term memory lasting days or weeks. Do these processes involve extension of preexisting mechanisms or novel mechanisms? Does long-term memory involve covalent modification of preexisting proteins or the synthesis of new proteins? Clearly, the analysis of long-term synaptic modulation is still in its early stages. As a result, some of the most exciting molecular linkages between synaptic transmission and learning still await exploration!

ACKNOWLEDGMENTS

This work was supported by the Howard Hughes Medical Institute and the National Institute of Mental Health. We thank Louise Katz for preparing the figures, and Harriet Ayers and Andrew Krawetz for typing.

REFERENCES

Abrams, T. W., and E. R. Kandel (1985) Roles of calcium and adenylate cyclase in activity-dependent facilitation: A cellular mechanism for classical conditioning in *Aplysia*. *J. Neurochem. Abstr.* **44**:S12.

Abrams, T. W., T. J. Carew, R. D. Hawkins, and E. R. Kandel (1983) Aspects of the cellular mechanism of temporal specificity in conditioning in *Aplysia*: Preliminary evidence for Ca^{2+} influx as a signal of activity. *Soc. Neurosci. Abstr.* **9**:168.

Abrams, T. W., L. Bernier, R. D. Hawkins, and E. R. Kandel (1984a) Possible roles of Ca^{2+} and cAMP in activity-dependent facilitation, a mechanism for associative learning in *Aplysia*. *Soc. Neurosci. Abstr.* **10**:269.

Abrams, T. W., V. F. Castellucci, J. S. Camardo, E. R. Kandel, and P. E. Lloyd (1984b) Two endogenous neuropeptides modulate the gill and siphon withdrawal reflex in *Aplysia* by presynaptic facilitation involving cAMP-dependent closure of a serotonin-sensitive potassium channel. *Proc. Natl. Acad. Sci. USA* **81**:7956–7960.

Adams, P. R., and D. A. Brown (1980) Luteinizing hormone-releasing factor and muscarinic agonists act on the same voltage-dependent K^+-current in bullfrog sympathetic neurons. *Br. J. Pharmacol.* **68**:353–355.

Adams, P. R., D. A. Brown, and A. Constanti (1982) M currents and other potassium currents in bullfrog sympathetic neurones. *J. Physiol. (Lond.)* **330**:537–572.

Altamirano, M., C. W. Coates, and H. Grundfest (1955) Mechanisms of direct and neural excitability in electroplaque of electric eel. *J. Gen. Physiol.* **38**:319–360.

Belardetti, F., S. Schacher, E. R. Kandel, and S. A. Siegelbaum (1986) The growth cones of *Aplysia* sensory neurons—Modulation by serotonin of action-potential duration and single potassium channel currents. *Proc. Natl. Acad. Sci. USA* **83**:7094–7098.

Bennett, M. V. L. (1960) Electrical connections between supramedullary neurons. *Fed. Proc.* **19**:282.

Bennett, M. V. L. (1979) Electrical transmission: A functional analysis and comparison to chemical transmission. *Handb. Physiol.* **1**:357–416.

Bernier, L., V. F. Castellucci, E. R. Kandel, and J. H. Schwartz (1982) Facilitatory transmitter causes a selective and prolonged increase in adenosine 3':5'-monophosphate in sensory neurons mediating the gill and siphon withdrawal reflex in *Aplysia*. *J. Neurosci.* **2**:1682–1691.

Boyle, M. B., M. Klein, S. J. Smith, and E. R. Kandel (1984) Serotonin increases intracellular Ca^{2+} transients in voltage-clamped sensory neurons of *Aplysia californica*. *Proc. Natl. Acad. Sci. USA* **81**:7643–7646.

Brostrom, M. A., C. O. Brostrom, B. M. Breckenridge, and D. J. Wolff (1978) Calcium-dependent regulation of brain adenylate cyclase. *Adv. Cyclic Nucleotide Res.* **9**:85–99.

Brown, D. A., and P. R. Adams (1980) Muscarinic suppression of a novel voltage-sensitive K^+ current in a vertebrate neurone. *Nature* **283**:673–676.

Brown, G. L., H. H. Dale, and W. Feldberg (1936) Reactions of the normal mammalian muscle to acetylcholine and to eserine. *J. Physiol. (Lond.)* **87**:394–424.

Brunelli, M., V. F. Castellucci, and E. R. Kandel (1976) Synaptic facilitation and behavioral sensitization in *Aplysia*: Possible role of serotonin and cAMP. *Science* **194**:1178–1181.

Byrne, J., V. F. Castellucci, and E. R. Kandel (1974) Receptive fields and response properties of mechanoreceptor neurons innervating siphon skin and mantle shelf in *Aplysia*. *J. Neurophysiol.* **37**:1041–1064.

Carew, T. J., and E. R. Kandel (1976) Two functional effects of decreased conductance EPSPs: Synaptic augmentation and increased electrotonic coupling. *Science* **192**:150–153.

Carew, T. J., V. F. Castellucci, and E. R. Kandel (1971) An analysis of dishabituation and sensitization of the gill-withdrawal reflex in *Aplysia*. *Int. J. Neurosci.* **2**:79–98.

Carew. T. J., E. T. Walters, and E. R. Kandel (1981) Classical conditioning in a simple withdrawal reflex in *Aplysia californica*. *J. Neurosci.* **1**:1426–1437.

Carew, T. J., R. D. Hawkins, and E. R. Kandel (1983) Differential classical conditioning of a defensive withdrawal reflex in *Aplysia californica*. *Science* **219**:397–400.

Castellucci, V. F., and E. R. Kandel (1976) Presynaptic facilitation as a mechanism for behavioral sensitization in *Aplysia*. *Science* **194**:1176–1178.

Castellucci, V. F., E. R. Kandel, J. H. Schwartz, F. D. Wilson, A. C. Nairn, and P. Greengard (1980) Intracellular injection of the catalytic subunit of cyclic AMP-dependent protein kinase simulates facilitation of transmitter release underlying behavioral sensitization in *Aplysia*. *Proc. Natl. Acad. Sci. USA* **77**:7492–7496.

Castellucci, V. F., A. Nairn, P. Greengard, J. H. Schwartz, and E. R. Kandel (1982) Inhibitor of adenosine 3':5'-monophosphate-dependent protein kinase blocks presynaptic facilitation in *Aplysia*. *J. Neurosci.* **2**:1673–1681.

Castellucci, V. F., L. Bernier, J. H. Schwartz, and E. R. Kandel (1983) Persistent activation of adenylate cyclase underlies the time course of short-term sensitization in *Aplysia*. *Soc. Neurosci. Abstr.* **9**:169.

Changeux, J.-P., T. Heidemann, and P. Patte (1984) Learning by selection. In *The Biology of Learning*, P. Marler and H. S. Terrace, eds., pp. 115–133, Springer, Berlin.

Clark, G. A. (1984) A cellular mechanism for the temporal specificity of classical conditioning of the siphon-withdrawal response in *Aplysia*. *Soc. Neurosci. Abstr.* **10**:268.

Dale, H. H. (1914) The action of certain esters and ethers of choline, and their relation to muscarine. *J. Physiol. (Lond.)* **6**:147–190.

Dale, H. H., W. Feldberg, and M. Vogt (1936) Release of acetylcholine at voluntary motor nerve endings. *J. Physiol. (Lond.)* **86**:353–380.

Dudai, Y., and S. Zvi (1984) Adenylate cyclase in the *Drosophila* memory mutant *rutabaga* displays an altered Ca^{2+} sensitivity. *Neurosci. Lett.* **47**:119–124.

Dudai, Y., Y.-N. Jan, D. Byers, W. G. Quinn, and S. Benzer (1976) *Dunce*, a mutant of *Drosophila* deficient in learning. *Proc. Natl. Acad. Sci. USA* **73**:1684–1688.

Dudel, J., and S. W. Kuffler (1961) Presynaptic inhibition at the crayfish neuromuscular junction. *J. Physiol. (Lond.)* **155**:543–562.

Eccles, J. C. (1936) Synaptic and neuromuscular transmission. *Ergeb. Physiol. Biol. Chem. Exp. Pharmakol.* **38**:339–444.

Eccles, J. C. (1949) A review and restatement of the electrical hypothesis of synaptic excitatory and inhibitory action. *Arch. Sci. Physiol.* **3**:567–584.

Eccles, J. C. (1953) *The Neurophysiological Basis of Mind*, Oxford Univ. Press, Oxford.

Eccles, J. C. (1957) *The Physiology of Nerve Cells*, Johns Hopkins Univ. Press, Baltimore.

Eccles, J. C. (1964) *The Physiology of Synapses*, Springer, Berlin.

Edelman, G. M. (1979) Group selection and phasic reentrant signaling: A theory of higher brain function. In *The Neurosciences: Fourth Study Program*, F. O. Schmitt and F. G. Worden, eds., pp. 1115–1140, MIT Press, Cambridge, Massachusetts.

Ehrlich, P. (1913) Chemotherapeutics: Scientific principles, methods, and results. *Lancet* **2**:445–451.

Eppler, C. M., M. J. Palazzolo, and J. H. Schwartz (1982) Characterization and localization of adenosine 3':5'-monophosphate-binding proteins in the nervous system of *Aplysia*. *J. Neurosci.* **2**:1692–1704.

Erlanger, J. (1939) The initiation of impulses in axons. *J. Neurophysiol.* **2**:370–379.

Fatt, P. (1954) Biophysics of junctional transmission. *Physiol. Rev.* **34**:674–710.

Fatt, P., and B. Katz (1951) An analysis of the end-plate potential recorded with an intra-cellular electrode. *J. Physiol. (Lond.)* **115**:320–370.

Feldberg, W., and J. H. Gaddum (1934) The chemical transmitter at synapses in a sympathetic ganglion. *J. Physiol. (Lond.)* **81**:205–319.

Frank, K., and M. G. F. Fuortes (1957) Presynaptic and postsynaptic inhibition of neurosynaptic reflex. *Fed. Proc.* **16**:39–40.

Freud, S. (1894) in Freud, S. (1950) *Aus den Anfängen der Psychoanalyse: Briefe an Wilhelm Fliess, Abhandlungen und Notizen aus den Jahre 1887–1902*, M. Bonaparte, A. Freud, and E. Kris, eds., Imago, London.

Frost, W. N., and E. R. Kandel (1984) Sensitizing stimuli reduce the effectiveness of the L30 inhibitory interneurons in the siphon withdrawal reflex circuit of *Aplysia*. *Soc. Neurosci. Abstr.* **10**:510.

Furshpan, E. J., and D. D. Potter (1957) Mechanism of nerve-impulse transmission at a crayfish synapse. *Nature* **180**:342–343.

Gasser, H. (1939) Axons as samples of nervous tissue. *J. Neurophysiol.* **2**:361–369.

Gingrich, K. J., and J. H. Byrne (1985) Simulation of synaptic depression, post-tetanic potentiation and presynaptic facilitation of synaptic potentials from sensory neurons mediating gill-withdrawal reflex in *Aplysia*. *J. Neurophysiol.* **53**:652–669.

Glanzman, D. L., T. W. Abrams, R. D. Hawkins, and E. R. Kandel (1984) Extracts of L29 interneurons produce spike-broadening in sensory neurons of *Aplysia*. *Soc. Neurosci. Abstr.* **10**:510.

Grundfest, H. (1952) General neurophysiology. In *Progress in Neurology and Psychiatry*, Vol. 7, E. A. Spiegel, ed., pp. 13–58, Grune & Stratton, New York.

Grundfest, H. (1956) Some properties of excitable tissue. In *Fifth Conference on the Nerve Impulse*, Davis Nachmansohn and H. Houston Merritt, eds., pp. 177–218, Josiah Macy, Jr. Foundation, New York.

Grundfest, H. (1957) The mechanisms of discharge of the electric organs in relation to general and comparative physiology. *Progr. Biophys.* **7**:1–85.

Grundfest, H. (1959) Synaptic and ephaptic transmission. *Handb. Physiol.* **1**:147–197.

Hawkins, R. D., T. W. Abrams, T. J. Carew, and E. R. Kandel (1983a). A cellular mechanism of classical conditioning in *Aplysia*: Activity-dependent amplification of presynaptic facilitation. *Science* **219**:400–405.

Hawkins, R. D., T. J. Carew, and E. R. Kandel (1983b) Effects of interstimulus interval and contingency on classical conditioning in *Aplysia*. *Soc. Neurosci. Abstr.* **9**:168.

Hochner, B., M. Klein, S. Schacher, and E. R. Kandel (1986a) Action-potential duration and the modulation of transmitter release from the sensory neurons of *Aplysia* in presynaptic facilitation and behavioral sensitization. *Proc. Natl. Acad. Sci. USA* **83**:8410–8414.

Hochner, B., M. Klein, S. Schacher, E. R. Kandel (1986b) Additional component in the cellular mechanism of presynaptic facilitation contributes to behavioral dishabituation in *Aplysia*. *Proc. Natl. Acad. Sci. USA* **83**:8794–8798.

Hodgkin, A. L. (1937) Evidence for electrical transmission in nerve. *J. Physiol. (Lond.)* **90**:183–232.

Jan, L. Y., and Y. N. Jan (1982) Peptidergic transmission in sympathetic ganglia of the frog. *J. Physiol. (Lond.)* **327**:219–246.

Jerne, N. K. (1967) Antibodies and learning: Selection versus instruction. In *The Neurosciences: A Study Program*, G. C. Quarton, T. Melnechuk, and F. O. Schmitt, eds., pp. 200–205, Rockefeller Univ. Press, New York.

Kamin, L. J. (1969) Predictability, surprise, attention and conditioning. In *Punishment and Aversive Behavior*, B. A. Campbell and R. M. Church, eds., pp. 279–296, Appleton-Century-Croft, New York.

Kandel, E. R., and L. Tauc (1965a) Heterosynaptic facilitation in neurones of the abdominal ganglion of *Aplysia depilans*. *J. Physiol. (Lond.)* **181**:1–27.

Kandel, E. R., and L. Tauc (1965b) Mechanism of heterosynaptic facilitation in the giant cell of the abdominal ganglion of *Aplysia depilans*. *J. Physiol. (Lond.)* **181**:28–47.

Kandel, E. R., T. M. Abrams, L. Bernier, T. J. Carew, R. D. Hawkins, and J. H. Schwartz (1983) Classical conditioning and sensitization share aspects of the same molecular cascade in *Aplysia*. *Cold Spring Harbor Symp. Quant. Biol.* **48**:821–830.

Karlin, A., R. Cox, R.-R. Kaldany, P. Lobel, and E. Holtzman (1983) The arrangement and functions of the chains of the acetylcholine receptor of *Torpedo* electric tissue. *Cold Spring Harbor Symp. Quant. Biol.* **48**:1–8.

Katz, B. (1939) *Mechanical Excitation of Nerve*, Oxford Univ. Press, London.

Katz, B. (1966) *Nerve, Muscle, and Synapse*, McGraw-Hill, New York.

Kistler, H. B., R. D. Hawkins, J. Koester, E. R. Kandel, and J. H. Schwartz (1983) Immunocytochemical studies of neurons producing presynaptic facilitation in the abdominal ganglion of *Aplysia californica*. *Soc. Neurosci. Abstr.* **9**:915.

Kistler, H. B., R. D. Hawkins, J. Koester, M. W. M. Steinbusch, E. R. Kandel, and J. H. Schwartz (1985) Distribution of serotonin-immunoreactive cell bodies and processes in the abdominal ganglion of mature *Aplysia*. *J. Neurosci.* **5**:72–80.

Klein, M., and E. R. Kandel (1978) Presynaptic modulation of voltage-dependent Ca^{2+} current: Mechanism for behavioral sensitization. *Proc. Natl. Acad. Sci. USA* **75**:3512–3516.

Klein, M., and E. R. Kandel (1980) Mechanism of calcium current modulation underlying presynaptic facilitation and behavioral sensitization in *Aplysia*. *Proc. Natl. Acad. Sci. USA* **77**:6912–6916.

Klein, M., E. Shapiro, and E. R. Kandel (1980) Synaptic plasticity and the modulation of the Ca^{2+} current. *J. Exp. Biol.* **89**:117–157.

Klein, M., J. Camardo, and E. R. Kandel (1982) Serotonin modulates a specific potassium current in the sensory neurons that show presynaptic facilitation in *Aplysia*. *Proc. Natl. Acad. Sci. USA* **79**:5713–5717.

Klein, M., B. Hochner, and E. R. Kandel (1986) Facilitatory transmitters and cAMP can modulate accommodation as well as transmitter release in *Aplysia* sensory neurons: Evidence for parallel processing in a single cell. *Proc. Natl. Acad. Sci. USA* **83**:7994–7998.

Langley, J. N. (1906) On nerve endings and on special excitable substances in cells. *Proc. R. Soc. Lond. (Biol.)* **78**:170–194.

Livingstone, M. S., P. P. Sziber, and W. G. Quinn (1984) Loss of calcium/calmodulin responsiveness in adenylate cyclase of *rutabaga*, a *Drosophila* learning mutant. *Cell* **37**:205–215.

Lloyd, P. E., A. C. Mahon, I. Kupfermann, J. L. Cohen, R. J. Scheller, and K. R. Weis (1985) Biochemical and immunocytological localization of molluscan small cardioactive peptides (SCRs) in the nervous system of *Aplysia californica*. *J. Neurosci.* **5**:1851–1861.

Loewi, O. (1921) Über humorale Übertragbarkeit der Herznervenwirkung. I. Mitteilung. *Pflügers Arch. Gesamte Physiol. Menschen Tiere* **189**:239–242.

Loewi, O., and E. Navratil (1926) Über humorale Übertragbarkeit der Herznervenwirkung. X. Mitteilung über das schickgal des vagusstoffs. *Pflügers Arch. Gesamte Physiol. Menschen Tiere* **214**:678–688.

Lorente de Nó, R. (1939) Transmission of impulse through cranial nerve nuclei. *J. Neurophysiol.* **2**:402–464.

Marnay, A., and D. Nachmansohn (1937) Sur la répartition de la cholinesterase dans la muscle couturier de la grenouille. *C. R. Soc. Biol.* (Paris) **125**:41–43.

Neher, E., and B. Sakmann (1976) Single-channel current recorded from membrane of denervated frog muscle fibres. *Nature* **260**:799–802.

Nestler, E. J., and P. Greengard (1984) *Protein Phosphorylation in the Nervous System*, Wiley, New York.

Nicoll, R. A. (1982) Neurotransmitters can say more than just "yes" or "no." *Trends Neurosci.* **5**:369–374.

Numa, S., M. Noda, H. Takahashi, T. Tanabe, M. Toyosato, Y. Furutani, and S. Kikyotani (1983) Molecular structure of the nicotinic acetylcholine receptor. *Cold Spring Harbor Symp. Quant. Biol.* **48**:57–69.

Ocorr, K. A., E. T. Walters, and J. H. Byrne (1985) Associative conditioning analog selectively increases cAMP levels of tail sensory neurons in Aplysia. *Proc. Natl. Acad. Sci. USA* **82**:2548–2552.

Paupardin-Tritsch, D., P. Deterre, and H. M. Gerschenfeld (1981) Relationship between two voltage-dependent serotonin responses of molluscan neurones. *Brain Res.* **217**:201–206.

Pennefather, P., B. Lancaster, P. R. Adams, and R. A. Nicholl (1985) Two distinct Ca-dependent K currents in bullfrog sympathetic ganglion cells. *Proc. Natl. Acad. Sci. USA* **82**:3040–3044.

Pinsker, H. M., W. A. Hening, T. J. Carew, and E. R. Kandel (1973) Long-term sensitization of a defensive withdrawal reflex in Aplysia. *Science* **182**:1039–1042.

Quinn, W. G. (1984) Work in invertebrates on the mechanisms underlying learning. In *The Biology of Learning*, P. Marler and H. S. Terrace, eds., pp. 197–246, Springer, Berlin.

Quinn, W. G., W. A. Harris, and S. Benzer (1974) Conditioned behavior in Drosophila melanogaster. *Proc. Natl. Acad. Sci. USA* **71**:708–712.

Ramón y Cajal, S. (1894) La fine structure des centres nerveux. *Proc. R. Soc. Lond. (Biol.)* **55**:444–468.

Rescorla, R. A. (1968) Probability of shock in the presence and absence of CS in fear conditioning. *J. Comp. Physiol. Psychol.* **66**:1–5.

Schramm, M., and Z. Selinger (1984) Message transmission: Receptor-controlled adenylate cyclase system. *Science* **225**:1350–1356.

Schwartz, J. H., L. Bernier, V. F. Castellucci, M. Palazzolo, T. Saitoh, A. Stapleton, and E. R. Kandel (1983) What molecular steps determine the time course of the memory for short-term sensitization in Aplysia? *Cold Spring Harbor Symp. Quant. Biol.* **48**:811–819.

Shuster, M., J. S. Camardo, S. A. Siegelbaum, and E. R. Kandel (1985) Cyclic AMP-dependent protein kinase closes the serotonin-sensitive K^+ channels of Aplysia sensory neurones in cell-free membrane patches. *Nature* **313**:392–395.

Siegelbaum, S. A., J. S. Camardo, and E. R. Kandel (1982) Serotonin and cyclic AMP close single K^+ channels in Aplysia sensory neurones. *Nature* **299**:413–417.

Weight, F. F., and J. Votava (1970) Slow synaptic excitation in sympathetic ganglion cells: Evidence for synaptic inactivation of potassium conductance. *Science* **170**:755–758.

Chapter 20

Calcium-Activated Proteases as Possible Mediators of Synaptic Plasticity

ROBERT SIMAN
MICHEL BAUDRY
GARY S. LYNCH

ABSTRACT

It is now established that the physiology and ultrastructure of synapses in adult mammalian brain can undergo long-lasting modification. In this chapter, we review the evidence that a calcium-activated proteolytic enzyme may be critically involved in synaptic modification. Synaptic membrane preparations from rat forebrain contain calpain I, a protease activated by micromolar calcium concentrations. Immunocytochemical studies confirm the neuronal localization of calpain I. Upon activation, calpain I degrades fodrin (brain spectrin), a major neuronal structural protein. It is shown that submembranous fodrin exerts transmembrane control over the distribution of proteins within the synaptic membrane, and that this control is modified by calpain I. This mechanism is postulated to be initiated by an activity-dependent postsynaptic calcium influx. Protease activation is also a candidate for the induction of changes in synaptic ultrastructure. In an erythrocyte ghost model system, calpain I activation produces structural protein breakdown and a shape change. It is proposed that the protease may function in a similar manner to modulate the shape of dendritic spines. The calpain I mechanism thus has properties expected of an inducer of synaptic modification: It is likely to be triggered by brief physiological events, it is specifically induced at intensely activated synapses, and it produces long-lived changes in synaptic membranes and perhaps ultrastructure.

In addition to possible mediation of synaptic plasticity in adulthood, the involvement of calpains in growth processes in developing neurons is considered. The idea is advanced that calpains may be determinants of dendritic growth, with respect to both its onset and its ultimate extent.

The idea that synapses are modifiable dates back to at least the early part of this century (e.g., Ramón y Cajal, 1929) and is so conceptually appealing that it is a common, if not ubiquitous, feature of ideas and hypotheses about memory (see Hinton and Anderson, 1981). The assumption that memory involves changes in neuronal connections seems all the more plausible in light of recent demonstrations that brief periods of physiological activity can produce stable modifications in the operating characteristics, ultrastructure, and chemistry of brain synapses. Understanding how transient events can have such long-term consequences represents a major challenge for neurobiology. Most cellular chemistries are concerned with processes that are rapid and fully reversible (e.g., transmitter release, ion fluxes) and a priori seem ill suited for a role in the production of effects like memory that can persist for extremely long periods. Nonetheless, ingenious hypotheses have been devised to explain long-term phenomena in terms of posttranslational covalent modifications of proteins and other reactions typically thought of as transient (Kandel and Schwartz, 1982). However, neurons also contain biochemical processes that produce essentially irreversible effects, and it is surprising that little attention has been given to the possibility that reactions of this type are involved in synaptic modification. This is the subject of the present review. We describe a proteolytic enzyme found in brain that degrades membrane-associated proteins that are likely to be critical for synaptic chemistry and ultrastructure. The argument is made that the conditions for the activation, the localization, and the substrates of this protease are such as to make it an excellent candidate for an agent that converts physiological activity into long-term alterations in synaptic connections. We begin with a short summary of the types of changes known to occur in brain synapses after brief periods of intense synaptic stimulation; this material will be used to suggest some limiting conditions for mechanisms of brain plasticity.

LASTING EFFECTS OF PHYSIOLOGICAL ACTIVITY ON THE STRUCTURE AND FUNCTION OF BRAIN SYNAPSES

Brief periods of electrical stimulation delivered at high frequencies to any of several pathways in hippocampus produce a potentiation of synaptic responses that can last for weeks (Bliss and Gardner-Medwin, 1973; Bliss and Lømo, 1973). This effect has been the subject of several reviews (see Swanson et al., 1982; Eccles, 1983; Lynch and Baudry, 1983; Seifert, 1983), and here we list only some of its prominent features:

Selectivity. Induction of long-term potentiation (LTP) in one group of synapses does not necessarily change responses in neighboring contacts (Andersen et al., 1977; Lynch et al., 1977; Dunwiddie and Lynch, 1978).

Cooperativity. LTP is more easily elicited and is greater in magnitude when large numbers of overlapping afferents are simultaneously stimulated at high frequencies (McNaughton et al., 1978; Levy and Steward, 1980; Barrionuevo and Brown, 1983; Lee, 1983).

Duration. There is evidence that at least two forms of LTP follow the high-frequency trains, one with a half-life of several hours, the other lasting for days or weeks (Racine et al., 1983). There is indirect evidence suggesting that these have different substrates (for a discussion, see Lynch and Baudry, 1984).

Additivity. Repeated episodes of high-frequency stimulation produce increasing degrees of potentiation; maximal effects are obtained only after several bursts of activity, even when these are widely separated in time (Bliss and Gardner-Medwin, 1973; Barnes, 1979).

As might be expected from its selectivity, LTP is not accompanied by changes in the resting membrane potentials or biophysical characteristics of the neuron, at least as recorded from the cell body (Andersen et al., 1977; Barrionuevo and Brown, 1983). It appears simply as an increase in the amplitude of the EPSP produced by the stimulation of a fixed population of axons.

Considerable work has been directed at identifying the triggers of LTP and establishing if LTP is due to changes in pre- and/or postsynaptic elements. Figure 1 summarizes a recent study from our laboratory that strongly suggests that the effect is due to dendritic modifications and that calcium is involved in its production. In this experiment, the calcium chelator EGTA was injected into hippocampal neurons and attempts were made to elicit LTP by high-frequency stimulation of the cell's afferents. In accord with previous work (Alger and Nicoll, 1980; Schwartzkroin and Stafstrom, 1980), EGTA had little discernable effect on the baseline properties of the cells, although it blocked a suspected calcium-mediated current. However, EGTA did greatly reduce the probability of eliciting LTP, this despite the fact that LTP was clearly observed in field potentials generated by neighboring neurons (Lynch et al., 1983).

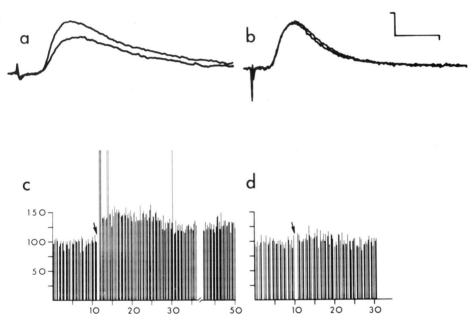

Figure 1.   *Excitatory postsynaptic potentials (EPSPs) recorded from hippocampal cells with a normal electrode (a) or one filled with EGTA (b). Two computer-averaged records are shown for each case; the first of these was collected immediately prior to a brief burst of high-frequency afferent stimulation and the second 20 min after the burst. The second response recorded from the control cell is potentiated; that from the EGTA-filled cell is unchanged. (Note that the two traces in b are virtually identical.) Calibration bars = 5 mV (vertical) and 20 msec (horizontal). c and d are graphs of the amplitudes of individual EPSPs collected from the two cells (expressed as percentage of the average for cell responses collected prior to the high-frequency burst). The X-axis is calibrated in minutes. The arrows indicate the point at which the high-frequency stimulation was applied. The extreme values seen in c immediately after the stimulation bursts are occasions on which the neurons emitted an action potential. As is evident, the control cell exhibited stable, long-term potentiation, whereas the EGTA-filled neuron did not. (From Lynch et al., 1983.)*

The long-lasting nature of LTP has suggested to many investigators that it is caused by some type of structural change. From the physiological work described immediately above, we should expect these changes to be found in the dendritic zones in the immediate vicinity of the synapses. These points have been confirmed. Electron microscope examination of the regions containing the potentiated connections resulted in the discovery that the dendritic spines had become rounder and that new synapses had formed on the shafts of the dendrites after the induction of LTP (Lee et al., 1980, 1981). Both effects were obtained in anesthetized rats and in *in vitro* slices of hippocampus. Recently, this pattern of results has been replicated by another laboratory, which made the additional observation that the number of small nub synapses was also increased (Chang and Greenough, 1984). These workers found that some of the structural modifications persisted through the longest time point tested (12 hours) and were highly correlated with the occurrence of LTP.

LTP is also associated with changes in synaptic chemistry. The transmitter used by hippocampal pathways remains uncertain, but considerable evidence points to an acidic amino acid (probably glutamate or aspartate); related to this, ligand binding experiments have identified a glutamate binding site that has characteristics expected of the postsynaptic receptor for the endogenous transmitter (Baudry and Lynch, 1981, 1984). Two studies have now shown that high-frequency stimulation of the type that produces LTP causes an increase in glutamate binding, apparently by increasing the number, but not the affinity, of the suspected receptor sites (Baudry et al., 1980; Lynch et al., 1982). Moreover, these effects were obtained only in preparations that exhibited physiological evidence of potentiation. Thus, high-frequency activity of very brief duration produces extremely persistent physiological, structural, and biochemical changes in hippocampal synapses, and the latter two effects are correlated with the first. Moreover, the physiological changes have been well defined and linked to what must be transient elevations of intracellular calcium levels in postsynaptic neurons.

This pattern of results tells us that hippocampus must possess cellular mechanisms capable of producing synaptic modification and moreover provides a reasonably precise description of this mechanism. That is, the chemistry underlying the effects under discussion appears to have the following features:

1. Localization in the region surrounding the synapses. This follows from the selectivity feature of LTP and from the restricted localization of the structural changes correlated with it.
2. Rapid action. The physiological, chemical, and structural changes described above develop within minutes of the high-frequency bursts of afferent activity.
3. Stimulated by transient changes in calcium levels. The EGTA experiments implicate calcium in the induction of LTP, while the selectivity and occurrence of LTP against a background of normal cell physiology indicate that the perturbations of cation levels must be extremely brief.
4. Produces structural modifications including shape change and new contacts, as well as reorganization of membrane surface receptors.

This is a demanding set of criteria, and it can be used to exclude a large number of biochemical mechanisms, but as reviewed in the following sections, it can be accommodated by a specific enzymatic process.

SOLUBLE AND MEMBRANE-ASSOCIATED CALCIUM-ACTIVATED PROTEASES IN BRAIN

Calcium-activated proteolytic enzymes are potentially important intraneuronal mediators of plasticity of the types described in the preceding section. Foremost among the characteristics that suggest such a function are the dual properties of inducing irreversible effects and strict dependence on the presence of calcium ions. Thus, in a relatively short burst of activity, proteases could bring about large-scale and long-lasting changes in structural or information-bearing proteins. In addition, even a protease requiring low micromolar calcium concentrations for activation would likely be inactive inside quiescent neurons, but could be activated under conditions that evoke a significant rise in intraneuronal free calcium levels.

Brain tissue has been known for a number of years to contain calcium-stimulated proteolytic activity (Guroff, 1964), but its requirement of millimolar calcium concentrations for activation called into question its possible physiological functions. However, more recent studies have demonstrated that rat brain contains a protease activated by low micromolar calcium concentrations (Baudry et al., 1981; Murachi et al., 1981a,b; Zimmerman and Schlaepfer, 1982; Siman et al., 1983a). This high-sensitivity enzyme is present not only in soluble fractions but also in synaptosomal plasma membrane (SPM) fractions prepared from rat forebrain.

Initial suggestions that rat forebrain SPMs contain a high-sensitivity, calcium-dependent protease were made on the basis of various indirect observations. Incubating rat forebrain SPMs in the presence of low micromolar concentrations of calcium resulted in two types of effects: (1) a decrease in the content of two high molecular weight polypeptides identified on SDS-polyacrylamide gels, and (2) an increase in the number of binding sites for the putative neurotransmitter L-glutamate (Baudry et al., 1981a). Both of these effects could be blocked by the thiol-protease inhibitor leupeptin when it is added before, but not after, calcium (Baudry et al., 1981a, 1983a). Additionally, both effects were rapid in onset, requiring less than 10 min for maximal expression, and were long-lasting in that they persisted after the removal of calcium. These experiments provided evidence that rat forebrain SPMs contain a protease that is activated by low micromolar calcium levels, induces the breakdown of endogenous polypeptides, and increases the number of available glutamate binding sites.

Direct evidence that SPMs contain a protease with the properties described above was obtained by extraction and partial purification of calcium-activated proteases from SPMs (Siman et al., 1983a). A low ionic strength extract from rat brain SPMs contained proteolytic activity against such exogenous substrates as casein. Although the caseinolytic activity primarily required 200 μM calcium or more, some activity could be detected at lower calcium concentrations. Similar observations have been made for protease activity in cytoplasmic fractions prepared from brain, liver, skeletal and heart muscle, and other tissues (Mellgren, 1980; Dayton et al., 1981; DeMartino, 1981; Murachi et al., 1981a). In these reports, multiple proteases with different sensitivities to activation by calcium could be separated by ion exchange chromatography on DEAE-cellulose. By using the same approach, we found that the SPM extract contained at least two proteases that had different requirements for calcium (Figure 2). One enzyme could be activated by the same low micromolar calcium levels that in SPMs were found to cause the polypeptide breakdown and the increase in glutamate binding site number. The other protease required more than 200 μM calcium for activation and accounted for more than 90% of the total protease activity in the extract.

The cytoplasmic proteases found in many mammalian cells and tissues share a number of properties and have been given the family name of "calpain," with the high and low calcium sensitivity forms (activated, respectively, by 5–30 μM

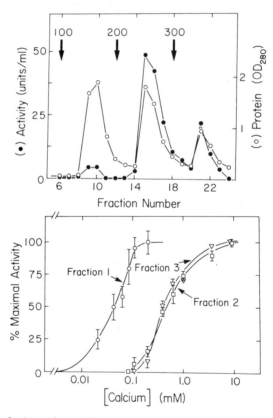

Figure 2. *Separation by ion exchange chromatography of multiple calcium proteases. Top: A low ionic strength extract of rat brain synaptosomal plasma membranes was fractionated on a DEAE-cellulose column. Aliquots of each fraction were assayed for calcium-stimulated (5 mM) proteolysis of a casein substrate. The amounts of sodium chloride (mM) included in the column buffer are indicated at the arrows. Bottom: Calcium sensitivities of proteases collected from the DEAE-cellulose column. Note that the peak of activity eluted at 100 mM sodium chloride (Fraction 1) is half-maximally active at about 30 μM calcium, a dose more than 10 times lower than that required for activation of the protease(s) eluted at 200–300 mM sodium chloride (Fractions 2 and 3).*

Table 1.   Similarities Between Membrane-
Associated Proteases and Calpains I and II

Calcium sensitivities
Cation selectivities
Inhibitors
Approx. molecular weights
DEAE-cellulose elution profiles
Autolysis
Reducing agent requirement
Neutral pH requirement

Source: From Murachi et al., 1981a; Siman; 1983a.

and 200–500 μM) designated as calpain I and calpain II (Murachi et al., 1981a).
The two calcium-stimulated proteases present in rat brain SPMs are also members
of this enzyme family. The similarities between the SPM-associated proteases
and cytoplasmic calpains I and II that have been uncovered to date are summarized
in Table 1. Their basic properties are similar in many respects, but the structural
details of the SPM-associated enzymes and of many of the cytoplasmic enzymes
from other tissues are not yet available. Best characterized among the calpain I-
type proteases are the erythrocyte, kidney, and skeletal muscle varieties, which
have been purified to homogeneity (Dayton, 1982; Melloni et al., 1982; Yoshimura
et al., 1983). Each of these is composed of two subunits of molecular weights
80–85 kD and 25–30 kD, with the higher molecular weight subunit possessing
the catalytic activity. Although the lower molecular weight subunit is of unknown
function, it is clearly a component of the native enzyme, as it copurifies with
the catalytic subunit in a stoichiometric amount (Dayton, 1982; Melloni et al.,
1982; Yoshimura et al., 1983) and can be immunoprecipitated by a monoclonal
antibody directed against and selective for the catalytic subunit (Siman et al.,
1985b). The catalytic subunits of calpain I-type proteases prepared from different
tissues of a single species are relatively similar, since they are all recognized by
antibodies against the kidney calpain catalytic subunit (Hatanaka et al., 1984).
On the other hand, such antibodies react only weakly or negligibly with calpain
II, and antibodies against calpain II do not recognize any of the calpain I-type
proteases (Sasaki et al., 1983; Hatanaka et al., 1984). In view of these apparent
structural differences, it is unlikely that calpains I and II are interconvertible
forms of a single protein. Preliminary evidence indicates that the SPM-associated
calpain I is similar to its cytoplasmic counterpart, as monoclonal antibodies
against the erythrocyte cytosolic catalytic subunit recognize the brain membrane
enzyme (Siman et al., 1985b). As these studies of calpain I are in their infancy,
it will be of interest in future work to detail structural and functional similarities
or differences between the enzymes from various species, tissues, and subcellular
compartments.

The presence of freely soluble as well as membrane-associated calcium-dependent proteases in neurons raises a number of important questions. In contrast
to proteases found in lysosomes that mainly degrade substrates transported
inside vesicles, the former proteases present a potential hazard for the normal

function of key cellular processes and constituents. Fortunately, several constraints restrict the destructive capabilities of these extralysosomal proteases. These are: (1) the absolute requirement of calpains for calcium for activation; (2) the coexistence in tissues of a specific inhibitor protein of the calpains, termed "calpastatin"; (3) the compartmentalization of calpains within cells, which limits the accessibility of the proteases to potential substrates; and (4) the restricted substrate specificities of the calpains.

Most prominent among the constraints listed above is the absolute need for free calcium to activate the enzyme, as mentioned previously. Other divalent cations are either weak or totally ineffective substitutes for calcium. Although few data are available for mammalian central neurons, intraneuronal free calcium levels are thought to be buffered to less than 1 μM (Dipolo et al., 1976), while even the high-sensitivity calpain I requires 5–30 μM calcium for activation. Thus, it is likely that calpains are inactive or only weakly active in neurons at rest. However, a number of observations suggest that a substantial rise in intraneuronal free calcium levels occurs during periods of intense neuronal activity. These

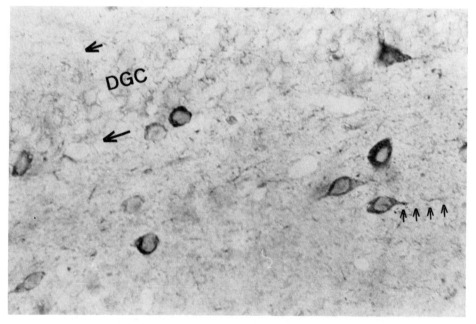

Figure 3. *Immunocytochemical localization of calpain I in rat dentate gyrus.* Monoclonal antibodies were prepared against rat erythrocyte cytosolic calpain I (Siman et al., 1985b). Hybridomas were selected that secreted antibodies which recognize the 80-kD catalytic subunit, as evidenced by immunoblotting. The antibody used in this experiment reacted on immunoblots with an 80-kD polypeptide in rat brain homogenate. The brain was fixed by intracardiac perfusion with 4% paraformaldehyde/0.1% glutaraldehyde. Transverse sections through the hippocampal formation, 40 μm thick, were treated with ascites fluid at 1:500 dilution. Bound antibody was visualized using an avidin–biotin–peroxidase method. Note the intense labeling of hilar polymorph neurons and the comparatively light annular staining of dentate granule cells (DGC; layer enclosed by *large arrows*). Glial cells are unstained. The dendritic processes of polymorph cells are distinctly stained (*small arrows*).

include the opening of voltage-sensitive calcium channels accompanying membrane depolarization (Hagiwara and Byerly, 1981), a substantial decline in extracellular calcium levels (Nicholson et al., 1977) and calcium accumulation in activated and postsynaptic structures (Fifková et al., 1983). Taken together, these studies point to a localized rise in intracellular calcium content at active synapses, and suggest that intense synaptic activity may provide sufficient calcium for at least transient calpain I activation.

In addition to those imposed by calcium levels, there are constraints placed on calpain activity by the coexistence in brain of calpastatin, a protein inhibitor of the calpains (Murachi et al., 1981a,b; Simonson et al., 1984). In some tissues, such as liver, calpastatin is prevalent to the extent that crude cytoplasmic preparations show no calpain activity. In rat brain, however, some proteolysis can be detected by the addition of as little as 5 μM calcium to crude cytoplasmic fractions, indicating that while calpastatin may dampen calpain activity in the brain, it may not suppress it completely (Simonson et al., 1984). Of importance for the present discussion are the localizations of calpains and calpastatin in neuronal populations and within individual neurons. Much of the brain calpastatin appears to be extracellular (Zimmerman and Schlaepfer, 1982). Conversely, calpains have been localized to the interiors of cell types such as erythrocytes (Murachi et al., 1981a; Melloni et al., 1982) and skeletal muscle (Barth and Elce, 1981), and immunocytochemical studies suggest a comparable localization in rat brain neurons (Figure 3) (Siman et al., 1985b). Furthermore, it has been suggested that when calpain I is associated with membranes, it is not sensitive to calpastatin inhibition (Siman et al., 1983a; Hatanaka et al., 1984). While more information is needed, the emerging picture is that calpastatin may not severely limit brain calpain activity, especially of the membrane-associated form.

CALPAIN SUBSTRATES

Compartmentalization of calpains within neurons will influence not only their susceptibility to activation by calcium and inhibition by calpastatin, but will restrict their accessibility to potential substrates. *In vitro* studies of calpain substrates conducted on brain subcellular fractions or on purified brain proteins are limited in that much of the inherent neuronal compartmentalization is not preserved. Nevertheless, they offer a means of identifying possible *in vivo* calpain substrates and as such can provide valuable information as to possible functional roles for the brain calpains.

These studies have revealed that calpain I has a capacity to use only a limited number of brain proteins as substrates. In SPM fractions prepared from adult rat forebrain, micromolar calcium concentrations promote the disappearance of only two polypeptides of the more than 40 that can be reliably detected on one-dimensional polyacrylamide gels (Baudry et al., 1981). The substrate polypeptides are large, having apparent molecular weights of approximately 240 kD and 235 kD, and occur in a one-to-one molar ratio (Figure 4). These properties are similar to those described for the subunits of the brain protein fodrin (Levine and Willard, 1981), suggesting that fodrin could serve as a substrate for calpain I.

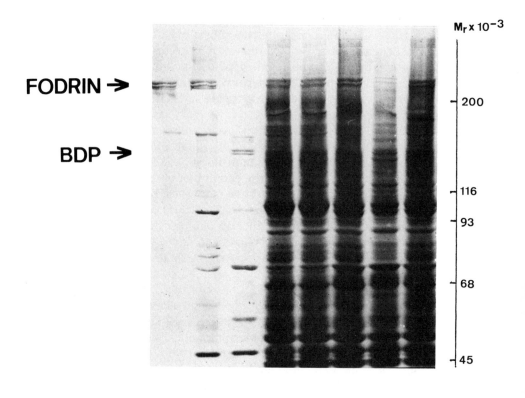

Figure 4. *Purified calpain I degrades purified and membrane-bound fodrin.* Calpain I, purified from rat erythrocyte cytosol, was incubated with purified rat brain fodrin (*lanes 2* and *3*) or synaptosmal plasma membranes (SPMs) prepared from rat hippocampus (*lanes 4–8*). *Lane 1,* purified fodrin; *lane 2,* fodrin plus calpain I preparation; *lane 3,* fodrin plus calpain I and 200 μM calcium; *lane 4,* SPMs; *lane 5,* SPMs plus 200 μM calcium; *lane 6,* SPMs plus calpain I; *lane 7,* SPMs plus calpain I and 200 μM calcium; *lane 8,* SPMs plus calpain I, 200 μM calcium, and 100 μM leupeptin. Purified calpain I degrades purified fodrin (compare *lanes 2* and *3*) and SPMs also degrade fodrin (compare *lanes 4* and *5*). The thiol-protease inhibitor leupeptin prevents calpain I-induced fodrin degradation (*lane 8*).

This suggestion is supported by a number of observations (Siman et al., 1984). First, the two polypeptide substrates comigrate on SDS-polyacrylamide gels with the two subunits of purified brain fodrin. Second, purified calpain I degrades purified brain fodrin, and this effect is blocked by calpain inhibitors. Purified fodrin is an excellent substrate for calpain I, as the enzyme has an affinity for the protein of about 50 nM and degrades it to near completion within 1 min. Third, the calpain preparation degrades the two SPM polypeptides that are substrates for the endogenous protease. Finally, antibodies to purified fodrin recognize only the SPM polypeptide substrates among all SPM proteins. Moreover, the antibodies recognize fodrin proteolytic fragments of identical molecular weights from purified fodrin and from the SPM polypeptide substrates. From these studies, it can be concluded that activation of SPM-associated calpain I leads to the selective degradation of fodrin.

Two cytoskeletal components, which are found principally in cytoplasmic fractions prepared from brain homogenates, are also excellent substrates for calpain I. The microtubule-associated protein MAP 2, which may provide cross-bridges that interconnect adjacent tubulin polymers, is degraded by calpain I (Klein et al., 1981; Baudry et al., 1983b). Additionally, the neurofilaments, and in particular the 200-kD and 150-kD component polypeptides, are substrates *in vitro* for calpain I (Zimmerman and Schlaepfer, 1982; R. Siman et al., unpublished observations). Interestingly, the functional role of the 200-kD neurofilament polypeptide is perhaps analogous to that of MAP 2, in the sense that, rather than being a core component of filaments, it serves as a bridge to interconnect neighboring filaments (Weber et al., 1983). Proteolytic modification of these bridge structures could be expected to influence the intricate organization of the neuronal cytoskeleton.

Fodrin can also be considered a part of the neuronal cytoskeleton. The protein in the native state is a filamentous rod that forms a submembranous lining in neurons (Levine and Willard, 1981; Glenney et al., 1982). Fodrin binds F-actin *in vitro* and has been suggested to provide a major point of linkage of actin filaments to neuronal membranes (for a review, see Lazarides and Nelson, 1982). With the potential to degrade fodrin, MAP 2, and two of the neurofilament polypeptides, calpain I conceivably could modify the structural organization of actin filaments, microtubules, and intermediate filaments, the three principal cytoskeletal systems found in neurons. Future investigations must address whether any or all of these proteins serve as calpain I substrates *in vivo*, and attempt to deduce the organizational changes in the cytoskeleton upon proteolysis of one or more of its component parts.

Calpain I substrates other than the ones mentioned above may exist. The protease may degrade proteins whose content or molecular weight places them below the sensitivity of detection by one-dimensional gel electrophoresis. Neural peptides, for example, would fall into this category. However, calpain I has proven notoriously poor at degrading small substrates such as peptides, and no convincing evidence has been presented to suggest that it plays a role in peptide processing in the brain. Thus, calpain I appears to have a relatively limited substrate specificity. This suggests that, rather than serving a general functional role, such as in the turnover of large numbers of neuronal proteins, the protease plays a part in specific cellular responses to elevated internal free calcium levels. As cytoskeletal proteins are the leading candidates for *in vivo* calpain I substrates, the enzyme may play a role in the dynamic organization of the neuronal cytoskeleton.

EFFECTS OF CALPAIN ACTIVATION ON CELLULAR PROCESSES

The identification of major cytoskeletal proteins such as calpain I substrates suggests that calpain I activation may have profound effects on neuronal function. We have used known functional properties of the major substrates to begin to assess the possible effects of calpain I activation at the cellular level. In particular, our functional studies thus far have focused on the high molecular weight protein fodrin. As mentioned previously, fodrin lines the cortical cytoplasm of neurons, and is present in dendritic as well as axonal processes (Levine and Willard, 1981;

Glenney and Glenney, 1983; Lazarides and Nelson, 1983). This places the protein in a key position from which it can control events at the cell surface as well as interactions between the plasma membrane and the cell interior. Intriguingly, ultrastructural studies have shown dendritic spines to be filled with 5–7-nm filaments that connect to the synaptic membrane and to the dendritic shaft (Landis and Reese, 1983). Since fodrin filaments *in vitro* have been found to possess such a diameter, it is tempting to speculate that they form these critically positioned filaments in spines. Consistent with this, postsynaptic density preparations contain abundant amounts of fodrin (Carlin et al., 1983). Certainly, an ultrastructural study localizing neuronal fodrin would reveal if indeed the protein is strategically placed in postsynaptic structures.

Fodrin has a number of interesting chemical and physical properties. The native molecule is a heterodimer consisting of two copies of each of the two subunits, and forms an extended rod about 200 nm in length. The higher molecular weight subunit binds calmodulin *in vitro*, and the head of the molecule binds filamentous actin. If the calmodulin and F-actin binding are also present *in vivo*, they may represent major mechanisms for the linkage of these two proteins to the membrane. Studies on two other cell types, fibroblasts and the intestinal epithelium, suggest an additional functional role for fodrin in regulating intermediate filament contact with both the plasma membrane and actin filaments (Hirokawa et al., 1983; Mangeat and Burridge, 1984).

In many of its properties, fodrin closely resembles spectrin, the principal component of the cytoskeleton of erythrocytes (Table 2). Brain fodrin and erythrocyte spectrin are part of a family of spectrinlike proteins that share a similar calmodulin-binding subunit (the 240-kD subunits of fodrin and spectrin) and have a variant, tissue-specific subunit (Glenney et al., 1982). Although functional studies of brain fodrin have just begun, considerable research effort has been directed toward understanding the function of erythrocyte spectrin. Like fodrin, spectrin forms a meshwork subjacent to the plasma membrane in which spectrin

Table 2.   Similarities Between Fodrin and Spectrin

Property	Fodrin	Spectrin
Subunit composition	Four subunits: $(\alpha\beta)_2$	Two or four subunits: $(\alpha\beta)$, $(\alpha\beta)_2$
Molecular weight	$\alpha \sim 240$ kD $\beta \sim 235$ kD	$\alpha \sim 240$ kD $\beta \sim 220$ kD
Shape	200-nm rod	100- or 200-nm rod
Localization	Cortical cytoplasm	Cortical cytoplasm
F-actin binding	Yes	Yes
Calmodulin binding	Yes, α-subunit	Yes, α-subunit
Peptide maps	Some similarities between α-subunits; β-subunits differ	
Immunological reactivity	Some cross-reactivity between α-subunits; little between β-subunits	
Membrane attachment	Unknown; can bind ankyrin	Via ankyrin

Source: Bennett et al., 1982; Glenney et al., 1982; Lazarides and Nelson, 1982.

filaments are interwoven with those of actin (for reviews, see Branton et al., 1981; Goodman and Shiffer, 1983). A number of studies have implicated the spectrin–actin cytoskeleton in the control of erythrocyte shape and deformability. A second established function of spectrin is to restrict the lateral mobility of proteins within the membrane. Thus, the model of integral membrane proteins floating freely in the lipid bilayer has been revised to include the transmembrane control on these proteins by the submembraneous cytoskeleton (Edelman, 1976; Nicolson, 1979; Branton et al., 1981). Proteolytic breakdown of part of the cytoskeleton, mediated by calpain I, could therefore have an effect both on cell shape and on the lateral mobility and distribution of integral membrane proteins.

EFFECT OF CALPAIN I ACTIVATION ON THE SHAPE OF ERYTHROCYTE GHOSTS

While we are most interested in the hypothesis that cytoskeletal proteolysis modifies the shape of neuronal processes, the erythrocyte offers a convenient model system with which to begin to investigate this idea. Advantages of the erythrocyte preparation include: (1) the ease of obtaining a virtually pure population of a single cell type; (2) their characteristic and uniform biconcave disk shape; (3) the possibility for visualization of shape by light microscopy; and (4) the ability to lyse and reseal their membranes in order to introduce various drugs and ions to act on the membrane inner face and cytoplasm.

We have made use of these advantages to test the hypothesis that calpain I activation can modify cell shape. Because the data have previously been presented only in a preliminary note (Siman et al., 1983b), we describe the experimental paradigm and results in detail. As shown in Table 3, freshly drawn and washed

Table 3. Erythrocyte Shape Change Methodology

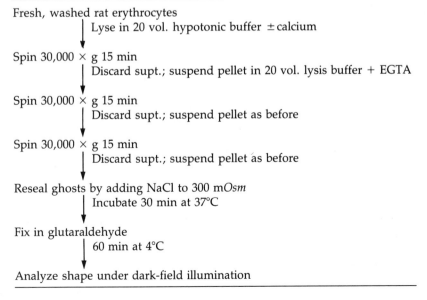

Fresh, washed rat erythrocytes
  Lyse in 20 vol. hypotonic buffer ± calcium

Spin 30,000 × g 15 min
  Discard supt.; suspend pellet in 20 vol. lysis buffer + EGTA

Spin 30,000 × g 15 min
  Discard supt.; suspend pellet as before

Spin 30,000 × g 15 min
  Discard supt.; suspend pellet as before

Reseal ghosts by adding NaCl to 300 mOsm
  Incubate 30 min at 37°C

Fix in glutaraldehyde
  60 min at 4°C

Analyze shape under dark-field illumination

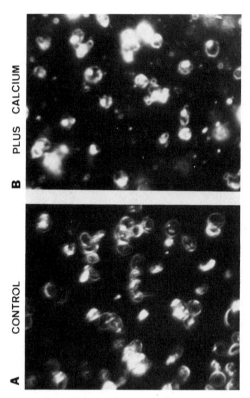

Figure 5. *Shape of the erythrocyte ghosts prepared in the absence* (A) *or presence* (B) *of calcium.* When prepared by lysis in a calcium-free buffer, ghosts are biconcave disks (A). However, when prepared by lysis in 100 μM calcium, ghosts take on a round shape, lack a central concavity, and frequently have a blebbed appearance (B).

rat erythrocytes are lysed in 20 volumes of hypotonic buffer. During this step, various calcium concentrations, protease inhibitors, and other drugs are included. Two minutes later, the lysate is centrifuged, and the membranes are washed three times in lysis buffer. For assessment of the effect of a treatment on the resealed membrane (ghost) shape, the tonicity is restored and the ghosts are incubated at 37°C. Next, the ghosts are either fixed and visualized under dark-field illumination for shape analysis or prepared for SDS-polyacrylamide gel electrophoresis for determination of the polypeptide composition.

Ghosts prepared from cells lysed in a calcium-free buffer will, upon resealing and incubation at 37°C, take on the concave disk shape characteristic of the intact erythrocyte. In contrast, the inclusion of micromolar calcium in the lysis buffer results in ghosts that are small, round, lacking a central concavity, and possessing blebs or spikes protruding from their surfaces (Figure 5). This discocyte–echinocyte transformation has been previously described both for calcium-treated ghosts (Palek et al., 1974) and for calcium-loaded intact erythrocytes (White, 1974). Free calcium concentrations of 30 μM produced a shape change in over 90% of the ghosts, while the half-maximal effect occurred at around 3 μM calcium.

The calcium levels that induce the discocyte–echinocyte transformation are similar to those concentrations known to activate calpain I. To determine if lysis conditions that caused a shape change also activated calpain I, the ghost poly-peptides were separated on polyacrylamide gels and quantified. As shown in Figure 6, lysis in micromolar calcium changed the content of a number of ghost polypeptides. The level of the predominant integral membrane protein, band 3 (Steck, 1974; Branton et al., 1981), was reduced by over 80%. Since no higher molecular weight bands appeared, the band 3 loss likely represented proteolytic cleavage (see also below). In addition, the two spectrin subunits and band 4.1 were degraded, whereas band 4.2 and actin (band 5) were relatively resistant

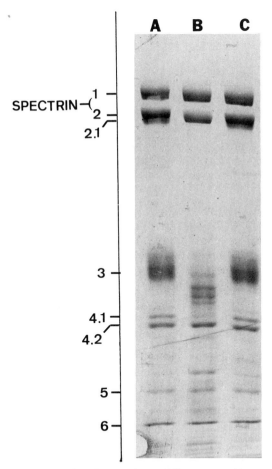

Figure 6. *Polypeptide composition of erythrocyte ghosts of discocyte or echinocyte configuration.* Ghosts prepared by lysis in the absence (discocytes) or presence (echinocytes) of 100 μM calcium chloride were run on a polyacrylamide gel (5–10% gradient). The gel was stained with Coomassie Blue. *A*, no calcium. *B*, plus 100 μM calcium. *C*, plus 100 μM calcium and 100 μM leupeptin. Inclusion of calcium in a lysis buffer causes the partial disappearance of four prominent bands: the two spectrin polypeptides (bands 1 and 2), band 3, and band 4.1. All of these bands are protected from proteolysis by leupeptin.

Table 4. Calpain Activation Induces Shape Change in Erythrocyte
Ghosts

Additions	Discocytes (%)	Band 3 Remaining (% Control)
No additions	95	100
Calcium 10 μM	35	57
30 μM	18	32
100 μM	7	18
Calcium 100 μM		
+ Leupeptin 3 μM	50	45
30 μM	83	86
+ Antipain 5 μM	59	48
50 μM	95	91
+ Iodoacetate 5 mM	78	87
+ N-ethylmaleimide 5 mM	62	73
+ Pepstatin A 500 μM	10	17
+ PMSF 1 mM	8	12
+ Trifluoperazine 50 μM	5	12

to calcium-induced proteolysis. These data show that those calcium levels that induce shape change also activate proteolysis and suggest that the proteolysis may bring about the shape change.

Direct support for the involvement of calpain I activation in the shape change was provided by the results of a study using protease inhibitors (Table 4). If the thiol-protease blockers leupeptin or antipain were included along with calcium during the lysis, the ghosts did not change to echinocytes. Furthermore, the concentrations of leupeptin or antipain that prevented the shape change also blocked the proteolysis of band 3, spectrin, and band 4.1. Partial blockade of the proteolysis was accompanied by a partial prevention of the shape change. If protease inhibitors were added at steps after the calcium treatment, they did not affect either the shape change or the proteolysis. The thiol-group alkylators N-ethylmaleimide and iodoacetate also prevented both the shape change and the proteolysis, whereas the serine protease inhibitor phenylmethylsulfonyl-fluoride, the pepsin blocker pepstatin A, and the calmodulin inhibitor trifluoperazine were without effect. The possible involvement of a calcium-stimulated protease other than calpain I in the observed changes can be ruled out for two reasons. First, purified calpain I degrades spectrin and bands 3 and 4.1, giving a pattern of proteolysis identical to that seen with cells lysed in the presence of calcium (Siman et al., 1984a). Secondly, calpain I appears to be the only calcium-dependent protease found in rat erythrocytes (Murachi et al., 1981a). These results indicate that calpain I activation can cause a shape change in erythrocyte membranes.

The mechanism by which calpain I-induced proteolysis causes shape change is important not only for understanding the molecular events in shape regulation in erythrocytes, but also for the assessment of possible generalized calpain I-induced shape changes in such other systems as neurons. In the case of the erythrocyte, the discocyte–echinocyte shape change has been considered to reflect a primary reorganization of the submembranous cytoskeleton (Branton et al., 1981; Goodman and Shiffer, 1983). Of relevance to the present discussion is the recent finding that a mild trypsinization detaches the cytoskeleton from the membrane and irreversibly locks the ghost in the echinocyte configuration (Jinbu et al., 1984). The calpain I-induced echinocyte formation may be an analogous process. After calpain I activation, the 90-kD band 3 is completely lost as a result of calpain-induced clipping off of the cytoplasmic domain of band 3 (R. Siman et al., unpublished observations). The cytoplasmic portion provides the major link for cytoskeletal attachment to the membrane (Branton et al., 1981). Thus, calpain I may induce shape change in erythrocyte ghosts by detaching the cytoskeleton from the membrane (Figure 7) via degradation of its major point of attachment.

Does calpain I mediate shape changes in neurons? To address this question, it is necessary to examine two conditions under which neurons change shape: (1) as a function of development; and (2) as a function of intense synaptic activity. Morphological changes in developing neurons are most certainly the result of modifications in the complement of proteins (and other components) that are synthesized and degraded, and changes in the organization of these components. The possible involvement of calpain I in morphological changes of this type is discussed in a later section. Here we consider alterations in the shape of a dendritic spine induced by changes in the activity of the synapse of which that spine is a part. Structural changes of this type have already been discussed and have been proposed to underlie long-term information storage (see above).

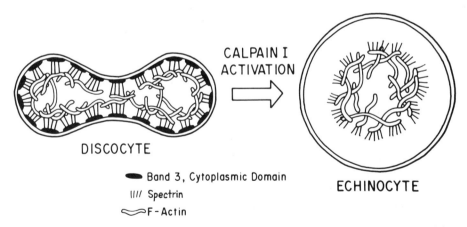

CALPAIN I
ACTIVATION

DISCOCYTE

● Band 3, Cytoplasmic Domain

||// Spectrin

F-Actin

ECHINOCYTE

Figure 7. *Proposed molecular mechanism underlying calpain I-induced shape change.* At the *left* is a schematic of the discocyte–erythrocyte ghost, whose shape is a property of the interaction of the submembraneous cytoskeleton with the plasma membrane. The shape change induced by calcium is indicated by the shift from the form on the *left* to that on the *right*. The round (echinocyte) ghost results from a detachment of the cytoskeleton from the plasma membrane, a consequence of calpain I-stimulated degradation of the major point of cytoskeletal attachment, the cytoplasmic domain of band 3. Surface blebs, which are also characteristic of the echinocyte, may not be the result of cytoskeletal detachment and are not presented in the figure.

The unusual shape of the dendritic spine is thought to be a manifestation of cytoskeletal organization within the spine (Fifková and Delay, 1982; Landis and Reese, 1983). Therefore, degradation of cytoskeletal components by calpain I activation could be expected to modify spine shape. Although cytoskeletal organization within dendritic spines is incompletely understood, in many respects the spine cytoskeleton resembles that of the erythrocyte. Like the red cell, dendritic spines are deficient in microtubules and intermediate filaments but do possess actin filaments (Peters et al., 1970; Fifková and Delay, 1982; Landis and Reese, 1983). Moreover, the spectrinlike protein fodrin may be present in spines, as discussed earlier, while an immunoreactive analogue of band 3 may be present as well (Kay et al., 1983). We hypothesize that intense synaptic stimulation, by promoting postsynaptic calcium influx, activates calpain I, leading to a reorganization (detachment from the membrane?) of the spine cytoskeleton and a consequent change in spine shape. It should be noted that the activity-dependent spine shape change consists of a rounding of the spines and a blebbing of new spines from the parent dendrites (Lee et al., 1980; Chang and Greenough, 1984). This is perhaps similar to the calcium-induced echinocyte formation in erythrocytes and would be expected to result from a partial detachment of the cytoskeleton from the dendritic spine or shaft plasma membrane. While speculative, this model must be considered as a candidate for mediating spine shape changes in view of its applicability in the erythrocyte system.

CALPAIN ACTIVATION AND SYNAPTIC MEMBRANE PROTEIN DISTRIBUTION

A second established function of the erythrocyte cytoskeleton is to control the position and lateral mobility of integral membrane proteins. Transmembrane control of cell surface proteins by the cytoskeleton may be a general mechanism for regulating cell surface interactions with the extracellular environment. Nowhere is this of greater importance than at synapses. The postsynaptic membrane is particularly specialized, in terms of its protein composition and organization, for extracellular signal recognition. In view of the capacity of neuronal calpain I to degrade cytoskeletal proteins, it is important to ask whether such structural protein breakdown might affect the distribution of proteins at the neuronal cell surface. We have tested the hypothesis that calpain I, by degrading cytoskeletal proteins underlying the postsynaptic membrane, modifies the distribution of proteins within the synaptic membrane. This hypothesis has implications for the adaptive capabilities of synapses.

We focused on possible calpain-mediated cytoskeletal control over synaptic membrane binding sites for the putative neurotransmitter L-glutamate. Glutamate binding sites were selected for the following reasons: (1) They very likely are integral membrane proteins, on the basis of direct evidence (Sharif and Roberts, 1980) and by analogy with other receptor binding sites. (2) The number of exposed glutamate binding sites is regulated by calpain I. Activation of the protease by micromolar calcium concentrations leads to a two- to threefold increase in the number of sodium-independent glutamate binding sites (Baudry et al., 1981). This effect is blocked by a large number of calpain inhibitors (Baudry et al., 1981), occurs within 5–10 min, and is not reversed by removal of calcium (Baudry and Lynch, 1981; Baudry et al., 1983a). Although high concentrations of the calcium chelator EGTA have been reported to reverse the calcium-induced increase (Fagg et al., 1983), this does not represent a true reversal of the calcium enhancement of binding, but rather is due to a nonspecific effect of high EGTA concentrations on neuronal membranes. When the EGTA is removed, calcium can no longer increase binding site number, indicating that EGTA has not reversed the calcium effect (M. Kessler, M. Baudry, and G. S. Lynch, unpublished observations). Furthermore, a variety of calpain inhibitors can prevent the calcium effect when added before, but not after, calcium. In conclusion, the data demonstrate that micromolar calcium increases the number of glutamate binding sites by activation of calpain I. The rapidity of the effect and its occurrence in washed membrane preparations rule out a role for *de novo* protein synthesis, but rather point to the uncovering of binding sites that were previously inaccessible to the ligand. Thus, calpain I activation causes a reorganization of glutamate binding sites within synaptic membranes. (3) Glutamate binding sites may play an essential role in synaptic communication, as L-glutamate or closely related compounds have been proposed to be transmitters at a large number of mammalian central synapses (for a review, see Di Chiara and Gessa, 1980). (4) The number of glutamate binding sites is increased by potentially important physiological stimuli, such as high-frequency synaptic stimulation (Lynch et al., 1982) or after classical conditioning (Mamounas et al., 1984). Since calpain I activation *in vitro* can increase the number of glutamate binding sites, it may mediate the increase in binding that follows synaptic stimulation or learning.

We tested the possibility that calcium increased glutamate binding by stimulating calpain-induced fodrin degradation. Fodrin likely plays a part in the calpain I-induced increase in glutamate binding, because it is the only protein that is detectably broken down under conditions in which the number of binding sites increases. We used polyclonal antibodies to fodrin in an attempt to block fodrin proteolysis without inhibiting calpain I activity per se (Siman et al., 1985a). Affinity-purified antibodies raised against purified rat brain fodrin recognized only fodrin among all rat brain membrane polypeptides (Figure 8, left). When cortical or hippocampal SPMs were first treated with antifodrin, calcium no longer induced fodrin degradation. Fodrin cross-linking was not necessary, because monovalent antifodrin Fab fragments were equally effective. Antifodrin thus blocks the calpain I-induced fodrin degradation.

With a method for preventing fodrin degradation without blocking calpain I activity against other potential substrates, we asked whether fodrin proteolysis was obligatory for uncovering new glutamate binding sites. As depicted in Figure 8 (right), antifodrin did not alter glutamate binding measured in the absence of calcium. However, the antibodies completely prevented the increase in binding caused by micromolar calcium. The blockade of calcium-stimulated glutamate binding depended on the concentration of antifodrin used. To assess the capacity of these concentrations of antifodrin to bind to the available fodrin, we measured the blockade by antifodrin of [^{125}I]antifodrin binding. There was an excellent correlation between the capacity of antifodrin to attach to fodrin (as determined from the blockade of [^{125}I]antifodrin binding) and to prevent the calcium stimulation of glutamate binding. Control experiments revealed that the antifodrin inhibition

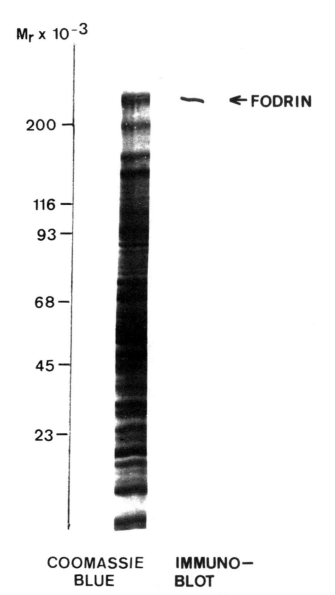

$M_r \times 10^{-3}$

200 —

116 —
93 —

68 —

45 —

23 —

← FODRIN

COOMASSIE   IMMUNO—
BLUE   BLOT

Figure 8. *Antibodies to fodrin block the calcium uncovering of hidden glutamate binding sites on synaptic membranes. Left*: Specificity of antifodrin for fodrin among all SPMs. At the *left* is a Coomassie Blue-stained gel lane of rat cerebral cortical synaptic membrane polypeptides. At the *right* is the immunoblot of an identical gel lane. Only the higher molecular weight fodrin subunit is recognized among all the polypeptides. *Right*: Antifodrin blocks the process by which calcium increases glutamate binding. Cerebral cortical SPMs were treated with (*stippled bars*) or without (*open bars*) 300 μM calcium chloride and then were assayed for specific sodium-independent binding of 100 nM [^{3}H]L-glutamate. Assays were conducted in a Tris-HCl buffer. In most cases, antifodrin or monovalent antifodrin Fab fragments (200 ng per μg membrane protein) were added 15 min prior to the calcium chloride. In the "delayed antifodrin" condition, membranes were treated first with calcium chloride and then with antifodrin. Since antifodrin must be present before the calcium chloride in order to block the calcium enhancement of binding, the antibodies do not directly modify glutamate binding, but rather interfere with the process by which calcium increases binding.

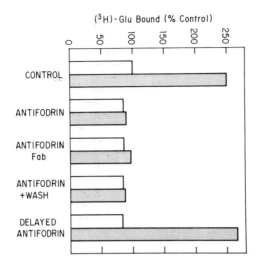

Figure 8. *(continued).*

of calcium-stimulated binding was not due to fodrin cross-linking, chelation of free calcium, or a direct effect on glutamate binding. Antifodrin thus prevented the calpain I-induced uncovering of hidden glutamate binding sites by blocking fodrin degradation.

These experiments demonstrate that submembranous fodrin exerts a trans-membrane control over glutamate binding sites. Degradation of fodrin by calpain I reorganizes the cytoskeleton in such a way that previously unexposed glutamate binding sites become accessible to glutamate. It is possible, although still inconclusive, that these binding sites may represent physiologically relevant neurotransmitter receptor binding sites. Consequently, calpain I-induced fodrin degradation may be of profound functional significance.

The precise way in which fodrin proteolysis reorganizes the cytoskeleton and uncovers glutamate binding sites is a subject for future investigation. Perhaps the situation is analogous to that of the erythrocyte, in which calpain I activation may detach the cytoskeleton from the plasma membrane. As fodrin is an F-actin-binding protein (Levine and Willard, 1981; Glenney et al., 1982; Goodman and Shiffer, 1983), it is possible that fodrin breakdown releases actin filaments from the membrane. An alternative possibility is that fodrin might control membrane proteins independently of its actin filament binding capability. In either case, the protein–protein interactions that link fodrin to the membrane and to other cytoskeletal components must be more completely understood.

Another area for further study is the nature of the reorganization within the membrane after calpain I-mediated cytoskeletal breakdown. It seems intuitively unlikely that glutamate binding sites are the sole synaptic proteins under cytoskeletal control, but the full extent of transmembrane control by fodrin is uncertain. It should be noted that while erythrocyte spectrin represents as much as 30% of the total protein in membrane fractions (Steck, 1974), the corresponding figure for neuronal fodrin is only 2–3% (Bennett et al., 1982). Although this makes fodrin one of the predominant synaptic membrane proteins, it implies that fodrin's control over integral membrane proteins may not be as pervasive as that of spectrin (see also Mangeat and Burridge, 1984). Nevertheless, if fodrin regulates even a few cell surface proteins at the synapse, then it may play a critical part in any of a number of interneuronal signaling phenomena.

SOME POSSIBLE ROLES OF SOLUBLE CALPAIN IN BRAIN DEVELOPMENT

As mentioned, calpain is both found in the cytoplasm and associated with synaptic membrane fractions. The possible involvement of SPM-associated calpain in the regulation of cell shape and protein distribution raises questions about the contributions of the larger, soluble fraction to neuronal functioning. Since calpain degrades structural cross-linking proteins, it presumably prevents the assembly of the cytoskeleton or causes the breakdown of part of the already assembled lattice. Indeed, Lasek and Hoffman (1976) proposed that calpain in the terminals of axons suppresses growth by degrading cytoskeletal elements needed for process elongation. According to their idea, the calcium needed for enzyme activation is supplied by calcium currents that develop with the formation of synapses. Because large, voltage-dependent calcium spikes are now known to occur in dendrites (Llinás and Hess, 1976; Wong et al., 1979), this hypothetical process could also be applicable to dendrites.

If calpain participates in the slowing and termination of process extension, we might expect its activity to bear a systematic relationship to the ultimate size achieved by dendritic and axonal arborizations. This can be approximated by assaying brains of different sizes, since the extent of dendritic and presumably axonal arborizations is highly correlated with brain volume (Jerison, 1973).

We first verified that the various endogenous substrates of endogenous soluble calpain were similar in different mammalian species (Figure 9). A similar pattern of protein degradation was observed when soluble fractions from forebrains of several species were incubated in the presence of calcium and the proteins were separated on SDS-polyacrylamide gels. Similar results were obtained from different brain regions. As previously discussed for the SPM-associated calpain I, the soluble enzyme used only a limited number of proteins as substrates, primarily MAP 2 ($\sim$300 kD), fodrin (240 kD and 235 kD), neurofilament polypeptides (200 kD and 160 kD), and tubulin ($\sim$53 kD). Although quantitative comparisons are difficult to obtain with this approach, it was nevertheless apparent that small-brained species exhibit much more calpain activity than do large-brained ones. More precise quantitation was obtained by determining the proteolytic activity of brain-soluble fractions from a variety of different mammalian species by using an exogenous substrate, [^{14}C]casein. With this assay, we found that calpain activity is negatively correlated with brain size with a slope of 0.4 on log/log representations. This is not greatly different from the relationship between neuron density (neurons per unit area) and brain size (slope of -0.3) previously reported by various authors and is the inverse of the allometric function relating dendritic length of brain size (exponent of 0.3; see Jerison, 1973, for a review). Thus, calpain activity appears to be inversely correlated with neuronal size—that is,

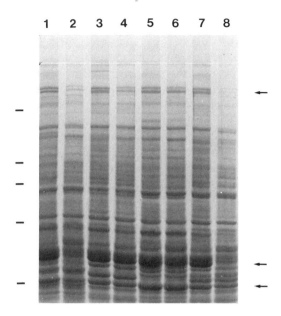

Figure 9. *Effect of calcium on cortical soluble proteins in different mammalian species.* Cortices from
different mammals were homogenized in 50 mM Tris-HCl buffer containing 5 mM 2-mercap-
toethanol. Homogenates were centrifuged at 48,000 × g for 30 min. Aliquots of the supernatants
were incubated in the absence (*odd numbers*) or presence (*even numbers*) of 500 μM calcium
chloride at 30°C for 30 min. The incubation was stopped by the addition of a solubilization
solution consisting of (final concentration): 50 mM Tris-PO₄ buffer ph 6.8, 2% sodium docecyl-
sulfate, 10% glycerol, and 33 mM dithiothreitol. After boiling for 3 min, aliquots of the solubilized
proteins (about 100 μg of protein) were subjected to electrophoresis on 3–10% gradient polyacrylamide sodium dodecylsulfate slab gels. The gels were stained with 0.1% Coomassie Brilliant
Blue-R in 50% trichloroacetic acid and de-stained in 7% acetic acid. *Lanes 1* and *2*, guinea pig;
3 and *4*, rat; *5* and *6*, pig; *7* and *8*, mouse. *Left bars*: Molecular weight standards (from *top* to
bottom): 200 kD; 116 kD; 93 kD; 68 kD; and 43 kD. *Right arrows* (from *top* to *bottom*): fodrin,
tubulin, and actin.

the larger the neurons become with increasing brain size, the less calpain activity
(expressed per unit of protein) is present in the soluble fraction.

Several lines of evidence indicate that the percentage of a constant cube of
cortex occupied by glial cells remains constant across various species of mammals
(Tower and Young, 1973), suggesting that most of the changes in calpain activity
with brain size are due to neuronal calpain. Immunocytochemical studies in rats
also point to a primarily neuronal localization of calpain I (Siman et al., 1985b).
If this is correct, the results described above lead to the unexpected conclusion
that total soluble calpain activity per cell is roughly the same across several
orders of mammals and therefore decreases progressively per unit cell volume
as the brain and neurons grows larger.

As mentioned, calpain activity is regulated by calpastatin, a high molecular
weight, heat-stable protein found in most mammalian tissues, but this is not
likely to be involved in the size–activity relationship described above, since we
could detect no significant differences in the amount of inhibitor in brains of
different size.

These comparative results provide some clues about the possible role of calpain in regulating the development of axonal and dendritic fields. Growth presumably reflects a disparity between the rates for synthesis and degradation of structural and other proteins, as well as the ontogenetic time required for these rates to become equal. It has been shown that protein synthesis and breakdown decline dramatically in rat brain postnatally, and that equivalence between the two is reached only weeks after birth (Dunlop et al., 1978). The pattern of results described above suggests that calpain levels are not greatly different on a per neuron basis in brains of different sizes, and that variations in its activity reflect the extent to which it is diluted by the axonal and dendritic arborizations of different sizes. If this is correct, then we might imagine that the variations in the extent of the field generated by neuronal processes are due to variations in the rate of synthesis or the rate at which synthesis declines toward the level of proteolysis. Hence, calpain might serve to terminate extension but would not determine *when* in development this occurs. Developmental studies of calpain activity in different species would serve to elucidate these issues. We have recently found that, in the rat, calpain I activity is robust at birth and then undergoes a drastic decline in the forebrain during the first postnatal week (Figure 10). Since cortical neurons elaborate their dendrites principally after birth, the drop in proteolysis may allow for the initiation of growth.

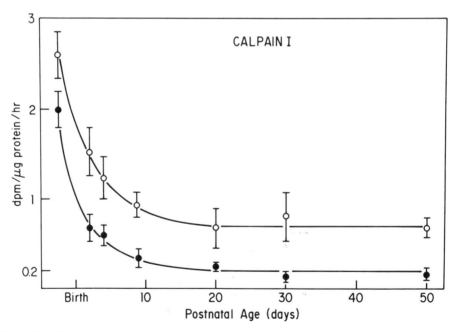

Figure 10. *Changes in calpain activity in rat forebrain and hindbrain during brain development.* Calcium-dependent caseinolytic activity in soluble fractions from rat forebrain and hindbrain was determined as described in Simonson et al. (1984). Calpain I was defined as the difference in activity measured in the presence of 30 μM calcium and in the absence of calcium. Results are means ± SEM of 4–5 experiments. *Closed circles,* forebrain; *open circles,* hindbrain. (From Simonson et al., 1985.)

The discussion to this point has been concerned with neurons in aggregate and has not dealt with the vast differences in size of the dendritic and axonal arborizations that exist between different types of neurons. This issue can be considered only after immunocytochemical mapping of brain calpain has been completed.

To summarize, soluble calpain activity is very high in the embryonic brain, declines rapidly in the postnatal period, and is negatively correlated with brain size in adulthood. We raised the possibility that it acts during development, as equilibrium with protein synthesis is reached, to slow or stop the extension of processes, and suggested that the rapid postnatal decrease might serve to initiate process growth (Lasek and Hoffman, 1976). As will be discussed, these observations may have implications for the understanding of the relationship of change and stability that surely are as much a part of plasticity as they are of development.

CONCLUSIONS

Membrane-associated calpain I meets many of the conditions required of an agent responsible for translating physiological events into lasting modifications of synapses. It is found associated with synaptic membrane fractions and therefore is positioned to produce local changes that would not necessarily disturb neighboring contacts (selectivity). The triggering step could be the opening of local ion channels in the spine, resulting in transient calcium accumulation and local activation of the enzyme in the vicinity of the synapse. Calpain's absolute requirement for calcium is also an ideal feature for a mediator of plasticity. Calcium has been strongly implicated in the production of long-lasting physiological changes, and its resting concentrations are well below those needed for activation of calpain. Physiological studies have shown that hippocampal neurons have voltage-sensitive calcium channels and that their dendrites exhibit calcium-driven action potentials (Wong et al., 1979).

The consequences of calpain activation also compare well with those expected for a substrate of plasticity. Its effects are irreversible and could only be readjusted by complex cellular events probably involving new protein synthesis and modification. Clearly, then, calpain meets the all-important requirement of producing modifications that persist for long, perhaps very long, periods of time. Moreover, while we still have only an imprecise understanding of the effects produced by the enzyme, what we do know indicates that calpain's actions should have important consequences for synaptic physiology. Fodrin, a prominent substrate for calpain I, can exert transmembrane control over integral synaptic membrane proteins, and this control is modified upon activation of the protease. Furthermore, if events in red blood cells can be used as a guide for small processes in brain, we can expect calpain to modify shape and ultrastructure as well. It will be recalled that high-frequency afferent activity resulted in changes in the binding of putative transmitters to membranes, as well as structural reorganization of connections.

The absence of an adequate pharmacology presents major problems in extending the calpain hypothesis to physiology and behavior. Very few inhibitors are known to penetrate brain cells, and where they do the extent of enzyme suppression can only be roughly approximated. It is also the case that these drugs block thiol (cysteine) -proteases other than calpain. These points, coupled with the fact that we have no idea how much enzyme activity might be needed to produce a given effect, preclude simple interpretations of drug studies.

Further difficulties are added by the complexity of the physiological and behavioral manifestations of plasticity. There is reason to suspect that long-term potentiation is not a unitary phenomenon (Racine et al., 1983), and we have argued elsewhere that only the variety lasting for several days and longer is likely to involve changes in membrane receptor binding (Lynch and Baudry, 1984). Fundamentally different versions of learning and memory are likewise now thought to coexist in the brains of mammals (cf. O'Keefe and Nadel, 1978; Squire, 1982). Whether these involve different cell chemistries is not known, but this is certainly a real possibility.

Despite these interpretative problems, drug studies have provided evidence implicating calpain in neuroplasticity. Infusion of leupeptin into the cerebral ventricles of rats produced substantial impairments in several tests requiring memory without causing apparent changes on a number of behavioral control measures (Staubli et al., 1984, 1985). As this material has been discussed elsewhere (Lynch and Baudry, 1984), we will not elaborate upon it here.

In an effort toward a broader perspective on brain calpain, we also briefly reviewed developmental and comparative studies of the soluble variant of the enzyme. This led to an admittedly speculative discussion of the possible contributions of the enzyme in neuronal growth. The negative relationship between calpain activity and brain size in adult mammals raises the intriguing possibility that the turnover of structural proteins proceeds at a much slower pace in mammals with bigger brains. Would this in turn mean that the stability of cell processes is greater as the brain increases in size? The question of how memories that last for years are encoded against a background of protein turnover, and perhaps the degeneration and replacement of anatomical elements, has not received the attention it deserves. If calpain activity can be taken as an index of the rate of turnover, then the described negative relationship may indicate that problems of relating storage to stability vary according to the size of the brain being considered.

REFERENCES

Alger, B. E., and R. A. Nicoll (1980) Epileptiform burst after hyperpolarization: Calcium-dependent potassium potential in hippocampal CA1 pyramidal cells. *Science* **210**:1122–1124.

Andersen, P. O., S. H. Sundberg, O. Sveen, and H. Wigstrom (1977) Specific long-lasting potentiation of synaptic transmission in hippocampal slices. *Nature* **6**:736–737.

Barnes, C. A. (1979) Memory deficits associated with senescence: A neurophysiological and behavioral study in the rat. *J. Comp. Physiol. Psychol.* **93**:74–104.

Barrionuevo, G., and T. H. Brown (1983) Associative long-term potention in hippocampal slices. *Proc. Natl. Acad. Sci. USA* **80**:7347–7351.

Barth, R., and J. S. Elce (1981) Immunofluorescent localization of a Ca^{2+}-dependent neutral protease in hamster muscle. *Am. J. Physiol.* **204**:E493–E498.

Baudry, M., and G. Lynch (1981) Hippocampal glutamate receptors. *Mol. Cell Biochem.* **38**:5–18.

Baudry, M., and G. Lynch (1984) Glutamate receptor regulation and the substrates of memory. In *The Neurobiology of Learning and Memory*, G. Lynch, J. M. McGaugh, and N. Weinberger, eds., pp. 431–451, Guilford, New York.

Baudry, M., M. Oliver, R. Creager, A. Wieraszko, and G. Lynch (1980) Increase in glutamate receptors following repetitive electrical stimulation in hippocampal slices. *Life Sci.* **27**:325–330.

Baudry, M., M. Bundman, E. Smith, and G. Lynch (1981) Micromolar levels of calcium stimulate proteolytic activity and glutamate receptor binding in rat brain synaptic membranes. *Science* **212**:937–938.

Baudry, M., K. Kramer, and G. Lynch (1983a) Irreversibility and time-course of the calcium stimulation of ^{3}H-glutamate binding to rat hippocampal membranes. *Brain Res.* **270**:142–145.

Baudry, M., R. Siman, E. K. Smith, and G. Lynch (1983b) Regulation by calcium ions of glutamate receptor binding in hippocampal slices. *Eur. J. Pharmacol.* **90**:161–168.

Bennett, V., J. Davis, and W. E. Fowler (1982) Brain spectrin, a membrane-associated protein related in structure and function to erythrocyte spectrin. *Nature* **299**:126–133.

Bliss, T. V. P., and A. T. Gardner-Medwin (1973) Long-lasting potentiation of synaptic transmission in the dentate area of the unanesthetized rabbit following stimulation of the perforant path. *J. Physiol. (Lond.)* **232**:357–374.

Bliss, T. V. P., and T. Lømo (1973) Long-lasting potentiation of synaptic transmission in the dentate area of the anesthetized rabbit following stimulation of the perforant path. *J. Physiol. (Lond.)* **232**:331–356.

Branton, D., C. M. Cohen, and J. Tyler (1981) Interaction of cytoskeletal proteins on the human erythrocyte membrane. *Cell* **24**:24–32.

Carlin, R. K., D. C. Bartelt, and P. Siekevitz (1983) Identification of fodrin as a major calmodulin-binding protein in postsynaptic density preparations. *J. Cell Biol.* **96**:443–448.

Chang, F. L. F., and W. T. Greenough (1984) Transient and enduring morphological correlates of synaptic activity and efficacy change in the rat hippocampal slice. *Brain Res.* **309**:35–46.

Dayton, W. R. (1982) Comparison of low- and high-calcium-requiring forms of the calcium-activated protease with their autocatalytic breakdown products. *Biochim. Biophys. Acta* **709**:166–172.

Dayton, W. R., J. V. Schollmeyer, R. A. Lepley, and L. R. Cortex (1981) A calcium-activated protease possibly involved in myofibrillar protein turnover: Isolation of a low-calcium-requiring form of the protease. *Biochim. Biophys. Acta* **659**:48–61.

DeMartino, G. N. (1981) Calcium-dependent proteolytic activity in rat liver: Identification of two proteases with different calcium requirements. *Arch. Biochem. Biophys.* **211**:253–257.

Di Chiara, G., and G. L. Gessa, eds. (1980) *Glutamate as a Neurotransmitter*, Raven, New York.

Dipolo, R., J. Requena, F. J. Brinley, L. J. Mullins, A. Scarpa, and T. Tiffert (1976) Ionized calcium concentrations in squid axons. *J. Gen. Physiol.* **67**:433–467.

Dunlop, D. S., W. Van Elden, and A. Lajtha (1978) Protein degradation rates in regions of the central nervous systems *in vivo* during development. *Biochem. J.* **170**:637–642.

Dunwiddie, T. V., and G. S. Lynch (1978) Long-term potentiation and depression of synaptic responses in the rat hippocampus: Localization and frequency dependency. *J. Physiol. (Lond.)* **276**:353–367.

Eccles, J. C. (1983) Calcium in long-term potentiation as a model for memory. *Neuroscience* **10**:1071–1081.

Edelman, G. M. (1976) Surface modulation in cell recognition and cell growth. *Science* **192**:218–226.

Fagg, G. E., E. E. Mena, and C. W. Cotman (1983) L-glutamate receptor populations in synaptic membranes: Effects of ions and pharmacological characteristics. *Adv. Biochem. Psychopharmacol.* **37**:199–209.

Fifková, E., and R. J. Delay (1982) Cytoplasmic actin in neuronal processes as a possible mediator of synaptic plasticity. *J. Cell Biol.* **95**:345–350.

Fifková, E., J. A. Markham, and R. J. Delay (1983) Calcium in the spine apparatus of dendritic spines in the dentate molecular layer. *Brain Res.* **266**:163–168.

Glenney, J. R., Jr., and P. Glenney (1983) Fodrin is the general spectrin-like protein found in most cells whereas spectrin and the TW protein have a restricted distribution. *Cell* **34**:503–512.

Glenney, J. R., P. Glenney, and K. Weber (1982) Erythroid spectrin, brain fodrin, and intestinal brush border proteins (TW-260/240) are related molecules containing a common calmodulin-binding subunit bound to a variant cell-type specific subunit. *Proc. Natl. Acad. Sci. USA* **79**: 4002–4005.

Goodman, S. R., and K. Shiffer (1983) The spectrin membrane skeleton of normal and abnormal human erythrocytes: A review. *Am. J. Physiol.* **244**:C121–C141.

Guroff, G. (1964) A neutral, calcium-activated proteinase from the soluble fraction of rat brain. *J. Biol. Chem.* **239**:149–155.

Hagiwara, S., and L. Byerly (1981) Calcium channel. *Annu. Rev. Neurosci.* **4**:69–125.

Hatanaka, M., N. Yoshimura, T. Murakami, R. Kannagi, and T. Murachi (1984) Evidence for membrane-associated calpain I in human erythrocytes: Detection by an immunoelectrophoretic blotting method using monospecific antibody. *Biochemistry* **23**:3272–3278.

Hinton, G. E., and J. A. Anderson (1981) *Parallel Models of Associative Memory*, Lawrence Erlbaum Associates, Hillsdale, New Jersey.

Hirokawa, N., R. E. Cheney, and M. Willard (1983) Location of a protein of the fodrin–spectrin–TW 260/240 family in the mouse intestinal brush border. *Cell* **32**:953–965.

Jerison, H. S. (1973) *Evolution of the Brain and Intelligence*, Academic, New York.

Jinbu, Y., S. Sato, T. Nakao, M. Nakao, S. Tsukita, and H. Ishikawa (1984) The role of ankyrin in shape and deformability change of human erythrocyte ghosts. *Biochim. Biophys. Acta* **773**:237–245.

Kandel, E. R., and J. H. Schwartz (1982) Molecular biology of learning: Modulation of transmitter release. *Science* **218**:433–443.

Kay, M. M. B., C. M. Tracey, J. R. Goodman, J. C. Cone, and P. S. Bassel (1983) Polypeptides immunologically related to band 3 are present in nucleated somatic cells. *Proc. Natl. Acad. Sci. USA* **80**:6882–6886.

Klein, I., D. Lehotay, and M. Godek (1981) Characterization of a calcium-activated proteinase that hydrolyzes a microtubule-associated protein. *Arch. Biochem. Biophys.* **208**:520–527.

Landis, D. M. D., and T. S. Reese (1983) Cytoplasmic organization in cerebellar dendritic spines. *J. Cell Biol.* **97**:1169–1178.

Lasek, R. J., and P. N. Hoffman (1976) The neuronal cytoskeleton, axonal transport and axonal growth. In *Cell Motility*, R. Goldman, T. Pollard, and J. Rosenbaum, eds., pp. 1021–1049, Cold Spring Harbor Laboratory, New York.

Lazarides, E., and W. J. Nelson (1982) Expression of spectrin in nonerythroid cells. *Cell* **31**:505–508.

Lazarides, E., and W. J. Nelson (1983) Erythrocyte and brain forms of spectrin in cerebellum: Distinct membrane cytoskeletal domains in neurons. *Science* **220**:1295–1296.

Lee, K. S. (1983) Cooperativity among afferents for the induction of long-term potentiation of the CA1 region of hippocampus. *J. Neurosci.* **3**:1369–1372.

Lee, K., F. Schottler, M. Oliver, and G. Lynch (1980) Brief bursts of high frequency stimulation produce two types of structural change in rat hippocampus. *J. Neurophysiol.* **44**:248–258.

Lee, K., M. Oliver, F. Schottler, and G. Lynch (1981) Electron microscopic studies of main slices: The effects of high frequency stimulation on dendritic ultrastructure. In *Electrical Activity in Isolated Mammalian CNS Preparations*, G. Kerkut, ed., pp. 189–212, Academic, New York.

Levine, J., and M. Willard (1981) Fodrin: Axonally transported polypeptides associated with the internal periphery of many cells. *J. Cell Biol.* **90**:631–643.

Levy, W. B., and O. Steward (1980) Synapses as associative memory elements in the hippocampal formation. *Brain Res.* **175**:233–245.

Llinás, R., and R. Hess (1976) Tetrodotoxin-resistant dendritic spikes in avian Purkinje cells. *Proc. Natl. Acad. Sci. USA* **73**:2520–2523.

Lynch, G., and M. Baudry (1983) Origins and manifestations of neuronal plasticity in the hippocampus. In *Clinical Neurosciences*, W. Willis, ed., Churchill-Livingstone, New York.

Lynch, G., and M. Baudry (1984) The biochemistry of memory: A new and specific hypothesis. *Science* **224**:1057–1063.

Lynch, G., T. Dunwiddie, and V. Gribkoff (1977) Heterosynaptic depression: A post-synaptic correlate of long-term potentiation. *Nature* **266**:737–739.

Lynch, G., S. Halpain, and M. Baudry (1982) Effects of high frequency synaptic stimulation on glutamate receptor binding studies with a modified *in vitro* hippocampal slice preparation. *Brain Res.* **244**:101–111.

Lynch, G., J. Larson, S. Kelso, G. Barrionuevo, and F. Schottler (1983) Intracellular injections of EGTA block the induction of hippocampal long-term potentiation. *Nature* **305**:719–721.

McNaughton, D. L., R. M. Douglas, and G. V. Goddard (1978) Synaptic enhancement in fascia dentata: Cooperativity among coactive afferents. *Brain Res.* **157**:277–293.

Mamounas, L., R. F. Thompson, G. Lynch, and M. Baudry (1984) Classical conditioning of the rabbit eyelid response increases glutamate receptor binding in hippocampal synaptic membranes. *Proc. Natl. Acad. Sci. USA* **81**:2478–2482.

Mangeat, P. H., and K. Burridge (1984) Immuno-precipitation of non-erythrocyte spectrin within live cells following microinjection of specific antibodies: Relation to cytoskeletal structures. *J. Cell Biol.* **98**:1363–1377.

Mellgren, R. L. (1980) Canine cardiac calcium-dependent proteases: Resolution of two forms with different requirements for calcium. *FEBS Lett.* **109**:129–133.

Melloni, E., B. Sparatore, F. Salamino, M. Michetti, and S. Pontremoli (1982) Cytosolic calcium-dependent proteinase of human erythrocytes: Formation of an enzyme–natural inhibitor complex induced by Ca^{2+} ions. *Biochem. Biophys. Res. Comm.* **106**:731–740.

Murachi, T., U. Tanaka, M. Hatanaka, and T. Muranami (1981a) Intracellular Ca^{2+}-dependent protease (calpain) and its high-molecular weight endogenous inhibitor (calpastatin). *Adv. Enzyme Regul.* **19**:407–424.

Murachi, T., M. Hatanaka, Y. Yasumoto, N. Nakayama, and K. Tanaka (1981b) A quantitative distribution study on calpain and calpastatin in rat tissues and cells. *Biochem. Int.* **2**:651–656.

Nicholson, C., G. Bruggencate, R. Steinberg, and H. Stockle (1977) Calcium modulation in brain extracellular microenvironment demonstrated with ion-selective micropipette. *Proc. Natl. Acad. Sci. USA* **74**:1287–1290.

Nicolson, G. L. (1979) Topographic display of cell surface components and their role in transmembrane signaling. *Curr. Top. Dev. Biol.* **13**:305–338.

O'Keefe, J., and L. Nadel (1978) *The Hippocampus as a Cognitive Map*, Oxford Univ. Press, London.

Palek, J., G. Stewart, and F. J. Lionetti (1974) The dependence of shape of human erythrocyte ghosts on calcium, magnesium, and adenosine triphosphate. *Blood* **44**:583–597.

Peters, A., S. L. Palay, and H. de F. Webster (1970) *Fine Structure of the Nervous System*, Hoeber, New York.

Racine, R. J., N. W. Milgram, and S. Hafner (1983) Long-term potentiation phenomenon in the rat limbic forebrain. *Brain Res.* **260**:217–231.

Ramón y Cajal, S. (1929) *Etude sur la Neurogenèse de Quelques Vertébrés*, trans. by L. Garth as *Studies on Vertebrate Neurogenesis*, Charles C Thomas, Springfield, Illinois, 1960.

Sasaki, T., N. Yoshimura, T. Kikuchi, M. Hatanaka, A. Kitahara, T. Sakihama, and T. Murachi (1983) Similarity and dissimilarity in subunit structures of calpains I and II from various sources as demonstrated by immunological cross-reactivity. *J. Biochem.* **94**:2055–2061.

Schwartzkroin, P. A., and C. E. Stafstrom (1980) Effects of EGTA on the calcium-activated after-hyperpolarization in hippocampal CA3 pyramidal cells. *Science* **210**:1125–1126.

Seifert, W., ed. (1983) *Neurobiology of the Hippocampus*, Academic, New York.

Shariff, N. A., and P. J. Roberts (1980) Effects of proteins and membrane-modifying agents on the binding of L-^{3}H-glutamate to cerebellar synaptic membranes. *Brain Res.* **194**:594–597.

Siman, R., M. Baudry, and G. Lynch (1983a) Purification from synaptosomal plasma membranes of calpain I, a thiol-protease activated by micromolar calcium concentrations. *J. Neurochem.* **41**:950–956.

Siman, R., M. Baudry, and G. Lynch (1983b) Possible molecular mechanism for modification of dendrite spine shape. *Soc. Neurosci. Abstr.* **9**:345.

Siman, R., M. Baudry, and G. Lynch (1984) Brain fodrin: Substrate for calpain I, an endogenous calcium-activated protease. *Proc. Natl. Acad. Sci. USA* **81**:3572–3576.

Siman, R., M. Baudry, and G. Lynch (1985a) Regulation of glutamate receptor binding by the cytoskeletal protein fodrin. *Nature* **313**:225–228.

Siman, R., C. Gall, L. S. Perlmutter, C. Christian, M. Baudry, and G. Lynch (1985b) Distribution of calpain I, an enzyme associated with degenerative activity, in rat brain. *Brain Res.* **347**:399–403.

Simonson, L., M. Baudry, R. Siman, and G. Lynch (1985) Regional distribution of soluble calcium-activated proteinase activity in neonatal and adult rat brain. *Brain Res.* **327**:153–159.

Squire, L. R. (1982) The neuropsychology of human memory. *Annu. Rev. Neurosci.* **5**:241–275.

Staubli, U., M. Baudry, and G. Lynch (1984) Leupeptin, a thiol-proteinase inhibitor, causes a selective impairment of spatial maze performance in rats. *Behav. Neural. Biol.* **40**:58–69.

Staubli, U., M. Baudry, and G. Lynch (1985) Olfactory discrimination learning is blocked by leupeptin, a thiol-proteinase inhibitor. *Brain Res.* **337**:333–336.

Steck, T. L. (1974) The organization of proteins in the human red blood cell membrane. *J. Cell Biol.* **62**:1–19.

Swanson, L. W., T. J. Teyler, and R. F. Thompson (1982) Hippocampal long-term potentiation: Mechanisms and implications for memory. *Neurosci. Res. Program Bull.* **20**:613–769.

Tower, D. B., and O. M. Young (1973) The activities of butyrylcholinesterase and carbonic anhydrase, the rate of anaerobic glycolysis, and the question of a constant density of glial cells in cerebral cortices of mammalian species from mouse to whale. *J. Neurochem.* **20**:269–278.

Weber, K., G. Shaw, M. Osborn, E. Debus, and N. Geisler (1983) Neurofilaments, a subclass of intermediate filaments: Structure and expression. *Cold Spring Harbor Symp. Quant. Biol.* **48**: 717–730.

White, J. G. (1974) Effects of an ionophore, A23187, on the surface morphology of normal erythrocytes. *Am. J. Pathol.* **77**:507–518.

Wong, R. K. S., D. A. Prince, and A. I. Basbaum (1979) Intradendritic recordings from hippocampal neurons. *Proc. Natl. Acad. Sci. USA* **76**:986–990.

Yoshimura, N., T. Kikuchi, T. Sasaki, A. Kitahara, M. Hatanaka, and T. Murachi (1983) Two distinct Ca^{2+} proteases (calpain I and calpain II) purified concurrently by the same method from rat kidney. *J. Biol. Chem.* **258**:8883–8889.

Zimmerman, U. J. P., and W. W. Schlaepfer (1982) Characterizations of a brain calcium-activated protease that degrades neurofilament protein. *Biochemistry* **21**:3977–3983.

Chapter 21

Allosteric Receptors and Molecular Models of Learning

JEAN-PIERRE CHANGEUX
THIERRY HEIDMANN

"Give me a nerve and a muscle and I make you a mind."

Unknown follower of Watson quoted by Piéron (1923)

ABSTRACT

Since its isolation and purification in the early seventies (for reviews, see Changeux, 1981; Conti-Tronconi and Raftery, 1982; Karlin, 1983; Stroud, 1983; Changeux et al., 1984a; Popot and Changeux, 1984; McCarthy et al., 1986), the nicotinic acetylcholine receptor has become one of the best-known neurotransmitter receptors for which complete primary structure data have been obtained (Noda et al., 1982, 1983a,b,c; Claudio et al., 1983; Devillers-Thiéry et al., 1983). In addition, it is one of the most thoroughly investigated membrane proteins with unambiguous allosteric properties (Changeux, 1981; Changeux et al., 1984a).

Because of their role in synaptic transmission, receptors for neurotransmitters may constitute critical targets for short- and long-term activity-dependent changes in synaptic efficacy. Thus, it appears timely to investigate to what extent realistic models for such material "learning traces" can be proposed on the basis of the known properties of the membrane-bound acetylcholine receptor. In this chapter, two groups of properties of the acetylcholine receptor are briefly analyzed and the relevant models discussed. First, characteristic allosteric properties of the receptor as a membrane-bound regulatory protein are briefly summarized. On the assumption that these properties hold for central receptors and ion channels, models for short-term learning at the postsynaptic level (see Changeux, 1981; Heidmann and Changeux, 1982; Changeux et al., 1984b) are presented. Then, data on the intrinsic and extrinsic modifications of the receptor molecule and of its metabolism in the course of synapse formation are reviewed and utilized to suggest models for long-term learning (see Changeux, 1981; Changeux et al., 1984b). As a prelude to these discussions, a history of learning theory and of the so-called Hebb synapse is briefly sketched, and a few experimental examples of short- and long-term learning at the cellular level are presented. In conclusion, the possible implications of the molecular models presented for the construction of large cooperative assemblies of neurons and for their storage by selection are mentioned.

HISTORICAL OVERVIEW OF CONNECTIONIST THEORIES
ON LEARNING AND MEMORY

The notion that learning and memory storage involve lasting changes in the strength and/or number of connections in neural networks is deeply rooted in history. Explicit mention of this concept can already be found in Descartes' *Traité de l'Homme* (1677), in which he writes "For instance, when the action of the object ABC, increasing the opening of the pipes 2, 4, 6, causes the spirits to enter in larger quantity than they would do without it, it also causes that, passing more toward N, they have the strength to form certain pathways which remain open still after the action of the object ABC has ceased." If one replaces "pipes" by nerve processes (axon and dendrites), and "openings" by synapses, then Descartes merely proposes that the "memory" trace in the brain consists of stable modifications of synapse efficacy! In the same chapter he also states that the "diverse openings of the pipes . . . trace figures [in the brain] which show analogies [*qui se rapportent*] with that of the objects," thus touching on an eventual isomorphism between the memory trace and the external object. Finally, Descartes, with regard to the evocation of memories, clearly states that "if one reopens only a few like a and b, that alone might cause the others like c and d to reopen also at the same time," the first allusion to an eventual "cooperative" character of neuronal assemblies. Little progress beyond Descartes' views on memory can be found in eighteenth- and early nineteenth-century writings, but the nomenclature changed. Descartes' "tube openings" became "contact barriers" (Freud, 1895) and finally synapses (Sherrington, 1897); "animal spirits" became electrical nerve impulses. Meanwhile, considerable progress was made in describing the anatomy of the nervous system at the cellular level (see Brazier, 1978), with detailed accounts of the axonal and dendritic arborizations of the diverse categories of neurons in the brain.

In 1895, the anatomist Ramón y Cajal proposed a theory on the "Increase of Interneuronal Connections as a Means to Improve Psychic Processes and Abilities." His idea was that "cellular expansions" were made and "orientate according to the major nerve currents or in the direction of the intercellular association which is the object of reiterated solicitations of the will." Nearly at the same time, the psychologist Thorndike, in his book *Animal Intelligence* (1898), postulated that the learning of a behavior, "the association between sense impressions and impulses to action," corresponds to the strengthening (or weakening) of a "bond" or "connection." According to him, learning occurred by trial and error ("selecting and connecting") and followed a number of laws. One of these is the classical "law of exercise," according to which practice strengthens connections (the "law of use"), while the weakening of connections or forgetting occurs when practice is discontinued (the "law of disuse"). Another is the well-known "law of effect," which relates the increase (or decrease) in associative strength with the "satisfying" (or "annoying") effect produced by the act. Thorndike's theoretical and experimental work established the foundations for subsequent research on animal learning.

In his "Lectures on the Work of the Cerebral Hemispheres," Pavlov (1927) (who explicitly referred to Thorndike) further developed a connectionist model to account for his data on the "conditioned reflex." He wrote: "The basic mechanism for the formation of the conditioned reflex is the encounter, the coincidence of the time of excitation of a given point of the cerebral cortex with a more intense excitation of another point, presumably also from the cortex, by which a bond, a facilitated pathway, forms more or less rapidly." Pavlov's followers in the United States (see Hilgard, 1948; for a review, see Terrace, 1984) have extensively utilized this theoretical model both with and without significant modification. In 1940, Hilgard and Marquis introduced the notion of a "transient trace mechanism," or short-term effect, linked with the self-excitation of closed circuits in which impulse activity persisted after stimulation had ceased. The trace was subsequently thought to be made permanent by an additional "structural change" or "growth process," which constituted the basis for long-term effects.

Hebb's book, *The Organization of Behavior* (1949), was primarily an attempt to interpret the problems of perception raised by the Gestalt psychologists in terms of neural mechanisms. His main proposal, following an "empiricist" scheme, was that "repeated stimulation of specific (sensory) receptors will lead slowly to the formation of an assembly of cells which can act briefly as a closed system after stimulation has ceased." According to Hebb, this constituted the "simplest instance of a representative process (image or idea)." The Pavlovian scheme of the conditioned reflex was extended at a more "molar" level to cooperative assemblies of neurons, and simultaneously, in the chapter entitled "The First Stage of Perception: Growth of the Assembly," a microscopic mechanism since then known as the "Hebb postulate" or "Hebb synapse" was proposed. It appeared, largely, as a restatement of Pavlov's views in connectionist terms: "When an axon of cell A is near enough to excite a cell B and repeatedly and persistently takes part in firing it, some growth process or metabolic change takes place in one or both cells so that A's efficiency as one of the cells firing B is increased." Hebb further mentions that "the details of these histological speculations are not important" and that "the general idea is an old one, that any two cells or systems of cells that are repeatedly active at the same time will tend to become associated so that the activity in one facilitates activity in the other." At the end of the same chapter, Hebb states that whatever the precise network of neurons involved, "the diagrams and discussion of the preceding section require the frequent existence of two kinds of coincidence: (1) the synchronization of firing in two or more converging axons and (2) the anatomical fact of convergence in fibers. . . . " We will refer to these propositions as *Hebb's laws of learning*.

Subsequent theoretical work has abundantly used (and sometimes misused) Hebb's postulate as a simple synaptic device to knot neurons under a variety of learning situations with adequate and most often arbitrary rules for relating the sign of the change in efficacy (increase/decrease) with the time relationships of pre- and postsynaptic activities (see, for instance, Marr, 1969; Albus, 1971; Sejnowski, 1977; Bienenstock et al., 1983; Carew et al., 1984). Stent's (1973) proposal of "a physiological mechanism" for Hebb's postulate appeared as an original attempt to interpret the change in synaptic efficacy in terms of the "stability" properties of the then recently discovered acetylcholine receptor. His assumption was that the "stability of the receptor protein in the cell membrane depends on the maintenance of an inward gradient of electrical potential," and that the sign reversal (of a few dozen millivolts) that occurred during the action potential impulse inactivated the molecule, while the neurally evoked postsynaptic potential prevented inactivation by "clamping" the membrane potential at -10 to -20 mV. Despite its elegance, the Stent model has not received experimental support. Subsequent studies have shown that the elimination of nonjunctional acetylcholine receptors occurs, not from a direct effect of electric fields on receptor stability, but from an activity-dependent repression of receptor biosynthesis. This justifies a reexamination of the Hebb postulate in terms of the most recent knowledge of acetylcholine receptor structure and metabolism.

CELLULAR AND SYNAPTIC EXAMPLES OF SHORT-TERM "LEARNING" AT THE POSTSYNAPTIC LEVEL

Diverse experimental systems, from both invertebrates and vertebrates, have been developed in the search for a cellular and even a molecular learning trace at either a presynaptic (Kandel, 1977; Hawkins and Kandel, 1984) or a postsynaptic (Andersen et al., 1980; Alkon, 1984; Lynch and Baudry, 1984) locus (for reviews, see Woody, 1982; Marler and Terrace, 1984; Changeux et al., 1987). The evident neuronal site that satisfies Hebb's law of "anatomical convergence" is, of course, the postsynaptic membrane on dendrites, somas, and even axons (in the case of axoaxonal synapses). At this level, signals which may, but also may *not*, include action potentials converge from the considered nerve terminal and from the rest of the postsynaptic cell and become integrated. On the other hand, the presynaptic membrane cannot simply be viewed as a site of convergence, except if it receives axoaxonal synapses (and then becomes postsynaptic) or if it is regulated by a transsynaptic transfer of signals (see Gouzé et al., 1983). In this chapter, a few examples of postsynaptic regulation have been selected and are briefly reviewed. Examples of homosynaptic regulation, the simplest instance of the regulation of a given synapse by its own state of activity, are presented first. Then, examples of heterosynaptic regulation in which convergent interaction takes place between different synapses are discussed.

Homosynaptic Regulation

Desensitization of the Response to Acetylcholine of Vertebrate Neuromuscular Junction. The simplest model of the regulation of synaptic efficacy at the postsynaptic level is the pharmacological desensitization of the end-plate postsynaptic membrane to the neurotransmitter acetylcholine. Prolonged application of acetylcholine to the end plate causes, within seconds to minutes, a decrease in the amplitude of the response to brief pulses of neurally evoked or ionophoretically applied acetylcholine (Katz and Thesleff, 1957). The phenomenon comprises two main kinetic processes (Feltz and Trautmann, 1980, 1982; Sakmann et al., 1980; Magleby and Pallotta, 1981) that are reversible.

At the frog neuromuscular junction, under voltage clamp conditions, blocking of acetylcholinesterase (by diisopropylfluorophosphate or neostigmine) causes desensitization to develop without the addition of exogenous acetylcholine. For instance, a 30-sec train of impulses in the motor nerve at 10 impulses/sec yields about a 50% desensitization of the response (Magleby and Pallotta, 1981). On the other hand, when the esterase is active, desensitization does not occur spontaneously, whatever the length of the stimulation period is, as long as the intervals between stimuli are 30 msec or greater. Shorter intervals between stimuli (20 msec), however, may lead to significant desensitization (Akasu and Karczmar, 1980). Desensitization occurs consistently when the motor nerve is submitted to pairs of stimuli (300–500) with an interval between impulses of 25 msec or less (Magleby and Pallotta, 1981). Desensitization may thus effectively play a role in the regulation of synaptic efficacy under adequate conditions of stimulation.

"Spontaneous" desensitization is enhanced by the noncompetitive blocker chlorpromazine and decreased when the postsynaptic membrane is depolarized (Magleby and Pallotta, 1981), as observed under conditions of iontophoretic application of acetylcholine (Magazanik and Vyskocil, 1975; Fiekers et al., 1980). Finally, calcium ions and other divalent cations accelerate the rate of desensitization (Magazanik and Vyskocil, 1970; Anwyl and Narahasi, 1980), when applied on the cytoplasmic side of the membrane (Miledi, 1980).

"Learning" in the physiological and behavioral sense is not expected to occur at the neuromuscular junction. Nevertheless, desensitization of the permeability response observed with this nerve–muscle preparation remains an excellent example of short-term change unambiguously localized on the postsynaptic side of the synapse and well understood in molecular terms. It serves as the basic mechanism on which our model of short-term learning is built.

Long-Term Potentiation of Synaptic Transmission in the Hippocampus. The phenomenon referred to as long-term potentiation was originally described (Bliss and Lømo, 1973) as a long-lasting enhancement, for hours or even days, of synaptic transmission in the perforant pathway–granule cell synapse elicited by a brief tetanic stimulation in the hippocampal formation. The phenomenon exists in all excitatory pathways of the hippocampus and has been extensively analyzed in hippocampal slices from the guinea pig (Andersen et al., 1980; Andersen, this volume). Changes at the presynaptic level (such as enhanced transmitter release) may occur, but significant effects at the postsynaptic level have been noted (see Teyler and Discenna, 1984; Sharfman and Sarvey, 1985).

Extracellular unit recordings of hippocampal pyramidal cells show that potentiation coincides with an increased probability of firing and a reduced firing latency of the recorded pyramidal cells. Intracellular recordings further disclose an increase in size of the excitatory postsynaptic potential (Andersen et al., 1980). Applications of the excitatory transmitter glutamate (Hvalby and Andersen, 1984), or of the agonist N-methyl-D-aspartate (NMDA) cause long-term potentiation in conjunction with low-frequency synaptic activation (Collingridge et al., 1983). On the other hand, the antagonist of the glutamate receptor, L-glutamic acid diethyl ester, reduces synaptic transmission without affecting long-term potentiation, while the NMDA receptor-blocking agent 2-amino-5-phosphonovalerate has the opposite effect, suggesting a primordial role for the NMDA receptor in long-term potentiation. Calcium ions are required for long-term potentiation to occur (see Lynch and Baudry, 1984) and may enter the dendrites of the pyramidal cell as a consequence of receptor activation. The NMDA receptor channel is blocked by extracellular magnesium, and this effect decreases with depolarization (Nowak et al., 1984). Such voltage-dependent blocking may lead to a long-term "regenerative potentiation" under conditions of glutamate-elicited depolarization (Ascher et al., 1986). An increase in the number of glutamate (?) receptors consecutive to a calcium-induced proteolytic degradation of cytoskeletal proteins has also been suggested as a molecular mechanism for long-term potentiation (see Lynch and Baudry, 1984), but additional (or alternative) mechanisms may still be considered.

Heterosynaptic Regulation

Cross-Desensitization and Cross-Potentiation Between Distinct Receptors. Interactions between the permeability responses elicited by different neurotransmitters have been reported in several instances at the level of the same postsynaptic neuron (see references in Ascher and Chesnoy-Marchais, 1982). In *Aplysia*, such interactions have been demonstrated for "slow" permeability changes. Yet these responses are less well understood than "fast" responses like those of the motor end plate to acetylcholine and may involve a number of successive steps after the binding of the agonist. Voltage clamp studies of the potassium ion permeability increase produced in identified *Aplysia* neurons from the cerebral ganglion by three distinct agonists, carbamylcholine, histamine, and dopamine, show that desensitization of the response may take place with any of the three. Moreover, prolonged exposure of the neurons to any one of the agonists reduces the response to the other agonists. Cross-desensitization occurs between agonists (Ascher and Chesnoy-Marchais, 1982). On the other hand, combined application of low doses of two of the agonists may give a supralinear summation of the response referred to as cross-potentiation.

In the *Aplysia* neurons investigated, such interactions between distinct neurotransmitter responses on the same postsynaptic soma do not seem to be mediated by the intracellular concentration of calcium ions, but may involve a common reaction step, possibly a common intracellular "messenger." Cross-potentiation has rarely been observed in other systems, in contrast to cross-desensitization, which has been reported, for instance, between histamine and carbamylcholine in guinea pig ileum (Hurwitz and McGuffee, 1979), and between β-agonists and prostaglandins in various other systems (see references in Ascher and Chesnoy-Marchais, 1982; Masters et al., 1985). Functional interactions between various neurotransmitter responses might thus be a rather widespread phenomenon of convergence, different of course from the straightforward "integration" of electrical signals by the neuronal membrane.

Heterosynaptic "Depression" in the Cerebellum. Purkinje cells in the vertebrate cerebellum receive two distinct synaptic inputs, one via numerous parallel fibers, the other via a unique, though extensively ramified, climbing fiber. Because of its simplicity and its eventual contribution to learning processes, this system has been investigated in great detail (see Eccles et al., 1967; Llinás, 1969; Marr, 1969; Ito et al., 1982; Ito, this volume). It exhibits, among other features, a particular cellular process, referred to as heterosynaptic depression, which is the following: The conjunction of parallel fiber stimulation at 20 impulses/sec (via a vestibular nerve) and of climbing fiber response (via stimulation of the inferior olive) for 25 sec depresses the parallel fiber response without a change in the spontaneous discharge of the Purkinje cells (Ito et al., 1982). The depression lasts several minutes and recovery is observed in about 10 min. The sites of modification are the parallel fiber–Purkinje cell synapses. Iontophoretic application of glutamate, the putative neurotransmitter of the parallel fibers, in conjunction with stimulation of the climbing fiber, depresses the response of the Purkinje cells to glutamate. The observed heterosynaptic depression would thus result from the enhanced desensitization of the glutamate receptor at the parallel fiber–Purkinje cell synapses as a consequence of the concomitant firing of the climbing fiber. The glutamate receptor present in the postsynaptic membrane of these synapses would thus be the site of geometrical and temporal integration of the afferent signals.

Heterosynaptic Regulation of the Siphon Withdrawal Reflex in Aplysia. Plausible models of elementary learning mechanisms in *Aplysia* neurons have been extensively investigated and reviewed (Kandel, 1977; Carew et al., 1984; Hawkins and Kandel, 1984; Quinn, 1984; Kandel et al., this volume), with a special emphasis given to *presynaptic* changes in synaptic efficacy. Indeed, "habituation" and "sensitization" of the gill withdrawal reflex have been shown to coincide with a change in sensorimotor synaptic efficacy entirely accounted for by a decrease (habituation) or an increase (sensitization) in the number of neurotransmitter quanta released by the nerve endings. Extension of the analysis to the siphon withdrawal reflex leads to an illustration of the law of convergence. Stimulation of the tail gives the unconditioned response (US); physiological or electrical stimulation of siphon sensory neurons from the abdominal ganglion gives the conditioned one (CS). Pairing of tail and siphon sensory neuron stimuli leads to a much greater siphon withdrawal when the sensory neurons are stimulated than in the control in which the stimuli are *not* paired. However, in *apparent* contradiction with the Hebb postulate, the prolonged depolarization of the motor neuron (which results in its firing) or its hyperpolarization (which abolishes firing) did not affect the change (Carew et al., 1984).

The actual sequence of synaptic modifications that takes place "upstream" of the sensorimotor synapse is not known. Yet the possibility has been considered (Hawkins et al., 1983) that one of them, issued from an interneuron [serotonergic (?) or peptidergic], is the convergence locus at which the primary modification takes place. This interneuron would be on line with the tail (US) sensory neuron and make an axoaxonal synapse (AA) on the nerve ending of the siphon (CS) sensory neurons. This sensory nerve ending itself would contact the motor neuron. Thus, according to the hypothetical scheme proposed, the integration of the convergent pathways would take place primarily on the *postsynaptic* side of AA. The firing of the siphon axon (CS) for instance, by stimulating the entry of calcium ions in conjunction with the activation of AA, would enhance the action of the neurotransmitter on its receptor located on the postsynaptic side of AA. Assuming this scheme correct, then, secondarily, the release of the neurotransmitter from the sensorimotor synapse would be modified as a consequence of a cascade of reactions involving cAMP and a cAMP-dependent protein kinase. These reasonings thus suggest that synapse AA would satisfy Hebb's law of anatomical convergence and coincidence of firing. Assuming the model correct, the primary target of the regulation would be the *postsynaptic* side of AA. Accordingly, as found by Carew et al. (1984), firing of the motor neuron would not be expected to modify the efficacy of AA except if a retrograde transfer of information from the motor neuron to the nerve ending was taking place. The authentic "associative" step would take place at the level of AA, its "readout" at the level of the sensorimotor synapse.

Synaptic Facilitation in the Neocortex.   Even though neurons from the neocortex, in particular the frontal cortex, should be the privileged target for activity-dependent changes of synaptic properties, only limited information is available as yet concerning these neurons (for a review, see Frégnac and Imbert, 1984). In the motor cortex of the cat, lasting changes in synaptic efficacy have been identified under various regimes of joint stimulation of convergent excitatory pathways (Baranyi and Feher, 1981a,b). For instance, in pyramidal motor cells (yielding pyramidal tract axons), the amplitude of excitatory postsynaptic potentials can be recorded intracellularly under conditions of classical conditioning. A typical example is the "facilitation" of the test postsynaptic potential elicited by the stimulation of the ventrolateral nucleus from the thalamus consecutive to pairing with "unconditioned" spikes from the callosal system (Baranyi and Feher, 1981b). Pairing of 60–90 stimuli at intervals between stimuli smaller than 100 msec yielded an approximately threefold increase in the amplitude of the postsynaptic response, which lasted for about 10–15 min (mean) and returned to the preconditioning level approximately 20 min after the training session. Few details are available as to the exact connectivity of the synapses involved and the pharmacology of their response.

Remarks About the Experimental Examples

The few model experiments briefly summarized illustrate that associative changes of membrane properties can be recorded at the *postsynaptic* level by electrophysiological techniques. These traces are elicited by chemical and/or electrical signals. In the original formulations of his postulate, Hebb exclusively mentioned "firing," that is, electrical impulses, as manifestations of "cellular activity." It should be recalled, however, that in 1949, when *The Organization of Behavior* was written, the existence of chemical transmission in the central nervous system was seriously challenged (for a historical account, see Eccles, 1964). It thus appears today legitimate to include both categories of signaling in our definition of "activity" and to refer to the more general Hebb's laws of synchronization and convergence as fundamental to the cellular and molecular mechanisms of learning. In these instances, short-term learning becomes a problem of regulation of membrane properties, and it is of course at the level of the molecular components of the postsynaptic membrane that such regulation should be investigated.

ALLOSTERIC PROPERTIES OF NEUROTRANSMITTER RECEPTORS

One of the outcomes of molecular biology from past decades has been the identification of the elementary mechanisms that underlie biological regulation. It is, nowadays, well established that in eukaryotic as well as in prokaryotic cells, regulatory circuits are built around two basic molecular components: (1) regulatory signals, in general, small diffusible molecules; and (2) specialized proteins that act as biological "transducers," recognize the regulatory signal, possess a biological activity, and mediate the interaction between the ligand binding site and the biologically active site. Extensive analysis of the structural and functional properties of this important class of intracellular proteins (regulatory enzymes, gene repressors, oxygen binding proteins, etc.) has led to the demonstration that the two categories of sites involved are topographically distinct. Their interaction is thus indirect or "allosteric" (Monod et al., 1963, 1965) and mediated by conformational transitions of the protein molecule between, in general, a small number of discrete states (Monod et al., 1965).

These concepts have been extended to the proteins involved in intercellular communication, typified in the nervous system by neurotransmitter receptors (Changeux, 1966, 1981; Changeux et al., 1967, 1984a; Karlin, 1967). In such a scheme, the neurotransmitter serves as a regulatory signal acting on the external face of the receptor molecule, and the biologically active site is either a transmembrane ion channel or an enzyme catalytic site, oriented toward the inside of the cell. Recent progress has been made regarding our knowledge of these membrane-bound regulatory proteins and may serve in the elaboration of models of regulation of synaptic efficacy. Only their most critical properties are briefly mentioned here.

Acetylcholine Receptor

Initially isolated and purified (Changeux et al., 1970; see Changeux, 1981) from the electric organ of fish with the help of snake venom α-toxins (Lee and Chang, 1966) as highly selective ligands, the acetylcholine receptor remains one of the best-characterized neurotransmitter receptors (Conti-Tronconi and Raftery, 1982; Karlin, 1983; Changeux et al., 1984a; Anholt et al., 1985; Stroud and Finer-Moore, 1985; McCarthy et al., 1986). Moreover, many of its structural and functional properties hold for the receptors of the neuromuscular junction from high vertebrates (in particular from humans; Noda et al., 1983c) and possibly for nicotinic receptors from the central nervous system (for a discussion, see Lindstrom et al., 1983; Jacob et al., 1986).

The smallest molecular weight unit of the molecule is a heterologous pentamer made up of four different subunits of exact protein molecular weight $\alpha = 50{,}116$ D, $\beta = 53{,}681$ D, $\gamma = 56{,}279$ D, $\delta = 57{,}565$ D (Noda et al., 1982, 1983a,b,c) with the stoichiometry $\alpha_2\beta\gamma\delta$ (Reynolds and Karlin, 1978; Raftery et al., 1980). The cDNAs coding for the four subunits have been cloned and sequenced in *T. californica* (Ballivet et al., 1982; Noda et al., 1982, 1983a,b; Claudio et al., 1983), in *T. marmorata* (Giraudat et al., 1982; Sumikawa et al., 1982; Devillers-Thiéry et al., 1983), and in high vertebrates (see references in Changeux et al., 1984a). The inferred amino acid sequences of the four chains show striking homologies

(10–60% identity, average 40%), suggesting an evolution by gene duplication from a common ancestral gene (Raftery et al., 1980; Noda et al., 1983b). Accordingly, the five subunits are viewed as making a transmembrane bundle with a rotational axis of pseudosymmetry perpendicular to the plane of the membrane. In *Torpedo*, the molecule may also exist as a dimer of two $\alpha_2\beta\gamma\delta$ oligomers cross-linked by a disulfide bridge between the δ-chains.

The two α-chains carry the acetylcholine α-toxin binding sites. These sites exhibit positive cooperative interactions, even though they differ in several of their pharmacological properties (such as inactivation by the coral diterpenoid lophotoxin (Culver et al., 1984) and are present on nonadjacent subunits within the $\alpha_2\beta\gamma\delta$ oligomer (Holtzman et al., 1982; Zingsheim et al., 1982a,b; Bon et al., 1984). These sites are part of a large amino-terminal hydrophilic domain that faces the synaptic cleft (see Wennogle and Changeux, 1980; Fairclough et al., 1983; Kao et al., 1984). Reconstitution experiments (for reviews, see Changeux, 1981; Anholt et al., 1983; Popot, 1983; Schindler et al., 1984; Montal et al., 1986) show that the $\alpha_2\beta\gamma\delta$ oligomer contains the ionic channel and all the structural elements required for the regulation of its opening.

The membrane-bound receptor carries, in addition, other categories of ligand binding sites that affect the properties of the acetylcholine binding sites and/or the opening of the ion channel. The most typical ones bind a rather heterogeneous group of pharmacologically active ligands referred to as noncompetitive blockers. These compounds, which include several local anesthetics, detergents, chlor-promazine, phencyclidine, and the frog toxin histrionicotoxin, are postulated to interfere directly and/or indirectly with the ion channel (for reviews, see Adams, 1981; Changeux, 1981). They bind to two main categories of sites: high-affinity sites, sensitive to histrionicotoxin and present as a unique copy per receptor pentamer, and low-affinity sites insensitive to histrionicotoxin, much more numerous (10–20 times the number of α-bungarotoxin sites) and lipid-dependent, that are most likely to be located at the interface of the receptor with membrane lipids (Heidmann et al., 1983b).

Binding of noncompetitive blockers to their site enhances, at equilibrium, the binding of cholinergic ligands to the acetylcholine binding site (Cohen et al., 1974; for reviews, see Heidmann et al., 1983b; Oswald et al., 1983). Conversely, cholinergic ligands potentiate their binding (Grünhagen and Changeux, 1976; Krodel et al., 1979; Heidmann et al., 1983b). Reciprocal allosteric interactions take place, under equilibrium conditions, between these two classes of sites. Binding sites for calcium and other multivalent cations (see Heidmann and Changeux, 1979; Rübsamen et al., 1978; Oswald, 1983a,b) have also been demonstrated on the *Torpedo* receptor. Finally, substance P affects the response of cells derived from the neural crest to acetylcholine (Stallcup and Patrick, 1980; Clapham and Neher, 1984).

Identification of the chain, or chains, of the receptor involved in the high-affinity site for noncompetitive blockers was done with photolabile derivatives of local anesthetics, quinacrine, and phencyclidine (Oswald et al., 1980; Oswald and Changeux, 1981a,b; Kaldany and Karlin, 1983; Muhn and Hucho, 1983; Haring et al., 1984), or under conditions of ultraviolet irradiation (Oswald and Changeux, 1981b). In a general manner, all four chains were labeled when the ligand occupied the unique high-affinity site but with a preferential incorporation of the label in the δ-chain with *T. marmorata* (Oswald et al., 1980) and of the α-chain with *T. californica* (Kaldany and Karlin, 1983; Muhn and Hucho, 1983). In all instances, the agonists potentiated the labeling.

The simplest location for this high-affinity site is the central hydrophilic funnel (visualized by electron microscopy in the pseudo-axis of symmetry of the molecule), where the distances to all five chains are minimum (Heidmann et al., 1983b). A similar location for an allosteric site has been described in hemoglobin for diphosphoglycerate (Arnone, 1972; see also Perutz et al., 1986). Since binding of ligands to this site blocks the ion channel when it opens, it appears likely, though still hypothetical, that it belongs to this channel. Models of transmembrane organization of the ion channel based on the sequence of defined segments of the four subunits have been discussed (see Changeux et al., 1984a; Popot and Changeux, 1984). In all of them, the peptide segment involved in acetylcholine binding differs from those that contribute to the ion channel (Giraudat et al., 1986; Oberthür et al., 1986) and, most likely, are coded by different exons of the chromosomic gene (Noda et al., 1983c). Accordingly, the interactions between the acetylcholine binding site and the ion channel would be indirect or *allosteric* and mediated by conformational transitions of the receptor molecule.

Rapid kinetic analysis in parallel with fluorescent (Heidmann and Changeux, 1979; Prinz and Maelicke, 1983) or radioactive (Boyd and Cohen, 1980; Neubig et al., 1982) agonist binding and analysis of channel opening (Heidmann and Changeux, 1980; Neubig and Cohen, 1980) leads to the distinction of two main categories of transitions: (1) the still unresolved reaction of activation, which results in the opening of the ion channel in the micro- to millisecond time scale; and (2) slower transitions that regulate the ability of the receptor molecule to be activated and are referred to as desensitization. Desensitization has been resolved into two processes (Feltz and Trautmann, 1980; Sakmann et al., 1980; Walker et al., 1981, 1982; Neubig et al., 1982; Heidmann et al., 1983a): a fast one, at the rate of $2–75 \text{ sec}^{-1}$ and a slow one, at the rate of $0.01–0.1 \text{ sec}^{-1}$. The rapid phase leads to a 1000-fold decrease in initial flux, the slow one to undetectable ion transport.

The simplest minimal model (Heidmann and Changeux, 1980; Neubig and Cohen, 1980) that fits the rapid binding and flux data is an adapted version of the concerted model for allosteric transitions (Monod et al., 1965) and of that proposed in a different context by Katz and Thesleff (1957) for pharmacological desensitization:

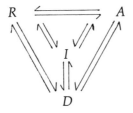

where *A* corresponds to the active state, with the channel open, and *I* and *D* correspond to the rapidly and slowly desensitized states, respectively. All these states are discrete and interconvertible, and at least two of them, *A* (Jackson,

1984) and D (Heidmann and Changeux, 1979), are accessible in the absence of agonist. Their respective dissociation constants are: 50–100 μM (R), less than 1 μM (I), and 5 nM (D) for the fluorescent agonist dansyl-6-choline (Heidmann and Changeux, 1979) and acetylcholine (Boyd and Cohen, 1980). Under resting conditions, in the absence of agonist, the R state would be the dominant state. During physiological transmission, the cleft concentration of acetylcholine jumps to 0.1–1 mM, yielding near saturation of the R state. Equilibration with acetylcholine yields the high-affinity D state, with a dissociation constant which, interestingly, falls in the range of the nonquantal leak concentration of acetylcholine in the synaptic cleft.

In agreement with the model, rapid mixing with agonists under conditions that populate in the A state enhances the association rate constant of the channel blockers perhydrohistrionicotoxin (Eldefrawi et al., 1980), phencyclidine (Oswald et al., 1983), and chlorpromazine (Heidmann and Changeux, 1984) to their high-affinity sites by a factor of 10^3–10^4. Conversely, the noncompetitive blockers shift the receptor toward the D state to greater or lesser extents, depending on the structure of the compound and of its relative affinity for the R and D states. Stabilization occurs either via their high-affinity site and/or their multiple, low-affinity, lipid-dependent sites (Heidmann et al., 1983b). In both cases, the non-competitive blockers behave as regulatory ligands of the permeability response to acetylcholine.

Calcium ions also play this role. At equilibrium, they stabilize preferentially the D state (Cohen et al., 1974; Heidmann and Changeux, 1979) but also accelerate the slow transition toward the same state (Oswald, 1983a). Electrical potentials affect the transition toward the D state: Hyperpolarization of the membrane accelerates rapid desensitization, while depolarization has the opposite effect (see references in Takeyasu et al., 1983).

Other Receptors for Neurotransmitters and Allosteric Ion Channels

Many receptors for neurotransmitters have been characterized by binding assays (Synder, 1984), but only a few of them are known protein species. They include the receptors for GABA (Olsen, 1981; Barnard et al., 1983), glycine (Pfeiffer et al., 1984), and the acetylcholine muscarinic receptor (Birdsall et al., 1983; Soko-lowsky, 1984). Electrophysiological recordings by standard or patch clamp techniques confirm the existence of desensitization of some glutamate (see references in Cull-Candy, 1983), and GABA (see references in Peck, 1980; Sakmann et al., 1983) receptors. Equilibrium binding studies with the GABA receptor reveal the unambiguous allosteric effects of pharmacologically active ligands such as the barbiturates or the benzodiazepines (Leeb-Lundberg et al., 1980; Olsen, 1981). Yet little information is available about the rapid binding of these compounds and about their eventual relationship to desensitization.

Binding interactions between different neurotransmitters have been demonstrated under equilibrium conditions with membrane preparations and referred to as receptor–receptor interactions (for reviews, see Fuxe et al., 1981, 1983; Birdsall, 1982; Agnati et al., 1983). The data available at this stage do not lead to an unambiguous distinction between interactions of allosteric sites on the same receptor molecule and actual interaction between different receptor molecules mediated, or not, by intracellular second (or even third) messengers.

Important structural differences exist between ion channel-linked and enzyme-linked receptor molecules that may be associated with different regulatory properties. For instance, at variance with what happens in the acetylcholine receptor, in the cyclase-linked adrenergic receptor (for reviews, see Schramm and Sillinger, 1984; Sibley and Lefkowitz, 1985) the phenomenon of desensitization seems to involve protein covalent modifications. Finally, in recent years, several nonsynaptic ion channels have been identified as proteins (see references in Agnew et al., 1983; Salkoff, 1983; Talvenheimo et al., 1983) and the cDNA for one of them, the voltage-sensitive sodium channel, has been cloned and sequenced (Noda et al., 1984). Moreover, binding studies with these membrane-bound channel proteins disclose (Agnew et al., 1983) typical allosteric interactions between pharmacologically active ligands (including animal toxins) (for reviews, see Catterall, 1980; Talvenheimo et al., 1983).

A MODEL FOR SHORT-TERM REGULATION OF SYNAPTIC EFFICACY BASED ON THE ALLOSTERIC PROPERTIES OF POSTSYNAPTIC RECEPTORS

The model (Heidmann and Changeux, 1982) discussed in this chapter was proposed for at least three reasons: (1) The acetylcholine receptor exhibits clear-cut allosteric transitions that take place in time scales orders of magnitude longer than synaptic transmission; (2) similar transitions have been recognized in other neurotransmitter receptors and may exist in nonsynaptic ion channels; and (3) the physiological role of these transitions is enigmatic and thus deserves interpretation.

Statements

The basic statements of the proposed model (Heidmann and Changeux, 1982) are the following:

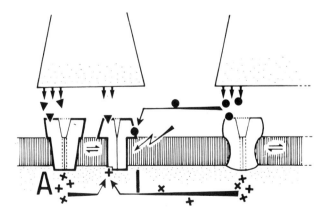

1. Receptors for neurotransmitters are transmembrane allosteric proteins with a fixed topological distribution in the adult neuron. They carry several distinct sets of sites for diverse categories of ligands such as neurotransmitters and nerve ending-released substances on their cleft face and internal second messengers on their cytoplasmic face.

2. The protein molecule exists under at least two interconvertible conformations, A and I, in reversible thermodynamic equilibrium. The A (activable) conformation gives the physiological response (channel opening, enzyme activation, etc.) in the presence of the neurotransmitter (or other physiological effector such as the membrane electrical potential), whereas the I (inactivable) conformation does not. The time scale of the $A \leftrightharpoons I$ transition is several orders of magnitude longer than that of the activation reaction.

3. The two conformations may differ by: (a) the affinities for the ligands l_i that bind to the various categories of sites carried by the receptor molecule; (b) the oriented electrical dipolar moment μ of the receptor protein; and (c) the reactivity to covalent bonding.

4. States A and I are discrete and interconvertible, and both may be present before ligand binding. In some systems prone to desensitization (or depression), the A state dominates at rest; in others prone to sensitization (or potentiation), the I state is spontaneously favored. Binding of the diverse categories of ligands to their respective sites stabilizes the receptor conformation for which they exhibit the highest affinity and shifts the $A \leftrightharpoons I$ equilibrium to an extent which is a function of the relative affinities of the considered ligand to the A and I state. Electric fields affect the transition as a function of the difference in dipole moment between the states. Covalent modification of the protein may also regulate the $A \leftrightharpoons I$ transition.

5. Initially proposed for neurotransmitter receptors, the model may be extended to other membrane-bound allosteric proteins such as nonsynaptic ion channels.

Basic Equations

Under conditions in which the binding of ligands l_i is rapid, compared to the rates of the conformational transitions between states A and I, the system can be entirely described by the reduced equation:

$$A \underset{k^- [V(t),\, l_i(t)]}{\overset{k^+ [V(t),\, l_i(t)]}{\rightleftharpoons}} I, \tag{1}$$

where k^+ and k^- are rate constants that depend on the transmembrane electrical potential V and on the concentrations of the effectors l_i at time t. For a given population of such proteins, the fraction $n_a(t)$ of molecules that are present at time t in the A conformation is the solution of the differential equation:

$$\frac{dn_a}{dt} + \{k^+[V(t),\, l_i(t)] + k^-[V(t),\, l_i(t)]\}n_a - k^-[V(t),\, l_i(t)] = 0 . \tag{2}$$

In general, resolution of Equation 2 requires numerical integration, but analytical solutions can be derived for simple cases.

Applications

Multiple Signals Integration. Bound to the neuronal membrane at a well-defined and fixed subcellular locus, the receptors for neurotransmitters (and also the allosteric ion channels) receive chemical signals from both the outside (e.g., from nerve terminals) and the inside (e.g., from the cytoplasm) of the cell. At this position, they are also submitted to the transmembrane electrical field.

When $V(t)$ and $l_i(t)$ are fixed, $n_a(t)$ reaches an equilibrium value $n_a(V, l_i)$ which can be analytically derived and is equal to

$$n_a(V, l_i) = (1 + L_0 \exp(V \delta \mu / MkT) \times \prod_i ((1 + l_i/K_{Ii})/(1 + l_i/K_{Ai}))^{n_i})^{-1} ,$$

$$(3)$$

where L_0 is a constant $[n_a(0,0)^{-1} - 1]$, M is the membrane thickness, k is the Boltzmann constant, T is the temperature, $\delta\mu$ is the change in dipole moment normal to the plane of the membrane associated with the $A \rightleftharpoons I$ transition, and K_{Ai} and K_{Ii} are the dissociation constants of the n_i sites carried by the receptor molecule for ligand l_i in the A and I conformations. The variations of n_a with l_i concentrations and membrane potential are illustrated in Figure 1. Several important features of allosteric receptors (some of which are well known in the case of allosteric enzymes) are the following:

Chemical Effectors. As typical allosteric proteins, receptors (and ion channels) may mediate interactions between identical (homotropic) and/or different (heterotropic) sites.

Homotropic Effects. The variation of n_a as a function of the concentration of a given effector l_i depends on the value of n_i, the number of identical sites for l_i. The concentration dependence before saturation can be quasi-linear ($n = 1$) or steplike for high values of n ($n = 10$); in the last case, almost no variation of n_a is observed until l_i reaches a critical value, above which n_a rises sharply.

Heterotropic Effects. The interaction between two different categories of ligands is illustrated by the upper graph in Figure 1. For example, l_2 changes both the domain of concentration in which l_1 is effective, and also the shape of the curve for the l_1 response; depending on the relative affinities of l_2 for the A and I conformations of the receptor, l_2 will shift the shape of the curve for the l_1 response to either more or less sigmoidicity.

Membrane Electrical Potential. If a net difference in the electrical dipole moment exists between A and I, a transmembrane electrical field may regulate the $A \rightleftharpoons I$ transition. However, the values of the parameters actually accessible in the cell impose severe constraints on regulation by the electrical potential. Physiologically significant values of the membrane potential range between

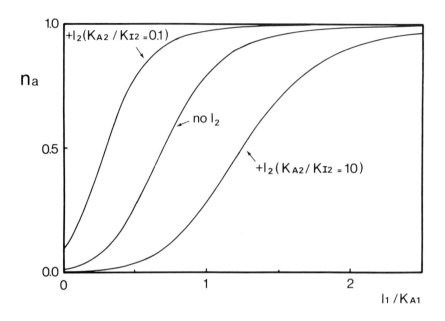

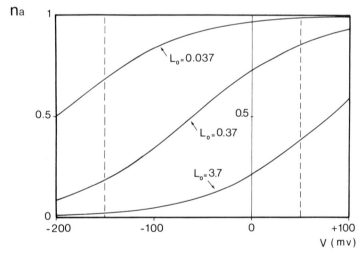

Figure 1. *Modulation of the fractional concentration* n_a *of receptors in the activable (A) conformation under steady-state conditions by allosteric effectors and transmembrane electrical potential. Upper graph*: Steplike variation of n_a as a function of the concentration l_1 of an allosteric effector, with $n_1 = 10$, $K_{A1}/K_{I1} = 0.1$, and $L_0 = 100$; modulation of the primary effect of l_1 in the presence of a second allosteric effector (l_2) with $K_{A2}/K_{I2} = 0.1$ *(left curve)* or 10 *(right curve)*. *Lower graph*: Variation of n_a as a function of the transmembrane electrical potential V, with $\delta\mu = 100$ D, $M = 50$ Å, and the values of L_0 indicated in the figure.

−150 and +50 mV and the differences in dipole moments accessible should be lower than the known dipole moment of proteins (200–500 D). These limitations restrict the maximal free energy U_{max} available for the shift of the $A \leftrightarrows I$ equilibrium, to approximately 1 kcal/mole ($U_{max} = E \cdot \delta\mu = V\delta\mu/M$). This value is smaller than that available from ligand binding ($U_{max} = -RT \ln K \sim 10$ kcal/mole for $K = 10^{-6}$ M). Accordingly, and as illustrated by the lower graph in Figure 1, the variation of n_a with membrane potential might be severely limited. For small variations ΔV of the applied transmembrane potential, the variation Δn_a of n_a is given by

$$\Delta n_a = n_a(1 - n_a)\delta\mu\,\Delta V/MkT , \qquad (4)$$

which shows that a significant variation of n_a takes place only when $n_a(1 - n_a)$ is not far from its maximum, which is reached when $n_a = 0.5$, that is, for $L_0 = 1$ ($n_a = (1 + L_0)^{-1}$ in the absence of effector l_i; see Equation 2). For instance, L_0 values outside the range 0.01–100 will result in a less than 1% variation of n_a in the 100-mV range of membrane potentials, with $\delta\mu = 100$ D. Interestingly, for the nicotinic cholinergic receptor where L_0 is known, L_0 equals 0.25, which is not far from 1 (Heidmann and Changeux, 1979). It can also be noted from Equations 3 and 4 that the presence of an effector l can a priori drive the $A \leftrightarrows I$ equilibrium in or out of the appropriate range in which membrane potential actually regulated n_a by shifting the initial L_0 value to L_0 $[(1 + l/K_I)^n/(1 + l/K_A)^n]$ (cf. Figure 1, lower graph).

Temporal Integration.   An important property of allosteric membrane-bound proteins appears when the set of fixed (V_1, l_{i1}) values is instantaneously changed to another set of fixed values (V_2, l_{i2}). Resolution of Equation 2 shows that $n_a(t)$ relaxes exponentially toward a new equilibrium value, given by Equation 3, with a time constant given by

$$\tau^{-1} = k^+ (V_2, l_{i2}) + k^- (V_2, l_{i2}) . \qquad (5)$$

Depending on the values of k^+ and k^-, and according to available data on classical allosteric enzymes and receptors, n_a may reach its final value within a fraction of a millisecond up to several seconds or minutes after the steplike perturbation; in the last instance, it is clear that n_a will be maintained apart from its equilibrium value for a long period of time. In other words, the allosteric membrane-bound protein will exhibit a "short-term memory" of its previous equilibrium state.

COMPARISON OF THEORY AND EXPERIMENTS

Parameters of Synaptic Efficacy at the Postsynaptic Level

For a given synapse, the most elementary experimental index of synaptic efficacy is the amplitude of the permeability (or conductance response) to the neurally released neurotransmitter, whatever the sign of the response (excitatory or in-hibitory) is. Difficulties appear in the more complex situation of the neuron which, in general, receives numerous nerve endings and possesses under each nerve terminal a fixed number of densely packed receptor molecules com-plementary to the neurotransmitter(s) released by each individual nerve end-ing.

The regulatory ligands that may affect the allosteric properties of the postsynaptic receptors may be: (1) presynaptic messengers such as the neurotransmitter itself, or neurotransmitters from different synapses, or any active compound co-released with the neurotransmitter(s) (such as ions, nucleotides, peptides, proteins; see Hökfelt et al., 1984); and (2) postsynaptic messengers produced on the postsynaptic side of the membrane as a consequence of receptor activation (entry of ions, such as calcium, by the open ion channel, enzymatic synthesis or degradation of cyclic nucleotides, diacylglycerol, inositol phosphates, and so forth). Each endogenous allosteric effector can be described by its point source s, in general a synapse, characterized by its distance r from the synapse under study and by a source–time function $S(t)$ describing the amount of effector produced, extra-cellularly or intracellularly, at the point source as a function of time.

Variations of the membrane electrical potential produced by the action of the neurotransmitters on their receptor propagate at the neuron surface, that is, between synapses and to the axon hillock, generally in a passive manner. In some cases, if they reach the threshold potential V_c for action potential generation, they may propagate in a nonattenuated form as action potentials (axonal spikes or calcium dendritic spikes). The efficacy of a given synapse either to cause the neuron to fire or to prevent its firing (for an inhibitory one) may be expressed as the extent to which this synapse will shift the membrane potential away from the membrane resting potential V_0, either beyond or below it, depending on whether the synapse is an excitatory or an inhibitory one.

The local change in membrane potential, $V - V_0$, associated with receptor activation can be expressed as

$$V - V_0 = (E_r - V_0)g/(g + G) , \tag{6}$$

where E_r is the reversal potential, V_0 is the membrane resting potential, G is the membrane resting conductance, and g is the membrane conductance change associated with receptor activation. Accordingly, g being an increasing function of the number n_a of *activable* receptors, the amplitude of the change in membrane potential for a given presynaptic stimulus is an increasing function of n_a. Then there will be a critical value n_{ac} above which the local change in membrane potential will be sufficient either to trigger or prevent action potential generation at the axon hillock. Computer simulations of the model may thus utilize, for a given synapse and a given neuron, n_{ac} as the reference value of synaptic efficacy. This does not exclude, however, that with real systems intermediate steps between the considered synapse and the axon hillock may be involved and eventually modified in the learning experience (see the concept of a "floating threshold" of synaptic efficacy by Bienenstock et al., 1982).

Parameters of Nerve Activity Expressed in Terms of Local Concentration of Diffusible Allosteric Effectors

Taking into consideration the simple scheme presented in the section above on homosynaptic regulation, the local concentration of l_i at a distance r from its point source is given by

$$l_i(t,r) = S_i(t) * P_i(t,r) , \tag{7}$$

where $*$ denotes convolution and $P_i(t,r)$ is equal to (D_i being the diffusion coefficient of l_i)

$$P_i(t) = \exp(-r^2/4D_it)/(4\pi D_it)^{3/2} \tag{8}$$

In a general manner, pre- and postsynaptic activity may be identified with repetitive sequences of frequency f of electrical or chemical pulses. Pulse duration being most often very brief (approximately 1 msec), the exact time course of the source function within a pulse need not be taken into consideration. Accordingly, Equation 7 reduces to

$$l_i(t,r) = l_{i0} \sum_n P_i(t - t_n,r) , \tag{9}$$

where t_n is the nth pulse position and l_{i0} is the amount of l_i released at the point source at each pulse. Plots of $l_i(t,r)$ as a function of time are given in Figure 2, for a value of D_i compatible with available data on the diffusion of small molecules and for physiologically relevant values of f (0–100 Hz). It can be observed that in some cases, the local l_i concentration globally increases to reach a plateau for a sufficiently long sequence of pulses. The mean plateau value can be derived analytically and is equal to

$$l_{i\ max} = l_{i0}f/4\pi D_ir , \tag{10}$$

that is, it is simply proportional to the *frequency* of the source function. From the knowledge of $l_i(t,r)$, it is clear from Equation 2 that $n_a(t)$ can then be derived.

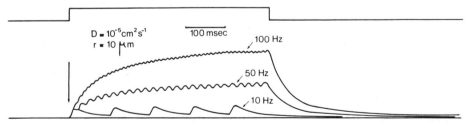

Figure 2. *Variation of the local concentration of a diffusible effector at a distance* r *from its point source.* $D = 10^{-5}$ cm^2 sec^{-1}; $r = 10$ µm; *frequencies of the source functions (see text) are indicated in the figure.*

Homosynaptic Regulation

The model can be applied, at our own risk, to fit the two experimental situations mentioned previously: neurally evoked desensitization of the acetylcholine receptor at the neuromuscular junction and long-term potentiation in the hippocampus. In the first case, the allosteric equilibrium is assumed to be spontaneously shifted in favor of the A state; in the second, it is assumed to be shifted in favor of the I state.

Desensitization at the Neuromuscular Junction.   Figure 3 (upper graph) shows that conditions can be found in which repetitive acetylcholine release for a sufficient period of time can cause a significant shift of the $A \rightleftharpoons I$ equilibrium of the acetylcholine receptor (initially set with A as the dominant state) in favor of the refractory I state. Situations exist where $n_a(t)$ reaches the critical value n_{ac} below which the muscle will not fire in response to the stimulation. For long-lasting stimulations, synaptic efficacy will be dependent only on the stimulation frequency, the synapse then acting as a high- (or low-) pass frequency filter.

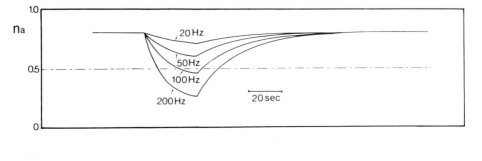

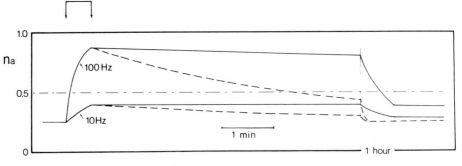

Figure 3.   *Homosynaptic regulation: Kinetics of the fractional concentration* n_a *of receptors in the A confor-mation, for a synapse stimulated at the frequencies indicated, under conditions leading to desensitization or facilitation. Upper graph;* Desensitization; k^+ and k^- values are 0.009 sec^{-1} and 0.036 sec^{-1}, respectively, in the absence of neurotransmitter and 0.18 sec^{-1} and 0.0027 sec^{-1} in its presence (values derived for the acetylcholine receptor in Heidmann and Changeux, 1979; pulse duration within the burst was selected equal to 2 msec). *Lower graph:* Facilitation; k^+ values are 0.025 sec^{-1} and 0.4 sec^{-1}, respectively, in the presence of the nerve-released effectors and 0.003 sec^{-1} and 0.001 sec^{-1} (*dashed lines*) or 310^{-4} sec^{-1} and 10^{-4} sec^{-1} (*solid lines*) in the absence of effector (values in the range of those reported in Heidmann and Changeux, 1979; Chang et al., 1984); pulse duration within the burst was selected equal to 2 msec.

Long-Term Potentiation in the Hippocampus. Assuming that the NMDA (or glutamate) receptor undergoes desensitization under similar conditions as the acetylcholine receptor, potentiation cannot be reached, solely as in the previous case, as a result of the binding of the excitatory neurotransmitter. Another allosteric effector has to be postulated in addition to the neurotransmitter. If before the learning experience the $A \rightleftharpoons I$ equilibrium is shifted in favor of the I state, and if the allosteric receptor stabilizes the A state, then, as illustrated in Figure 3 (lower graph), a potentiation of the response to the neurotransmitter might take place. Under these conditions, the synapse may act, again, as a frequency filter, and as such may be involved in signal recognition processes and resonance mechanisms. In both cases, as illustrated in Figure 3, the change of n_a resulting from the stimulations persists a given period of time after the last pulse. Such short-term change can be made to persist longer if subsequent steps of perpetuation, such as an interaction with the cytoskeleton (Lynch and Baudry, 1984; Yeramian and Changeux, 1986), or voltage-dependent unblocking of the ion channel by magnesium (Nowak et al., 1984), follow the initial allosteric transition of the receptor.

Heterosynaptic Regulation

The heterosynaptic regulation of a given synapse σ by neighboring synapses is formally equivalent to that analyzed above, except that the distance r of synapse σ from the point source (the other synapses in this case) has to be taken into consideration. In other words, the condition of anatomical convergence (Hebb's first law) becomes critical.

Heterosynaptic Depression in the Cerebellum. The model simply accounts for the situation described by Ito et al. (1982) if one assumes that: (1) The postsynaptic receptor (for glutamate?) at the parallel fiber–Purkinje cell synapse does not desensitize significantly (n_a remains above n_{ac}) under conditions of homosynaptic stimulation; (2) its desensitization is enhanced by a second messenger produced by the stimulation of the climbing fibers. The internal allosteric effector might be calcium ions if they stabilize (directly or via covalent modification) the I state (as in the case of the acetylcholine receptor) of the postsynaptic receptor that underlies the parallel fibers. Figure 4 shows that a reasonable simulation of the experimental situation can be achieved under these conditions. Clearly a time coincidence has to exist between the stimulations of σ and s for a significant shift of $A \rightleftharpoons I$ to occur (Hebb's first law).

Heterosynaptic Facilitation in Aplysia *Ganglion and in the Neocortex: Models of Classical Conditioning.* Instead of heterosynaptic depression, the experimental situations considered in the case of *Aplysia* and of the neocortex are heterosynaptic facilitations. The regulated synapse σ is that impinging on the axon terminal of the siphon sensory neuron in *Aplysia* (Hawkins et al., 1983) or the thalamocortical pathway or synapse in the neocortex (Baranyi and Feher, 1981a,b), the regulating stimulus being propagated by the axon of the sensory neuron in *Aplysia* or by the callosal axons in the neocortex. The scheme is exactly the same as that described above except that at the level of the regulated synapse the receptor

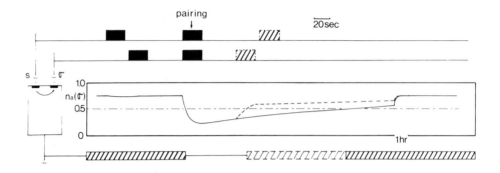

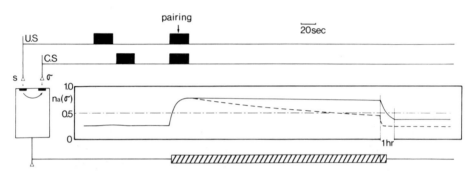

Figure 4. *Heterosynaptic regulation: Kinetics of the fractional concentration* n_a *of receptors in the* A *conformation under conditions of heterosynaptic regulation for the indicated patterns of firing of the presynaptic* s *and* σ *nerve endings.* The period of time when synapse σ is activable is indicated by a *striped bar* beneath each set of records. *Top*: Heterosynaptic depression, as in the cerebellum (Ito et al., 1982), where s is the parallel fiber–Purkinje cell synapse, and σ is the climbing fiber–Purkinje cell synapse. Receptors at synapse σ are regulated: (1) in a homosynaptic manner by a nerve-released effector l_1; k^+ and k^- values are selected equal to 0.001 sec^{-1} and 0.003 sec^{-1}, respectively, in the absence of effector and 0.020 sec^{-1} and 0.001 sec^{-1} in the presence of l_1; and (2) in a heterosynaptic manner by a diffusible effector l_2 released at synapse s. Diffusion coefficient and distance between synapses s and σ as in Figure 2; k^+ and k^- values are selected equal to 0.01 sec^{-1} and 0.03 sec^{-1}, respectively, in the presence of l_2 and 2.0 sec^{-1} and 0.1 sec^{-1} in the presence of both l_1 and l_2. Pulse duration within the burst at both synapses is selected equal to 3 msec, and the frequency of stimulation is 20 Hz. *Bottom*: Heterosynaptic facilitation under conditions of classical conditioning in which US is the unconditioned stimulus, and CS is the conditioned stimulus. Same conditions as above, with the following numerical values: k^+ and k^- are equal to 0.003 sec^{-1} and 0.001 sec^{-1} (*dashed lines*) or 10^{-4} sec^{-1} and 10^{-4} sec^{-1} (*solid lines*) in the absence of effector; 0.001 sec^{-1} and 0.02 sec^{-1} in the presence of l_1; 0.03 sec^{-1} and 0.01 sec^{-1} in the presence of l_2; and 0.1 sec^{-1} and 2.0 sec^{-1} in the presence of both l_1 and l_2.

is spontaneously present in the *I* state, and the second messenger produced by the other synapse favors the *A* state instead of the *I* one. This could be achieved by an internal effector such as calcium, which in the *Aplysia* case would activate the receptor-linked cyclase in the *A* state (Kandel et al., 1983) and/or by the membrane electrical potential, which when it decreases might also favor the *A* state as it does in the case of the acetylcholine receptor at the neuromuscular junction.

Regulation of Synaptic Efficacy by the Electrical Activity of the Target Neuron: A Plausible Mechanism for Resonance

The temporal integration properties of allosteric receptors can be utilized for the regulation of synaptic efficacy by the electrical activity of the postsynaptic target neuron (the Hebb postulate in its strict definition). As long as the rates of the $A \leftrightharpoons I$ transition are slower than those of the action potential rise and fall, important regulations might take place. For the sake of simplicity, the activity of the postsynaptic neuron will be considered as a periodic sequence of square pulses of 2-msec duration and fixed amplitude, $V_{max} - V_{min}$. Equation 3 can then be resolved for each time interval during which V is constant, and plots of n_a as a function of time are given in Figure 5 (upper graph). Two essential features can be noted:

1. Transiently, that is, between two successive pulses or action potentials, n_a may be significantly shifted, provided that the $A \leftrightharpoons I$ transition is rapid, and reach for a period of time larger than the action potential duration values significantly different from its initial value. As a consequence, the probability that an aleatory synaptic stimulation falls within a period of time during which n_a has a sufficient value for the neuron to fire in response to the stimulation is de facto much higher than the probability calculated above, assuming a direct modulation of synaptic efficacy by membrane potential. In the mean, the spontaneous firing activity of the neuron, even if of short duration, has increased the efficacy of the synapse.

2. For long-lasting signals, n_a globally increases (Figure 5, lower graph). The value $n_a(i)$ of n_a at the ith pulse can be analytically derived and is equal to:

$$n_a(i) = n_a(0) + [n_a(\infty) - n_a(0)] k^i , \qquad (11)$$

where $n_a(\infty)$ is the plateau n_a value for a signal of infinite duration and k is a constant. The rate at which n_a increases with f, but is limited by the maximal accessible $(V_{max} - V_{min})$ and $\delta\mu$ values (which limit the ratio of the rate constants k_r and k_f for the rising and falling phases of the interpulse n_a variation, respectively, to approximately 10). The value of the plateau $n_a(\infty)$ varies monotonically with the frequency of the electrical signal (see the insert in Figure 5). Clearly, for long-lasting signals of sufficient duration, n_a can be maintained continuously above a critical n_{ac} value, and therefore synaptic efficacy will be modulated not only in the mean as above, but also continuously.

An interesting consequence of the observed effect of the firing activity of the neuron on the efficacy of its synapses may concern the possible role of spontaneous oscillatory processes that are commonly observed in central neurons (see Berridge and Rapp, 1979). According to the proposed scheme, efficacy of afferent synapses might be modulated by the intrinsic spontaneous activity of the neuron. Conditions may be defined in which the correlation between the state of activity of the afferent (e.g., sensory) synapses and the spontaneous firing of the target neuron is such that it shifts synaptic contacts into a responsive state of resonance, or

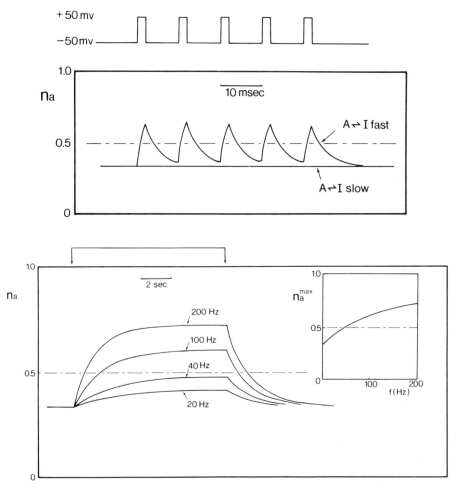

Figure 5. *A mechanism for "resonance": Kinetics of heterosynaptic regulation by the transmembrane electrical potential of the fractional concentration* n_a *of receptors in the A conformation. Upper graph*: Variation of n_a for the firing pattern indicated in the figure, with $\delta\mu = 100$ D and fast or slow $A \rightleftharpoons I$ interconversion (300 sec^{-1} and 0.3 sec^{-1}, respectively, at -50-mV membrane potential). *Lower graph*: Variation of n_a for long-lasting firing patterns as above, with frequencies as indicated in the figure; $\delta\mu = 150$ D, and a rate of $A \rightleftharpoons I$ interconversion of 0.3 sec^{-1} at -50-mV membrane potential. *Inset*: Variation of the plateau n_a value for long-lasting signals as a function of frequency. Same conditions as above.

alternatively into a silent state of dissonance (see Changeux et al., 1984b; Heidmann et al., 1984).

LONG-TERM CHANGES OF ACETYLCHOLINE RECEPTOR PROPERTIES

The short-term changes in synaptic efficacy associated with the slow and reversible interconversions of the postsynaptic receptor between the activable and inactivable allosteric states may become long term if additional mechanisms make irreversible and/or perpetuate the activity-linked changes. Data on the acetylcholine receptor again suggest plausible molecular models for such mechanisms. Most of them derive from studies on the evolution of the acetylcholine receptor in the course of end-plate formation and/or maturation (for reviews, see Fambrough, 1979; Changeux, 1981); others derive from structural investigations on the adult receptor from *Torpedo* electric organ, mostly in its native membrane environment.

In embryonic muscle fiber, the acetylcholine receptor is diffusely distributed all along the fiber and exhibits significant lateral motion (Axelrod et al., 1976) and rapid turnover time (half-life 17–22 hours) (Berg and Hall, 1975; Chang and Huang, 1975; Devreotes and Fambrough, 1975); the mean open time of its ionic channel is 3–10 msec (Katz and Miledi, 1972; Neher and Sakmann, 1976). In contrast, in adult muscle, the acetylcholine receptor is highly localized at the end plate, with a density about 1000 times higher than in nonsynaptic areas, is immobile (Bourgeois et al., 1973, 1978b; Frank et al., 1975; Rousselet et al., 1979, 1982), and turns over slowly (half-life of approximately 10 days or more); the mean open time of its channel is 3–5 times shorter than that of the embryonic receptor (except in the chick), and its intrinsic conductance is significantly larger. The transition from the embryonic receptor (mobile, labile, with long openings) to the adult one (immobile, stable, with short openings) may thus serve to elaborate models for long-term changes of receptor functional properties.

Several possibilities have been considered to account for this evolution. One is that embryonic and adult receptors possess different primary structures and thus result from the expression of different chromosomal genes (or of the differential splicing of a unique gene complex). Southern blot hybridization of genomic DNA with specific cDNA probes is consistent with the existence of a single gene for the α-chain in *Torpedo* (Klarsfeld et al., 1984) and in the mouse (Merlie et al., 1983a; Olson et al., 1984), and for the δ-chain in *Torpedo* (Hershey et al., 1983). On the other hand, a novel subunit referred to as ε in the adult (Takai et al., 1985) may replace the γ-subunit and account for the transition from long to short mean channel times (Mishina et al., 1985).

Alternatively, the differences between embryonic and adult receptors might be posttranscriptional and concern either intrinsic modifications of the molecule and/or extrinsic differences of its membrane environment. Attempts have been made to identify these posttranscriptional events. Several changes in the chemical and/or physicochemical properties of the receptor and of its membrane environment have been identified. Yet their correlation with the evolution of the physiological properties of the receptor has not been established for most of them. One fact nevertheless is clear: The different features that distinguish embryonic and/or adult receptors develop not simultaneously but successively during the formation and maturation of the end plate, and thus are most likely accounted for by a cascade of different molecular events. In addition, changes in the biosynthesis and turnover rate of the receptor may play a critical role in this evolution. These possibilities are briefly reviewed and discussed below.

Intrinsic Modifications of the Acetylcholine Receptor

Several groups of covalent modifications of the receptor protein have been identified in the *Torpedo* electromotor synapse (for reviews, see Changeux, 1981; Changeux et al., 1984a) and mammalian motor end plate (for a review, see Hall et al., 1983) and have been suggested to take part in synapse formation and maturation.

Disulfide Bonding of the Receptor Light Form into Heavy Form Dimer. Early experiments with the acetylcholine receptor heavy and light forms reconstituted into liposomes did not reveal any significant functional difference between the two forms (Anholt et al., 1980). Recently, however, their reconstitution into planar lipid bilayer suggests that the two oligomers may cooperate within the dimer and undergo all-or-none channel openings and closings with a conductance approximately twice that of the single $\alpha_2\beta\gamma\delta$ oligomer (Schindler et al., 1984). Also, during embryonic and postnatal development of the electric organ, the ratio of the light to heavy form, initially strongly in favor of the light form, subsequently shifts toward the heavy form dimer that is almost exclusively present in the adult electric organ (Holton et al., 1984). The formation of the covalent dimer may thus account for significant changes in the permeability response to acetylcholine during development but may also contribute to the aggregation and stabilization of the receptor at the end plate (see below). Yet, conclusive evidence in favor of such roles is missing, and no evidence exists for an effect of activity on dimer formation, even if disulfide bond formation and maintenance are expected to be directly regulated by the energy metabolism of the muscle cell.

Phosphorylation. Early experiments with *E. electricus* crude receptor extracts revealed sodium fluoride-sensitive interconversion between the two isoelectric forms of the receptor protein, suggesting a contribution of phosphorylation–dephosphorylation reactions in this interconversion (Teichberg and Changeux, 1976, 1977). Direct *in vitro* incorporation of phosphorous-32 into the receptor polypeptides was subsequently demonstrated by autoradiography after immunoelectrophoresis (Gordon et al., 1977; Teichberg et al., 1977). Phosphoserines have also been identified by chemical analysis of the purified chains of *T. californica* receptor (Vandlen et al., 1979). Finally, several protein kinases have been isolated from extracts of electric organ and shown to phosphorylate various subunits of the acetylcholine receptor (for a review, see Nestler and Greengard, 1984). At least in the case of the δ-subunit, phosphorylation takes place at the level of a peptide located in the carboxy-terminal region of the chain and most likely is included in the small hydrophilic domain (Devillers-Thiéry et al., 1983; Noda et al., 1983b) exposed to the cytoplasmic face of the membrane (Wennogle et al., 1981). Potassium ions enhance phosphorylation *in vitro* while sodium ions give the opposite result, but cholinergic ligands and local anesthetics have no significant effect under these conditions (Saitoh and Changeux, 1980; see, however, Gordon et al., 1977). Phosphorylation has been suggested as a plausible mechanism for the regulation of ion channel properties (see Nestler and Greengard, 1984) and shown to enhance desensitization of the acetylcholine receptor from *Torpedo* (Huganir et al., 1986).

Phosphorylation also affects structural parameters of the receptor protein. Treatments at acid pH or by *E. coli* alkaline phosphatase under conditions known to dephosphorylate phosphoproteins enhance the susceptibility to heat inactivation of the receptor protein in its membrane-bound and detergent-extracted forms

(Saitoh et al., 1979; Saitoh and Changeux, 1981). The state of phosphorylation of the membrane-bound receptor changes during the maturation of the electric organ. Nevertheless, the actual participation of phosphorylation in the assembly and stabilization of the acetylcholine receptor in the postsynaptic membrane remains to be established.

Glycosylation. Like many membrane proteins, the acetylcholine receptor is a glycoprotein. It reacts with concanavalin A and other plant lectins (Meunier et al., 1974; Brockes and Hall, 1975; Boulter and Patrick, 1977) and contains chemically identified mannose, galactose, glucose, and N-acetyl-D-galactosamine (Mattson and Heilbronn, 1975; Raftery et al., 1976). All four subunits carry glycosyl residues, but interestingly, the δ-polypeptide reacts with phytohemagglutinin A, whereas the α-subunit does not (Wennogle and Changeux, 1980). Glycosylation may be required for the folding and assembly of the subunits (Merlie et al., 1983b). Moreover, different reactivities toward sera from myasthenic patients have been noticed between junctional and extrajunctional receptors (Almon and Appel, 1975; Weinberg and Hall, 1979; Dwyer et al., 1981) and assigned to a differential glycosylation of the two α-subunits (Hall et al., 1983).

Lipid Binding. The covalent attachment of lipids has been shown to be critical for the correct folding of the α-subunit (Olson et al., 1984).

Extrinsic Modifications of the Membrane-Bound Receptor

The membrane-bound receptor interacts on the cleft side with the basal lamina within the postsynaptic membrane, with the lipid bilayer, and on the cytoplasmic side with the cytoskeleton. Modifications in this local environment may alter the functional and/or structural parameters of the molecule (for reviews, see Changeux, 1981; Changeux et al., 1983, 1984a).

Lipid Bilayer. In the postsynaptic membrane, despite their very high surface density (15,000–20,000 per μm^2), the receptor molecules are embedded in the lipid bilayer and are accessible to spin-labeled (Brisson et al., 1975; Bienvenue et al., 1977; Marsh et al., 1981; Ellena et al., 1983) or photoreactive (Giraudat et al., 1985) lipids. The lipid composition of this membrane is characterized by a high content of unesterified cholesterol and the predominance of long-chain, highly unsaturated fatty acids that are precisely those with which the purified receptor reacts preferentially in pure lipid monolayers (Popot et al., 1978). Functional reconstitution of detergent-purified receptor into lipid vesicles (Epstein and Racker, 1978; Changeux et al., 1979; Wu and Raftery, 1979, 1981; Gonzalez-Ros et al., 1980; Lindstrom et al., 1980) and planar bilayers (Nelson et al., 1980; Schindler and Quast, 1980) reveal a strong dependence on the presence of lipids throughout the isolation and purification procedure.

Fatty acids added to the membrane (Brisson et al., 1975) or generated by phospholipase A action (Andreasen and MacNamee, 1977, 1980; Andreasen et al., 1979), detergents (Brisson et al., 1975), or local (see references in Heidmann et al., 1983b) and general (Young and Sigman, 1982, 1983) anesthetics strongly block the permeability response to agonists and modify the rapid binding kinetics (possibly via allosteric effects mediated by the multiple low-affinity and histrio-nicotoxin-insensitive sites for noncompetitive blockers possibly located at the boundary between the transmembrane α-helices and the lipid bilayer). Reciprocal effects of agonist binding on the relations of the receptor with the neighboring lipid phase have also been suggested (Gonzalez-Ros et al., 1983). The lipid environment of the receptor thus exerts a critical, although mostly permissive, action on the regulatory properties of the receptor. Its contribution to the change of receptor properties in the course of synapse formation and/or its activity dependence remain to be tested.

Basal Lamina. Early ultrastructural studies on mammalian neuromuscular junction pointed to the presence of a dense coating of the extracellular matrix on the cleft face of the folded postsynaptic membrane, referred to as the basement membrane or basal lamina (see Couteaux, 1981). Immunocytochemical techniques (see Sanes and Hall, 1979) using antisera directed against purified basal lamina components revealed at this level laminin (Timpl et al., 1979), collagen type IV (Orkin et al., 1977), heparin sulfate proteoglycan (Hassel et al., 1980), collagen type V, and fibronectin (Daniels et al., 1984, and the references therein). The enzyme acetylcholinesterase and its high molecular weight form (16–19.5 S) is also primarily associated with the basal lamina, possibly by its collagen tail (for a review, see Massoulié and Bon, 1982). In adult frog muscle, regeneration of muscle fibers after degeneration of the afferent motor nerve leads to the formation of acetylcholine receptor aggregates at the level of the basal lamina differentiation that initially marked the location of the neuromuscular junction (Sanes et al., 1978). Also, components of the basal lamina such as laminin (Vogel et al., 1983) or still unidentified high molecular weight substances (Podleski et al., 1978; Schaffner and Daniels, 1982) cause the appearance (or increase the number) of acetylcholine receptor aggregates on the surface of cultured myotubes.

The contribution of the basal lamina to the localization of the acetylcholine receptor at the end-plate level thus looks plausible. Experiments in which the developing muscle fibers were destroyed by toxins and were subsequently allowed to regenerate further suggest that the characteristic basal lamina topology of the end plate becomes stable within a few days after the initial motor nerve–muscle contact (Slater et al., 1985). At this stage of development, the turnover of the receptor protein is still fast. This suggests that the basal lamina plays the role of a stable organizing matrix or "sticky zone" under which the labile receptor molecules are continuously replaced (see Poo et al., 1985). This suggestion is supported by the observation that while denervation in the adult maintains a local high density of receptors within the postsynaptic membrane (Bourgeois et al., 1973, 1978b; Frank et al., 1975), the stable receptor molecules are locally replaced by ones that turn over rapidly (Loring and Salpeter, 1980; Levitt and Salpeter, 1981; Brett et al., 1982; see references in Salpeter and Harris, 1983; Salpeter and Loring, 1985). Yet the specificity of the basement membrane components can be questioned, since positively charged latex beads trigger cluster formation and even postsynaptic specializations (for a review, see Peng, 1984).

The establishment of this organizing matrix does not seem linked to the activity of the developing end plate, even though at this stage neurally evoked end-plate potentials can be recorded (Cohen, 1980), and calcium ions (which may enter the open voltage-dependent ion channel) appear necessary for the formation of receptor clusters (Peng, 1984). In any case, the differences in turnover rates noticed between the acetylcholine receptor and the basal lamina components (in particular that of the collagens) may serve to build models of long-term traces at the postsynaptic level.

43-kD Protein and Cytoskeleton. On the cytoplasmic side of the synaptic membrane at the motor end plate or the electromotor synapse, electron microscopy reveals "condensations" beneath the receptor layer (Rosenbluth, 1975; Cartaud et al., 1978; Sealock, 1980) in morphological relationships with the cytoskeleton (see references in Couteaux, 1981; Cartaud et al., 1982, 1983). Similarly, postsynaptic densities have been identified in central synapses and their rather complex protein composition described (see references in Carlin and Siekewitz, 1983). In the electric organ, proteins with an apparent molecular weight of 43 kD on SDS-polyacrylamide gels purify together with the receptor-rich membranes (Sobel et al., 1977, 1978) and give, on two-dimensional gels (Saitoh and Changeux, 1981), one major component referred to as the 43-kD protein and at least two others identified as cytosolic creatine phosphokinase (Barrantes et al., 1983; Gysin et al., 1983; Giraudat et al., 1984) and cytoplasmic actin, respectively (Gysin et al., 1983; Porter and Froehner, 1983).

Selective proteolysis (Wennogle and Changeux, 1980), labeling with isotopic iodine (St. John et al., 1982), and gold labeling with specific monoclonal antibodies (Nghiêm et al., 1983; Sealock et al., 1984) have shown that the 43-kD protein exclusively faces the cytoplasmic side of the membrane and distributes along with the acetylcholine receptor. Brief exposure of the receptor-rich membrane to pH 11 (Neubig et al., 1979) or lithium diiodosalicylate (Elliott et al., 1980) releases the 43-kD and other peripheral proteins without significant changes of the receptor functional properties monitored by ion flux measurements and rapid binding of agonists or noncompetitive blockers (Neubig et al., 1979; Elliott et al., 1980; Heidmann et al., 1980).

In contrast, elimination of the 43-kD protein destabilizes the receptor to heat treatment (Saitoh et al., 1979) or proteolytic attack (Klymkowsky et al., 1980) and enhances its motion, as monitored with spin-labeled (Rousselet et al., 1979, 1980, 1982) or phosphorescent (Lo et al., 1980) derivatives of α-bungarotoxin and by electron microscopy (Barrantes et al., 1980; Cartaud et al., 1981). Its binding to the cytoplasmic domain of the receptor, at least by way of the β-subunit (Burden et al., 1983), thus strongly immobilizes the molecule. A contribution of the heavy-form dimer to this process has been suggested (Holton et al., 1984). The close relationship between intermediate filaments and the 43-kD protein suggests that this highly insoluble, cysteine-rich molecule (Sobel et al., 1978) may serve as an "intermediate piece" between the cytoskeleton and the postsynaptic membrane (Cartaud et al., 1983). The precise stage of development at which the 43-kD protein attaches to the acetylcholine receptor is not yet known (see, however, Burden, 1985); neither is its eventual contribution to the metabolic stabilization of the receptor and/or to its change of channel mean open time. The 43-kD protein can be phosphorylated *in vitro* (Saitoh and Changeux, 1980). This opens the possibility of a regulation of the 43-kD protein attachment to the receptor and/or the cytoskeleton by phosphorylation–dephosphorylation reactions

(Saitoh and Changeux, 1981; Gordon et al., 1983; Yeramian and Changeux, 1986). Still no data are available regarding this question.

Biosynthesis and Turnover of the Acetylcholine Receptor

The biosynthesis of the acetylcholine receptor and its regulation have been thoroughly investigated in developing embryos, in cell cultures, and in adult denervated muscle (for reviews, see Fambrough, 1979; Changeux, 1981; Merlie et al., 1985). In chick embryo, the receptor is detected as soon as day five (Giacobini et al., 1973), its content increases markedly during the following days, reaches a peak at day 14 (in breast muscle), and subsequently decreases to 95% of its maximal value (Burden, 1977a,b; Betz et al., 1977, 1980; Bourgeois et al., 1978a). Throughout this evolution, the degradation rate of the receptor protein does not change, thus supporting the view that a regulation of its biosynthesis accounts for the change in its content during embryonic development (Merlie et al., 1975, 1978; Fambrough, 1979).

Chronic injection of neuromuscular blocking agents *in ovo* shows that the initial onset of receptor biosynthesis does not require muscle activity, while the late decline results from an activity-linked repression of receptor biosynthesis (Giacobini-Robecchi et al., 1975; Burden, 1977a,b; Bourgeois et al., 1978a; Betz et al., 1980). This evolution in total receptor content parallels that of the extrajunctional receptor and thus does not concern the late maturation of the end plate. A similar regulation can be reproduced in the adult muscle as a consequence of denervation (for a review, see Fambrough, 1979). In this case, the electrical activity of the muscle has also been shown to regulate the biosynthesis of the receptor rather than its degradation rate (Hogan et al., 1976; Linden and Fambrough, 1979). This activity-dependent regulation of receptor biosynthesis may thus serve as a model for lasting changes of receptor content on the time scale of 10–20 hours (the range of the metabolic half-life of the surface receptor).

The observed changes of receptor content have been related to that of its specific mRNA by using α-subunit cDNA probes. With the two systems used, adult rat muscle under conditions of denervation (Merlie et al., 1985), and spontaneously contracting myotubes in culture in the presence or in the absence of tetrodotoxin (Klarsfeld and Changeux, 1985), an increase in α-subunit-specific mRNA is noticed when the content of surface receptor increases. However, in both cases, the content of mRNA increases to a much larger extent (approximately 13- to 17-fold) than that of the surface receptor (severalfold). The activity-dependent regulation of receptor biosynthesis thus primarily affects mRNA production (and/or stability) but may also involve posttranscriptional events such as assembly, maturation, and transport of the oligomeric receptor (see Merlie, 1984).

The intracellular second messenger(s) that links the electrical activity of the cell with gene expression is (are) not yet identified. Studies with the mouse mutant *muscular dysgenesis*, in which electrical activity still regulates receptor biosynthesis despite uncoupling of the excitation–contraction process, exclude a contribution of muscle mechanical activity to this regulation (Powell and Friedman, 1977). A role for calcium (Birnbaum et al., 1980; Forrest et al., 1981) and/ or sodium (Weidoff et al., 1979) ions that enter the voltage-sensitive sodium channel during activity has been suggested but still deserve further exploration. Aggregation of the acetylcholine receptor under motor nerve endings and the subsequent evolution of the subsynaptic membrane during embryonic and post-natal development have been described in detail in mammalian skeletal muscle (for a review, see Matthews-Bellinger and Salpeter, 1983). Strong evidence indicates that the aggregated receptor is gathered from diffusely distributed and mobile, embryonic, nonjunctional receptors (Anderson and Cohen, 1977; Stya and Axel-rod, 1983). Subsequently, the density of receptor molecules increases from 2000 to about 9000 $[^{125}I]\alpha$-bungarotoxin sites per μm^2 at the tip of the subsynaptic folds, and concomitantly the overall surface of the end plate grows, the total number of receptors increasing up to about 30-fold until the adult stage (Matthews-Bellinger and Salpeter, 1983). Newly synthesized receptor molecules become incorporated into the subsynaptic membrane, possibly as coated vesicles (Burstajn and Fischbach, 1984; however, see Matthews-Bellinger and Salpeter, 1983).

In the rat, the metabolic degradation rate of the subsynaptic receptor slows down before birth (see Reiness and Weinberg, 1981; Steinbach, 1981) and precedes the shortening of the mean channel open time that takes place between the first and second postnatal weeks (see Brenner and Sakmann, 1981, 1983). In the chick, the mean channel open time does not change (Fischbach and Schuetze, 1980), and the metabolic degradation rate of the localized receptor begins to slow down only about 23 days after hatching (Burden, 1977a,b; Betz et al., 1980). In the adult, the turnover of the receptor molecules is uniform throughout the end plate, the new molecules being inserted anywhere in the membrane and exhibiting already long half-lives (Salpeter and Harris, 1983). Similarly, once the shortening of the mean channel open time has occurred, the newly inserted receptor molecules display the short channel open time, even 42 days after denervation (Brenner and Sakmann, 1983). During formation of ectopic end plates in the adult, the conversion of the receptor channel from a long to a short mean open time is greatly accelerated by muscle activity but once established no longer depends on it (Brenner and Sackmann, 1983; Brenner et al., 1983). In other words, there is an activity-dependent, long-term perpetuation of the short channel feature of the acetylcholine receptor.

In conclusion, much remains to be done about the identification of the molecular mechanisms that contribute to the localization, stabilization, and maturation of the acetylcholine receptor in the postsynaptic membrane and in particular to those that regulate the turnover of the receptor molecule. Their understanding is expected to offer mechanisms for long-term changes of membrane properties.

Localization of Acetylcholinesterase

Acetylcholinesterase is a polymorphic protein that may exist in at least six forms (three globular and three collagen-tailed), the distribution of which varies with species, physiological state, and localization (see Massoulié and Bon, 1982). In the adult end plate, acetylcholinesterase is not an integral component of the subsynaptic membrane but is primarily associated with the basal lamina (for a review, see Massoulié and Bon, 1982). Its evolution during development is not, at all stages, coordinated with that of the acetylcholine receptor (Betz et al.,

1977; Rubin et al., 1979); its accumulation at the end plate follows with some delay that of the receptor and does not obey the same rules.

The spontaneous activity of the embryo affects the localization of the esterase. In the chick, paralysis of the embryo by injection of snake venom α-toxin into the egg yolk from days 3 to 12 causes a disappearance of end-plate acetylcholinesterase detected by the Koelle method (Giacobini et al., 1973; see also Bourgeois et al., 1978a; Oppenheim et al., 1978; Betz et al., 1980). After chronic paralysis *in vivo* or paralysis of motor neuron–muscle cocultures *in vitro* (Vigny et al., 1976a,b; Rubin et al., 1978, 1980; Rieger et al., 1980) the heavy 16–19.5 S collagen-tailed form of the enzyme [primarily associated with end plates (Hall, 1973) but also present in aneural muscle (Sohal and Wrenn, 1984)] disappears (however, see Sohal and Wrenn, 1984). Conversely, electrical stimulation of the muscle (Rubin et al., 1978, 1980; see also Lømo and Slater, 1976, 1980) or application of dibutyryl cGMP (Rubin et al., 1980) reverses this effect.

Activity of the muscle thus regulates the production and localization of acetylcholinesterase, though in a direction opposite to that of the extrajunctional receptor. Differences have, however, been noticed in this respect between primary cultures and some muscle cell lines from mouse (Inestrosa et al., 1983) such as line C_2, which may, for instance, conserve acetylcholinesterase repression by tetrodotoxin but loses the enhanced synthesis of acetylcholine receptors. Since chronic blocking of the end plate does not interfere with the localization of the receptor but only with that of the esterase (Bourgeois et al., 1978; Betz et al., 1980; Rubin et al., 1980), it yields functional junctions with a "modified" end-plate potential (Rubin et al., 1980; see also Kullberg et al., 1980). This regulation can be taken as a model for the lasting effects of disuse or experience on the efficacy of the neuromuscular junction.

PERSPECTIVES: MODELS OF LONG-TERM LEARNING AT THE POSTSYNAPTIC LEVEL

The distinction between short- and long-term learning is not as clear-cut as it may look. If one considers that the traffic of postsynaptic potentials in the dendrites and their integration takes place in the millisecond-to-second time scale, reversible traces lasting longer than this time scale may be considered as short term. Long-term storage is in general viewed as lasting for days, weeks, or even years and as requiring protein synthesis for consolidation. However, even though the adult neuron no longer divides, its cellular and molecular components turn over. Thus, models for long-term learning hinge upon the lifetime of the synapse and of its constituent macromolecules. Long-term modifications that involve changes in the number of connections have already been extensively discussed (see Changeux et al., 1973; Changeux and Danchin, 1976; Purves and Lichtman, 1980; Changeux, 1983; Gouzé et al., 1983; Cowan et al., 1984) and are not considered further here.

An approximate half-life of 18 days has been evaluated for the whole synaptic junction with the ciliary muscle (see Cotman and Nieto-Sampedro, 1984), but longer half-lives (several months) have been suggested for the skeletal muscle end plate (Barker and Ip, 1966). Turnover times in the range of one month look plausible for central synapses (see Cotman and Nieto-Sampedro, 1984). Yet it is not known if all brain synapses turn over at such a fast rate. In the adult motor end plate, the turnover time of the acetylcholine receptor, as already discussed, is about one and a half weeks, that is, only 2–4 times faster than that of the entire synapse. One thus is led to distinguish "traces" shorter than the half-lives of the synapse and of its components from those that persist beyond these limits and thus should be considered self-perpetuating.

To the extent that the intrinsic and extrinsic modifications mentioned in the case of the acetylcholine receptor also hold for central receptors (see Barnard et al., 1983; Snyder, 1984), such modifications may prolong the short-term changes of efficacy mentioned previously. As a consequence, the degradation rate of the protein may also change, and an activity-dependent stabilization of the receptor may thus occur. Also, regulation of the number of receptor molecules and thus, most likely, of their biosynthesis has been extensively reported in the peripheral and central nervous system (for reviews, see Schwartz et al., 1983; Fuxe et al., 1984). Nevertheless, these changes alone are not expected to persist beyond the metabolic lifetime of the modified receptor molecule. Additional mechanisms must be added that make them self-perpetuating. Examples of such self-perpetuating systems are the following:

Self-Sustained Metabolic Steady States

The postsynaptic side of the synapse (or dendritic spine) can be viewed as an open thermodynamic system that may exist under multiple steady states (Prigogine, 1961). The logical structures that make such a system able to generate multiple steady states have been analyzed in detail (Thomas, 1981). The simplest case is pure autocatalysis: a loop with only one positive element. For instance, in addition to the allosteric receptor there may exist nearby in the cytoplasm an enzyme E, such that one has the following sequence of reactions:

$$X_o \xrightarrow{\ receptor\ } X_i \xrightarrow{\ enzyme\ E\ } P \ ,$$

where X is a permeant ion that enters the cytoplasm by the open receptor ion channel ($X_o \rightarrow X_i$) and serves as a substrate (or activator) of the enzyme yielding the compound P. If P stabilizes the receptor in the A state, a positive feedback loop is established which, after a conditioning train of impulses, may shift synaptic efficacy to a stable state robust to molecular turnover (as long as the steady-state input and the concentrations of enzymes and receptors remain constant). Other mechanisms may be invented that include negative feedback loops, but in even numbers (Delbrück, 1949; Thomas, 1981).

No experimental evidence exists for such a long-term, self-sustained mechanism under unambiguous learning conditions. To make it more plausible, one may illustrate it with concrete examples. For instance, X_i could be calcium, the hypothetical "enzyme" a calcium-activated nucleotide cyclase, and P a cyclic nucleotide that would stabilize the A state of the postsynaptic membrane. [The scheme might be made even more complex by intercalating a cyclic nucleotide-dependent protein kinase (and diesterase) that would selectively phosphorylate and dephosphorylate the *A* state (see Nestler and Greengard, 1984; see also Lisman, 1985).]

   Examples of self-sustained steady states have already been discussed extensively in the case of the regulation of gene expression in bacteria (see Monod and Jacob, 1961; Thomas, 1981) and in the course of the differentiation of eukaryotic cells (Britten and Davidson, 1969). Such discussions may legitimately be extended to the synapse, as long as one is aware that all synaptic proteins are coded by the unique nucleus present in the neuronal soma. The activity-dependent regulation of the synaptic cleft content in acetylcholinesterase and of brain receptor numbers (see Schwartz et al., 1983; Fuxe et al., 1984) may be relevant to such mechanisms.

Perpetuation of Protein Structural Changes

Discussions concerning the self-reproduction of protein patterns can be traced back to the origins of molecular biology in the 1940s. Several possibilities may be reasonably considered in the case of the postsynaptic membrane. All of them as yet are entirely hypothetical.

Allotropic Crystalline States of the Postsynaptic Membrane. According to this hypothesis, the postsynaptic membrane is viewed as a two-dimensional lattice of, for instance, receptor molecules (see Changeux, 1969). The difference in conformation of the *A* and *I* states would affect, in addition to the susceptibility of channel opening by acetylcholine, the near-neighbor relationships between receptor molecules within the crystal. The "learning" impulse would then trigger a "phase transition" (see Changeux et al., 1967) toward a stable (but not necessarily equilibrium) allotropic state that may propagate its own structure by "crystal growth."

   A lattice cooperativity has been shown to occur in the case of the purple membrane (Blaurock and Stoeckenius, 1971; Henderson and Unwin, 1975; Korenstein et al., 1979). Evidence for long-range cooperative effects in the case of the postsynaptic membrane of the cholinergic synapse is lacking, despite the fact that such effects might occur with purified acetylcholine receptors reconstituted into planar lipid bilayers (H. G. Schindler, unpublished observations). Also, the dense aggregates of acetylcholine receptors revealed by electron microscopy in the native postsynaptic membrane appear closely packed (without preferential orientation of the receptor molecules in the plane of the membrane) rather than organized into an authentic two-dimensionally oriented lattice (see Brisson, 1980; Kistler and Stroud, 1981).

Conservation of Symmetry in Oligomeric Protein Molecules. Molecular mechanisms have been identified (Razin and Friedman, 1981) or postulated (Brown, 1984) for the maintenance (or propagation) of a determined (or differentiated) state of DNA through molecular turnover and/or DNA replication. For instance, propagation of the methylated state of DNA occurs via an enzyme that methylates the "new" strand of the DNA molecule exclusively when the complementary "old" one is methylated (Razin and Friedman, 1981). A similar mechanism (Crick, 1984) has been proposed for " . . . a protein molecule, that is an essential part of a synapse and can exist in two states: active and inactive. . . . the molecule forms a dimer, probably with a twofold rotation axis, that can be modified chemically by, for example, the attachment of a phosphate group." Without being named, the acetylcholine receptor seems behind this portrait! In short, a protein kinase would exist that exclusively phosphorylates a freshly replaced monomer in a dimer when the complementary monomer from the same dimer is in a phosphorylated state, for instance, as a consequence of a previous activity-dependent step. Experimental demonstration of the relative enrichment in dimers of the population of receptor molecules during maturation of the electric organ (Holton et al., 1984) does not yet suffice to bring support to this still hypothetical mechanism.

"Protein Template." Strong evidence exists for a role of the basal lamina as an organizing matrix of the underlying postsynaptic membrane. Let us assume first that one of its long-lived components, X, selectively immobilizes or "grasps" one of the two states of the receptor, for instance A, and that its synthesis by the muscle depends on the state of activity of the postsynaptic cell. Then, as long as the replacement by turnover of X and of the receptor takes place at random, conditions may be found in which a self-sustained change in the complex (postsynaptic membrane plus basal lamina) becomes robust to turnover (see Yeramian and Changeux, 1986). The brain lacks a typical basal lamina, but proteoglycans, laminin, and/or cell adhesion molecules (Edelman, 1983) may have an equivalent role. A similar mechanism can be imagined on the cytoplasmic side of the postsynaptic membrane in which the complex (43-kD protein–cytoskeleton) may play a role equivalent to that of the basal lamina on the cleft side.

Autoreproduction **En Bloc** *of Activity-Modified Synapses.* An eventual turnover of the entire synapse has been considered and recently discussed (Cotman and Nieto-Sampedro, 1984). Two possibilities may be envisioned. One is that the pre- and postsynaptic elements turn over independently. Then each element may serve as a matrix for the other, in particular if it contains cell adhesion molecules, which may bridge the two faces of the synapse in its modified versus unmodified state. An alternative model (Carlin and Siekevitz, 1983) is that the synapse splits longitudinally before one of the daughter synapses regresses while the other becomes stable. The division would begin by the perforation of the junction, yielding two postsynaptic junctions, then two spines, and finally two nerve endings. A perpetuation of activity-dependent postsynaptic changes may take place with any of the mechanisms mentioned above. Yet, direct evidence in favor of such schemes based upon synaptic "fission" and turnover is lacking.

CONCLUSIONS

The scope of this chapter was deliberately limited to models of short- and long-term postsynaptic changes in synaptic efficacy based on a number of known properties of the acetylcholine receptor from fish electric organ and vertebrate neuromuscular junction. The explicit assumption is that the functional and structural properties of this particular peripheral receptor can be extended to other neurotransmitter receptors, in particular to those from central neurons. Investigations of the central receptors for glycine, GABA, and possibly acetylcholine have indeed revealed rather similar allosteric properties (e.g., regulation by heterotropic ligands, desensitization, etc.), but differences may exist and may have to be taken into consideration. Also, the molecular architecture of the receptors, coupled with enzymes such as nucleotide cyclase, may follow different rules and thus possess allosteric properties of its own (see Schramm and Sillinger, 1984).

On the other hand, the ion channels involved in electrical signaling and usually considered as molecular entities only distantly related to receptors for neurotransmitters may in fact share with them rather similar allosteric and even structural properties (for the sodium channel, see Talvenheimo et al., 1983; Noda et al., 1984). Some of the models proposed for the acetylcholine receptor may thus also be reasonably extended to these nonsynaptic ion channels (see, e.g., Finkel and Edelman, 1985, and this volume) even though the endogenous ligands for these "channel receptors" are less identified than in the case of typical neurotransmitter "receptor channels" (see, however, Fosset et al., 1984). Nonsynaptic areas on dendrites, somas, and even axon terminals may thus become loci for short-term changes as long as they possess membrane-bound allosteric proteins able to integrate different categories of signals in both space and time, thus satisfying Hebb's laws of convergence and time coincidence. Experimental tests for such short-term modifications of membrane properties should be provided by joint microphysiological recordings of membrane properties under well-identified "learning" conditions and molecular investigations on the allosteric transitions of the relevant receptors (or ion channels) by physicochemical techniques.

Models for long-term changes have been discussed on the basis of observations about the acetylcholine receptor and its membrane environment. In a general manner, short-term changes might be made to last longer by covalent intrinsic modifications, by changes in the extrinsic environment of the membrane (lipid and protein), or by regulation of the metabolism (biosynthesis, degradation, distribution) of the receptor (and of the corresponding neurotransmitter degradative enzyme) both during development and in the adult synapse. Additional models have been discussed for the self-perpetuation of activity-dependent changes of membrane properties through the turnover of the macromolecular components of the synapse or of whole synapses. A large variety of plausible mechanisms for long-term learning are thus available and might be amenable to experimental test.

One should not forget, however, that the information presented in this chapter about the acetylcholine receptor concerns a protein produced by multinucleated muscle cells. Differential regulation of gene expression in a distinct population of nuclei (junctional vs. nonjunctional) may have to be taken into consideration (Merlie and Sanes, 1985). On the other hand, in nerve cells, the regulation of receptor biosynthesis by innervation (for reviews, see Kuffler et al., 1971; Schwartz et al., 1983; Fuxe et al., 1984) and by activity (Betz, 1983; Schwartz et al., 1983; Fuxe et al., 1984) has been demonstrated, even though these cells possess a single nucleus. Specific mechanisms might thus be involved in these systems. Also, nerve cells are expected to synthesize a large variety of receptor molecules, and still unknown mechanisms of segregation and stabilization of receptors according to the neurotransmitter liberated by each particular nerve ending have to be postulated.

In addition to the postsynaptic mechanisms extensively discussed in this chapter, neuron activity may regulate the content of the cell in neuropeptides and in enzymes specifically involved in the biosynthesis of neurotransmitters (see Mallet et al., 1983; Black et al., 1984). Such a mechanism may, of course, play a fundamental role in the regulation of synaptic efficacy at the presynaptic level, in addition to a direct regulation of the neurotransmitter release mechanism (Kandel et al., this volume). A drawback of such regulation at the gene level is that it may concern equally all the nerve endings issued from a given neuronal soma rather than being specific to a given synapse. The contribution of cytoplasmic allosteric proteins (e.g., protein kinases, phosphatases, diesterases) may have to be taken into consideration at the postsynaptic level in addition to the contribution of membrane-bound proteins (see Hemmings et al., this volume).

From a more general point of view, the molecular models for short- and long-term changes in synaptic efficacy considered in this chapter might be utilized to create large-scale "assemblies of neurons" (Hebb, 1949) or "mental objects" (Changeux, 1983; Bienenstock, 1985). They can also be applied to the storage of such mental objects by selection on the basis of a resonance between spontaneously generated "prerepresentation" and externally evoked percepts (Changeux, 1983; Changeux et al., 1984b; Heidmann et al., 1984; see also Edelman, 1978, 1981; Finkel and Edelman, 1985, and this volume). Mechanisms of learning by selection may operate at various levels of organization: (1) at the level of large assemblies of neurons, as mentioned above; (2) at the neuronal level, for instance, via selective neuronal death (see Hamburger and Levi-Montalcini, 1949; Cowan, 1973; Cowan et al., 1984); (3) at the synaptic level, for instance, via selective stabilization—regression of synaptic connections (Changeux et al., 1973; Changeux and Danchin, 1976; Purves and Lichtman, 1980; Gouzé et al., 1983; Cowan et al., 1984); and (4) at the molecular level.

In the case of the immune response, mechanisms of selection have been demonstrated at the molecular level after variations of gene structure and organization. Such mechanisms, which involve a differential proliferation of cells, cannot be simply applied to the nervous system, where the number of neurons no longer increases in the adult. On the other hand, within the framework of the models discussed, the various allosteric states of the receptor (Heidmann and Changeux, 1979) may preexist with respect to the binding of ligands, and regulation thus operates via the selection of the state that exhibits the highest affinity for the ligand (see Katz and Thesleff, 1957; Monod et al., 1965). Also, during end-plate formation, the receptor molecules that become clustered under the motor axons are initially present over the surface of the muscle cell before the arrival of the growth cone. Subsequently, more than 95% of the receptor synthesized by the muscle cell becomes eliminated. The assembly of the postsynaptic membrane thus may itself involve, at the molecular level, mechanisms of selection.

In his inspired paper on "Antibodies and Learning: Selection versus Instruction," Jerne (1967) quotes Socrates' conclusion that "all learning consists of being reminded of what is preexisting in the brain" and further states that "in all processes resembling learning, a discussion of instruction versus selection serves only to determine the organizational level of the elements upon which selective mechanisms operate." The present speculations on allosteric receptors and models of short- and long-term learning in the nervous system are in harmony with these views and further suggest that, because of the complexity of the central nervous system, learning by selection in the brain may operate at several levels of its organization.

REFERENCES

Adams, P. R. (1981) Acetylcholine receptor kinetics. *J. Membr. Biol.* **58**:161–174.

Agnati, L., K. Fuxe, F. Benfenati, L. Calza, N. Battistini, and S. O. Ogren (1983) Receptor–receptor interactions: Possible new mechanisms for the reaction of some antidepressant drugs. In *Frontiers in Neuropsychiatric Research*, E. Usdin, M. Goldstein, A. T. Friedhoff, and A. Gergotas, eds., pp. 301–318, Macmillan, London.

Agnew, W. S., J. A. Miller, M. H. Ellisman, R. L. Rosenberg, S. A. Tomiko, and S. R. Levinson (1983) The voltage-regulated sodium channel from the electroplax of *Electrophorus electricus. Cold Spring Harbor Symp. Quant. Biol.* **48**:165–180.

Akasu, T., and A. G. Karczmar (1980) Effects of anticholinesterases and of sodium fluoride on neuromyal desensitization. *Neuropharmacology* **19**:393–403.

Albus, J. G. (1971) Theory of cerebellar function. *Math. Biosci.* **10**:25–61.

Alkon, D. L. (1984) Calcium-mediated reduction of ionic currents: A biophysical memory trace. *Science* **226**:1037–1045.

Almon, R. R., and S. H. Appel (1975) Interactions of myasthenic serum globulin with the acetylcholine receptor. *Biochim. Biophys. Acta* **393**:66–77.

Andersen, P. O., S. Sundberg, O. Sveen, J. W. Swann, and H. Wigström (1980) Possible mechanisms for long-lasting potentiation of synaptic transmission in hippocampal slices from guinea-pigs. *J. Physiol. (Lond.)* **302**:463–482.

Anderson, M. J., and M. W. Cohen (1977) Nerve-induced and spontaneous redistribution of acetylcholine receptors on cultured muscle cells. *J. Physiol. (Lond.)* **268**:757–773.

Andreasen, T. J., and M. G. McNamee (1977) Phospholipase A inhibition of acetylcholine receptor function in *Torpedo californica* membrane vesicles. *Biochem. Biophys. Res. Commun.* **79**:958–965.

Andreasen, T. J., and M. G. McNamee (1980) Inhibition of ion permeability control properties of acetylcholine receptor from *Torpedo californica* by long-chain fatty acids. *Biochemistry* **19**:4719–4726.

Andreasen, T. J., D. R. Doerge, and M. G. McNamee (1979) Effects of phospholipase A_2 on the binding and ion permeability control properties of the acetylcholine receptor. *Arch. Biochem. Biophys.* **194**:468–480.

Anholt, R., J. Lindstrom, and M. Montal (1980) Functional equivalence of monomeric and dimeric forms of purified acetylcholine receptors from *Torpedo californica* in reconstituted lipid vesicles. *Eur. J. Biochem.* **109**:481–487.

Anholt, R., M. Montal, and J. Lindström (1983) Incorporation of acetylcholine receptors in model membranes: An approach aimed at studies of the molecular basis of neurotransmission. In *Peptide and Protein Reviews*, Vol. 1, M. Hearn, ed., pp. 95–137, Marcel Dekker, New York.

Anholt, R., J. Lindström, and M. Montal (1985) The molecular basis of neurotransmission: Structure and function of the nicotinic acetylcholine receptor. In *The Enzymes of Biological Membranes*, Vol. 3, A. N. Martonosi, ed., pp. 335–401, Plenum, New York.

Anwyl, R., and T. Narahashi (1980) Desensitization of the acetylcholine receptor of denervated rat soleus muscle and the effect of calcium. *Br. J. Pharmacol.* **69**:91–98.

Arnone, A. (1972) X-ray diffraction study of binding of 2,3-diphosphoglycerate to human deoxy-haemoglobin. *Nature* **231**:146–149.

Ascher, P., and D. Chesnoy-Marchais (1982) Interactions between three slow potassium responses controlled by three distinct receptors in *Aplysia* neurons. *J. Physiol. (Lond.)* **324**:67–92.

Ascher, P., L. Nowak, and J. S. Kehoe (1986) Glutamate-activated channels in molluscan and vertebrate neurons. In *Ion Channels in Neural Membranes*, J. M. Ritchie, R. D. Keynes, and L. Bolis, eds., pp. 283–293, Alan R. Liss, New York

Axelrod, D., P. M. Ravdin, D. E. Koppel, J. Schlessinger, W. W. Webb, E. L. Elson, and T. R. Podleski (1976) Lateral motion of fluorescently labeled acetylcholine receptors in membranes of developing muscle fibers. *Proc. Natl. Acad. Sci. USA* **73**:4594–4595.

Ballivet, M., J. Patrick, J. Lee, and S. Heinemann (1982) Molecular cloning of cDNA coding for the α-subunit of *Torpedo* acetylcholine receptor. *Proc. Natl. Acad. Sci. USA* **79**:4466–4470.

Baranyi, A., and O. Feher (1981a) Synaptic facilitation requires paired activation of convergent pathways in the neocortex. *Nature* **290**:413–415.

Baranyi, A., and O. Feher (1981b) Selective facilitations of synapses in the neocortex by heterosynaptic activation. *Brain Res.* **212**:164–168.

Barker, D., and M. C. Ip (1966) Sprouting and degenerations of mammalian motor axons in normal and deafferented skeletal muscle. *Proc. R. Soc. Lond. (Biol.)* **163**:538–554.

Barker, J. L., and R. N. McBurney (1979) GABA and glycine may share the same conductance channel on cultured mammalian neurones. *Nature* **277**:234–235.

Barnard, E. A., D. Beeson, G. Bilbe, D. A. Brown, A. Constanti, B. M. Conti-Tronconi, J. O. Dolly, S. M. J. Dunn, F. Mehraban, B. M. Richards, and T. G. Smart (1983) Acetylcholine and GABA receptors: Subunits of central and peripheral receptors and their encoding nucleic acids. *Cold Spring Harbor Symp. Quant. Biol.* **48**:109–124.

Barrantes, F. J., D. C. Neugebauer, and H. P. Zingsheim (1980) Peptide extraction by alkaline treatment is accompanied by rearrangement of the membrane-bound acetylcholine receptor from *Torpedo marmorata*. *FEBS Lett.* **112**:73–78.

Barrantes, F. J., G. Mieskes, and T. Wallimann (1983) A membrane-associated creatine kinase (EC 2.7.3.2) identified as an acidic species of the non-receptor, peripheral ν-proteins in *Torpedo* acetylcholine receptor membranes. *FEBS Lett.* **152**:270–276.

Berg, D. K., and Z. M. Hall (1975) Loss of alpha-bungarotoxin from junctional and extrajunctional acetylcholine receptors in rat diaphragm muscle *in vivo* and in organ culture. *J. Physiol. (Lond.)* **252**:771–789.

Berridge, M., and P. Rapp (1979) A comparative survey of the function, mechanism and control of cellular oscillations. *J. Exp. Biol.* **81**:217–280.

Betz, H. (1983) Regulation of α-bungarotoxin receptor accumulation in chick retina cultures: Effects of membrane depolarization, cyclic nucleotide derivatives, and Ca^{2+}. *J. Neurosci.* **3**:1333–1341.

Betz, H., and J.-P. Changeux (1979) Regulation of muscle acetylcholine receptor synthesis *in vitro* by derivatives of cyclic nucleotides. *Nature* **278**:749–752.

Betz, H., J. P. Bourgeois, and J.-P. Changeux (1977) Evidence for degradation of the acetylcholine (nicotinic) receptor in skeletal muscle during the development of the chick embryo. *FEBS Lett.* **77**:219–224.

Betz, H., J. P. Bourgeois, and J.-P. Changeux (1980) Evolution of cholinergic proteins in developing slow and fast skeletal muscles from chick embryo. *J. Physiol. (Lond.)* **302**:197–218.

Bienenstock, E. (1985) Une approche topologique de l'objet mental. In *Colloque de Cerisy: "Les Théories de la Complexité,"* F. Fogelman and S. Milgram, eds., Le Seuil, Paris.

Bienenstock, E., Y. Frégnac, and S. Thorpe (1983) Iontophoretic clamp of activity in visual cortical neurons in the cat: A test of Hebb's hypothesis. *J. Physiol. (Lond.)* **345**:123P.

Bienvenue, A., A. Rousselet, G. Kato, and P. F. Devaux (1977) Fluidity of lipids next to acetylcholine-receptor protein of *Torpedo* membrane fragments—use of amphiphilic reversible spin-labels. *Biochemistry* **16**:841–848.

Birdsall, N. J. M. (1982) Can different receptors interact directly with each other? *Trends Neurosci.* **5**:137–138.

Birdsall, N. J. M., E. C. Hulme, and J. M. Stockton (1983) Muscarinic receptor subclasses: Allosteric interactions. *Cold Spring Harbor Symp. Quant. Biol.* **48**:53–56.

Birnbaum, M., M. Reiss, and A. Shainberg (1980) Role of calcium in the regulation of acetylcholine receptor synthesis in cultured muscle cell. *Pfluegers Arch.* **385**:37–43.

Black, I. B., J. E. Adler, C. F. Dreyfus, G. M. Jonakait, D. M. Katz, E. F. Lagamma, and K. M. Markey (1984) Neurotransmitter plasticity at the molecular level. *Science* **225**:1266–1270.

Blaurock, A. E., and W. Stoeckenius (1971) Structure of the purple membrane. *Nature New Biol.* **233**:152–155.

Bliss, T. V. P., and T. Lømo (1973) Long-lasting potentiation of synaptic transmission in the dentate area of the anaesthesized rabbit following stimulation of the perforant path. *J. Physiol. (Lond.)* **232**:331–356.

Bon, F., E. Lebrun, J. Gomel, R. Van Rappenbusch, J. Cartaud, J. L. Popot, and J.-P. Changeux (1984) Image analysis of the heavy form of the acetylcholine receptor from *Torpedo marmorata*. *J. Mol. Biol.* **176**:205–237.

Boulter, J., and J. Patrick (1977) Purification of an acetylcholine receptor from a non-fusing muscle cell line. *Biochemistry* **16**:4900–4908.

Bourgeois, J. P., J. L. Popot, A. Ryter, and J.-P. Changeux (1973) Consequences of denervation on the distribution of the cholinergic (nicotinic) receptor sites from *Electrophorus electricus* revealed by high resolution autoradiography. *Brain Res.* **62**:557–563.

Bourgeois, J. P., H. Betz, and J.-P. Changeux (1978a) Effets de la paralysie chronique de l'embryon de poulet par le flaxedil sur le développement de la jonction neuromusculaire. *C. R. Seances Acad. Sci. (Paris)* **286D**:773–776.

Bourgeois, J. P., J. L. Popot, A. Ryter, and J.-P. Changeux (1978b) Quantitative studies on the localization of the cholinergic receptor protein in the normal and denervated electroplaque from *Electrophorus electricus*. *J. Cell. Biol.* **79**:200–216.

Boyd, N. D., and J. B. Cohen (1980) Kinetics of binding of [^{3}H]acetylcholine and [^{3}H]carbamoylcholine to *Torpedo* postsynaptic membranes: Slow conformational transitions of the cholinergic receptor. *Biochemistry* **19**:5344–5358.

Brazier, M. (1978) Architectonics of the cerebral cortex: Research in the 19th century. In *Architectonics of the Cerebral Cortex*, M. Brazier and H. Petsche, eds., pp. 9–29, Raven, New York.

Brenner, H. R., and B. Sakmann (1981) Neural control of end-plate channel gating in rat muscle. *J. Physiol. (Lond.)* **318**:44–45.

Brenner, H. R., and B. Sakmann (1983) Neurotrophic control of channel properties at neuromuscular synapses of rat muscle. *J. Physiol. (Lond.)* **337**:159–171.

Brenner, H. R., T. Meier, and B. Widmer (1983) Early action of nerve determines motor endplate differentiation in rat muscle. *Nature* **395**:536–537.

Brett, R. S., S. G. Youkin, M. Konieczkowski, and R. M. Slugg (1982) Accelerated degradation of junctional acetylcholine receptor–α-bungarotoxin complexes in denervated rat diaphragm. *Brain Res.* **233**:133–142.

Brisson, A. D. (1980) Thèse de doctorat d'état, Université de Grenoble, France.

Brisson, A. D., P. F. Devaux, and J.-P. Changeux (1975) Effet anesthésique local de plusieurs composés liposolubles sur la réponse de l'électroplaque de Gymnote à la carbamylcholine et sur la liaison de l'acétylcholine au récepteur cholinergique de Torpille. *C. R. Seances Acad. Sci. (Paris)* **280D**:2153–2156.

Britten, R., and E. Davidson (1969) Gene regulation for higher cells: A theory. *Science* **165**:349–357.

Brockes, J. P., and Z. W. Hall (1975) Acetylcholine receptors in normal and denervated rat diaphragm muscle. I. Purification and interaction with [^{125}I]-α-bungarotoxin. *Biochemistry* **14**:2092–2106.

Brown, D. (1984) The role of stable complexes that repress and activate eucaryotic genes. *Cell* **38**:359–365.

Burden, S. J. (1977a) Development of the neuromuscular junction in the chick embryo. The number, distribution and stability of the acetylcholine receptor. *Dev. Biol.* **57**:317–329.

Burden, S. J. (1977b) Acetylcholine receptors at the neuromuscular junction: Developmental change in receptor turnover. *Dev. Biol.* **61**:79–85.

Burden, S. J. (1985) The subsynaptic 43 kD protein is concentrated at developing nerve–muscle synapses *in vitro*. *Proc. Natl. Acad. Sci. USA* **82**:7805–7809.

Burden, S. J., R. L. De Palma, and G. S. Gottesman (1983) Cross-linking of proteins in acetylcholine receptor-rich membranes: Association between the β-subunit and the 43-kD subsynaptic protein. *Cell* **35**:687–692.

Bursztajn, S., and G. D. Fischbach (1984) Evidence that coated vesicles transport acetylcholine receptors to the surface membrane of chick myotubes. *J. Cell. Biol.* **98**:498–506.

Carew, T., R. Hawkins, T. W. Abrams, and E. Kandel (1984) A test of Hebb's postulate at identified synapses which mediate classical conditioning in *Aplysia*. *J. Neurosci.* **4**:1217–1224.

Carlin, R. K., and P. Siekevitz (1983) Plasticity in the central nervous system: Do synapses divide? *Proc. Natl. Acad. Sci. USA* **80**:3517–3521.

Cartaud, J., L. Benedetti, A. Sobel, and J.-P. Changeux (1978) A morphological study of the cholinergic receptor protein from *Torpedo marmorata* in its membrane environment and in its detergent-extracted purified form. *J. Cell Sci.* **29**:313–337.

Cartaud, J., A. Sobel, A. Rousselet, P. F. Devaux, and J.-P. Changeux (1981) Consequences of alkaline treatment for the ultrastructure of the acetylcholine-receptor-rich membranes from *Torpedo marmorata* electric organ. *J. Cell. Biol.* **90**:418–426.

Cartaud, J., R. Oswald, G. Clément, and J.-P. Changeux (1982) Evidence for a skeleton in acetylcholine receptor-rich membranes from *Torpedo marmorata* electric organ. *FEBS Lett.* **145**:250–257.

Cartaud, J., C. Kordeli, H. O. Nghiêm, and J.-P. Changeux (1983) La proteine 43000 daltons: Pièce intermédiaire assurant l'ancrage du recepteur cholinergique au cytosquelette sous-neural? *C. R. Seances Acad. Sci. (Paris)* **297**:285–289.

Catterall, W. A. (1980) Neurotoxins that act on voltage-sensitive sodium channels. *Annu. Rev. Pharmacol. Toxicol.* **20**:15–43.

Chang, C. C., and M. C. Huang (1975) Turnover of junctional and extrajunctional acetylcholine receptors of the rat diaphragm. *Nature* **253**:643–644.

Chang, H. W., E. Bock, and E. Neumann (1984) Long-lived metastable states and hysteresis in the binding of acetylcholine to *Torpedo californica* acetylcholine receptor. *Biochemistry* **23**:4546–4556.

Changeux, J.-P. (1966) Responses of acetylcholinesterase from *Torpedo marmorata* to salts and curarizing drugs. *Mol. Pharmacol.* **2**:369–392.

Changeux, J.-P. (1969) Remarks on the symmetry and cooperative properties of biological membranes. *Nobel Symp.* **11**:235–256.

Changeux, J.-P. (1981) The acetylcholine receptor: An "allosteric" membrane protein. *Harvey Lect.* **75**:85–254.

Changeux, J.-P. (1983) Concluding remarks on the "singularity" of nerve cells and its ontogenensis. *Prog. Brain Res.* **58**:465–478.

Changeux, J.-P., and A. Danchin (1976) Selective stabilization of developing synapses as a mechanism for the specification of neuronal networks. *Nature* **264**:2712.

Changeux, J.-P., J.-P. Thiéry, T. Tung, and C. Kittel (1967) On the cooperativity of biological membranes. *Proc. Natl. Acad. Sci. USA* **57**:335–341.

Changeux, J.-P., M. Kasai, and C. Y. Lee (1970) The use of a snake venom toxin to characterize the cholinergic receptor protein. *Proc. Natl. Acad. Sci. USA* **67**:1241–1247.

Changeux, J.-P., P. Courrège, and A. Danchin (1973) A theory of the epigenesis of neuronal networks by selective stabilization of synapses. *Proc. Natl. Acad. Sci. USA* **70**:2974–2978.

Changeux, J.-P., T. Heidmann, J. L. Popot, and A. Sobel (1979) Reconstitution of a functional acetylcholine regulator under defined conditions. *FEBS Lett.* **105**:181–187.

Changeux, J.-P., F. Bon, J. Cartaud, A. Devillers-Thiéry, J. Giraudat, T. Heidmann, B. Holton, H. O. Nghiêm, J. L. Popot, R. Van Rapenbusch, and S. Tzartos (1983) Allosteric properties of the acetylcholine receptor protein from *Torpedo marmorata*. *Cold Spring Harbor Symp. Quant. Biol.* **48**:35–52.

Changeux, J.-P., A. Devillers-Thiéry, and P. Chemouilli (1984a) Acetylcholine receptor: An allosteric protein. *Science* **225**:1335–1345.

Changeux, J.-P., T. Heidmann, and P. Patte (1984b) Learning by selection. In *The Biology of Learning*, P. Marler and H. Terrace, eds., pp. 115–139, Springer, Berlin.

Changeux, J.-P., A. Klarsfeld, and T. Heidmann (1987) The acetylcholine receptor and molecular models for short- and long-term learning. In *Molecular and Cellular Bases of Learning*, J.-P. Changeux and M. Konishi, eds., pp. 31–83, Wiley, Chichester.

Clapham, D. E., and E. Neher (1984) Substance P reduces acetylcholine-induced current in isolated bovine chromaffin cells. *J. Physiol. (Lond.)* 347:255–277.

Claudio, T., M. Ballivet, J. Patrick, and S. Heinemann (1983) Nucleotide and deduced amino acid sequences of *Torpedo californica* acetylcholine receptor subunit. *Proc. Natl. Acad. Sci. USA* 80:1111–1115.

Cohen, J. B., M. Weber, and J.-P. Changeux (1974) Effects of local anesthetics and calcium on the interaction of cholinergic ligands with the nicotinic receptor protein from *Torpedo marmorata*. *Mol. Pharmacol.* 10:904–932.

Cohen, S. A. (1980) Early nerve muscle synapses *in vitro* release transmitter over post-synaptic membrane having low acetylcholine sensitivity. *Proc. Natl. Acad. Sci. USA* 77:644–648.

Collingridge, G. L., S. J. Kehl, and H. McLennan (1983) The antagonism of amino-acid induced excitations of rat hippocampal CA1 neurons *in vitro*. *J. Physiol. (Lond.)* 334:19–31.

Conti-Tronconi, B. M., and M. A. Raftery (1982) The nicotinic cholinergic receptor: Correlation of molecular structure with functional properties. *Annu. Rev. Biochem.* 51:491–530.

Cotman, C. W., and M. Nieto-Sampedro (1984) Cell biology of synaptic plasticity. *Science* 225:1287–1294.

Couteaux, R. (1981) Structure of the subsynaptic sarcoplasm in the interfolds of the frog neuro-muscular junction. *J. Neurocytol.* 10:947–962.

Cowan, M. W. (1973) Neuronal death as a regulative mechanism in the control of cell number in the nervous system. In *Development and Aging in the Nervous System*, M. Rockstein and M. L. Sussman, eds., pp. 19–41, Academic, New York.

Cowan, M. W., J. W. Fawcett, D. O'Leary, and B. B. Stanfield (1984) Regressive events in neurogenesis. *Science* 225:1258–1270.

Crick, F. (1984) Memory and molecular turnover. *Nature* 312:101.

Cull-Candy, S. G. (1983) Glutamate and GABA-receptor channels at the locust nerve–muscle junction: Noise analysis and single channel recording. *Cold Spring Harbor Symp. Quant. Biol.* 48:269–278.

Culver, P., W. Fenical, and P. Taylor (1984) Lophotoxin irreversibly inactivates the nicotinic acetylcholine receptor by preferential association at one of the two primary agonist sites. *J. Biol. Chem.* 259:3763–3770.

Daniels, M., M. Vigny, P. Sonderegger, H. C. Bauer, and Z. Vogel (1984) Association of laminin and other basement membrane components with regions of high acetylcholine receptor density on cultured myotubes. *Int. J. Dev. Neurosci.* 2:87–99.

Delbrück, M. (1949) *Unités Biologiques Douées de Continuité Génétique*, Publication of the Centre National Recherche Scientifique, Paris.

Descartes, R. (1677) *Traité de l'Homme*, 2nd Ed., C. Angot, Paris.

Devillers-Thiéry, A., J. Giraudat, M. Bentaboulet, and J.-P. Changeux (1983) Complete mRNA coding sequence of the acetylcholine binding α-subunit of *Torpedo marmorata* acetylcholine receptor: A model for the transmembrane organization of the polypeptide chain. *Proc. Natl. Acad. Sci. USA* 80:2067–2071.

Devreotes, P. N., and D. M. Fambrough (1975) Acetylcholine receptor turnover in membranes of developing muscle fibers. *J. Cell. Biol.* 65:335–358.

Dwyer, D. S., R. L. Bradley, L. Furner, and G. E. Kemp (1981) Immunochemical properties of junctional and extrajunctional acetylcholine receptor. *Brain Res.* 217:23.

Eccles, J. (1964) *The Physiology of Synapses*, Springer, Berlin.

Eccles, J., M. Ito, and J. Szentagothai (1967) *The Cerebellum as a Neuronal Machine*, Springer, Berlin.

Edelman, G. M. (1978) Group selection and phasic reentrant signaling: A theory of higher brain function. In *The Mindful Brain: Cortical Organization and the Group-Selective Theory of Higher Brain Function*, by Gerald M. Edelman and Vernon B. Mountcastle, pp. 58–100, MIT Press, Cambridge, Massachusetts.

Edelman, G. M. (1981) Group selection as the basis for higher brain function. In *The Organization of the Cerebral Cortex*, F. G. Worden, G. Adelman, and S. G. Dennis, eds., pp. 535–563, MIT Press, Cambridge, Massachusetts.

Edelman, G. M. (1983) Cell adhesion molecules. *Science* **219**:450–457.

Eldefrawi, M. E. (1983) The acetylcholine receptor of electric organs. In *Myasthenia Gravis*, E. X. Albuquerque and A. T. Eldefrawi, eds., pp. 189–203, Chapman and Hall, London.

Eldefrawi, M. E., M. S. Aronstam, N. M. Bakry, A. T. Eldefrawi, and E. X. Albuquerque (1980) Activation, inactivation, and desensitization of acetylcholine receptor channel complex detected by binding of perhydrohistrionicotoxin. *Proc. Natl. Acad. Sci. USA* **77**:2309–2313.

Ellena, J. F., M. A. Blazing, and M. G. McNamee (1983) Lipid–protein interactions in reconstituted membranes containing acetylcholine receptor. *Biochemistry* **22**:5523–5535.

Elliott, J., S. G. Blanchard, W. Wu, J. Miller, C. D. Strader, P. Hartig, H. P. Moore, J. Racs, and M. A. Raftery (1980) Purification of *Torpedo californica* post-synaptic membranes and fractionation of their constituent proteins. *Biochem. J.* **185**:667–677.

Epstein, M., and E. Racker (1978) Reconstitution of carbamylcholine-dependent sodium ion flux and desensitization of the acetylcholine receptor from *Torpedo californica*. *J. Biol. Chem.* **253**:6660–6662.

Fairclough, R. H., J. Finer-Moore, R. A. Love, D. Kristofferson, P. J. Desmeules, and R. M. Stroud (1983) Subunit organization and structure of an acetylcholine receptor. *Cold Spring Harbor Symp. Quant. Biol.* **48**:9–20.

Fambrough, D. (1979) Control of acetylcholine receptors in skeletal muscle. *Physiol. Rev.* **59**:165–227.

Feltz, A., and A. Trautmann (1980) Interaction between nerve-released acetylcholine and bath-applied agonists at the frog end plate. *J. Physiol. (Lond.)* **299**:533–552.

Feltz, A., and A. Trautmann (1982) Desensitization at the frog neuromuscular junction: A biphasic process. *J. Physiol. (Lond.)* **322**:257–272.

Fiekers, J. F., P. M. Spannbauer, B. Scubon-Mulieri, and R. L. Parsons (1980) Voltage dependence of desensitization. Influence of calcium and activation kinetics. *J. Gen. Physiol.* **75**:511–529.

Finkel, L., and G. M. Edelman (1985) Interaction of synaptic modification rules within populations of neurons. *Proc. Natl. Acad. Sci. USA* **82**:1291–1295.

Fischbach, G. D., and S. M. Schuetze (1980) A postnatal decrease in acetylcholine channel open time at rat end-plates. *J. Physiol. (Lond.)* **303**:125–137.

Forrest, J. W., R. G. Mills, J. J. Bray, and J. I. Hubbard (1981) Calcium-dependent regulation of the membrane potential and extrajunctional acetylcholine receptors of rat skeletal muscle. *Neuroscience* **6**:741–749.

Fosset, M H. Schmid-Antomarchi, M. Hugues, G. Romey, and M. Lazdunski (1984) The presence in pig brain of an endogenous equivalent of apamin, the bee venom peptide that specifically blocks Ca^{++}-dependent K^+ channels. *Proc. Natl. Acad. Sci. USA* **81**:7228–7233.

Frank, E., K. Gautvik, and H. Sommer-Schild (1975) Cholinergic receptors at denervated mammalian endplates. *Acta Physiol. Scand.* **95**:66–76.

Frégnac, Y., and M. Imbert (1984) Development of neuronal selectivity in primary visual cortex of cat. *Physiol. Rev.* **64**:325–434.

Freud, S. (1895) Project for a scientific psychology. In *The Complete Psychological Works: Standard Edition*, 24 vols., J. Strachey, ed., published in 1976 by Hogarth, London.

Fuxe, K., F. L. Agnati, F. Benfenati, M. Cimmino, S. Algeri, T. Hökfelt, and V. Mutt (1981) Modulation by cholecystokinins of ^3H-spiroperidol binding in rat striatum: Evidence for increased affinity and reduction in the number of binding sites. *Acta Physiol. Scand.* **113**:567–569.

Fuxe, K., L. Agnati, F. Benfenati, M. Celani, I. Zini, M. Zoli, and V. Mutt (1983) Evidence for the existence of receptor–receptor interaction in the central nervous system. Studies on the regulation of monoamine receptors by neuroleptics. *J. Neuronal Trans.* **18**:165–179.

Fuxe, K., L. Agnati, K. Andersson, M. Martire, S. O. Ogren, L. Giardino, N. Battistini, R. Grimaldi, C. Farabegoli, A. Härfstrand, and G. Toffano (1984) Receptor–receptor interactions in the central nervous system: Evidence for the existence of heterostatic synaptic mechanisms. In *Regulation of Transmitter Function: Basic and Clinical Aspects*, E. S. Vizi and K. Magyars, eds., Elsevier, New York.

Giacobini, G., G. Filogamo, M. Weber, P. Boquet, and J.-P. Changeux (1973) Effects of a snake-neurotoxin on the development of innervated motor muscles in chick embryo. *Proc. Natl. Acad. Sci. USA* **70**:1708–1712.

Giacobini-Robecchi, M. G., G. Giacobini, G. Filogamo, and J.-P. Changeux (1975) Effect of the type A toxin from *C. botulinum* on the development of skeletal muscles and of their innervation in chick embryo. *Brain Res.* **83**:107–121.

Giraudat, J., A. Devillers-Thiéry, C. Auffray, F. Rougeon, and J.-P. Changeux (1982) Identification of a cDNA clone coding for the acetylcholine binding subunit of *Torpedo marmorata* acetylcholine receptor. *EMBO J.* **1**:713–717.

Giraudat, J., A. Devillers-Thiéry, J. C. Perriard, and J.-P. Changeux (1984) Complete nucleotide sequence of *Torpedo marmorata* mRNA coding for the 43,000 daltons v_2 protein: Muscle specific creatine kinase. *Proc. Natl. Acad. Sci. USA* **81**:7313–7317.

Giraudat, J., C. Montecucco, R. Bisson, and J.-P. Changeux (1985) Transmembrane topology of acetylcholine receptor subunits probed with photoreactive phospholipids. *Biochemistry* **24**: 3121–3127.

Giraudat, J., M. Dennis, T. Heidmann, J.-Y. Chang, and J.-P. Changeux (1986) Structure of the high affinity binding site for noncompetitive blockers of the acetylcholine receptor: Serine 262 of the δ-subunit is labeled by [^{3}H]chlorpromazine. *Proc. Natl. Acad. Sci. USA* **83**:2719–2723.

Gonzalez-Ros, J. M., A. Paraschos, and M. Martinez-Carrion (1980) Reconstitution of functional membrane-bound acetylcholine receptor from isolated *Torpedo californica* receptor protein and electroplax lipids. *Proc. Natl. Acad. Sci. USA* **77**:1796–1800.

Gonzalez-Ros, J. M., M. C. Farach, and M. Martinez-Carrion (1983) Ligand-induced effects at regions of acetylcholine receptor accessible to membrane lipids. *Biochemistry* **22**:3807–3811.

Gordon, A. S., G. Davis, and I. Diamond (1977) Phosphorylation of membrane proteins at a cholinergic synapse. *Proc. Natl. Acad. Sci. USA* **74**:263–267.

Gordon, A. S., D. Milfay, and I. Diamond (1983) Identification of a molecular weight 43,000 protein kinase in acetylcholine receptor-enriched membranes. *Proc. Natl. Acad. Sci. USA* **80**:5862–5865.

Gouzé, J. L., J. M. Lasry, and J.-P. Changeux (1983) Selective stabilization of muscle innervation during development: A mathematical model. *Biol. Cybern.* **46**:207–215.

Grünhagen, H. H., and J.-P. Changeux (1976) Studies on the electrogenic action of acetylcholine with *Torpedo marmorata* electric organ. Quinacrine: A fluorescent probe for the conformational transitions of the cholinergic receptor protein in its membrane-bound state. *J. Mol. Biol.* **106**: 497–516.

Gysin, R., B. Yost, and S. D. Flanagan (1983) Immunochemical and molecular differentiation of 43,000 molecular weight proteins associated with *Torpedo* neuroelectrocyte synapses. *Biochemistry* **22**:5781–5789.

Hall, Z. W. (1973) Multiple forms of acetylcholinesterase and their distribution in endplate and non-endplate regions of rat diaphragm muscle. *J. Neurobiol.* **4**:343–361.

Hall, Z. W., M. P. Roisin, Y. Gu, and P. D. Gorin (1983) A developmental change in the immunological properties of acetylcholine receptors at the rat neuromuscular junction. *Cold Spring Harbor Symp. Quant. Biol.* **48**:101–108.

Hamburger, V., and R. Levi-Montalcini (1949) Proliferation, differentiation and degeneration in the spinal ganglia of the chick embryo under normal and experimental conditions. *J. Exp. Zool.* **111**:457–502.

Haring, R., Y. Kloog, and M. Sokolovsky (1984) Localization of phencyclidine binding sites on α- and β-subunits of the nicotinic acetylcholine receptor from *Torpedo ocellata* electric organ using azido phencyclidine. *J. Neurosci.* **4**:627–637.

Hassel, J. R., P. G. Robey, H. J. Barrach, J. Wilczek, S. I. Rennard, and G. R. Martin (1980) Isolation of a heparan sulfate-containing proteoglycan from basement membrane. *Proc. Natl. Acad. Sci. USA* **77**:4494–4498.

Hawkins, R. D., and E. Kandel (1984) Is there a cell-biological alphabet for simple forms of learning? *Psychol. Rev.* **91**:375–391.

Hawkins, R. D., S. W. Abrahms, T. J. Carew, and E. R. Kandel (1983) A cellular mechanism of classical conditioning in *Aplysia*: Activity-dependent enhancement of presynaptic facilitation. *Science* **219**:400–405.

Hebb, D. O. (1949) *The Organization of Behavior: A Neuropsychological Theory*, Wiley, New York.

Heidmann, T., and J.-P. Changeux (1979) Fast kinetic studies on the interaction of a fluorescent agonist with the membrane-bound acetylcholine receptor from *Torpedo marmorata*. *Eur. J. Biochem.* **94**:281–296.

Heidmann, T., and J.-P. Changeux (1980) Interaction of a fluorescent agonist with the membrane-bound acetylcholine receptor from *Torpedo marmorata* in the millisecond time range: Resolution of an "intermediate" conformational transition and evidence for positive cooperative effects. *Biochem. Biophys. Res. Commun.* **97**:889–896.

Heidmann, T., and J.-P. Changeux (1982) Un modèle moléculaire de régulation d'efficacité d'un synapse chimique au niveau postsynaptique. *C. R. Seances Acad. Sci. (Paris)* **295**:665–670.

Heidmann, T., and J.-P. Changeux (1984) Time-resolved photolabeling by chlorpromazine of the acetylcholine receptor ion channel in its transiently open and closed conformations. *Proc. Natl. Acad. Sci. USA* **81**:1897–1901.

Heidmann, T., A. Sobel, J. L. Popot, and J.-P. Changeux (1980) Reconstitution of an acetylcholine receptor. Conservation of the conformational and allosteric transition and recovery of the permeability response; role of lipids. *Eur. J. Biochem.* **110**:35–55.

Heidmann, T., J. Bernhardt, E. Neumann, and J.-P. Changeux (1983a) Rapid kinetics of agonist binding and permeability response analyzed in parallel on acetylcholine receptor-rich membranes from *Torpedo marmorata*. *Biochemistry* **22**:5452–5459.

Heidmann, T., R. E. Oswald, and J.-P. Changeux (1983b) Multiple sites of action for noncompetitive blockers on acetylcholine receptor-rich membrane fragments from *Torpedo marmorata*. *Biochemistry* **22**:3112–3127.

Heidmann, A., T. Heidmann, and J.-P. Changeux (1984) Stabilisation-selective de représentations neuronales par résonance entre "pré-représentations" spontanées du réseau cérébral et "percepts" évoqués par interaction avec le monde extérieur. *C. R. Seances Acad. Sci. (Paris)* **299**:839–844.

Henderson, R., and P. N. T. Unwin (1975) Three-dimensional model of purple membrane obtained by electron microscopy. *Nature* **257**:28–32.

Hershey, N. D., D. J. Noonan, K. S. Mixter, T. Claudio, and N. Davidson (1983) Structure and expression of genomic clones coding for the α-subunit of the *Torpedo* acetylcholine receptor. *Cold Spring Harbor Symp. Quant. Biol.* **48**:79–82.

Hilgard, E. (1948) *Theories of Learning*, Appleton-Century, New York.

Hilgard, E., and D. Marquis (1940) *Conditioning and Learning*, Appleton-Century, New York.

Hogan, P. G., J. M. Marshall, and Z. Hall (1976) Muscle activity decreases rate of degradation of α-bungarotoxin bound to extrajunctional acetylcholine receptors. *Nature* **261**:328–330.

Hökfelt, T., O. Johansson, and M. Goldstein (1984) Chemical anatomy of the brain. *Science* **225**:1326–1334.

Holton, B., S. J. Tzartos, and J.-P. Changeux (1984) Comparison of embryonic and adult *Torpedo* acetylcholine receptor by sedimentation characteristics and antigenicity. *Dev. Neurosci.* **2**:549–555.

Holtzman, E., D. Wise, J. Wall, and A. Karlin (1982) Electron microscopy of complexes of isolated acetylcholine receptor, biotinyl-toxin, and avidin. *Proc. Natl. Acad. Sci. USA* **79**:310–314.

Huganir, R. L., A. H. Delcour, P. Greengard, and G. P. Hess (1986) Phosphorylation of the nicotinic acetylcholine receptor regulates its rate of densensitization. *Nature* **321**:774–776.

Hurwitz, L., and L. J. McGuffee (1979) Desensitization phenomena in smooth muscle. In *Trends in Autonomic Pharmacology*, Vol. 1, S. Kalsner, ed., pp. 251–265, Urban and Schwarzenberg, Baltimore.

Inestrosa, N., J. Miller, L. Silberstein, L. Ziskind-Conhaim, and Z. W. Hall (1983) Developmental regulation of 16S acetylcholinesterase and acetylcholine receptors in a mouse muscle cell line. *Exp. Cell Res.* **147**:393–405.

Ito, M., M. Sakurai, and P. Tongroach (1982) Climbing fibre-induced depression of both mossy fibre responsiveness and glutamate sensitivity of cerebellar Purkinje cells. *J. Physiol. (Lond.)* **324**: 113–134.

Jackson, M. (1984) Spontaneous openings of the acetylcholine receptor channel. *Proc. Natl. Acad. Sci. USA* **81**:3901–3904.

Jacob, M., J. M. Lindstrom, and D. K. Berg (1986) Surface and intracellular distribution of a putative neuronal nicotinic receptor. *J. Cell Biol.* **103**:205–214.

Jerne, N. (1967) Antibodies and learning: Selection versus instruction. In *The Neurosciences: A Study Program*, G. C. Quarton, T. Melnechuck, and F. O. Schmitt, eds., pp. 200–205, Rockefeller Univ. Press, New York.

Kaldany, R. R. J., and A. Karlin (1983) Reaction of quinacrine mustard with the acetylcholine receptor from *Torpedo californica*: Functional consequences and sites of labeling. *J. Biol. Chem.* **258**:6232– 6242.

Kandel, E. R. (1977) Cellular insights into behavior and learning. *Harvey Lect.* **73**:19–32.

Kandel, E. R., T. Abrams, L. Bernier, T. J. Carew, R. D. Hawkins, and J. H. Schwartz (1983) Classical conditioning and sensitization share aspects of the same molecular cascade in *Aplysia*. *Cold Spring Harbor Symp. Quant. Biol.* **48**:821–830.

Kao, P., A. Dwork, R. Kaldany, M. Silver, J. Wideman, S. Stein, and A. Karlin (1984) Identification of the α-subunit half-cystine specifically labeled by an affinity reagent for the acetylcholine receptor binding site. *J. Biol. Chem.* **258**:11662–11665.

Karlin, A. (1967) On the application of "a plausible model" of allosteric proteins to the receptor for acetylcholine. *J. Theor. Biol.* **16**:306–320.

Karlin, A. (1983) Anatomy of a receptor. *Neurosci. Comment.* **1**:111–123.

Katz, B., and R. Miledi (1972) The statistical nature of the acetylcholine potential and its molecular components. *J. Physiol. (Lond.)* **224**:665–699.

Katz, B., and S. Thesleff (1957) A study of the "desensitization" produced by acetylcholine at the motor end-plate. *J. Physiol. (Lond.)* **138**:63–80.

Kistler, J., and R. M. Stroud (1981) Crystalline arrays of membrane-bound acetylcholine receptor. *Proc. Natl. Acad. Sci. USA* **78**:3678–3682.

Klarsfeld, A., and J.-P. Changeux (1985) Activity regulates the level of acetylcholine receptor α-subunit mRNA in cultured chick myotubes. *Proc. Natl. Acad. Sci. USA* **82**:4558–4562.

Klarsfeld, A., A. Devillers-Thiéry, J. Giraudat, and J.-P. Changeux (1984) A single gene codes for the nicotinic acetylcholine receptor α-subunit in *Torpedo marmorata*: Structural and developmental implications. *EMBO J.* **3**:35–41.

Klymkowsky, M. W., J. E. Heuser, and R. M. Stroud (1980) Protease effects on the structure of acetylcholine receptor membranes from *Torpedo californica*. *J. Cell Biol.* **85**:823–838.

Korenstein, R., B. Hess, and N. Markus (1979) Cooperativity in the photocycle of purple membrane of *Halobacterium halobium* with a mechanism of free energy transduction. *FEBS Lett.* **102**:155– 161.

Krodel, E. K., R. A. Beckman, and J. B. Cohen (1979) Identification of a local anesthetic binding site in nicotinic post-synaptic membranes isolated from *Torpedo marmorata* electric tissue. *Mol. Pharmacol.* **15**:294–312.

Kuffler, S. W., M. J. Dennis, and A. J. Harris (1971) The development of chemosensitivity in extrasynaptic areas of the neuronal surface after denervation of parasympathetic ganglion cells in the heart of the frog. *Proc. R. Soc. Lond. (Biol.)* **177**:555.

Kullberg, R. W., F. S. Mikelberg, and M. W. Cohen (1980) Contribution of cholinesterase to developmental decrease in the time course of synaptic potentials at an amphibian neuromuscular junction. *Dev. Biol.* **75**:255–267.

Lee, C. Y., and C. C. Chang (1966) Modes of actions of purified toxins from elapid venoms on neuromuscular transmission. *Memoires Institut Butantan (São Paulo)* **33**:555–572.

Leeb-Lundberg, F., A. Snowman, and R. W. Olsen (1980) Barbiturate receptors are coupled to benzodiazepine receptors. *Proc. Natl. Acad. Sci. USA* **77**:7468–7472.

Levitt, T. A., and M. M. Salpeter (1981) Denervated endplates have a dual population of junctional acetylcholine receptors. *Nature* **291**:239–241.

Linden, C. D., and D. Fambrough (1979) Biosynthesis and degradation of acetylcholine receptors in rat skeletal muscles. Effects of electrical stimulation. *Neuroscience* 4:527–538.

Lindstrom, J., R. Anholt, B. Einarson, A. Engel, M. Osame, and M. Montal (1980) Purification of acetylcholine receptors, reconstitution into lipid vesicles and study of agonist-induced cation channel regulation. *J. Biol. Chem.* 255:8340–8350.

Lindstrom, J., S. Tzartos, W. Gullick, S. Hochschwender, L. Swanson, P. Sargent, M. Jacob, and M. Montal (1983) Use of monoclonal antibodies to study acetylcholine receptors from electric organs, muscle, and brain and the autoimmune response to receptor in myasthenia gravis. *Cold Spring Harbor Symp. Quant. Biol.* 48:89–99.

Lisman, J. (1985) A mechanism for memory storage insensitive to molecular turnover: A bistable autophosphorylating kinase. *Proc. Natl. Acad. Sci. USA* 82:3055–3057.

Llinás, R., ed. (1969) *Neurobiology of Cerebellar Evolution and Development*, American Medical Association/ Education and Research Foundation, Chicago.

Lo, M. M. S., P. B. Garland, J. Lamprecht, and E. A. Barnard (1980) Rotational mobility of the membrane-bound acetylcholine receptor of *Torpedo* electric organ measured by phosphorescence depolarisation. *FEBS Lett.* 111:407–412.

Lømo, T., and C. R. Slater (1976) Control of neuromuscular synapse formation. In *Synaptogenesis*, L. Tauc, ed., pp. 9–31, Naturalia and Biologia.

Lømo, T., and C. R. Slater (1980) Control of junctional acetylcholinesterase by neural and muscular influences in the rat. *J. Physiol. (Lond.)* 303:191–202.

Loring, R. H., and M. M. Salpeter (1980) Denervation increases turnover rate of junctional acetylcholine receptors. *Proc. Natl. Acad. Sci. USA* 77:2293–2297.

Lynch, G., and M. Baudry (1984) The biochemistry of memory: A new and specific hypothesis. *Science* 224:1057–1063.

McCarthy, M. P., J. P. Earnest, E. F. Young, S. Choe, and R. M. Stroud (1986) The molecular biology of the acetylcholine receptor. *Annu. Rev. Neurosci.* 9:383–413.

Magazanik, L. G., and F. Vyskocil (1970) Dependence of acetylcholine desensitization on the membrane potential of frog muscle fibre and on the ionic changes in the medium. *J. Physiol. (Lond.)* 210:507–518.

Magazanik, L. G., and F. Vyskocil (1975) The effect of temperature on desensitization kinetics at the post-synaptic membrane of the frog muscle fibre. *J. Physiol. (Lond.)* 249:285–300.

Magleby, K. L., and B. S. Pallotta (1981) A study of desensitization of acetylcholine receptors using nerve-released transmitter in the frog. *J. Physiol. (Lond.)* 316:225–250.

Mallet, J., N. Faucon, M. Buda, A. Lamouroux, and D. Samolyk (1983) Detection and regulation of the tyrosine hydroxylase mRNA levels in rat adrenal medulla and brain tissues. *Cold Spring Harbor Symp. Quant. Biol.* 48:305–308.

Marler, P., and H. Terrace, eds. (1984) *The Biology of Learning*, Springer, Berlin.

Marr, D. (1969) A theory of cerebellar cortex. *J. Physiol. (Lond.)* 202:437–470.

Marsh, D., A. Watts, and F. J. Barrantes (1981) Phospholipid chain immobilization and steroid rotational immobilization in acetylcholine receptor-rich membranes from *Torpedo marmorata*. *Biochim. Biophys. Acta.* 645:97–101.

Massoulié, J., and S. Bon (1982) The molecular forms of cholinesterase and acetylcholinesterase in vertebrates. *Annu. Rev. Neurosci.* 5:57–106.

Masters, S. B., M. T. Quinn, and J. H. Brown (1985) Agonist-induced desensitization of muscarinic receptor-mediated calcium efflux without concomitant desensitization of phosphoinositide hydrolysis. *Mol. Pharmacol.* 27:325–332.

Matthews-Bellinger, J. A., and M. M. Salpeter (1983) Fine structural distribution of acetylcholine receptors at developing mouse neuromuscular junctions. *J. Neurosci.* 3:644–657.

Mattson, C., and E. Heilbronn (1975) The nicotinic acetylcholine receptor: A glycoprotein. *J. Neurochem.* 25:899–901.

Merlie, J. P. (1984) Biogenesis of the acetylcholine receptor, a multisubunit integral membrane protein. *Cell* 36:573–575.

Merlie, J. P., and J. R. Sanes (1985) Concentration of acetylcholine receptor mRNA in synaptic regions of adult muscle fibers. *Nature* 317:66–68.

Merlie, J. P., A. Sobel, J.-P. Changeux, and F. Gros (1975) Synthesis of acetylcholine receptor during differentiation of cultured embryonic muscle cells. *Proc. Natl. Acad. Sci. USA* **72**:4028–4032.

Merlie, J. P., J.-P. Changeux, and F. Gros (1978) Skeletal muscle acetylcholine receptor. Purification, characterization, and turnover in muscle cell cultures. *J. Biol. Chem.* **253**:2882–2891.

Merlie, J. P., R. Sebbane, S. Gardner, and J. Lindstrom (1983a) cDNA clone for the α-subunit of the acetylcholine receptor from the mouse muscle cell line BC3H-1. *Proc. Natl. Acad. Sci. USA* **80**:3845–3849.

Merlie, J. P., R. Sebbane, S. Gardner, E. Olson, and J. Lindstrom (1983b) The regulation of acetylcholine receptor expression in mammalian muscle. *Cold Spring Harbor Symp. Quant. Biol.* **48**:135–146.

Merlie, J. P., K. E. Isenberg, S. D. Russell, and J. R. Sanes (1985) Denervation supersensitivity in skeletal muscle: Analysis with a cloned cDNA probe. *J. Cell Biol.* **99**:332–335.

Meunier, J. C., R. Olsen, R. Sealock, and J.-P. Changeux (1974) Purification and properties of the cholinergic receptor protein from *Electrophorus electricus* electric tissue. *Eur. J. Biochem.* **45**:371–394.

Miledi, R. (1980) Intracellular calcium and desensitization of acetylcholine receptors. *Proc. R. Soc. Lond. (Biol.)* **209**:447–452.

Mishina, M., T. Takai, K. Imoto, M. Noda, T. Takahashi, S. Numa, C. Methfessel, and B. Sakmann (1986) Molecular distinction between fetal and adult forms of muscle acetylcholine receptor. *Nature* **321**:406–411.

Monod, J., and F. Jacob (1961) General conclusions: Teleonomic mechanisms in cellular metabolism, growth and differentiation. *Cold Spring Harbor Symp. Quant. Biol.* **26**:389–401.

Monod, J., J.-P. Changeux, and F. Jacob (1963) Allosteric proteins and cellular control systems. *J. Mol. Biol.* **6**:306.

Monod, J., J. Wyman, and J.-P. Changeux (1965) On the nature of allosteric transitions: A plausible model. *J. Mol. Biol.* **12**:88–118.

Montal, M., R. Anholt, and P. Labarca (1986) The reconstituted acetylcholine receptor. In *Ion Channel Reconstitution*, C. Miller, ed., pp. 157–204, Plenum, New York.

Muhn, P., and F. Hucho (1983) Covalent labeling of the acetylcholine receptor from *Torpedo* electric tissue with the channel blocker [^{3}H]triphenylmethylphosphonium by ultraviolet irradiation. *Biochemistry* **22**:421–425.

Neher, E., and B. Sakmann (1976) Single channel currents recorded from membrane of denervated frog muscle fibres. *Nature* **260**:799–802.

Nelson, N., R. Anholt, J. Lindstrom, and M. Montal (1980) Reconstitution of purified acetylcholine receptor with functional ion channels in planar lipid bilayers. *Proc. Natl. Acad. Sci. USA* **77**: 3057–3061.

Nestler, E., and P. Greengard (1984) *Protein Phosphorylation in the Nervous System*, Wiley, New York.

Neubig, R. R., N. D. Boyd, and J. B. Cohen (1982) Conformations of *Torpedo* acetylcholine receptor associated with ion transport and desensitization. *Biochemistry* **21**:3460–3467.

Neubig, R. R., and J. B. Cohen (1980) Permeability control by cholinergic receptors in *Torpedo* postsynaptic membranes: Agonist dose–response relations measured at second and millisecond times. *Biochemistry* **19**:2770–2779.

Neubig, R. R., E. K. Krodel, N. D. Boyd, and J. B. Cohen (1979) Acetylcholine and local anesthetic binding to *Torpedo* nicotinic postsynaptic membranes after removal of nonreceptor peptides. *Proc. Natl. Acad. Sci. USA* **76**:690–694.

Nghiêm, H. O., J. Cartaud, C. Dubreuil, C. Kordeli, G. Buttin, and J.-P. Changeux (1983) Production and characterization of a monoclonal antibody directed against the 43,000 M.W. v_1 polypeptide from *Torpedo marmorata* electric organ. *Proc. Natl. Acad. Sci. USA* **80**:6403–6407.

Noda, M., H. Takahashi, T. Tanabe, M. Toyosato, Y. Furutani, T. Hirose, M. Asai, S. Inayama, T. Miyata, and S. Numa (1982) Primary structure of α-subunit precursor of *Torpedo californica* acetylcholine receptor deduced from cDNA sequence. *Nature* **299**:793–797.

Noda, M., H. Takahashi, T. Tanabe, M. Toyosato, S. Kikyotani, T. Hirose, M. Asai, H. Takashima, S. Inayama, T. Miyata, and S. Numa (1983a) Primary structures of β- and δ-subunit precursors of *Torpedo californica* acetylcholine receptor deduced from cDNA sequences. *Nature* **301**:251–255.

Noda, M., H. Takahashi, T. Tanabe, M. Toyosato, S. Kikyotani, Y. Furutani, T. Hirose, H. Takashima, S. Inayama, T. Miyata, and S. Numa (1983b) Structural homology of *Torpedo californica* acetylcholine receptor subunits. *Nature* **302**:528–532.

Noda, M., Y. Furutani, H. Takahashi, M. Toyosato, T. Tanabe, S. Shimizu, S. Kikyotani, T. Kayano, T. Hirose, S. Inayama, and S. Numa (1983c) Cloning and sequence analysis of calf cDNA and human genomic DNA encoding α-subunit precursor of muscle acetylcholine receptor. *Nature* **305**:818–823.

Noda, M., S. Shimizu, T. Tanabe, T. Takai, T. Kayano, T. Ikeda, H. Takahashi, H. Nakayama, Y. Kanaoka, N. Minamino, K. Kangawa, H. Matsuo, M. A. Raftery, T. Hirose, S. Inayama, H. Hayashida, T. Miyata, and S. Numa (1984) Primary structure of *Electrophorus electricus* sodium channel deduced from cDNA sequence. *Nature* **312**:121–127.

Nowak, L., P. Bregetovski, P. Ascher, A. Herbet, and A. Prochiantz (1984) Magnesium gates glutamate-activated channels in mouse central neurones. *Nature* **307**:462–465.

Oberthür, W., P. Muhn, H. Baumann, F. Lottspeich, B. Wittmann-Liebold, and F. Hucho (1986) The reaction site of a noncompetitive antagonist in the δ-subnit of the nicotinic acetylcholine receptor. *EMBO J.* **5**:1815–1819.

Olsen, R. W. (1981) GABA–benzodiazepine–barbiturate receptor interactions. *J. Neurochem.* **37**:1–13.

Olson, E. N., L. Glaser, J. P. Merlie, and J. Lindstrom (1984) Expression of acetylcholine receptor α-subunit mRNA during differentiation of the BC_3Hl muscle cell line. *J. Biol. Chem.* **259**:3330–3336.

Oppenheim, R. W., R. Pittman, M. Gray, and J. L. Madredrut (1978) Embryonic behavior, hatching and neuromuscular development in the chick following a transient reduction of spontaneous mobility and sensory input by neuromuscular blocking agents. *J. Comp. Neurol.* **179**:619–640.

Orkin, R. W., P. Gehron, E. B. McGoodwin, G. R. Martin, T. Valentine, and R. Swarm (1977) A murine tumor producing a matrix of basement membrane. *J. Exp. Med.* **145**:204–220.

Oswald, R. E. (1983a) Effects of calcium on the binding of phencyclidine to acetylcholine receptor-rich, membrane fragments from *Torpedo californica* electroplaque. *J. Neurochem.* **41**:1077.

Oswald, R. E. (1983b) Binding of phencyclidine to the detergent-solubilized acetylcholine receptor from *Torpedo marmorata*. *Life Sci.* **32**:1143–1149.

Oswald, R. E., and J.-P. Changeux (1981a) Ultraviolet light-induced labeling by noncompetitive blockers of the acetylcholine receptor from *Torpedo marmorata*. *Proc. Natl. Acad. Sci. USA* **78**:3925–3929.

Oswald, R. E., and J.-P. Changeux (1981b) Selective labeling of the δ-subunit of the acetylcholine receptor by a covalent local anesthetic. *Biochemistry* **20**:7166–7174.

Oswald, R. E., A. Sobel, G. Waksman, B. Roques, and J.-P. Changeux (1980) Selective labeling by [³H]trimethisoquinazide of polypeptide chains present in acetylcholine receptor-rich membranes from *Torpedo marmorata*. *FEBS Lett.* **111**:29–34.

Oswald, R. E., T. Heidmann, and J.-P. Changeux (1983) Multiple affinity states for noncompetitive blockers revealed by ³H-phencyclidine binding to acetylcholine receptor-rich membrane fragments from *Torpedo marmorata*. *Biochemistry* **22**:3128–3136.

Pavlov, I. P. (1927) *Conditioned Reflexes: An Investigation of the Physiological Activity of the Cerebral Cortex*, trans. by G. V. Anrep, Oxford Univ. Press, Oxford. Reprinted by Dover, New York.

Peck, E. J. (1980) Receptors for amino-acids. *Annu. Rev. Physiol.* **42**:615–627.

Peng, H. B. (1984) Participation of calcium and calmodulin in the formation of acetylcholine receptor clusters. *J. Cell Biol.* **98**:550–557.

Perutz, M., G. Fermi, D. A. Abraham, C. Poyart, and E. Bursaux (1986) Hemoglobin as a receptor of drugs and peptides: X-ray studies of the stereochemistry of binding. *J. Am. Chem. Soc.* **108**:1064–1078.

Pfeiffer, K., R. Simler, G. Grenningloh, and H. Betz (1984) Monoclonal antibodies and peptide mapping reveal structural similarities between the subunits of the glycine receptor of rat spinal cord. *Proc. Natl. Acad. Sci. USA* **81**:7224–7227.

Piéron, H. (1923) *Le Cerveau et la Pensée*, Alcan, Paris.

Podleski, T. R., D. Axelrod, P. Ravdin, I. Greenberg, M. M. Johnson, and M. M. Salpeter (1978) Nerve extract induces increase and redistribution of acetylcholine receptors on cloned muscle cells. *Proc. Natl. Acad. Sci. USA* **75**:2035–2039.

Poo, M., Y. Sun, and S. H. Young (1985) Three types of transmitter secretion from embryonic neurons. *J. Physiol. (Paris)* **80**:283–289.

Popot, J. L. (1983) Structural and functional properties of the acetylcholine receptor: Studies using reconstituted vesicles. In *Basic Mechanisms of Neuronal Hyperexcitability*, H. H. Jasper and N. M. Van Gelder, eds., pp. 137–170, Alan R. Liss, New York.

Popot, J. L., and J.-P. Changeux (1984) The nicotinic acetylcholine receptor: Structure of an oligomeric integral membrane protein. *Physiol. Rev.* **64**:1162–1184.

Popot, J. L., R. A. Demel, A. Sobel, L. L. M. Van Deenen, and J.-P. Changeux (1978) Interaction of the acetylcholine (nicotinic) receptor protein from *Torpedo marmorata* electric organ with monolayers of pure lipids. *Eur. J. Biochem.* **85**:27–42.

Porter, S., and S. C. Froehner (1983) Characterization and localization of the $M_r = 43,000$ proteins associated with acetylcholine receptor-rich membranes. *J. Biol. Chem.* **258**:10034–10040.

Powell, J. A., and B. A. Friedman (1977) Electrical membrane activity: Effect on distribution incorporation and degradation of acetylcholine receptors in the membranes of cultured muscle. *J. Cell Biol.* **75**:321a.

Prigogine, I. (1961) *Introduction to the Thermodynamics of Irreversible Processes*, Wiley, New York.

Prinz, H., and A. Maelicke (1983) Interaction of cholinergic ligands with the purified acetylcholine receptor protein: Equilibrium binding studies. *J. Biol. Chem.* **258**:10263–10271.

Purves, D., and J. Lichtman (1980) Elimination of synapses in the developing nervous system. *Science* **210**:153–157.

Quinn, W. G. (1984) Work in intervertebrates on the mechanisms underlying learning. In *The Biology of Learning*, P. Marler and H. S. Terrace, eds., pp. 197–248, Springer, Berlin.

Raftery, M. A., R. L. Vandlen, K. L. Reed, and T. Lee (1976) Characterization of *Torpedo californica* acetylcholine receptor: Its subunit composition and ligand-binding properties. *Cold Spring Harbor Symp. Quant. Biol.* **40**:193–202.

Raftery, M. A., M. W. Hunkapiller, C. D. Strader, and E. L. Hood (1980) Acetylcholine receptor: Complex of homologous subunits. *Science* **208**:1454–1457.

Ramón y Cajal, S. (1895) Consideraciones sobre la morphologia della celula nerviosa, quoted in *Histologie du Système Nerveux de l'Homme et des Vertébrés*, Vol. 2, p. 887, Maloine, Paris, 1909.

Razin, A., and J. Friedman (1981) DNA methylation and its possible logical roles. *Prog. Nucleic Acid Res. Mol. Biol.* **25**:33–52.

Reiness, C. G., and C. B. Weinberg (1981) Metabolic stabilization of acetylcholine receptors at newly formed neuromuscular junction in rat. *Dev. Biol.* **84**:247–254.

Reynolds, J. A., and A. Karlin (1978) Molecular weight in detergent solution of acetylcholine receptor from *Torpedo californica*. *Biochemistry* **17**:2035–2038.

Rieger, F., M. Vigny, and J. Koenig (1980) Spontaneous contractile activity and the presence of 16-S form acetylcholinesterase in rat muscle cells in culture. Reversible suppressive action of tetrotoxin. *Dev. Biol.* **76**:358–365.

Rosenbluth, J. (1975) Synaptic membrane structure in *Torpedo* electric organ. *J. Neurocytol.* **4**:697–712.

Rousselet, A., J. Cartaud, and P. F. Devaux (1979) Importance des interactions protéine–protéine dans le maintien de la structure des fragments excitables de l'organe électrique de *Torpedo marmorata*. *C. R. Seances Acad. Sci. (Paris)* **289**:461–463.

Rousselet, A., J. Cartaud, T. Saitoh, J.-P. Changeux, and P. Devaux (1980) Factors influencing the rotational diffusion of the major proteins of the acetylcholine receptor-rich membranes from *Torpedo marmorata* investigated by saturation-transfer electron-spin resonance spectroscopy. *J. Cell Biol.* **90**:418–426.

Rousselet, A., J. Cartaud, P. F. Devaux, and J.-P. Changeux (1982) The rotational diffusion of the acetylcholine receptor in *Torpedo marmorata* membrane fragments studied with a spin-labelled α-toxin: Importance of the 43,000 protein(s). *EMBO J.* **1**:439–445.

Rubin, L. L., S. M. Schuetze, C. Weill, and G. D. Fischbach (1978) The appearance of acetylcholinesterase at newly formed neuromuscular junctions is regulated by nerve–muscle activity. *Soc. Neurosci. Abstr.* **4**:1193.

Rubin, L. L., S. M. Schuetze, and G. D. Fischbach (1979) Accumulation of acetylcholinesterase at newly formed nerve–muscle synapses. *Dev. Biol.* **69**:46–58.

Rubin, L. L., S. M. Schuetze, C. L. Weill, and G. D. Fischbach (1980) Regulation of acetylcholinesterase appearance at neuromuscular junctions *in vitro*. *Nature* **283**:264–267.

Rübsamen, H., A. T. Eldefrawi, M. E. Eldefrawi, and G. P. Hess (1978) Characterization of the calcium-binding sites of the purified acetylcholine receptor and identification of the calcium binding subunit. *Biochemistry* **17**:3818–3825.

Saitoh, T., and J.-P. Changeux (1980) Phosphorylation *in vitro* of membrane fragments from *Torpedo marmorata* electric organ. *Eur. J. Biochem.* **105**:51–62.

Saitoh, T., and J.-P. Changeux (1981) Change in state of phosphorylation of acetylcholine receptor during maturation of the electromotor synapse in *Torpedo marmorata* electric organ. *Proc. Natl. Acad. Sci. USA* **78**:4430–4434.

Saitoh, T., L. P. Wennogle, and J.-P. Changeux (1979) Factors regulating the susceptibility of the acetylcholine receptor protein to heat inactivation. *FEBS Lett.* **108**:489–494.

Sakmann, B., J. Patlak, and E. Neher (1980) Single acetylcholine activated channels show burst-kinetics in presence of desensitizing concentrations of agonist. *Nature* **286**:71–73.

Sakmann, B., J. Bormann, and O. P. Hamill (1983) Ion transport by single receptor channels. *Cold Spring Harbor Symp. Quant. Biol.* **48**:247–258.

Salkoff, L. (1983) Genetic and voltage clamp analysis of a *Drosophila* potassium channel. *Cold Spring Harbor Symp. Quant. Biol.* **48**:221–232.

Salpeter, M., and R. Harris (1983) Distribution and turnover rate of acetylcholine receptors throughout the junction folds at a vertebrate neuromuscular junction. *J. Cell Biol.* **96**:1781–1785.

Salpeter, M., and R. Loring (1985) Nicotinic acetylcholine receptors in invertebrate muscle: Properties, distribution, and neural control. *Progr. Neurobiol.* **25**:297–325.

Sanes, J. R., and Z. W. Hall (1979) Antibodies that bind specifically to synaptic sites on muscle fiber basal lamina. *J. Cell Biol.* **83**:357–370.

Sanes, J. R., L. M. Marshall, and U. J. McMahan (1978) Reinnervation of muscle fiber basal lamina after removal of myofibers. Differentiation of regenerating axons at original synaptic sites. *J. Cell Biol.* **78**:176–198.

Schaffner, A., and M. P. Daniels (1982) Conditioned medium from cultures of embryonic neurons contains a high molecular weight factor which induces acetylcholine receptor aggregation on cultured myotubes. *J. Neurosci.* **2**:623–632.

Scharfman, H. E., and J. M. Sarvey (1985) Postsynaptic firing during repetitive stimulation is required for long-term potentiation in hippocampus. *Brain Res.* **331**:267–274.

Schindler, H., and U. Quast (1980) Functional acetylcholine receptor from *Torpedo marmorata* in planar membranes. *Proc. Natl. Acad. Sci. USA* **77**:3052–3056.

Schindler, H., F. Spillecke, and E. Neumann (1984) Different channel properties of *Torpedo* acetylcholine receptor monomers and dimers reconstituted in planar membranes. *Proc. Natl. Acad. Sci. USA* **81**:6222–6226.

Schramm, M., and Z. Sillinger (1984) Message transmission: Receptor-controlled adenylate cyclase system. *Science* **225**:1350–1356.

Schwartz, J. C., C. Llorens Cortes, C. Rose, T. T. Quach, and H. Pollard (1983) Adaptive changes of neurotransmitter receptor mechanisms in the central nervous system. *Prog. Brain Res.* **58**:117–130.

Sealock, R. (1980) Identification of regions of high acetylcholine receptor density in tannic acid-fixed postsynaptic membranes from electric tissue. *Brain Res.* **199**:267–281.

Sealock, R., B. E. Wray, and S. C. Froehner (1984) Ultrastructural localization of the Mr. 43,000 protein and the acetylcholine receptor in Torpedo post-synaptic membranes using monoclonal antibodies. *J. Cell Biol.* **98**:2239.

Sejnowski, T. J. (1977) Storing covariance with nonlinearly interacting neurons. *J. Math. Biol.* **4**: 303–321.

Sherrington, C. S. (1897) The central nervous system. In *A Textbook of Physiology*, Part III, 7th Ed., M. Foster, ed., Macmillan, London.

Sibley, D. R., and R. J. Lefkowitz (1985) Molecular mechanisms of receptor desensitization using the β-adrenergic-coupled adenylate cyclase system as a model. *Nature* **317**:124–129.

Slater, C. R. (1985) Acetylcholine-receptor distribution on regenerating mammalian muscle-fibers at sites of mature and developing nerve–muscle junctions. *J. Physiol. (Paris)* **80**:238–246.

Snyder, S. (1984) Drug and neurotransmitter receptors in the brain. *Science* **224**:22–31.

Sobel, A., T. Heidmann, J. Hofler, and J.-P. Changeux (1978) Distinct protein components from *Torpedo marmorata* membranes carry the acetylcholine receptor site and the binding site for local anesthetics and histrionicotoxin. *Proc. Natl. Acad. Sci. USA* **75**:510–514.

Sobel, A., M. Weber, and J.-P. Changeux (1977) Large-scale purification of the acetylcholine receptor protein in its membrane-bound and detergent-extracted forms from *Torpedo marmorata* electric organ. *Eur. J. Biochem.* **80**:215–224.

Sohal, G. S., and R. W. Wrenn (1984) Appearance of high-molecular-weight acetylcholinesterase in aneural muscle developing *in vivo*. *Dev. Biol.* **101**:229–234.

Sokolowsky, M. (1984) Muscarinic receptors in the central nervous system. *Int. Rev. Neurobiol.* **25**: 139–183.

St. John, P. A., S. C. Froehner, D. A. Goodenough, and J. B. Cohen (1982) Nicotinic postsynaptic membranes from *Torpedo*: Sidedness, permeability to macromolecules, and topography of major polypeptides. *J. Cell Biol.* **92**:333–342.

Stallcup, W. B., and J. Patrick (1980) Substance P enhances cholinergic receptor desensitization in a clonal nerve cell line. *Proc. Natl. Acad. Sci. USA* **77**:634–638.

Steinbach, J. H. (1981) Developmental changes in acetylcholine receptor aggregates at rat skeletal neuromuscular junctions. *Dev. Biol.* **84**:267–276.

Stent, G. (1973) A physiological mechanism for learning. *Proc. Natl. Acad. Sci. USA* **70**:997–1001.

Stroud, R. M. (1983) Acetylcholine receptor structure. *Neurosci. Comment.* **1**:124–138.

Stroud, R. M., and J. Finer-Moore (1985) Acetylcholine receptor structures, function and evolution. *Annu. Rev. Cell Biol.* **1**:317–351.

Stya, M., and D. Axelrod (1983) Diffusely distributed acetylcholine receptors can participate in cluster formation on cultured rat myotubes. *Proc. Natl. Acad. Sci. USA* **80**:449–453.

Sumikawa, K., M. Houghton, J. C. Smith, L. Bell, B. M. Richards, and E. A. Barnard (1982) The molecular cloning and characterization of cDNA coding for the alpha subunit of the acetylcholine receptor. *Nucleic Acids Res.* **10**:5809–5822.

Takai, T., M. Noda, M. Mishina, S. Shimizu, Y. Furutani, T. Kayano, T. Ikeda, T. Kubo, H. Takahashi, M. Kuno, and S. Numa (1985) Cloning, sequencing and expression of cDNA for a novel subunit of acetylcholine receptor from calf muscle. *Nature* **315**:761–764.

Takeyasu, K., J. B. Udgaonkar, and G. P. Hess (1983) Acetylcholine receptor: Evidence for a voltage-dependent regulatory site for acetylcholine. Chemical kinetic measurements in membrane vesicles using a voltage clamp. *Biochemistry* **22**:5973–5978.

Talvenheimo, J. A., M. M. Tamkun, R. P. Hartshorne, D. J. Messner, R. G. Sharkey, M. R. C. Costa, and W. A. Catterall (1983) Structure and functional reconstitution of the voltage-sensitive sodium channel from rat brain. *Cold Spring Harbor Symp. Quant. Biol.* **48**:155–164.

Teichberg, V., and J.-P. Changeux (1976) Presence of two forms with different isoelectric points of the acetylcholine receptor in the electric organ of *Electrophorus electricus* and their catalytic interconversion *in vitro*. *FEBS Lett.* **67**:264–268.

Teichberg, V., and J.-P. Changeux (1977) Evidence for protein phosphorylation and dephosphorylation in membrane fragments isolated from the electric organ of *Electrophorus electricus*. *FEBS Lett.* **74**:71–76.

Teichberg, V., A. Sobel, and J.-P. Changeux (1977) *In vitro* phosphorylation of the acetylcholine receptor. *Nature* **267**:540–542.

Terrace, H. S. (1984) Animal learning, ethology and biological constraints. In *The Biology of Learning*, P. Marler and H. S. Terrace, eds., pp. 15–46, Springer, Berlin.

Teyler, T. J., and P. Discenna (1984) Long-term potentiation as a candidate mnemonic device. *Brain Res. Rev.* **7**:15–28.

Thomas, R. (1981) On the relation between the logical structure of systems and their ability to generate multiple steady-states or sustained oscillations. *Springer Ser. Synergetics* **9**:180–193.

Thorndike, E. (1898) and (1911) *Animal Intelligence*, Macmillan, New York.

Timpl, R., H. Rohde, P. G. Robey, S. I. Rennard, J. M. Foidart, and G. R. Martin (1979) Laminin: A glycoprotein from basement membrane. *J. Biol. Chem.* **254**:9933–9937.

Vandlen, R. L., W. C. S. Wu, J. C. Eisenach, and M. A. Raftery (1979) Studies of the composition of purified *Torpedo californica* acetylcholine receptor and its subunits. *Biochemistry* **10**:1845–1854.

Vigny, M., L. Di Giamberardino, J. Y. Couraud, F. Rieger, and J. Koenig (1976a) Molecular forms of chicken acetylcholinesterase: Effect of denervation. *FEBS Lett.* **69**:277–280.

Vigny, M., J. Koenig, and F. Rieger (1976b) The motor endplate specific form of acetylcholinesterase: Appearance during embryogenesis and reinnervation of rat muscle. *J. Neurochem.* **27**:1347–1353.

Vogel, Z., C. N. Christian, M. Vigny, H. C. Bauer, P. Sonderegger, and M. P. Daniels (1983) Laminin induces acetylcholine receptor aggregation on cultured myotubes and enhances the receptor aggregation activity of a neuronal factor. *J. Neurosci.* **3**:1058–1068.

Walker, J. W., M. G. McNamee, E. Pasquale, D. J. Cash, and G. P. Hess (1981) Acetylcholine receptor inactivation in *Torpedo californica* electroplax membrane vesicles. Detection of two processes in the millisecond and second time region. *Biochem. Biophys. Res. Comm.* **100**:86–90.

Walker, J. W., K. Takeyasu, and M. G. McNamee (1982) Activation and inactivation kinetics of *Torpedo californica* acetylcholine receptor in reconstituted membranes. *Biochemistry* **21**:5384–5389.

Weidoff, P. M., M. G. McNamee, and B. W. Wilson (1979) Modulation of cholinergic proteins and RNA by ouabain in chick muscle cultures. *FEBS Lett.* **100**:389–393.

Weinberg, C. B., and Z. Hall (1979) Antibodies from patients with *myasthenia gravis* recognize determinants unique to extra junctional acetylcholine receptors. *Proc. Natl. Acad. Sci. USA* **76**: 504–508.

Wennogle, L. P., and J.-P. Changeux (1980) Transmembrane orientation of proteins present in acetylcholine receptor-rich membranes from *Torpedo marmorata* studied by selective proteolysis. *Eur. J. Biochem.* **106**:381–393.

Wennogle, L. P., R. Oswald, T. Saitoh, and J.-P. Changeux (1981) Dissection of the 66,000-dalton subunit of the acetylcholine receptor. *Biochemistry* **20**:2492–2497.

Woody, C. D. (1982) Memory learning and higher function: A cellular view. Springer, New York.

Wu, W. C. S., and M. Raftery (1979) Carbamylcholine-induced rapid cation efflux from reconstituted membrane vesicles containing purified acetylcholine receptor. *Biochem. Biophys. Res. Commun.* **89**:26–35.

Wu, W. C. S., and M. Raftery (1981) Functional properties of acetylcholine receptor monomeric and dimeric forms in reconstituted membranes. *Biochem. Biophys. Res. Commun.* **99**:436–444.

Yeramian, E., and J.-P. Changeux (1986) Un modèle de changement d'efficacité synaptique à long terme fondé sur l'interaction du recepteur de l'acetylcholine avec la protéine sous-synaptique de 43 000 daltons. *C. R. Seances Acad. Sci. (Paris)* **302**:609–616.

Young, A. P., and D. S. Sigman (1982) Allosteric effects of volatile anesthetics on the membrane-bound acetylcholine receptor protein. I. Stabilization of the high-affinity state. *Mol. Pharmacol.* **20**:498–505.

Young, A. P., and D. S. Sigman (1983) Conformational effects of volatile anesthetics on the membrane-bound acetylcholine receptor protein: Facilitation of the agonist-induced affinity conversion. *Biochemistry* **22**:2154–2161.

Zingsheim, H. P., F. J. Barrantes, J. Frank, W. Hänicke, and D. C. Neugebauer (1982a) Direct structural localization of two toxin-recognition sites on an ACh receptor protein. *Nature* **299**: 81–84.

Zingsheim, H. P., D. C. Neugebauer, J. Frank, W. Hänicke, and F. J. Barrantes (1982b) The arrangement and structure of the membrane-bound acetylcholine receptor studied by electron microscopy. *EMBO J.* **1**:541–547.

Section 5

Theoretical Models of Synaptic Function

Given the diversity of pre- and postsynaptic mechanisms and the variety of anatomical networks within which synaptic modifications occur, the need for theoretical approaches is apparent. In this section, four different salients are investigated.

Rall's early analysis of the passive properties of dendritic trees laid the groundwork for the current generation of network models. In their chapter, Rall and Segev review the current state of dendritic modeling and propose a new model for the function of synaptic spines. They carefully consider the potential effect of active membrane in the spine head, which because of high input impedance in the spine neck allows propagated dendritic spikes leading to the notion "spiking spines." This model has important consequences for neuronal function and plasticity.

Koch and Poggio consider how the biophysics of synaptic interactions may account for the neuronal processing of inputs. They show how neurons can act as logic gates, and how circuits of these neurons can implement algorithms for motion detection and stereopsis. They present a view of computation in the nervous system based on the known mechanisms of ion channels, receptors, and dendritic integration.

Stevens addresses the question of whether there are any specific properties of neural structures that arise solely from a consideration of the general similarity among various nervous tissues. The constraints of development and evolution necessarily lead to certain commonalities among the regions of the nervous system. Using the formulations of functional calculus, Stevens argues that such properties include the center–surround of organization receptive fields and the inherently limited accuracy of neuronal computations.

In the final chapter, Finkel and Edelman integrate recent biophysical and molecular understanding of synaptic function into a population model of synaptic change leading to network plasticity. They argue that presynaptic and postsynaptic modifications should be treated independently and go on to propose detailed realistic rules for both. Their postsynaptic rule relates directly to the findings of Andersen, Changeux and Heidmann, and Kandel et al. presented in earlier chapters and their presynaptic rule to those of Magleby. The authors then study the interaction of short-term postsynaptic changes with long-term presynaptic changes and show that the interaction critically depends upon network architecture. Their population model has several implications for the relationship between neuroanatomy and synaptic mechanisms, particularly as it applies to learning and memory.

Chapter 22

Functional Possibilities for Synapses
on Dendrites and Dendritic Spines

WILFRID RALL
IDAN SEGEV

ABSTRACT

Most neurons exhibit extensive dendritic branching, and several important cell types have their dendrites studded with thousands of spines. Each neuron also receives thousands of synaptic contacts, and (where spines are present) most synaptic contacts are upon spines. To understand the functional possibilities of such synapses requires theoretical and computational studies. Here we review earlier results for passive dendrites and passive dendritic spines, and then explore both the implications of assuming excitable spine head membrane and of assuming clusters of excitable spines for the integrative properties of neurons. (1) When an excitable spine head membrane fires an action potential, this amplifies the synaptic response relative to the passive case. (2) Excitable channels produce much more dendritic depolarization when they are allocated to several spine heads rather than to one; this may partially account for the large numbers of spines. (3) For distal dendritic locations, the firing of one (or a few) excitable spines may trigger (through the spread of sufficient depolarization along the dendritic shaft) the firing of neighboring excitable spines and thus produce significant amplification of the somatic excitatory postsynaptic potential. (4) Such a chain reaction will usually spread (and fire) only a subset of the available excitable spine clusters. Such spread is more secure toward distal branches, and usually blocks proximally; this asymmetry can fractionate a dendritic tree into many regions of spine clusters (arbors) that can fire almost independently. (5) Whether a spine cluster or region fires or not depends (with nonlinear sensitivity) upon changes in synaptic excitation and inhibition and changes in spine stem resistance or other spine parameters. (6) The thousands of spines and synaptic contacts per neuron can provide a rich repertoire of logical operations implemented by excitable spine clusters.

Transient computations with excitable dendritic spines were reported in November, 1983 at a symposium of the Society for Neuroscience by two independent research groups: Miller, Rall and Rinzel, and Perkel and Perkel. Both groups reported that significant synaptic amplification results when an excitable spine head membrane is used with a suitable combination of dendritic spine parameters (geometric, electric, and ionic). Optimal conditions were characterized, physical intuitive explanations were provided, and some interesting functional implications were pointed out. Because their new results were independent and complementary, these two groups agreed to cooperate in seeking early paired publication of two brief reports. These reports were submitted to *Nature* (January, 1984) and to *Science* (April and June, 1984), but the editors judged our reports to be of insufficient interest to a wide audience and recommended publication in a specialized journal. Subsequently both reports were accepted (August, 1984) for publication together in *Brain Research* (Miller et al., 1985; Perkel and Perkel, 1985).

Meanwhile, an ongoing exploration of various functional implications and possibilities has continued, stimulated by collaborative discussions (with John Miller, John Rinzel, and Gordon Shepherd) of our various computations. Miller has focused upon conditions under which excitable dendritic spine interactions could generate bursts of spikes (Malinow and Miller, 1984). Shepherd has focused more upon the possibility of saltatory propagation in distal dendrites from one excitable spine head to another (Shepherd et al., 1984). Here we focus our attention upon clusters of spines in distal dendritic arbors, and upon the variety of synaptic input conditions for which various excitable spine clusters, or combinations of such clusters, can deliver significant membrane depolarization to the neuron. This can provide highly nonlinear and contingent processing of synaptic input patterns.

THEORETICAL BACKGROUND

A theoretical treatment of the passive electrical response in an extensively branched neuron to synaptic inputs at different dendritic locations was begun about twenty-five years ago. This resulted in a number of useful biophysical insights relevant to synaptic processing (Rall, 1957, 1960, 1962, 1964, 1967; see also Rall et al., 1966, 1967; Rall and Shepherd, 1968; Jack and Redman, 1971; Dodge and Cooley, 1973; Rall and Rinzel, 1973; Barrett and Crill, 1974; Butz and Cowan, 1974; Rinzel and Rall, 1974; Jack et al., 1975; Redman, 1976; Rall, 1977; Traub, 1977; Horwitz, 1981; Carnevale and Johnston, 1982; Brown and Johnston, 1983; Finkel and Redman, 1983; Redman and Walmsley, 1983; Rall and Segev, 1985); some of these are summarized in Figures 3 and 4. The extension of this analysis to passive dendritic spines began over ten years ago (Rall and Rinzel, 1971a,b; see also Rall, 1974, 1978; Jack et al., 1975; Shepherd and Brayton, 1979; Rinzel, 1982; as well as Koch and Poggio, 1983; Kawato and Tsukahara, 1984; Turner, 1984; Wilson, 1984); some of the resulting insights into synaptic efficacy and its possible contribution to plasticity in nervous systems are summarized in Figures 5 and 6. The possibility that the membrane of dendritic spine heads might be excitable was tossed about in conversation, but only Julian Jack published an early and astute discussion of this possibility (Jack et al., 1975). Not until 1983, to the best of our knowledge, did anyone carry out detailed transient computations for the response of an excitable spine head to synaptic input.

Dendrites and Dendritic Spines

The extensiveness of dendritic branching, and the large numbers of spines on the dendrites of some neuron types, were seen and illustrated about one hundred years ago by Ramón y Cajal, using the reduced silver method of Golgi (see Figure 1A). An early study in experimental neuropathology (on the effects of

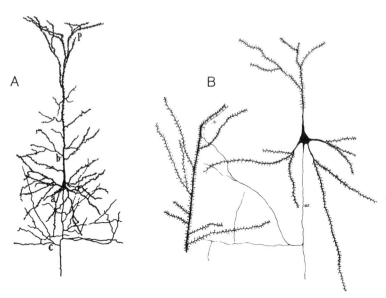

Figure 1.   *Dendrites with spines. A* shows a pyramidal cell of rabbit cortex drawn by Ramón y Cajal
(1909), using the Golgi method. Spines can be seen on the distal branches (P) of the apical
dendrite (b) and on the basilar dendrites (a), but not on the axon collaterals (c). *B* shows two
cortical cells drawn by Berkley (1897). The branches at *left* belong to an apical dendrite of a
pyramidal cell and show many spines; the cell at *right* also shows spines on its dendrites, but
not on the axon whose collateral contacts spines of the other neuron at (b).

chronic alcohol and other poisons) by Berkley (1897) devoted particular attention
to dendrites and spines. See Figure 1B, which shows an axon collateral (from
the neuron on the right) making contacts with several spines of a different
neuron; Berkley considered these to be important functional contacts.

However, it was 60 years before Gray (1959) reported electron microscope
evidence of synaptic contacts upon dendritic spines; since then, the existence
and variety of such synaptic contacts have been verified by many investigators,
who have found that some cortical neurons receive nearly all of their synaptic
contacts upon their dendritic spines (Colonnier, 1968; Scheibel and Scheibel,
1968; Diamond et al., 1970). Some of the variety in spine size, shape, and synaptic
contact configuration is illustrated in Figure 2; this variety should be kept in
mind as a warning against limiting spine calculations to some "standard" or
"average" spine.

It was probably first pointed out by Chang (1952) that the high ohmic resistance
of a thin spine stem would attenuate the effect delivered to the postsynaptic
neuron from a synaptic input to the spine head. He concluded that the summation
of many such inputs would be needed for effective excitation of such neurons.
He did not introduce the idea that changing spine stem resistance values could
change the relative weighting of synapses. That idea was introduced by Rall
and Rinzel (1971a,b), who pointed out the possible contribution of such changing
synaptic weights to plasticity and learning (see also Rall, 1970, 1974, 1978; Jack
et al., 1975; Rinzel, 1982). Because dendritic spines are too small for present
microelectrode techniques, we suggest that biophysical computations provide

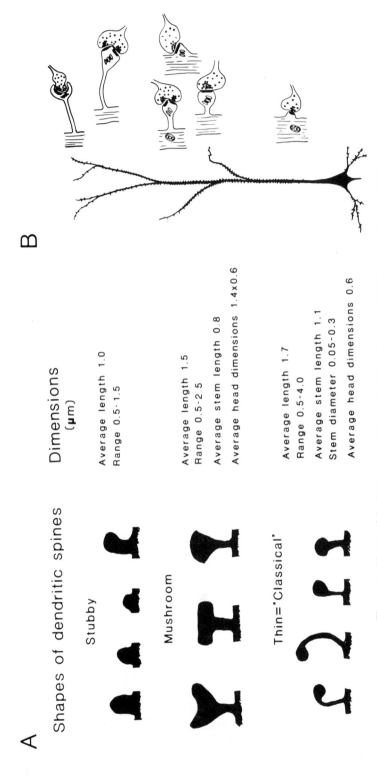

A

Shapes of dendritic spines

Stubby

Mushroom

Thin="Classical"

Dimensions
(μm)

Average length 1.0
Range 0.5-1.5

Average length 1.5
Range 0.5-2.5
Average stem length 0.8
Average head dimensions 1.4x0.6

Average length 1.7
Range 0.5-4.0
Average stem length 1.1
Stem diameter 0.05-0.3
Average head dimensions 0.6

B

Figure 2. *Variety of dendritic spines. A* is modified from Peters and Kaiserman-Abramof (1970) and shows a variety of spine shapes, calibers, and lengths; the dimensions are from the same authors, and these have been confirmed by others and have been used to estimate ranges of spine parameters. *B* is from Jones and Powell (1969) and shows a pyramidal cell together with enlarged drawings of spines and synaptic contacts based upon electron microscope observations.

perhaps the best means to explore dendritic spine function at this time. It is important, however, to emphasize that experimental testing is possible in principle and may soon be available; we refer to antibody markers for ionic channels, voltage-sensitive dyes for spine head voltage transients, and specialized patch clamping of spine head membrane.

INSIGHTS FOR PASSIVE DENDRITIC TREES

The application of cable theory to dendritic trees has been presented, discussed, and reviewed in a book by Jack et al. (1975) and in chapters by Rall (1964, 1977), by Redman (1976), and most recently (with application to voltage clamping) by Rall and Segev (1985). Definitions of symbols, statements of simplifying assumptions, derivations of equations, formulation and solution of appropriate boundary value problems, methods of estimating geometric and membrane parameters, and comments about the results can be found there. Here we summarize some of the concepts that resulted from the interplay of theory and experiment.

Dendritic Tree Length Moderate (L from 1 to 2)

Because of an earlier dogma that dendritic distances were too long and tenuous for distally located synapses to have any effect upon the neuron soma, it was important to estimate the dimensionless electrotonic length, L, along a path from the soma to an average dendritic terminal: $L = \Sigma (\Delta x_j / \lambda_j)$, where Δx_j is the actual length and λ_j is the characteristic length constant (depending upon membrane resistance, core resistance, and branch diameter) of the jth branch along that path. One method of estimating L depends upon computing this sum from the detailed anatomy and from known or estimated resistance values (Rall, 1959, 1964). Another method depends upon a theoretical analysis of voltage transients and consists of peeling the slowest two exponential time constants (Rall, 1969). In many laboratories, both methods have been found to yield values between 1 and 2 for cat spinal motoneurons; values close to 1 have been reported for several cell types in hippocampus. The resulting insight was that distal dendritic locations are not functionally as remote as was once supposed, and that distal synaptic inputs are attenuated less than had been supposed (Rall, 1964, 1970, 1977; Jack et al., 1975; Redman, 1976). The extension to different neuron types in different animals depends upon good data and careful estimation of L for each case.

Dendritic Synaptic Preponderance

For the neuron types most studied, it has been found that the dendritic surface area is 20–100 times the soma surface area. Given that the surface density of synapses is comparable for dendrites and soma, it follows that dendritic synapses represent 95–99% of the synapses upon such a neuron. Given also that the moderate L values of 1 to 2 imply only moderate attentuation of effects from distal synapses, it follows that the large population of dendritic synapses can play a dominant role in the integrative processes of such a neuron (Rall, 1959, 1964, 1977).

Contrasting Dendritic and Somatic Synaptic Function

These insights, together with the differences in excitatory postsynaptic potential (EPSP) time course (see the fast time course for the proximal input versus the slow time course for the distal input at the upper left in Figure 3) led to the early recognition of a possible functional distinction between dendritic and somatic synaptic activity. In contrast to the relatively sluggish and finely graded depolarization that would spread to the soma from distal dendritic synapses, brief synchronous activity of a few synapses at or near the soma could produce precisely timed and relatively sharp depolarizations. These would be well suited for precisely timed triggering of axonal impulses—their amplitudes might well be too small to reach threshold without the help of earlier dendritic synaptic activity. Thus, the dendritic activity could determine success or failure in the onward transmission of temporal synaptic patterns delivered at the soma (Rall, 1959, 1964). A different mode of behavior would result when sustained dendritic synaptic activity was sufficient to cause a rhythmic discharge of impulses (similar to the action of a generator potential in a sensory neuron). In such a case, synaptic inhibition at the soma could block the discharge of impulses over specific periods, or it could reduce the frequency of rhythmic discharge (Rall, 1964). Also, the degree of nonlinearity in the combined effects of several excitatory, and possibly inhibitory, synaptic inputs depends upon the relative locations of these synapses and the spatiotemporal pattern of the synaptic activation (Rall, 1964; Rall et al., 1967). Such problems are best analyzed with the help of computations made with a compartmental model, to be described next.

Compartmental Model Specifies Different Regions of Neuron

A compartmental model of a dendritic neuron offers a number of important advantages. It depends neither upon assuming uniform membrane properties nor upon assuming branching that corresponds to an equivalent cylinder. It permits computation of voltage transients in response to any specified spatiotemporal pattern of synaptic inputs to the compartmental regions. A single compartment may correspond to a single dendritic branch, a group of branches, or just a segment of a trunk or branch element, according to the needs of a given problem. For problems compatible with the equivalent cylinder constraints, the compartmental model is simply a straight chain of compartments of equal size. This case permits a comparison of predictions made with both kinds of models. Branching chains of compartments of unequal size can be used to approximate an unlimited variety of dendritic branching systems and of synaptic activity patterns (Rall, 1964). Computations with compartmental models did lead to important functional insights, which are reviewed in the next few paragraphs.

EPSP Shape Depends upon Spatiotemporal Pattern of Input

The voltage transients (A, B, C, and D in Figure 3, upper left) illustrate the effect of input location when exactly the same square synaptic conductance change is applied to different pairs of dendritic compartments, in a chain of ten compartments, extending from the soma (compartment 1) to all dendritic terminal branches (compartment 10). The most proximal input location (case A: compartments 2 and 3) results in a simulated EPSP (at the soma), which has the earliest peak and the most rapid early decay. With more distal input locations (B, C, and D), there is a delayed rise to a later, lower, and more rounded peak with slower early decay. Such shape differences were later explored more fully with smooth, brief synaptic conductance transients and were compared with experimental results by means of shape index plots (Rall et al., 1967). Given restricted synaptic inputs having the same time course, and given an L value around 1.8, good agreement between theory and experiment was found and subsequently confirmed by other laboratories. The evidence for significant dendritic synaptic input was recognized (Rall et al., 1967; Jack et al., 1975; Redman, 1976; Rall, 1977). The upper right part of Figure 3 demonstrates the different results found for two different spatiotemporal input patterns: input pattern ABCD consists of the four input locations used already at the upper left, activated in the temporal sequence, first A, then B, then C, then D. Input pattern DCBA represents the same input locations activated in reversed time sequence. The resulting composite EPSP shapes are significantly different: ABCD shows that subsequent distal synaptic input does not increase the EPSP peak amplitude from A alone, but does contribute to a sustained plateau of depolarization: DCBA shows that earlier distal synaptic input provides a depolarization upon which the proximal input can build to a larger peak amplitude. Relative to an appropriate threshold for neuronal firing (say a normalized value of 0.12 in this figure) DCBA would succeed while ABCD would fail to fire the neuron. When the total synaptic input is smeared uniformly over the time and locations of these two sequences, the intermediate curve results. These three curves represent perhaps the first theoretical demonstration of an effect of spatiotemporal pattern in passive dendritic trees (Rall, 1964). On the basis of these differences, Erulkar et al. (1968) suggested a possible mechanism for the directional selectivity of neurons in the cochlear nucleus.

Linearity and Nonlinearity in Summation of Synaptic Excitation

The compartmental model is a linear system, with the consequence that when electrodes inject specified current input at several locations, the resulting transient is a linear superposition of the separate responses for separate current inputs. However, because we model synaptic input as a synaptic conductance change (following Fatt and Katz, 1953; Coombs et al., 1955), we can show that such conductance changes perturb the linear system and that such inputs do not, in general, combine linearly. A physiological basis for this is that when the membrane depolarization caused by one input reaches the location of a second input during the time of its conductance change, the reduced synaptic driving potential (the difference between local membrane potential and synaptic equilibrium potential) results in a reduced amount of synaptic current flow through the second synaptic conductance (Rall et al., 1967; Rall, 1970).

Figure 3 (lower left) shows both linear and nonlinear summation in a dendritic tree that was not equivalent to a cylinder. In contrast to the linear summation shown by curves A, B, and C for instantaneous inputs to distal dendritic com-partments 1, 2, and 4, curves D–H show different degrees of nonlinear summation

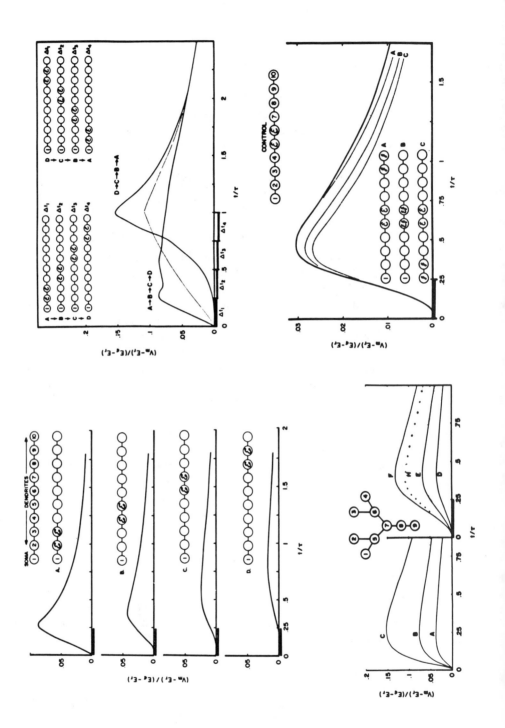

Figure 3. *Spatiotemporal patterns and nonlinear combinations of dendritic synaptic excitation and inhibition.* This montage is based upon Figures 6, 7, 8, and 9 of Rall (1964). The *upper left graphs* show how the shape of a computed excitatory postsynaptic potential (EPSP) at the soma, designated compartment 1, depends upon the dendritic location of equal synaptic conductance input delivered to two dendritic compartments. *Insets* show the following input locations: Compartments 2 and 3 for case A; 4 and 5 for case B; 6 and 7 for case C; and 8 and 9 for case D. The *upper right graph* contrasts two different spatiotemporal synaptic input sequences composed of the same four input locations; thus ABCD means first A, then B, then C, and then D, while DCBA indicates the reverse spatiotemporal sequence. The resulting curves, so labeled, differ from each other and from the intermediate *broken line* curve that corresponds to the same amount of synaptic excitatory input spread evenly over the space and time of the two sequences. The *lower left graph* summarizes computations that demonstrate linear and nonlinear summation of EPSP amplitudes (at the soma, regarded as compartment 8 for inputs to different distal dendritic regions designated compartments 1, 2, 3, and 4). *Curves A, B,* and *C* show linear summation for instantaneous inputs to 1, 2, and 4, respectively, of these distal compartments, or, in this case of instantaneous inputs, to 1, 2, and 4 quanta to any one of the distal compartments. *Curves D–H* show different degrees of nonlinear summation for finite duration synaptic conductance (0.25 τ, as indicated by the *heavy bar*). *Curve D* is the reference EPSP for input to any one distal compartment; *curve E* is for simultaneous input to two sibling compartments, showing 1.94 of the reference amplitude; *curve F* is for simultaneous input to all four distal compartments, showing 3.84 of the reference amplitude; *curve H* is for four simultaneous inputs to a single distal compartment, showing 3.12 of reference amplitude. The *lower right graph* shows the effects of synaptic inhibitory input location upon a reference EPSP produced by synaptic excitatory input in compartments 5 and 6. The *uppermost curve* is the reference EPSP; *curve A* shows the effect of sustained inhibitory input at distal dendritic locations 9 and 10; *curve B* shows sustained inhibitory input at the same locations (5 and 6) as the excitatory input; *curve C* shows sustained inhibitory input more centrally located at the soma (1) and proximal dendrites (2).

for synaptic conductance inputs. Relative to curve D for input to one distal compartment, curve F shows an amplitude 3.84 times as great for the same conductance input to all four distal compartments, while curve H shows an amplitude 3.12 times reference when the four conductance inputs are simultaneous in a single distal compartment. There is a 22% loss in summation when synaptic conductances are localized to the same compartment (significant nonlinearity), while there is only a 4% loss when these synaptic conductances are separated into distinct distal compartments of one tree (small nonlinearity). Predictably, it was found that when brief synaptic conductances are separated into distal compartments of different dendritic trees belonging to the same neuron, their EPSP contributions at the soma do add linearly, because negligible depolarization from one reaches the location of the other (Rall, 1970).

Nonlinear Effect of Synaptic Inhibition

The fact that synaptic inhibition, treated as a conductance increase coupled with an equilibrium potential near the resting potential, must have a nonlinear shunting effect upon nearby synaptic excitation was recognized by Fatt and Katz (1953). Also, Lettvin and his collaborators often referred to this as a multiplicative effect. Whenever synaptic shunting inhibition occurs at a location whose membrane potential happens to be at the inhibitory equilibrium potential, no inhibitory postsynaptic potential (IPSP) should be expected, even though a powerful inhibition would be revealed when this is combined with nearby synaptic excitation. Rall et al. (1967) pointed out that when synaptic excitation and inhibition occur at widely separated locations (as in different dendritic trees of the same neuron), the IPSP and EPSP at the soma sum linearly, as is sometimes observed experimentally. On the other hand, very large nonlinearity can result when the excitatory and inhibitory conductances are located near each other, especially in distal dendritic locations where larger depolarizations are expected (Rall et al., 1967). The effects of different amounts of temporal overlap between synaptic excitation and inhibition have been examined by Segev and Parnas (1983).

Location of Synaptic Inhibition

We have already noted that synaptic inhibition is particularly effective when it is located at the same place and time as synaptic excitation. Synaptic inhibition delivered to the soma is effective against all excitatory inputs, provided that the timing is correct, while synaptic inhibition delivered to a dendritic branch is selectively effective against excitatory inputs in the same branch. The computations summarized at lower right in Figure 3 were designed to compare the effectiveness of sustained synaptic input when located more distally, or more proximally, than the middendritic location assumed for the synaptic excitation. Curve A shows that a significantly more distal location (compartments 9 and 10, distal to compartments 5 and 6) produces no reduction of the EPSP peak (from control) but that the sustained distal inhibition does cause more rapid EPSP decay. Curve B shows significant reduction of the EPSP peak when the inhibitory location is the same middendritic compartments 5 and 6 as the excitation. Curve C shows that the proximal location (compartments 1 and 2) is the most effective. On the basis of similar results obtained for different amounts of inhibitory conductance, a generalization was noted at that time. The transient EPSP peak at the soma is reduced in amplitude (relative to control) when the sustained synaptic inhibitory input location is identical with or proximal to (but not distal to) the excitatory input location (Rall, 1964). A careful further exploration of such synaptic interactions has been provided by Jack (Jack et al., 1975). Recently, Poggio and his collaborators have restated the treatment of synaptic input to dendritic trees using different symbols and terminology: They present "main results" (Koch et al., 1982) that implicitly confirm the earlier results and observations reviewed above, especially those of Rall (1964).

Arbitrary Branching Can Be Treated

For passive trees with arbitrary branch lengths and diameters, a general method of solution involving iterative computations was demonstrated early for steady states (Rall, 1959) and then generalized for transients (Barrett and Crill, 1974) using complex admittances. A closely related approach using Laplace transforms (Butz and Cowan, 1974) is formally valid but difficult to implement; progress with this problem has been achieved by Horwitz (1981, 1983), by Koch (personal communication), and by Holmes (personal communication). However, an alternative method for solving transient problems with arbitrary branching, and with specified distributions of synaptic input and of nonuniform and even voltage-dependent membrane properties, is provided by the compartmental model (Rall, 1964) already noted above. This can be effectively implemented with high-speed computers, by using programs (such as SPICE) designed by electrical engineers for the simulation of complex circuits. Two points may be noted: (1) Arbitrary branching and complex membrane properties can be treated whenever necessary; and (2) much information can be gained by taking advantage of the mathematical simplification available when branching is constrained to the class of trees transformable to an equivalent cylinder.

Class of Dendritic Trees Equivalent to Cylinder

Although implicit in Rall (1959), it was later made explicit (Rall, 1962, 1964) that a particular class of dendritic branching permits an entire dendritic tree to be reduced to an equivalent cylinder. Given the usual simplifying assumptions of cylindrical branches with uniform membrane and with extracellular isopotentiality, the essential additional conditions are: (1) at every branch point, the diameters d_1 and d_2 of the two daughter branches, when raised to the $3/2$ power and then added, equal the $3/2$ power of the parent cylinder diameter, d_p, thus, $d_p^{3/2} = d_1^{3/2} + d_2^{3/2}$, where the daughter branch diameters and lengths need not be equal, but (2) terminal branches are all terminated with the same boundary condition (usually a sealed end, $dV/dx = 0$), and (3) the dimensionless electrotonic distance, L, from the soma to all terminals is the same. Clearly, no actual dendritic tree will exactly satisfy these constraints, but some trees do provide approximate agreement; consequently, the idealized class yields important mathematical and physical intuitive advantages. The explicit analytical solutions (steady-state and transient) for the equivalent cylinder can be mapped onto the branches of such idealized dendritic trees. Equal increments of electrotonic distance ($\Delta x/\lambda$) in the whole tree correspond to equal amounts of dendritic surface area and, given uniform synaptic density, correspond to equal numbers of synapses. When synaptic input has the same value for all branches at the same dimensionless electrotonic distance from the soma, such synaptic patterns can be formulated and solved for the equivalent cylinder (Rall, 1962, 1964). However, when synaptic input is restricted to certain branches, the resulting complications can be studied by means of superposition methods for current injection inputs (Rall and Rinzel, 1973). Rinzel and Rall (1974) also treat synaptic conductance input by means of a linear Volterra integral equation.

Input to One Terminal Branch

Figure 4 illustrates an idealized neuron having six equal dendritic trees, but with steady current injected at only one terminal branch of one symmetric dendritic tree (Rall and Rinzel, 1973). We distinguish the input branch (I) from its sibling branch (S), its first cousin branches (C-1), and second cousin branches (C-2). The steady-state voltage distribution in the various branches of the input tree has been plotted in Figure 4. Because the input branch and its sibling have exactly the same length and diameter, it is interesting to contrast the steep voltage decrement along the input branch with the very small voltage decrement along the sibling branch. Such a contrast must seem paradoxical to those who thought that steady voltage decrement along a neurite is simply proportional to $\exp(-x/\lambda)$, and, for given materials, would depend only upon cylinder length and diameter. The key to understanding this contrast lies in the importance of the boundary condition at the other end of each cylinder (Rall, 1959, 1977). For the sibling branch, current flow is in the distal direction toward a sealed terminal where the boundary condition, $dV/dX = 0$, means that no current leaks out of that end. Little current flows into this branch along the core and out across the cylindrical membrane, resulting in a very small voltage decrement.

In contrast, the current flow in the input branch is in the central direction toward a branch point, where the sum of $d^{3/2}$ of the parent cylinder plus the sibling branch is three times that of the input branch, while the combined input conductance $G_p + G_s$ into parent and sibling is nearly five times the reference value, G_∞ (for an infinite extension of input branch length); this very "open" end corresponds to a boundary condition, $(-dV/dX)/V = (G_p + G_s)/G_\infty \approx 5$, which means that so much current flows along the core that the current leak across the cylindrical membrane is relatively negligible, resulting in a steep and essentially linear voltage decrement. [The steepness of the voltage gradient (with respect to x/λ) in the parent branch is about half that in the input branch, because $d^{3/2}$ is doubled.] Very briefly, the overall point is that the asymmetry of the boundary conditions is responsible for the asymmetry of voltage decrement in these two branches of identical length, diameter, and resistivities of core and membrane.

Asymmetric Decrement Relevant to Dendritic Spines

One reason for emphasizing the asymmetry of the voltage decrement in the input and sibling branches of Figure 4 is that this same kind of asymmetry is

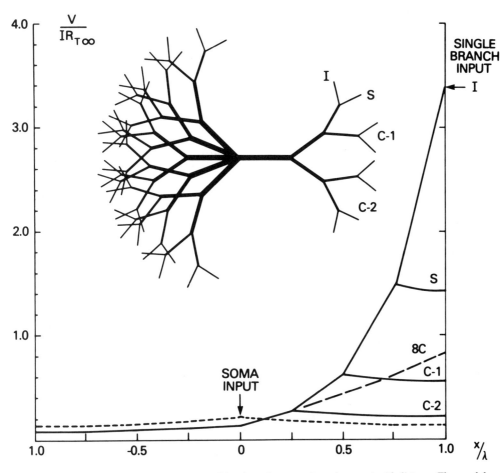

Figure 4. *Diagram of multipolar neuron model and steady-state voltage decrement with distance.* The model shows six dendritic trees, one of which is labeled to distinguish an input branch (I), its sibling branch (S), its first cousin branches (C-1), and second cousin branches (C-2). The *dashed curve* shows steady voltage decrement with distance when a steady current is injected at the neuron soma (taken as the origin of the six dendritic trees). The *solid curve* shows the very different voltages calculated when the same steady input current is injected into the end of one terminal branch of one tree of the same neuron model. The voltage scale is expressed relative to the product of the injected current and $R_{T\infty}$, which is the input resistance of a dendritic trunk cylinder when extended to semi-infinite length. (Equations and quantitative details can be found in Rall and Rinzel, 1973, from which this figure was modified.)

highly relevant to dendritic spines. When the parent dendrite of a spine is depolarized by spread from neighboring regions, this depolarization spreads with very little decrement into the spine head, because the high resistance of the spine head membrane is very similar to a sealed end; little current flow is required to bring that spine head voltage very close to that of the parent dendrite. On the other hand, when depolarization is initiated in the spine head, most of the current flows from the spine head to the parent dendrite and this usually produces a significant voltage decrement from spine head to spine base, as is discussed further below.

SPINE DEFINITIONS AND PARAMETERS

Basic Concepts

A spine can be schematized, as in Figure 5A, but there is no need to idealize the spine head as a sphere or the spine stem as a cylinder. What is essential is that the neuronal cytoplasm extends continuously from the dendrite, through the spine stem, into the spine head. Upon synaptic excitation, the spine head membrane becomes depolarized and we regard the spine head interior to be isopotential at a voltage V_{SH} expressed relative to rest. If the corresponding intracellular voltage at the spine base is designated V_{SB}, then the intracellular voltage drop that drives current from the spine head into the dendrite can be expressed as

$$(V_{SH}) - (V_{SB}) = (I_{SS}) \cdot (R_{SS}) , \tag{1}$$

where I_{SS} represents the spine stem current (from spine head to spine base) and R_{SS} represents spine stem resistance. This application of Ohm's law is valid because a more detailed analysis shows that negligible current leaks out across the spine stem membrane for the range of parameters (geometric and electric) relevant to dendritic spines.

Spine Stem Resistance

The spine stem resistance is a key parameter in the theory and computations involving spines. Although no one has yet measured this resistance directly, such measurement may become possible in the future. Meanwhile, we can estimate likely ranges of values. This lumped resistance can be expressed as the sum of incremental resistances, $(R_i/A)\Delta x$, along the length of a stem whose area of cross section, A, and intracellular resistivity, R_i, may both vary with distance, x, along the spine stem. Where the cytoplasm contains significant inhomogeneities (such as the spine apparatus, which presumably offers higher resistance to electric current), their effect can be approximated by increasing the effective R_i value or decreasing the effective area of cross section for one or more increments of stem length and resistance. The important point here is that a constriction or partial occlusion can increase the value of R_{SS} significantly above that calculated for a homogeneous cylindrical stem (Wilson et al., 1983; Miller et al., 1985).

For example, using a value of 63 Ωcm for R_i, a simple cylindrical stem 0.1 μm in diameter and 1 μm in length has a spine stem resistance of 80 MΩ; tripling the stem length yields 240 MΩ; adding a stem constriction 0.05 μm in diameter and 0.5 μm in length adds 160 MΩ. If this constricted area of cross section is 84% occluded by an insulating body, the combined effect of constriction and occlusion corresponds to 1000 MΩ.

Ranges of Spine Parameter Values

We define no standard or typical spine. It is important to emphasize estimated ranges of values for the various spine parameters, and to explore their consequences in biophysical computations.

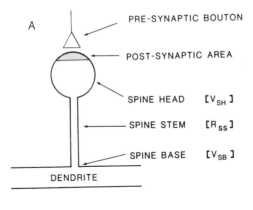

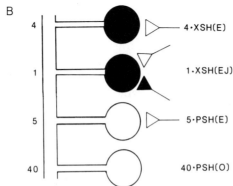

Figure 5. *Diagram showing spine components and symbolic notation.* A: The principal components are the spine head, spine stem, and spine base (where the stem attaches to the dendrite shaft). The synaptic contact consists of a presynaptic bouton and a postsynaptic area. For Figures 7 and 8, the whole spine head area was 1.5 μm^2, of which 12.5% was designated postsynaptic, and the remaining 1.31 μm^2 was available for voltage-gated ion channels. The synaptic excitatory conductance had a peak value of 0.37 nS, with a reversal potential of 100 mV and a time course proportional to $t \cdot \exp(-t/t_p)$, where the peak time was $t_p = 0.035$ msec (corresponding to a value of 40 for the usual parameter, $\alpha = \tau/t_p$, for $\tau = 1.4$ msec); the voltage-gated ion channel density corresponded to either 5 or 10 times the reference case of Hodgkin and Huxley (for the squid axon at 22°C), implying that the 10 · (H–H) for Figure 7 used $\bar{g}_{Na} = 1200$ mS/cm^2, $\bar{g}_K = 360$ mS/cm^2, and $\bar{g}_L = 3$ mS/cm^2. The dendritic shaft was usually assumed to be 0.63 μm in diameter, with $R_m = 1400$ Ωcm^2, $C_m = 1$ $\mu F/cm^2$, and $R_i = 70$ Ωcm. Such a cylinder implies an input resistance $R_{\pm\infty}$, for doubly infinite length, of 200 MΩ; however, we assumed finite length equal to the length constant λ in both directions, implying an input resistance of 262 MΩ. B: The four examples of symbolic spine diagrams and notation have the following meanings: 4 · *XSH(E)* means that four excitable spine heads receive synaptic excitatory input; 1 · *XSH(EJ)* means that one excitable spine receives both excitatory and inhibitory synaptic input; 5 · *PSH(E)* means that five passive spine heads receive synaptic excitatory input; while 40 · *PSH(0)* means that 40 passive spine heads receive no synaptic input at the time in question. A FORTRAN program was used (Parnas and Segev, 1979) for the results shown in Figures 7 and 8; SPICE, an electrical analysis program (Vladimirescu et al., 1980), was used for Figure 10.

The ranges of spine stem dimensions reported by Peters and Kaiserman-Abramof (1970) are summarized in Figure 2. These ranges (also confirmed by Wilson et al., 1983) suggest spine stem resistance values between 10^7 and 10^9 Ω, except for unusually thick or short spines whose resistance values can be around 10^5 and 10^6 Ω; these ranges are the same as those estimated over ten years ago (Rall and Rinzel, 1971a,b; Rall, 1974, 1978) and agree with other recent estimates (Koch and Poggio, 1983; Kawato and Tsukahara, 1984; Wilson, 1984; Miller et al., 1985).

PASSIVE SPINE RESULTS AND INSIGHTS

Our early computations of synaptic conductance input to passive dendritic spines (Rall and Rinzel, 1971a,b; Rall, 1974, 1978; Rinzel, 1982) included both steady-state and transient examples, with a primary emphasis upon changing the value of spine stem resistance relative to the dendritic input resistance and the spine head resistance (illustrations are provided in Figure 6, p. 622). Having reviewed the range of anatomical values (e.g., Figure 2), we estimated that the resistance R_{SH} of passive spine head membrane probably lies between 10^{10} and 10^{12} Ω. This is usually several orders of magnitude greater than the spine stem resistance R_{SS}, estimated to range between 10^5 and 10^9 Ω. From such estimates, we gained the insight that essentially all of the synaptic current generated at the spine head would flow through the spine stem, for steady states; this is essentially true also for transients because the spine head capacity is small.

We also realized that when synaptic input is very small, the spine head depolarization is very small and linear behavior can be expected; however, such small inputs did not interest us because they are ineffective. We focused our attention on larger input conductance values (e.g., steady-state synaptic conductances something like 10 times the reciprocal of R_{SS}), which cause a large depolarization of the spine head membrane involving significant nonlinearity (near saturation) as V_{SH} approaches the synaptic equilibrium value, V_{EQ}. This is explained in detail by Equations 1–3 of Rall (1978). The observation we made was that under such conditions, the depolarization delivered by the spine to its parent dendritic branch depends on the ratio of the spine stem resistance R_{SS} to the input resistance R_{BI} of the parent branch.

In Figure 6, the left side summarizes this result for steady-state conditions (note that V_{BI} at the branch input point is equivalent to V_{SB} at the spine base, bringing Figure 6 into agreement with Figure 5 and Equation 1 above). When R_{SS} equals R_{BI}, it follows that V_{BI} is half of V_{SH}; when $R_{SS}/R_{BI} = 0.1$, then $V_{BI}/V_{SH} = 1/1.1 = 0.91$. These values lie in what we designated an optimal "operating range" over which small changes in the value of R_{SS} (or the ratio R_{SS}/R_{BI}) produce a significant change in the depolarization delivered to the dendrite and soma (i.e., in the weight or potency of that synapse).

The dendritic depolarization, V_{BI} at the spine base, corresponds to less depolarization than would result when the same synaptic conductance is placed directly on the parent dendrite; the operating range necessarily involves some attenuation of synaptic weight. The principle involved is to sacrifice some power in order to gain flexibility. Adjustable synaptic weights could either increase or decrease relative to the average weight. Thus, we thought of delicate adjustments of the relative weights of many different synapses to any given neuron. Such changes would be responsible for changes in dynamic patterns of activity in the assemblies of neurons organized with convergent and divergent connective overlaps.

It was also pointed out that such an operating range would imply that thin or distal dendritic branches, which have higher input resistance values, would be matched with larger spine stem resistance values, such as those for the longer and thinner spine stems. This theoretical expectation is in agreement with the experimental correlation reported by both Jones and Powell (1969) and Peters and Kaiserman-Abramof (1970) for the pyramidal cells in their studies.

The right side of Figure 6 summarizes results from early transient computations for both large (solid curves) and small (dashed curves) synaptic conductance transients. Several useful points can be verified by inspection. The smallest R_{SS} value offers negligible separation between the spine head and the spine base; the resulting weight is at its saturated maximum value for that synaptic input and that dendritic location. For $R_{SS} = R_{BI}$, V_{SB} is significantly less than V_{SH}, and the resulting synaptic weight at the soma is somewhat less than maximum. For the largest R_{SS} value, the spine head is almost isolated from the dendrite; V_{SH} saturates, V_{SB} attenuates more than 100-fold, and V_{soma} attenuates at least 10-fold, where it may be noted that different attenuation factors occur for different transient shapes (Rinzel and Rall, 1974).

Additional computation and discussion for passive dendritic spines have been provided by Koch and Poggio (1983), Kawato and Tsukahara (1984), and Wilson (1984). Also, many control computations for passive spines are included with the new results computed for active spines.

EXCITABLE SPINE CONTRASTED WITH PASSIVE SPINE

Spine Stem Resistance and Critical Combinations of Parameters

The computed results shown in Figure 7 are intended to correspond to a thin spine stem located on a distal dendritic branch. A dendritic diameter of 0.63 μm (together with the geometry and resistivities specified in the Figure 5 legend) yields a dendritic input resistance (from the spine base into the dendrite) of 262 MΩ. The right side of Figure 7 summarizes the results computed for 45 different values of spine stem resistance; the left side of this figure shows them in greater detail (i.e., the voltage time course) for just two values of spine stem resistance, namely, 630 MΩ in case (a) and 1000 MΩ in case (b). Inspection of the voltage time course for case (a) in the spine head (upper left) reveals a combination of conditions corresponding to just above threshold for generating an action potential in the spine head; near failure to fire an action potential is indicated by the plateau and dip (near 20 mV) and by the subsequently delayed rise to peak voltage. The hesitation and delay are especially clear when curve (a) is compared with curve (b), which is securely above threshold. These impressions are confirmed by the right side of Figure 7 where cases (a) and (b) correspond to points (a) and (b) on these curves. Threshold corresponds to the very steep nonlinearity

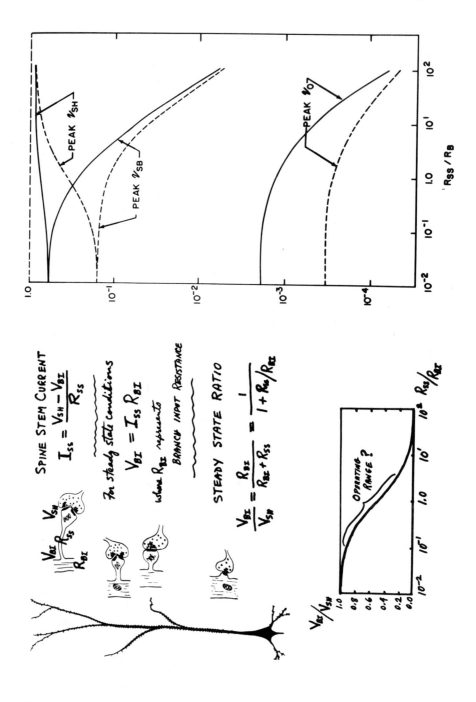

SPINE STEM CURRENT

$$I_{ss} = \frac{V_{SH} - V_{BI}}{R_{ss}}$$

For steady state conditions

$$V_{BI} = I_{ss} R_{BI}$$

where R_{BI} represents

BRANCH INPUT RESISTANCE

STEADY STATE RATIO

$$\frac{V_{BI}}{V_{SH}} = \frac{R_{BI}}{R_{BI} + R_{ss}} = \frac{1}{1 + R_{ss}/R_{BI}}$$

OPERATING RANGE?

Figure 6. *Diagram and results for passive dendritic spines.* At *left*, the diagram summarizes the steady-state implications of Ohm's law for the depolarizing voltage at the spine base, V_{BI}, relative to that at the spine head, V_{SH}, in terms of the spine stem resistance, R_{SS}, and the input resistance of the dendritic branch, R_{BI}, at the spine base. The *curves* at *right* summarize peak voltage values obtained in 1970 from transient computations for two different values of peak synaptic conductance, which differed by a factor of 10. Voltages are plotted on a normalized log scale, where 1.0 represents the synaptic reversal potential; V_{SH} represents normalized depolarization at the spine head; V_{BI} the corresponding depolarization at the spine base; and V_0 the corresponding depolarization at the soma. (From Rall and Rinzel, 1971a,b; Rall, 1974; Rinzel, 1982.)

between 620 and 630 MΩ of spine stem resistance. When all other parameters are held the same, spine stem resistance values less than 600 MΩ are too small for an action potential to be generated (i.e., the conditions are below threshold).

The dotted curves in Figure 7 correspond to passive membrane in the spine head. For spine stem resistance values less than 400 MΩ, the voltage in the excitable spine head (*VXSH*) differs negligibly from that in a passive spine head (*VPSH*); this means that such spine stem resistances are too small for the synaptic current generated to cause depolarization of the excitable channels sufficient for generating a significant (nonlinear) local response. However, as spine stem resistance is increased from 400 to 600 MΩ, a larger depolarization is produced at the spine head, and current loss from the excitable spine head membrane is decreased. This results in a subthreshold local response that is indicated by *VXSH* growing slightly larger than *VPSH* in the upper right quadrant. Because such excitable local response also broadens the peak and thus increases the time integral of *VXSH* even more than the peak amplitude, more current flows from the spine head to the spine base, and the result is a larger deviation of the solid curve from the dotted curve at the spine base (see the lower right quadrant of Figure 7) over the range of 400–600 MΩ.

Next, we need to understand why the solid curve in the lower right quadrant decreases so significantly as the spine stem resistance is increased from 640 to 1000 MΩ. First, we note that in the spine head (upper left), although peak (b) is higher than peak (a), the areas under these two action potential curves are almost the same. It is this area (the time integral of spine head voltage) that drives current from the spine head to the dendrite, according to Equation 1. But if these spine head voltage integrals are almost equal, why is significantly less current (and hence less depolarization) delivered to the spine base in case (b) compared to case (a)? The answer is that less current flows in case (b) because of the larger spine stem resistance and the Ohm's law relation expressed in Equation 1; using a simplifying approximation (that the time integral of the voltage drop ($V_{SH} - V_{SB}$) remains constant), an increase of the spine stem resistance from 700 to 1000 MΩ (a factor of about 1.4) implies that the total current and the resulting dendritic depolarization are divided by this factor. Then the 6.6-mV peak at 700 MΩ drops to about 4.7 mV at 1000 MΩ, and this estimate agrees roughly with the peak at 5.1 mV that was found in Figure 7.

Optimal Spine Stem Resistance for Maximal Amplification

Because spine stem resistance values less than 600 MΩ are below threshold and values above 700 MΩ produce significantly less dendritic depolarization, we can bracket an optimal value of spine stem resistance between these two values. In fact, the optimal range can be narrowed to something like 630–670 MΩ for the conditions and parameter values used in Figure 7. The maximal factor of amplification of dendritic depolarization can be expressed as 6.8/1.1 ≈ 6.2 for the excitable case (6.8) relative to the passive case (1.1) under these conditions. Such optimal conditions were previously noted by Jack et al. (1975), Miller et al. (1985), and Perkel and Perkel (1985).

This optimum differs from the optimal range designated for passive spines;

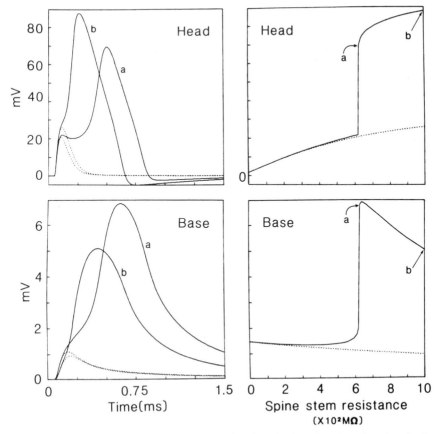

Figure 7. *Depolarizing voltages at the spine head and at the spine base depend on the value of spine stem resistance. Left:* The voltage time course is shown for two values of spine stem resistance, 630 MΩ for case (a) and 1000 MΩ for case (b); the *solid lines (upper left quadrant)* represent action potentials in excitable spine heads, while the *dotted lines* show responses for the same synaptic input to a passive spine head. The voltage transients at the spine base *(lower left quadrant)* are attenuated more than 10-fold in amplitude and are shown with a different voltage scale. *Right: Curves* summarize the peak values of voltages computed for 45 different spine stem resistance values; the particular points (a and b) correspond to the two cases shown at left. Computations were done with the parameter values specified in the Figure 5 legend, with voltage-gated ion conductances corresponding to $10 \cdot$ (H–H).

that range involved no amplification, but it did involve sensitivity to changes in spine stem resistance and centered about the value of spine stem resistance that equaled the dendritic input resistance (Rall and Rinzel, 1971a,b; Rall, 1974, 1978; Rinzel, 1982; see also Figure 6).

Advantage of Increasing the Number of Spines

The best way to add more excitable ion channels is to add more spines that satisfy the critical parameter combination requirement. This is because adding more excitable channels to an already effective excitable spine head results in voltage saturation and consequent nonlinear summation. This point can be demonstrated by means of the computations summarized in Figure 8.

In Figure 8, we compare a reference spine, at left, with two different ways of doubling the number of excitable channels: the middle case corresponds to doubling the number of excitable channels in a single spine head, while the other case (at right) corresponds to a pair of spines, each having the original reference number of excitable channels, and each having a small distance between their spine bases (less than 0.1 of the length constant, λ, of this dendritic cylinder).

Inspection of the voltage transients in Figure 8 shows that doubling the number of excitable channels in the single spine head does increase the voltage peak in the spine head; however, it cannot double the peak because of nonlinear voltage saturation with approach to the reversal potential. Also, given the earlier peak time, there is little change in area under the curve. The result at the spine base is a less than 20% increase from a voltage peak of 4.3 mV to one of 5.1 mV. In contrast to this middle case, the case of two spines (shown at right) nearly doubles the depolarization of the dendrite at the base of both spines. Here, the voltage transient at each spine head differs negligibly from the reference case, and each of the two spines delivers almost as much current to the dendrite as the single reference spine. The resulting peak voltage of 8.4 mV at the base of each spine is about 1.95 times the reference peak. To understand why this factor

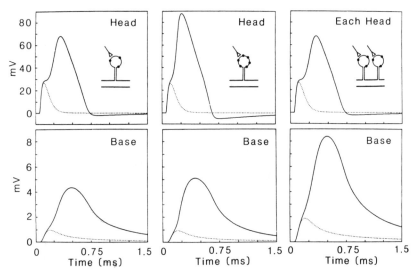

Figure 8. *A pair of excitable spines is shown to be more effective than doubling excitable channels in one spine.* It is assumed that the two spine bases are located near each other (less than 0.1 λ apart, where λ is the length constant of the dendritic shaft). The *left graphs* show the reference case of one excitable spine, with its number of excitable channels (schematically shown as *three dots*) corresponding to 5 · (H–H). The *middle graphs* show increased voltage at the spine head and spine base when the number of channels in one spine head is doubled (schematically shown as *six dots*). The *graphs* at *right* correspond to simultaneous synaptic input to a pair of spines having the same number of channels (schematically shown as *three dots* each) as the reference case; the voltage in each spine head is almost unchanged from the reference case, but the voltage at their common spine base is nearly doubled.

is slightly less than 2.0, we note that the voltage drop from spine head to spine base ($V_{SH} - V_{SB}$) that drives the spine stem current into the dendrite (see Equation 1) is slightly reduced because of the greater dendritic depolarization; for example, at the time of spine head peak voltage, this voltage drop is about $(68 - 3) = 65$ mV in the reference case compared to about $(68 - 7) = 61$ mV in the paired spine case, suggesting about a 6% reduction in the peak current but a smaller reduction in total current delivered per spine.

The comparison provided by Figure 8 shows clearly that doubling the numbers of excitable channels is much more effective using two spines (factor 1.95) than doubling the channel number in one spine (factor about 1.19). Furthermore, our understanding that the larger deficit (in one spine) is due to large nonlinear loss of summation in the spine head, while the smaller deficit (for two spines) is due to small nonlinear loss in the summed synaptic current delivered by the two spines, permits us to generalize this result. A severalfold increase in the number of excitable channels will produce much more dendritic depolarization by means of several spines (provided that they are synaptically activated or brought to threshold by neighboring activity) than by increasing the number of excitable channels of a single spine beyond that needed for just above threshold conditions.

Remark Regarding Amplification Factor

The dotted curves in Figure 8 show the results for passive spine heads with a spine head peak voltage of about 26 mV in all cases and a spine base peak voltage of about 0.9 mV for one spine and about 1.8 mV for the pair of spines. Thus, the factor of amplification can be expressed $4.3/0.9 \cong 4.8$ for the reference case, $5.1/0.9 \cong 5.7$ for the middle case, and about $8.4/1.8 \cong 4.7$ for the paired spines, excitable relative to passive. Although the paired spines do yield the largest depolarization, they do not yield the largest amplification factor.

Remark Regarding Combinations of Parameters

Note that the middle case of Figure 8 is equivalent to case (b) of Figure 7. This provides an easy illustration of the point that the optimal value of spine stem resistance depends upon other parameters, such as the amount of the synaptic input, or, as in the present comparison, the amount of peak Hodgkin–Huxley (H–H; 1952) ionic conductance. In Figure 7, where the computations used 10 times the standard H–H peak conductance density for the squid at 22°C, the optimal spine stem resistance range was close to 630 MΩ, and the value of 1000 MΩ (case b) was much larger than optimal. However, in Figure 8, the reference case (at left) was computed with half as much H–H ionic conductance (corresponding to five times the standard for squid at 22°C), and we can deduce from the plateau and delay of this voltage time course that these conditions are only slightly above threshold. Therefore, for these conditions, the optimal spine stem resistance range is close to 1000 MΩ. However, if the amount of synaptic current were increased significantly, thus increasing the early rate of spine head depolarization, it would be found that smaller values of spine stem resistance would be sufficient for threshold conditions, and the optimal range of values would be significantly less than 1000 MΩ.

SPINE CLUSTERS

Clusters of Passive and Excitable Spines on Distal Branches

We introduce the concept of spine clusters with Figure 9. This neuron model
has six equal dendritic trees, but the branching is shown explicitly for only one
of these trees; it has a trunk and five orders of branching. Next, we focus in
greater detail upon one pair of terminal branches (A and B), together with their
parent branch (C). From careful spine counting, Wilson et al. (1983) reported
linear densities of spines along distal branches that usually range between one
and two spines per micron of branch length; thus, for the branch lengths of
35–44 µm assumed for the distal branches of Figure 9, it is quite reasonable to
suppose that each branch would have a cluster of spines numbering about 50;
an even larger number could be justified on the basis of the spine count corrections
presented in and illustrated by Feldman and Peters (1979). For our computations,
we assumed clusters of exactly 50 spines per branch; for each such cluster, we
assumed that 45 spines were passive and that 5 were excitable. Such spine counts
are shown in Figure 9, using the symbols and notation defined earlier in Figure
5B. The particular details shown in Figure 9 signify an occasion when only two
of the excitable spines of the branch A spine cluster receive excitatory synaptic
input, while only three of the passive spines of the branch B spine cluster receive
excitatory synaptic input, and none of the spines of the branch C spine cluster
receives any synaptic input; this set of input conditions corresponds to case (4)
of the five cases illustrated in Figure 10. There the symbolic notation has been
further simplified by showing only those particular spines of each cluster that
receive synaptic input (column at left) or those that generate action potentials
(middle column); the remaining spines of each cluster of 50 are present, but not
shown.

Contingency of Spine Cluster Firing upon Input Conditions

We have computed many more cases than those shown in Figure 10; however,
these five cases simplify the task of presenting this rich domain of distal dendritic
synaptic processing. Case 1 shows excitatory synaptic input to only one excitable
spine. For the set of parameters used in these computations, that spine head
membrane does generate an action potential, and the current supplied by that
spine to branch A causes an 8.5-mV peak depolarization at the midpoint of
branch A and a 2.7-mV peak depolarization at the midpoint of branch C, resulting,
after electrotonic attenuation to the soma, in a 24-µV peak EPSP at the soma.
The same synaptic input to a single passive spine on branch A would produce
only a 12-µV peak EPSP at the soma; thus, the single excitable spine is responsible
for an amplification factor of two in this example (we note that the same synaptic
conductance at the soma produces a 73-µV peak).

   What is most important about case 1 is that the local membrane depolarization
at branch A is not sufficient to bring the four other excitable spines on branch
A to threshold. However, in case 2, where two excitable spines receive simultaneous
synaptic input, the depolarization of branch A is sufficient to bring the three
other excitable spines on branch A to threshold. These three spines generate

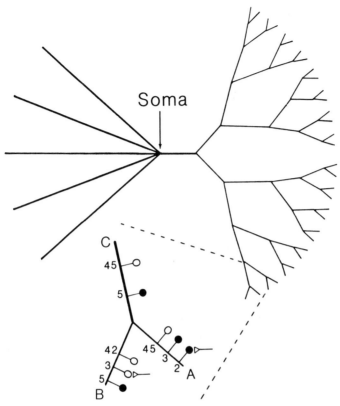

Figure 9. *Branched neuron model showing details of dendritic branching in one tree and details of spine clusters for three distal branches.* The tree has five orders of symmetric bifurcations that preserve a constant sum of $d^{3/2}$. The branch lengths (not drawn to scale) are all meant to correspond to dimensionless length increments ($\Delta X = \Delta x/\lambda$) of 0.2, implying a value of 1.2 for the dimensionless (electrotonic) length of the tree. The enlargement provides schematic information about the clusters of spines assumed for branches A, B, and C; each of these three branches has 50 dendritic spines, of which five are excitable (indicated by the *filled heads*) and 45 are passive (*open heads*); the *triangular* synaptic bouton shown for branch A indicates that this branch receives excitatory synaptic input delivered simultaneously to two of its excitable spine heads, which is also expressed as $2 \cdot XSH(E)_A$ (see also Figure 5B), while the synaptic bouton shown for branch B indicates that excitatory synaptic input is delivered simultaneously to three of its passive spine heads, which is expressed as $3 \cdot PSH(E)_B$. These particular input conditions correspond to case 4 of Figure 10. Some parameters differ here from Figures 5, 7, and 8: $R_m = 2500\ \Omega\mathrm{cm}^2$, implying $\tau_m = 2.5$ msec; also, a terminal branch diameter of 0.36 µm implies a λ value of about 180 µm, with a branch length of 36 µm; the trunk diameter then corresponds to 3.6 µm, implying a whole neuron input resistance of $R_N = 7.8$ MΩ. The synaptic reversal potential and peak conductance are the same as in Figures 5, 7, and 8, but the peak time is changed to 0.2 msec (implying $\alpha = 12.5$, with $\tau = 2.5$ msec). The excitable membrane uses conductances that are five times the standard H–H for 22°C. Spine head area was 1.5 µm^2 without subtraction for a postsynaptic area.

action potentials that peak only about 0.68 msec later than in the synaptically excited spine pair. The not quite synchronous firing of these five excitable spines generates a 25.5-mV peak depolarization at the midpoint of branch A, an 11.7-mV peak for branch B, an 8.6-mV peak for branch C, and an 84-μV peak EPSP at the soma. The same synaptic input to two passive spines on branch A would produce a 24-μV peak EPSP at the soma; thus, this pair of inputs to this pair of excitable spines is responsible for an amplification factor of 3.5.

What is fascinating about case 2 is that the local depolarization is sufficient to fire all five excitable spines in branch A but none of those on branches B and C. However, only a little help is needed to fire excitable spines in these neighboring clusters. Case 3 shows that when all five of the excitable spines in branch A receive synchronous synaptic excitation, the local depolarization of branch B is sufficient to fire all five excitable spines of this cluster, but none of those in branch C. To understand why branch B is more depolarized than branch C, we need only look again at Figure 4, which clearly shows that voltage attenuation into a sibling terminal branch is small (because of the sealed end boundary condition), while the voltage attenuation in the parent branch is much larger (because the boundary condition at its other end corresponds to a relatively large input conductance). The 140-μV peak EPSP at the soma, compared to about 60 μV for five passive spines, implies an amplification factor of about 2.3.

Case 4 differs from case 2 only by the addition of synchronous excitatory synaptic inputs to any three of the 45 passive spines on branch B. Not only does this added depolarization of branch B help the excitable spines of branch B to reach threshold, but it helps these five spines to fire earlier than in case 3; this more nearly synchronous firing of the 10 excitable spines of branches A and B results in a larger peak depolarization in branch C for case 4 compared to case 3, and this is sufficient to fire (with a delay) the five excitable spines of branch C. Together, these 15 spine firings (plus three passive spines with synaptic input) produce a 230-μV peak EPSP at the soma, implying an amplification factor of about 3.8 for this case. It may be noted that 230 μV is almost three times the 84 μV of case 2, but it is about 10 times (not 15 times) the 24 μV of case 1. Case 5 shows one of many possible examples of how synaptic inhibition delivered to one or two spines could make all the difference between success or failure of the kind of multiple cluster firing shown in cases 3 and 4.

More Results with Clusters

Looking back at cases 3 and 4 in Figure 10, it is natural to consider some other closely related cases. For example, suppose synchronous synaptic excitation is delivered to five excitable spines of branch C, instead of branch A. This can be expressed as $5 \cdot XSH(E)_C$ in the notation of Figure 5B; our computation shows that this fires all 15 of the XSH of branches A, B, and C. The spine head voltage peaks in A and B were 0.78 msec later than in C, and there was a 207-μV peak EPSP at the soma, attributable to 15 excitable distal spine heads. It may be noted that the depolarization that spread into neighboring branches (the sibling branch of C and two first cousin branches of A and B) was not sufficient to fire the excitable spines there. However, a consideration of case 4 in Figure 10 should make it obvious that a small assist by synaptic input to only a few spines in

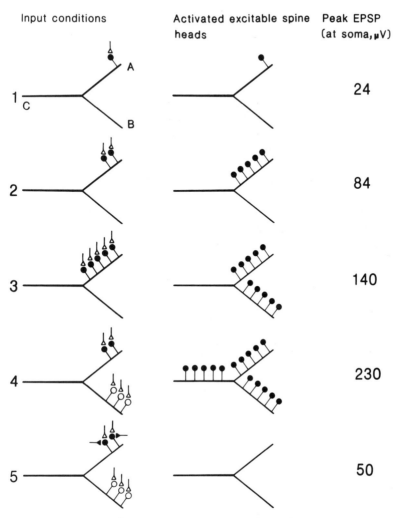

Figure 10. *Spine cluster firing contingencies: Schematic summary of five different input combinations to the spine clusters of distal branches A, B, and C of Figure 9. Left column schematizes the five different cases of synaptic input conditions (cf. Figures 5B and 9). Middle column shows only those excitable spine heads that fired an action potential in each case. Right column lists the peak amplitude of the resulting EPSP at the soma in microvolts for each case. In case 5, black synaptic boutons indicate synchronous inhibitory synaptic input; its conductance time course was assumed to be the same as that for synaptic excitation (in this case), with a peak conductance of 1.5 nS and a reversal potential of −10mV from rest.*

those branches could easily result in the firing of 15 additional excitable spines, for a total of 30 spine firings in this dendritic arbor. The larger EPSP at the soma could be designated a composite EPSP because of the explosive firing of several spine clusters belonging to a distal dendritic arbor. It could also be called a "prepotential" because of "distal arbor spine cluster firing." Whatever we call it, such near-synchronous firing is noteworthy for three different reasons: (1) It can make a significant contribution to the EPSP at the soma and (2) to depolarization in neighboring dendritic arbors; and (3) the conditions for it to occur correspond to multiple and alternative contingencies, such as $5 \cdot XSH(E)_C + 3 \cdot PSH(E)_C^*$, provided that there is no inhibition to any of these particular spines. If one or two of these spines were inhibited, it would be necessary to add synaptic excitatory input to several more spines in this arbor.

Other computations, in which synaptic input was restricted to spines of branch D, showed that $5 \cdot XSH(E)_D$ was not sufficient to fire any neighboring excitable spines. To understand why, we note that this branch has a lower input resistance value and larger capacitance (because of its larger diameter and the flow of current into several attached branches; see Figure 4 and the mathematical solution of this problem in Rall and Rinzel, 1973). This smaller input resistance and larger capacitance means that the current delivered to the dendrite by the activated spines produces significantly less local membrane depolarization, and this is insufficient to fire excitable spine heads in neighboring branches. We found that if 12 excitable spines were available and were provided with synchronous synaptic excitation, $12 \cdot XSH(E)_D$, this would produce sufficient local depolarization to fire the cell's distal arbor; such a firing of 42 excitable spines produced a 515-μV EPSP at the soma.

From such results, we conclude that (for given input conditions) usually only some of the spine clusters will fire. In general, those clusters that are distal to the cluster that receives the input will fire more readily than will more proximal clusters. One can see the rich number of possibilities for fractionating the dendritic tree into functionally (almost independent) regions; and that different input conditions can result in different logical operations, implemented by dendritic trees with excitable spine clusters.

DISCUSSION

Economy of Excitable Channels

Based upon our computations, we can see that concentrating adequate numbers of excitable channels in the spine heads of a limited number of distal dendritic spines can be particularly effective. This provides efficient and economical use of a finite number of such channels. Many more channels (with much higher densities over much larger areas) would be needed to generate action potentials in the membrane of the dendritic shafts for two reasons. (1) Because of the relatively low input resistance at the shaft, the local dendritic membrane depolarization would not be boosted at shaft locations, compared to active spine head locations where the large spine stem resistance boosts the spine head depolarization that results from both synaptic and active currents. This must be compensated for by much higher densities of both synaptic and active channels in order to reach action potential threshold conditions. (2) Compared to an isolated membrane patch, a membrane cylinder has both a higher voltage threshold and a minimal active length requirement for the generation and propagation of an action potential (Rushton, 1937; Jack et al., 1975). As a consequence, dendritic shaft action potentials would require much larger numbers of both synaptic and active channels. However, even more important than such consideration of channel economics is the difference in richness of the logic repertoire for the processing of many different synaptic input combinations: Fully propagating dendritic action potentials would seem to provide a much more limited all-or-nothing type of repertoire, compared to the many different contingencies for success or failure in spine clusters of various distal branches and arbors, of which only a few were described in Figure 10 and its associated explanation.

Plasticity by Changes in Spine Parameters

The results obtained above for individual excitable spines and for clusters of excitable spines provide a basis for very significant (nonlinear) sensitivity to small changes in one or more spine parameters. These could underlie the functional plasticity of synapses, spatiotemporal patterns, and dynamic activity in overlapping multineuronal pathways. For example, if the values of the spine stem resistance, the synaptic conductance, and the excitability of the spine head membrane happen to be a combination that is just below threshold, then an increase in one of these parameters can be responsible for shifting conditions from below threshold to above threshold. One or more spine heads fire now that did not fire before, and this may shift the balance for an entire cluster of excitable spines, which in turn can shift the set of contingencies for neuronal firing. Conversely, a decrease in one of these parameters can bring conditions below threshold and prevent that cascade of consequences.

CONCLUDING REMARKS

Because we have explored the possibilities of excitable spines so recently, it will obviously be some time before the last word will be said on this subject. Further theoretical studies are needed to explore more of the many interesting possibilities. Also, in view of past technical advances there is reason to suppose that some of these ideas can be tested experimentally in the not distant future. At this early time it seems safe to say that we have achieved a number of insights related to the dendritic processing of many different synaptic inputs.

REFERENCES

Barrett, J. N., and W. E. Crill (1974) Influences of dendritic location and membrane properties on the effectiveness of synapses on cat motoneurones. *J. Physiol. (Lond.)* **239**:325–345.

Berkley, H. J. (1897) Studies on the lesions produced by the action of certain poisons on the cortical nerve cell. *Johns Hopkins Hosp. Reports* **6**:1–93.

Brown, T. H., and D. Johnston (1983) Voltage-clamp analysis of mossy fiber synaptic input to hippocampal neurons. *J. Neurophysiol.* **50**:487–507.

Butz, E. G., and J. D. Cowan (1974) Transient potentials in dendritic systems of arbitrary geometry. *Biophys. J.* **14**:661–689.

Carnevale, N. T., and D. Johnston (1982) Electrophysiological characterization of remote chemical synapses. *J. Neurophysiol.* **47**:606–621.

Chang, H. T. (1952) Cortical neurons with particular reference to the apical dendrites. *Cold Spring Harbor Symp. Quant. Biol.* **17**:189–202.

Colonnier, M. (1968) Synaptic patterns on different cell types in the different laminae of the cat visual cortex. An electron microscope study. *Brain Res.* **9**:268–287.

Coombs, J. S., J. C. Eccles, and P. Fatt (1955) The inhibitory suppression of reflex discharges from motoneurones. *J. Physiol. (Lond.)* **130**:396–413.

Diamond, J., E. G. Gray, and G. M. Yasargil (1970) The function of the dendritic spines: An hypothesis. In *Excitatory Synaptic Mechanisms*, P. O. Andersen and J. K. S. Jansen, eds., pp. 213–222, Universitetsforlaget, Oslo.

Dodge, F. A., Jr., and J. W. Cooley (1973) Action potential of the motoneuron. *IBM J. Res. Dev.* **17**:219–229.

Erulkar, S. D., R. A. Butler, and G. L. Gerstein (1968) Excitation and inhibition in cochlear nucleus. II. Frequency-modulated tones. *J. Neurophysiol.* **31**:537–548.

Fatt, P., and B. Katz (1953) The effect of inhibitory nerve impulses on a crustacean muscle fibre. *J. Physiol. (Lond.)* **121**:374–389.

Feldman, M. L., and A. Peters (1979) A technique for estimating total spine numbers on Golgi-impregnated dendrites. *J. Comp. Neurol.* **118**:527–542.

Finkel, A. S., and S. J. Redman (1983) The synaptic current evoked in cat spinal motoneurones by impulses in single group Ia axons. *J. Physiol. (Lond.)* **342**:615–632.

Gray, E. G. (1959) Axo-somatic and axo-dendritic synapses of the cerebral cortex: An electron microscopic study. *J. Anat.* **93**:420–433.

Hodgkin, A. L., and A. F. Huxley (1952) A quantitative description of membrane current and its application to conduction and excitation in nerve. *J. Physiol. (Lond.)* **117**:500–544.

Horwitz, B. (1981) An analytical method for investigating transient potential in neurons with branching dendritic trees. *Biophys. J.* **36**:155–192.

Horwitz, B. (1983) Unequal diameters and their effect on time varying voltages in branched neurons. *Biophys. J.* **41**:51–66.

Jack, J. J. B., and S. J. Redman (1971) An electrical description of the motoneurone and its application to the analysis of synaptic potentials. *J. Physiol. (Lond.)* **215**:321–352.

Jack, J. J. B., D. Noble, and R. W. Tsien (1975) *Electric Current Flow in Excitable Cells*, Oxford Univ. Press, London.

Jones, E. G., and T. P. S. Powell (1969) Morphological variations in the dendritic spines of the neocortex. *J. Cell Sci.* **5**:509–519.

Kawato, M., and N. Tsukahara (1984) Electrical properties of dendritic spines with bulbous end terminals. *Biophys. J.* **46**:155–166.

Koch, C., and T. Poggio (1983) A theoretical analysis of electrical properties of spines. *Proc. R. Soc. Lond. (Biol.)* **218**:455–477.

Koch, C., T. Poggio, and V. Torre (1982) Retinal ganglion cells: A functional interpretation of dendritic morphology. *Philos. Trans. R. Soc. Lond. (Biol.)* **298**:227–264.

Malinow, R., and J. P. Miller (1984) Interactions between active dendritic spines could generate bursts of spikes. *Soc. Neurosci. Abstr.* **10**:547.

Miller, J. P., W. Rall, and J. Rinzel (1985) Synaptic amplification by active membrane in dendritic spines. *Brain Res.* **325**:325–330.

Parnas, I., and I. Segev (1979) A mathematical model for conduction of action potentials along bifurcating axons. *J. Physiol. (Lond.)* **295**:323–343.

Perkel, D. H., and D. J. Perkel (1985) Dendritic spines: Role of active membrane in modulating synaptic efficacy. *Brain Res.* **325**:331–335.

Peters, A., and I. R. Kaiserman-Abramof (1970) The small pyramidal neuron of the rat cerebral cortex. The perikaryon, dendrites and spines. *Am. J. Anat.* **127**:321–356.

Rall, W. (1957) Membrane time constant of motoneurons. *Science* **126**:454.

Rall, W. (1959) Branching dendritic trees and motoneuron membrane resistivity. *Exp. Neurol.* **1**:491–527.

Rall, W. (1960) Membrane potential transients and membrane time constant of motoneurons. *Exp. Neurol.* **2**:503–532.

Rall, W. (1962) Theory of physiological properties of dendrites. *Ann. N.Y. Acad. Sci.* **96**:1071–1092.

Rall, W. (1964) Theoretical significance of dendritic trees for neuronal input–output relations. In *Neural Theory and Modeling*, R. Reiss, ed., pp. 73–97, Stanford Univ. Press, Stanford, California.

Rall, W. (1967) Distinguishing theoretical synaptic potentials computed for different soma-dendritic distributions of synaptic input. *J. Neurophysiol.* **30**:1138–1168.

Rall, W. (1969) Time constants and electrotonic length of membrane cylinders and neurons. *Biophys. J.* **9**:1483–1508.

Rall, W. (1970) Cable properties of dendrites and effect of synaptic location. In *Excitatory Synaptic Mechanisms*, P. O. Andersen and J. K. S. Jansen, eds., pp. 175–187, Universitetsforlaget, Oslo.

Rall, W. (1974) Dendritic spines, synaptic potency and neuronal plasticity. *Brain Info. Service Res. Report* **3**:13–21.

Rall, W. (1977) Core conductor theory and cable properties of neurons. *Handb. Physiol., Cellular Biology of Neurons* **1**:39–97.

Rall, W. (1978) Dendritic spines and synaptic potency. In *Studies in Neurophysiology*, R. Porter, ed., Cambridge Univ. Press, New York.

Rall, W., and J. Rinzel (1971a) Dendritic spines and synaptic potency explored theoretically. *Proc. IUPS (XXV Int. Congr.)* **IX**:466.

Rall, W., and J. Rinzel (1971b) Dendritic spine function and synaptic attenuation calculations. *Soc. Neurosci. Abstr.* **1**:64.

Rall, W., and J. Rinzel (1973) Branch input resistance and steady attenuation for input to one branch of a dendritic neuron model. *Biophys. J.* **13**:648–688.

Rall, W., and I. Segev (1985) Space clamp problems when voltage clamping branched neurons with intracellular microelectrodes. In *Voltage and Patch Clamping with Microelectrodes*, T. G. Smith, Jr., H. Lecar, S. J. Redman, and P. Gage, eds., pp. 191–215, American Physiological Society, Bethesda, Maryland.

Rall, W., and G. M. Shepherd (1968) Theoretical reconstruction of field potentials and dendrodendritic synaptic interactions in olfactory bulb. *J. Neurophysiol.* **31**:884–915.

Rall, W., G. M. Shepherd, T. S. Reese, and M. W. Brightman (1966) Dendro-dendritic synaptic pathway in the olfactory bulb. *Exp. Neurol.* **14**:44–56.

Rall, W., R. E. Burke, T. G. Smith, P. G. Nelson, and K. Frank (1967) Dendritic location of synapses and possible mechanisms for the monosynaptic EPSP in motoneurons. *J. Neurophysiol.* **30**:1169–1193.

Ramón y Cajal, S. (1909) *Histologie du Système Nerveux de l'Homme et des Vertébrés*, Vol. 1, trans. by L. Azoulay, Maloine, Paris.

Redman, S. J. (1976) A quantitative approach to the integrative function of dendrites. *Int. Rev. Physiol.* **10**:1–36.

Redman, S. J., and B. Walmsley (1983) The time course of synaptic potentials evoked in cat spinal motoneurones at identified group Ia synapses. *J. Physiol. (Lond.)* **343**:117–133.

Rinzel, J. (1982) Neuronal plasticity (learning). In *Some Mathematical Questions in Biology–Neurobiology*, Vol. 15, R. M. Miura, ed., pp. 7–25, American Mathematical Society, Providence, Rhode Island.

Rinzel, J., and W. Rall (1974) Transient response in a dendritic neuron model for current injected at one branch. *Biophys. J.* **14**:759–790.

Rushton, W. A. H. (1937) Initiation of the propagated disturbance. *Proc. R. Soc. Lond. (Biol.)* **124**:210.

Scheibel, M. E., and A. B. Scheibel (1968) On the nature of dendritic spines—Report of a workshop. *Commun. Behav. Biol.* **IA**:231–265.

Segev, I., and I. Parnas (1983) Synaptic integration mechanisms. Theoretical and experimental investigation of temporal postsynaptic interaction between excitatory and inhibitory inputs. *Biophys. J.* **41**:41–50.

Segev, I., and W. Rall (1984) EPSP shape indices when dendritic trees have unequal length. *Soc. Neurosci. Abstr.* **10**:734.

Shepherd, G. M., and R. K. Brayton (1979) Computer simulation of a dendro-dendritic synaptic circuit for self- and lateral-inhibition in the olfactory bulb. *Brain Res.* **175**:377–382.

Shepherd, G. M., R. K. Brayton, A. Belanger, J. P. Miller, R. Malinow, I. Segev, J. Rinzel, and W. Rall (1984) Interactions between active dendritic spines could augment impact of distal dendritic synapses. *Soc. Neurosci. Abstr.* **10**:547.

Traub, R. D. (1977) Motorneurons of different geometry and the size principle. *Biol. Cybern.* **25**: 163–176.

Turner, D. A. (1984) Conductance transients onto dendritic spines in a segmental cable model of hippocampal neurons. *Biophys. J.* **46**:85–96.

Wilson, C. J. (1984) Passive cable properties of dendritic spines and spiny neurons. *J. Neurosci.* **4**: 281–297.

Wilson, C. J., P. M. Groves, S. T. Kitai, and I. C. Linder (1983) Three dimensional structure of dendritic spines in the rat neostriatum. *J. Neurosci.* **3**:383–398.

Vladimirescu, A., A. R. Newton, and D. O. Pederson (1980) SPICE version 26.0 *User's Guide*, EECS Dept., Univ. of California, Berkeley.

Chapter 23

Biophysics of Computation: Neurons, Synapses, and Membranes

CHRISTOF KOCH
TOMASO POGGIO

ABSTRACT

Synapses, membranes, and transmitters play an important role in processing information in the nervous system. We do not know, however, what biophysical mechanisms are critical for neuronal computations, what elementary information processing operations they implement, and which sensory or motor computations they underlie. In this chapter, we outline an approach to these problems. More precisely: (1) We review the mechanisms underlying impulse initiation and conduction, repetitive firing of impulses, and the failure of impulses to propagate past axonal branch points, analyzing some of the underlying operations. (2) We discuss chemical and electrical transduction at the synapse. The operation performed by a chemical synapse is nonlinear amplification and is equivalent to a nonreciprocal electrical element. Electrical synapses are equivalent to linear and nonlinear resistances, such as diodes. (3) We introduce postsynaptic interaction between conductance changes. In the specific case of excitation and silent (or shunting) inhibition, the operation implemented is the analog equivalent of an AND–NOT gate or a veto operation. This mechanism may be the key component in the circuitries computing the direction of motion in the retina and visual depth in cortical cells. (4) We analyze the function of dendritic spines. Two of the operations that may be implemented by dendritic spines are changing the weight of a synapse and subserving a very local interaction between excitation and inhibition. Examples of possible computations are information storage in the cortex and the selective suppression of visual input in the lateral geniculate nucleus. (5) We consider the role of quasi-active membranes, that is, time- and voltage-dependent channels. Short of underlying spiking behavior, they can perform different filtering operations, acting as resonant filters. An example of a specific computation is the tuning of hair cells to acoustic frequencies. (6) Finally we consider transmitter regulation of voltage-dependent channels and the action of neurotransmitters at large distances. We discuss how the nonclassical action of these neuromodulatory substances may affect the circuitry in a very specific manner over long time courses. We conclude by discussing a possible distinction between biophysical mechanisms acting over short and long time ranges. Finally, we will present a new biophysical model of analog computation that is very different from the model of computation provided by present digital computers and appears to be very suggestive in terms of the nervous system.

This chapter is based on the belief that brains are very sophisticated computing machines, and that one of the ultimate goals of brain science is to understand the computations and information processing they perform. A study of the role of synapses, membranes, and cells in information processing tasks is therefore part of this broad enterprise. But this is not the only motivation for such a study. In recent years, computational studies have provided promising—although far from complete—theories of the computations necessary for sensory processing (for partial reviews, see Marr, 1982; Poggio, 1984a; Poggio et al., 1985). Despite their initial success, we have now come to realize that computational theories, even complemented by psychophysical experiments, have inherent limitations with regard to understanding the brain. A given computation, for instance, the computation of stereo depth or motion, can in general be performed by several different algorithms. These algorithms depend not only on the nature of the computation itself but also on the properties and limitations of the hardware in which the algorithm is implemented.

As a consequence, to bridge the gap between computational theories and the biological data, we must first understand how the elementary computations are performed in neural hardware. In recent years, neurobiologists have shown, through such experimental findings as dendrodendritic synapses, gap junctions, dendritic spikes, nonsynaptic release of neural transmitters, and a variety of voltage- and transmitter-dependent channels, that the complexity of the processing that takes place within a single neuron may be far greater than previously presumed (see Schmitt and Worden, 1979, for a thorough review of this development). An understanding of the role of these biophysical mechanisms in biological information processing is necessary in order to understand the implementation of specific computations in neuronal hardware.

In computer science, work on the physics of computation attempts to characterize the physical mechanisms that can be exploited to perform elementary information processing operations in technical systems (Mead and Conway, 1980). These mechanisms constrain in turn the types of operation that can be exploited for computing. A case in point is the so-called metal oxide semiconductor (MOS) technology used in integrated circuits. Because of the physics of the MOS transistor, the basic logic circuit is an inverter, whose output is the complement of its input. NAND and NOR logic circuits can be constructed as simple expansions of the basic inverter circuit. Therefore, very large scale integrated (VLSI) systems in MOS technology use NAND and NOR logic (Mead and Conway, 1980). We believe that a biophysics of computation is now needed for understanding the role of neurons, synapses, and membranes in information processing in biological systems.

Simply stated, the questions we are asking are: What is the hardware of the brain? Where are the elementary information processing operations performed? What is the equivalent in nervous systems of transistors and gates? In this chapter, we outline our initial approach to these questions. We review briefly some of the biophysical mechanisms, both in synapses and membranes, that may have a role in information processing. For each one, we discuss the information processing operations that may be implemented. In some cases, we will also suggest specific computations, such as the computation of the direction of visual motion, where the given operation may have an important role. Table 1 gives a list of biophysical mechanisms of corresponding information processing op-

Table 1. Some Neuronal Operations and the Underlying Biophysical Mechanisms

Biophysical Mechanism	Neural Operation	Example of Computation
Action potential initiation	Analog OR/AND one-bit analog-to-digital converter	
Repetitive spiking activity	Current-to-frequency transducer	
Action potential conduction	Impulse transmission	Long-distance communication in axons
Conduction failure at axonal branch points	Temporal/spatial filtering of impulses	Opener muscle in crayfish
Chemically mediated synaptic transduction	Nonreciprocal two-port "negative" resistance Sigmoid "threshold"	
Electrically mediated synaptic transduction	Reciprocal one-port resistance	Coupling of rod photoreceptors to enhance detection of signals
Distributed excitatory synapses in dendritic tree	Linear addition	α, β cat retinal ganglion cells Bipolar cells
Interaction between excitatory and (silent) inhibitory conductance inputs	Analog AND-NOT, veto operation	Directional-selective retinal ganglion cells Disparity-selective cortical cells
Excitatory synapse on dendritic spine with calcium channels	Postsynaptic modification in functional connectivity	Short- and long-term information storage
Excitatory and inhibitory synapses on dendritic spine	Local AND-NOT "presynaptic inhibition"	Enabling/disabling retinal input to geniculate X-cells
Quasi-active membranes	Electrical resonant filter analog Differentiation delay	Hair cells in lower vertebrates
Transmitter regulation of voltage-dependent channels (M-current inhibition)	Gain control	Midbrain sites controlling gain of retinogeniculate transmission
Calcium sensitivity of cAMP-dependent phosphorylation of potassium channel protein	Functional connectivity	Adaptation and associative storage of information in *Aplysia*
Long-distance action of neurotransmitter	Modulating and routing transmission of information	

erations and of specific examples of computations in which each mechanism may be used. The list is not intended to be exhaustive.

The main goal here is to state the problem—what are the biophysical mechanisms underlying information processing and how are these mechanisms used to perform specific computations—and to stimulate experimental and theoretical research that can lead to its answer. As we discuss later, many biophysical mechanisms may have only an indirect role in computations in the nervous system and be, so to speak, side effects of a cell's properties. The situation is not much different in our present computers: Many of the components are dedicated to functions, such as supplying power, that are only indirectly relevant to the elementary information processing operations. Ultimately, only experimental work can answer which biophysical mechanisms are used in information processing and how. Computational considerations in conjunction with computer simulations can help, however, to direct experimental work effectively.

We consider several biophysical mechanisms of neuronal membranes and synapses. For each one we discuss the information processing operation that it may implement. For instance, the mechanism leading to action potentials performs a threshold operation similar to the analog–digital conversion performed by a Schmitt trigger. A subset of these operations is sufficient to synthesize a universal computer. Together they provide the nervous system with a powerful set of basic hardware operations in terms of which simple and complex computations and algorithms can be implemented. Whenever possible, we speculate about a specific instance of computation where the biophysical mechanism may play a central role. The best example is probably the computation of the direction of motion in retinal ganglion cells. We suggest that the underlying mechanism is the interaction of excitatory and inhibitory conductance changes of postsynaptic origin.

The first section considers the biophysical mechanisms of spike initiation and conduction and the corresponding information processing operations. It also describes a specific example of a computation (for motor control) that exploits the mechanism of differential spike conduction in branching axonal trees. Synapses are discussed next. We first characterize, from the point of view of information processing, chemical synapses, then electrical synapses, and finally the postsynaptic interactions between synaptic conductance changes. Several examples of computations are suggested. We explore in considerable detail the biophysical mechanisms and the possible anatomical pathways underlying direction selectivity in neurons of the vertebrate retina. Experiments for testing these hypotheses are also described. Dendritic spines and their possible role in information storage and processing are the subject of the following section. The mechanisms of nonspiking voltage- and time-dependent channels are introduced in the first part of this chapter. As an example of a computation, we describe the resonant electrical tuning of hair cells in the vertebrate cochlea. Transmitter regulation of voltage-dependent channels and the functional role of neuropeptides make up the rest of the chapter. The final section discusses the distinction between biophysical mechanisms acting in the millisecond range, such as conductance changes and impulse initiation, and the class of mechanisms that modulate the processing of information via these fast mechanisms on a long time sale. We will also briefly allude to a novel model of information processing in analog electrical or chemical networks. Such a model could be easily implemented in neuronal hardware, suggesting a style of neuronal computation very different from the threshold models of the McCulloch and Pitts (1943) type.

IMPULSE INITIATION AND CONDUCTION

Action potential initiation and propagation were among the first biophysical mechanisms that were elucidated. Action potentials and their generation are such a dominant feature of the nervous system that for a considerable amount of time it was widely held that they underlie all information processing in the nervous system. In the next four sections, we provide a brief overview of their possible role in information processing.

Impulse Initiation

Biophysical Mechanism. The first quantitative analysis of the ionic currents underlying the action potential was done on the squid giant axon (Hodgkin and Huxley, 1952; for a summary, consult Hodgkin, 1964; Katz, 1966). The responsible agents are time- and voltage-dependent sodium channels, described by the variables m and h. The inward current flowing through these channels is given by $I_{Na}(t) = \bar{g}_{Na}m^3h(V(t) - E_{Na})$, where $V(t)$ is the voltage across the membrane, E_{Na} is the reversal potential associated with the sodium ions, and $\bar{g}_{Na}$ is a constant. The activation variable, m, increases with increasing depolarization, while h, the inactivation variable, decreases. When the membrane is depolarized, the sodium conductance begins to increase, depolarizing the membrane further, and so on. This cycle proceeds until the membrane approaches the potential at which there is no more driving potential for the sodium ions, that is, $V = E_{Na}$, and until voltage-dependent inactivation sets in. In the meantime a counteracting outward current, mediated by the outflow of potassium, is activated. It is usually described by $I_K(t) = \bar{g}_K n^4(V(t) - E_K)$, where n is the corresponding activation variable. Concurrent with the activation of the outward potassium current, the inward sodium current begins to inactivate, reducing the voltage to levels slightly below the initial resting level (see Figure 1). Action potentials are all-or-none events, and therefore highly nonlinear. Below threshold, a stimulus elicits only a local graded response; above threshold, the membrane goes through its stereotyped voltage change independent of the stimulus intensity. Action potentials are all-pervasive, occurring in both vertebrates and invertebrates (Hagiwara, 1983).

Calcium currents are also known to trigger all-or-none electrical events (Kleinhaus and Prichard, 1975; Schwartzkroin and Slawsky, 1977; Wong et al., 1979; Llinás and Sugimori, 1980; Llinás and Yarom, 1981; Jahnsen and Llinás, 1984). Since most calcium channels do not inactivate readily, their time course is usually longer than the time course of sodium spikes. Moreover, while the sodium conductances giving rise to spikes are predominately found in cell bodies and axons, high-threshold calcium spikes are believed to originate in the dendritic trees of neurons of the vertebrate central nervous system.

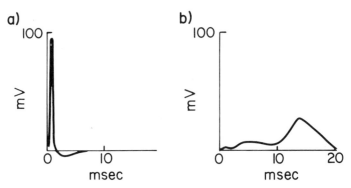

Figure 1. *Typical axonal sodium* (a) *and dendritic calcium* (b) *action potential.* Axonal spikes, in this
case from the squid axon, display amplitudes of about 100 mV and have a pulse width of about
1 msec. Dendritic spikes typically have lower amplitudes and are more "smeared out." Shown
is a Purkinje cell dendritic spike following blockage of sodium current with tetrodotoxin (TTX).
Note the humps in the curve that suggest the presence of multiple sites for spike initiation.
(Modified from Llinás, 1979.)

Neuronal Operation.   The basic operation implemented by such a threshold
mechanism is a digital OR or AND gate. If the threshold is low enough, a single
input will be able to surpass the threshold and trigger a spike. For larger threshold
values, two or more converging inputs may be required to elicit a spike. The
dependence of this operation on the value of the threshold seems important in
light of the observation that the threshold for eliciting spikes is known to depend
on the prior spiking history. Thus, the firing threshold in frog sciatic nerve fibers
and in cat motoneurons can increase by a factor of two for prolonged spiking
activity (Raymond, 1979; Schwindt and Crill, 1982). The threshold scheme underlies
a second operation: converting an analog graded signal, the intracellular current
or membrane potential, into a digital event, the spike. It is thus similar to a one-
bit analog–digital converter.

An Example of a Computation.   The early and influential view of information
processing in neurons was expressed well in the threshold neuron model of
McCulloch and Pitts (1943). In the most common version of this model, the
neuron is considered as the elementary processing unit that receives excitatory
and inhibitory inputs leading to depolarizing and hyperpolarizing dendritic potentials. These are subsequently propagated to the soma where they contribute—in a linear fashion—to the somatic potential. If the somatic potential
exceeds a given threshold, a spike is initiated and transmitted along the axon.
Otherwise the neuron remains silent. It is fairly straightforward to show that a
set of these threshold neurons is complete, that is, every input–output behavior
can be reproduced by appropriate combinations of threshold neurons (given a
fixed input–output coding in some fixed alphabet like {0,1}; Kleene, 1956; Palm,
1982).

Repetitive Spiking Activity

Biophysical Mechanism.   One distinguishing characteristic of different types of
neurons is their response to prolonged current injections or synaptic input.

Responses range from a single burst to tonic, continuous spiking that can increase linearly or nonlinearly with increasing stimulus amplitude. If the average firing frequency in response to a prolonged current pulse in cat spinal motoneurons is plotted against the injected current strength, the resulting plot, the f–I curve, is best described by two linear segments (Figure 2). The steeper linear segment has been termed the secondary range and the shallower segment the primary range (Kernell, 1970; Schwindt and Crill, 1982). For cat extraocular motoneurons and frog lumbar motoneurons, the f–I curve is best described by only one linear segment.

The underlying biophysical mechanisms are a slow, outward, calcium-dependent potassium current I_{KS}, a persistent calcium current I_i, and the accommodative properties of the axon initial segment, which lead to a rise in firing threshold with increasing firing rate (Schwindt and Crill, 1982; Crill and Schwindt, 1983). The potassium current is activated at 10 mV or greater (relative to the resting potential of the cell) and is partially responsible for the long afterhyperpolarization present in motoneurons. I_i is a steady inward current activated at voltages traversed by the cell during steady rhythmic firing and showing little evidence of voltage-dependent inactivation. Depolarizing the membrane activates I_i, adding a substantial inward current and increasing the firing rate. I_{KS} and the increase in firing threshold have the converse effect, reducing the f–I slope. Thus, the relative strengths of the tonic inward current and the outward current are the major determinant of the f–I relationship.

It is easy to imagine a calcium current that is already activated near the resting potential and that inactivates for depolarization. Injecting more and more current into the cell would then cause a "compensatory" decrease in this calcium current through voltage-dependent inactivation of the calcium currents. The net effect may be a roughly constant firing frequency, relatively independent of the injected current. Calcium channels in egg cell membrane do inactivate for increasing levels of membrane depolarization (Fox, 1981). The inactivation kinetics of the calcium current in this case are similar to, but slower than, the kinetics of the sodium channel.

Neuronal Operation.   A single action potential carries only one bit of information if its timing is irrelevant. Information is most likely coded in terms of the interval between successive action potentials. In many instances, the nervous system

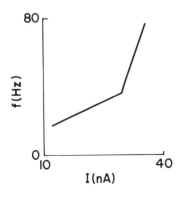

Figure 2.   *Average steady-state impulse frequency* (f), *plotted against the intensity of injected current* (I) *in a spinal* α-*motoneuron. There is an approximately linear relation between I and f over a range of lower and higher discharge frequencies (termed "primary" and "secondary" range). (Modified from Kernel, 1970.)*

might well use the average spiking frequency as a convenient measure of information. The $f–I$ relationship discussed above would then serve as a current–frequency transducer, converting one sort of graded signal, current, into another, spike frequency. Note that at this level of description, the code used is no longer digital but analog. The slope of the $f–I$ relationship is primarily governed by two currents, I_{KS} and I_i. Reducing or enhancing their amplitude, by applying, for instance, a neurotransmitter or a neuropeptide to the cell, may change the slope of the input–output relationship.

Impulse Conduction

Biophysical Mechanism.   In a cable with a sufficient number of voltage-dependent sodium and potassium channels, electrical impulses can propagate in a nondecremental fashion. Once an action potential has been initiated, the initial sodium current will spread to neighboring membrane patches, depolarizing the membrane and going through exactly the same cycle, and so on, down the length of the axon (Katz, 1966; Jack et al., 1975). Since the shape of the spike remains constant over the whole length of the axon, the conduction is nondecremental. There are two different groups of spike-conducting fibers, myelinated and nonmyelinated fibers.

In myelinated axons found only in vertebrates, conduction does not proceed continuously along the fiber, but jumps, as it were, from node to node. The channels responsible for the regenerative action potential concentrate at these small specialized sites (called the nodes of Ranvier). This is known as saltatory conduction. The space between the nodes, the internodal segment, is covered by several hundred layers of myelin, what amounts to a high-resistance and low-capacity insulating substance (see, however, Funch and Faber, 1984). While the two dominant currents for nonmyelinated axons are sodium and potassium carried, the impulse at the mammalian node of Ranvier is generated almost exclusively by sodium currents (Chiu et al., 1979). Potassium channels may, however, be present below the internodal axonal membrane where they normally do not subserve any function in action potential regeneration or propagation (Chiu and Ritchie, 1982, 1984; Kocsis and Waxman, 1980). Because ionic currents flow only at the node in myelinated fibers, saltatory conduction is favorable from a metabolic point of view. Less energy must be expended by the sodium–potassium pump in restoring the sodium and potassium concentration gradients, which tend to run down as a result of prolonged spike activity in small fibers.

Since axons can be up to several meters long, the conduction time of the electrical impulses is of crucial importance. In nonmyelinated fibers, the conduction times of action potentials is proportional to the square root of the fiber diameter (Figure 3). In myelinated fibers, the conduction times are considerably increased, being directly proportional to the diameter (Rushton, 1951; Pickard, 1969; Ritchie, 1982). Propagation velocity also depends on the number of active channels. If their number drops below a critical value, nondecremental propagation ceases (Sabah and Leibovic, 1972).

Neuronal Operation.   The axon is the equivalent of the wire or interconnect between (and not so much within) silicon chips, connecting the different com-

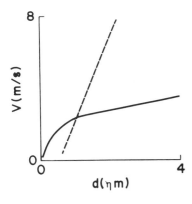

Figure 3. *Relation between the conduction velocity of action potentials (v) and fiber diameter (d) for small myelinated and nonmyelinated fibers. (Modified from Waxman and Bennett, 1972.)*

putational devices, neurons, with a high-speed pathway. Thus, its main function is the transmission of impulses, namely, the transmission of information. The reliability of transmission depends on a number of factors, most notably the spike frequency and the specific morphology of the axon (see next section). Axons can have an extensive fan-out, making contact with a multitude of post-synaptic targets via highly branched axonal trees (for an example in the visual cortex of the cat, see Gilbert and Wiesel, 1983).

Axonal Trees

The all-or-none nature of action potentials has led to the idea that the axon serves mainly as a reliable transmission line, connecting two or more information processing devices. The axon itself is assumed to lack any processing function. This view may have to be broadened with the findings that, in regions of membrane and geometrical inhomogeneities, the transmission of action potentials depends on a number of parameters, such as the geometry of the axon and the previous spiking history (for instance, Krnjević and Miledi, 1959; Tauc and Hughes, 1963; Bittner, 1968; Chung et al., 1970; Grossman et al., 1979a,b).

Biophysical Mechanism. It has been shown both theoretically and experimentally that action potentials may fail to successfully invade the daughter branches of a bifurcating axon. As the theoretical analysis of Goldstein and Rall (1974) pointed out, the single most important parameter upon which propagation depends is the geometric ratio,

$$GR = \frac{d_1^{3/2} + d_2^{3/2}}{d_0^{3/2}},$$

where d_1 and d_2 are the diameters of the daughter branches, d_0 is the diameter of the main axon, and the membrane is homogeneous across the branch point. GR equals the impedance ratio for branches of semi-infinite length. The use of the geometrical ratio assumes that the specific membrane properties are the same in all branches. For $GR = 1$, the action potential does not "see" the branching (i.e., perfect impedance match), and it propagates without perturbation past the branch point. $GR = 1$ essentially captures Rall's equivalent tree concept (Rall, 1964). If $GR < 1$, the action potential behaves as if the axon tapers and it speeds up. The more interesting situation occurs if $GR > 1$, that is, if the combined load of the daughter branches is larger than the load of the main branch. When $1 < GR < 10$, the action potential is delayed at the branch point and a "reflection potential" appears (Parnas and Segev, 1979). If GR is about 10 (e.g., $GR = 10$ if $d_1 = d_2 = 4.6 \, d_0$), propagation into both branches fails simultaneously, since the electrical load of the daughter branches has increased beyond the point at which the initiation of the action potential in the daughter branches can be supported. Parnas and Segev (1979) emphasize that for each constant geometric ratio, changes in the diameter ratio between the daughter branches never yield differential conduction into the daughter branches if the membrane properties are identical in both branches.

In a study of conduction failure in a branching axon of the lobster, Grossman et al. (1979a) report that, although the geometrical ratio is close to one, conduction across the branch point fails at stimulation frequencies above 30 Hz. Moreover, the conduction block appeared first in the thicker daughter branch and only later in the thin branch, thus calling for an extension of the Goldstein and Rall (1974) model. By increasing the extracellular potassium concentration, Grossman et al. (1979b) could mimic the block of conduction, suggesting that a differential buildup of extracellular potassium can account for the blockage. For prolonged trains of action potentials, sodium accumulates faster in the small diameter daughter branch, triggering the electrogenic sodium–potassium pump earlier than in the thick branch. Therefore, the extracellular potassium accumulation will be reduced faster than for the thick branch, preventing the early onset of conduction block. A further factor known to affect the conduction of action potentials is the average interspike interval (Chung et al., 1970).

Neuronal Operation. Little if anything is known about the possible relevance of action potential conduction failures for information processing. Although it seems possible to control the conduction of action potentials into different branches, such a mechanism may not be robust enough to be widely applied in the nervous system. One could even argue that conduction block is an undesirable property of the system. One possible physiological function could be the protection of the system from overexcitation by limiting the total number of spikes transmitted. One possible role of this phenomenon for information processing could be the following: Virtually all axons, like those in the motor neuron or the geniculocortical projection cells, branch frequently before forming their final synaptic processes. In these structures, filtering may occur, in which the pattern of impulses in the parent axon diverges into different patterns in its daughter branches (Chung et al., 1970; I. Segev, personal communication). The filtering may be temporal, in which the frequency of the impulses in the daughter branches is different from that in the parent axon. On the other hand, the filtering could be spatial, in which temporal patterns are resolved into spatial ones, that is, different daughter branches show different firing behavior.

Example of a Computation. One instance in which such a mechanism might be used to perform a specific function is in the excitatory motor axon innervating the muscle used for opening the claw in the crayfish. This axon branches to different regions of the opener muscle, two of which are called superficial distal and superficial central fibers. When the axon is stimulated at a frequency of 1 Hz or less, junctional potentials (JPs) recorded from the distal fibers are up to 50 times larger than JPs in central fibers. At 80 Hz, central JPs are up to four times larger than those observed in distal fibers. Since equal amounts of depolarization produce equal amounts of tension in both fiber types, it follows that distal fibers produce almost all of the total muscle tension at low frequencies of stimulation. Central fibers add an increasingly greater contribution to the total muscle tension as the corresponding nerve terminals begin to receive action potentials in response to higher firing frequencies. The mechanism underlying this behavior is thought to be the more efficient invasion of action potentials into distal terminals at low firing frequencies (Bittner, 1968).

SYNAPSES

Specialized sites of contact between neurons, called synapses, represent one of the major means of communicating information between cells. In this respect, they can be compared to the pins on silicon chips, through which information is relayed to and from the chip. There are, of course, several critical differences. Today's LSI chips have, at most, approximately 100 pins (see Blodgett and Barbour, 1982); the dendritic tree of a neuron may carry up to 10^5 (morphological) synapses. The synapses themselves not only transmit information from the presynaptic to the postsynaptic neuron, using a chemical or electrical transducing mechanism, but may also process information, that is, perform some computation. In the following, we consider the possible role of chemical and electrical synapses in information processing.

Chemical Synapses

Biophysical Mechanism.   We do not attempt to review the literature concerning the biophysical and molecular mechanisms underlying synaptic transmission and release (see Katz, 1966; for a good overview see Shepherd, 1979b). Suffice it to say that the release of a chemical substance, the neurotransmitter, which crosses the space between the pre- and postsynaptic membrane, is essentially controlled by the amount of depolarization of the presynaptic terminal. The higher the presynaptic depolarization, the stronger the postsynaptic response, which can be either hyper- or depolarization. The transduction between presynaptic and postsynaptic voltage, V_{pre} and V_{post}, is usually described as either an almost linear or a sigmoidal transformation (Figure 4).

The neurotransmitter diffusing across the synaptic cleft activates specific ion-specific channels in the postsynaptic membrane, resulting in a change in membrane conductance $g(t)$ in series with the ionic battery E. The conductance change induces in turn a voltage change $V_{post}(t)$ (relative to the resting potential of the cell, E_{rest}). The change in potential is given by the Volterra equation, $V_{post}(t) = \{g(t) \cdot (E - V_{post}(t))\} * K_{ii}(t)$, where $K_{ii}(t)$ is the input impedance (Green function) at the postsynaptic location and $*$ represents convolution (see, e.g., Rall, 1967).

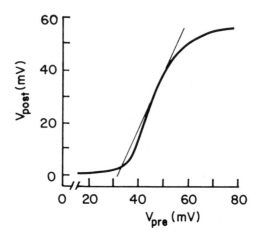

Figure 4. *Input–output relationship for a "typical" synapse from a spiking neuron, in this case the giant synapse in the squid stellate ganglion.* The voltages are given with respect to the resting potential. The maximum value of the dynamic gain is $dV_{post}/dV_{pre} \approx 3$. (Modified from Katz and Miledi, 1967.)

For stationary inputs, or when the input changes slowly in comparison with the membrane time constant, this equation reduces to

$$V_{post} = \frac{g\tilde{K}_{ii}E}{1 + g\tilde{K}_{ii}} \, ,$$

where $\tilde{K}_{ii}$ is the steady-state real input impedance at location i (essentially, the DC component of the complex Fourier transform of $K_{ii}(t)$). For a hyperpolarizing synapse, in which an increased level of presynaptic potential leads to an increase in the postsynaptic hyperpolarization, the sigmoid relation, as illustrated in Figure 4, will be inverted (Graubard et al., 1980).

The rolloff at large depolarizations is expected in part from the finite number of receptors in the postsynaptic membrane and partly from the postsynaptic saturation effect, that is, when the change in voltage V_{post} approaches the synaptic reversal potential E (see, for instance, Figure 13). Subsequent increases in the presynaptic voltage, that is, in the conductance $g(t)$, will fail to evoke larger potential responses. Synaptic saturation can be an important factor in limiting the total dynamic range of the system. For instance, the dynamic range in insect monopolar cells is 10^1–10^2, in contrast to the range of the presynaptic photoreceptor, 10^5 (Shaw, 1981). One way to avoid having synapses with a low dynamic range is to distribute the synapses in the postsynaptic dendritic tree, thus minimizing synaptic saturation and avoiding the early onset of postsynaptic saturation (see below).

A postsynaptic response graded by the amount of presynaptic depolarization is a crucial property for many synapses. While an axodendritic or axosomatic synapse is normally activated by an action potential invading the terminal, a dendrodendritic synapse from a dendrite may be activated by the graded depolarization of synaptic potentials within that dendrite (Graubard, 1978). In fact, graded synaptic transmission may even occur between spiking neurons: Thus, neurons in the lobster stomatogastric ganglion, in addition to eliciting spike-evoked inhibitory potentials in the postsynaptic cell, also release functionally significant amounts of transmitter below the threshold for action potential (Graubard et al., 1980, 1983; see also Llinás, 1979).

One way of characterizing chemical synapses is to measure the synaptic amplification, called sensitivity or dynamic gain, by recording the change in postsynaptic voltage in response to a small change in the presynaptic voltage, that is, dV_{post}/dV_{pre} (for a good exposition of this method see Shaw, 1981, or Llinás, 1979). The maximum value of the dynamic gain identifies the most effective operating range at a particular synapse. For the chemical synapse between the photoreceptors and the lamina monopolar cells in the dragonfly retina, the maximum dynamic gain is about 34 at presynaptic depolarizations of only 0.7 mV (Laughlin, 1973). This system, functioning without action potentials, can optimally signal the potential evoked by a single photon in the photoreceptor. Estimations of the dynamic gain in a homologue system, the rod–bipolar synapse in the dogfish, give similar numbers (at least 50; Ashmore and Falk, 1976, 1979; for more details, see Koch et al., 1986b). By contrast, values for impulse-transmitting, nonsensory synapses are considerably less: 0.3 at a lamprey central synapse (Martin and Ringham, 1975) or approximately three at the squid giant synapse (Katz and Miledi, 1967; see Figure 4). Both cases are optimized at presynaptic depolarizations of 60–80 mV, with little observable transmission taking place below 30 mV. The dichotomy between high and low dynamic gains suggests that in both vertebrates and invertebrates, synapses may be specialized in transmitting either very small voltages with no obvious threshold—converting one type of an analog signal into another analog signal—or in transmitting unitary impulses in a noise-free manner, that is, converting a digital signal into an analog signal.

Neuronal Operation. A chemical synapse converts V_{pre} into V_{post} (via a chemical process) and corresponds to a nonreciprocal two-port in the sense of Brayton and Moser (1964) or Oster et al. (1971). It can be described as a two-port element, since current and voltage can be varied independently at two sites, pre- and postsynaptically. Chemical synapses are nonreciprocal, since the input and output variables cannot be exchanged. Synapses decouple neuronal elements from each other, rather like operational amplifiers, since the postsynaptic current can be varied without any change in presynaptic current. Reciprocal synapses, like those found between mitral and granule cells in the olfactory bulb (Shepherd, 1979a) or between bipolar and amacrine cells in the vertebrate retina (Dowling and Boycott, 1966; Ellias and Stevens, 1972), may reintroduce reciprocity. Since V_{post} may well be larger in amplitude than V_{pre}, chemical synapses may amplify. Moreover, synapses can mimic positive or negative resistances, depending on whether their postsynaptic action is excitatory or inhibitory (Poggio and Koch, 1985).

Electrical Synapses

Biophysical Mechanism. Interaction between neurons mediated by electrical coupling is a common feature of the nervous system in both invertebrates and vertebrates, including mammals (Bennett, 1977; Korn and Faber, 1979). Effective electrical coupling between cells is achieved through specialized low-resistance connections—the gap or electrotonic junction. A gap junction consists of two closely apposed membranes of adjacent cells, with the two membranes separated by a 2–4 nm space or gap. The junction itself allows the passage of ions or small molecules (of roughly 300–1500 D). Usually, gap junctions can be represented by an electrical resistance constant over a range of ±25 mV (Bennett, 1977). Note that because of different values of the input resistances on the two sides of the junction, this does not necessarily imply symmetrical propagation of impulses. Gap junctions can be strongly unidirectional or rectifying. In their study of electrical transmission at the giant motor nerve synapse of the crayfish, Furshpan and Potter (1959) showed that with small potentials across the junction, conductance was rather symmetric, but with potentials exceeding a few millivolts it was markedly nonlinear and asymmetric (Figure 5). It has been possible to demonstrate that junctional permeability can be reversibly modulated by intra-cellular pH (Spray et al., 1981), by voltage across the junction (Harris et al., 1983), and, possibly of great functional consequence, by inhibitory synapses (Spira and Bennett, 1972).

   An important difference in comparison to chemically mediated synapses is the lack of a substantial delay between the "presynaptic" depolarization and the "postsynaptic" response, usually averaging about 0.25 msec at chemical synapses in warm-blooded animals.

Neuronal Operation.   Electrical synapses correspond to reciprocal one-ports in the sense of Brayton and Moser (1964). Varying the potential on one side of an electrical junction leads to a change in the potential at the other side of the junction. Many electrical synapses can be described over a large voltage range by a constant, positive resistance. Thus, different from chemical synapses, they serve to couple cells electrically with little delay. Some electrical synapses behave

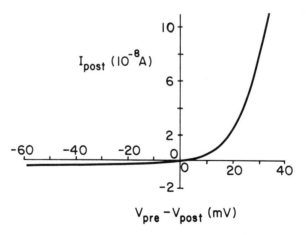

Figure 5.   *Current–voltage relationship of an electrical rectifying junction in the crayfish giant motor nerve synapse. Such a synapse mimics a diode. (Modified from Furshpan and Potter, 1959.)*

like a typical rectifier device, implementing the biological analog of a diode. Moreover, they serve to synchronize the firing of nearby cells. An instance of such an operation is cardiac muscle cells, which are electrically coupled in an electrical syncytium (Torre, 1976).

An Example of a Computation. In the vertebrate retina, cone photoreceptors of the same spectral sensitivity have been shown to be electrically coupled via nonrectifying gap junctions, as have the rods and horizontal cells of teleosts and turtles (Copenhagen and Owen, 1976; Kaneko, 1976; Detwiler and Hodgkin, 1979; Attwell and Wilson, 1980; Torre and Owen, 1983). It can be shown that when the membrane impedance of the photoreceptors can be linearized to a satisfactory approximation, analytical solutions to the network equations can be found that describe the dynamics of the response of any given cell to a variety of one- or two-dimensional visual stimuli (Torre et al., 1983). Such an analysis seems of particular importance when one realizes that under conditions of dark adaptation, for instance at night, the rod response to the absorption of single photons lies well within the linear response range of the cell. As a result of their analysis, Torre et al. suggest, following an idea of Hodgkin, that one functional role of coupling is to enhance the detection of signals. In particular, the signal-to-noise ratio decreases for small spots of light, resulting, for instance, from the random capture of photons, while the ratio increases for diffuse or long, narrow patterns of light. Moreover, the coupling may serve to avoid aliasing because of the discrete sampling lattice of the photoreceptors. The Shannon sampling theorem (Shannon and Weaver, 1949) requires the spatial frequencies in the image to be below a critical frequency in order for perfect reconstruction to occur subsequent to the sampling process. If higher frequencies are present, aliasing occurs, degrading the effective spatial resolution. Since the coupling can be equated with low-pass filtering of the image falling upon the retina prior to sampling, it may help to reduce aliasing (Poggio et al. 1982; Torre et al., 1983).

Interaction Between Synaptic Inputs

When two neighboring regions of a dendritic tree undergo simultaneous conductance changes—induced by synaptic inputs—the resulting postsynaptic potential is in general not the sum of the potentials generated by each synapse alone. The postsynaptic potential induced by one synapse will propagate to the other synaptic site and change the driving potential at that location, that is, the difference between the current postsynaptic potential and the reversal potential of the synapse. Thus, a different amount of current flows as a result of the "interfering" synapse nearby, allowing for the possibility that synapses situated "close" to each other may interact in a highly nonlinear way. We briefly examine two different cases: the synaptic interaction between synapses of the same sign and the interaction between excitatory and inhibitory synapses.

Biophysical Mechanism. *Nonlinear Saturation.* Let us consider an excitatory synapse that modulates the conductance g to a particular ion with an associated reversal potential $E > 0$ (relative to E_{rest}). In the steady-state case, the change in somatic potential is given by

$$V_s = \frac{g\tilde{K}_{is}E}{1 + g\tilde{K}_{ii}} ,$$

where $\tilde{K}_{is}$ is the steady-state transfer impedance between the location i and the soma, and $\tilde{K}_{ii}$ is the input impedance at location i. For small values of g, V_s is proportional to $g\tilde{K}_{is}E$, and for very large values of g, V_s saturates at $\tilde{K}_{is}E/\tilde{K}_{ii}$. This value therefore represents—under the assumption of a passive membrane— the maximal somatic depolarization evoked by a single synapse. We will now assume that the same synaptic input is spread among N identical synapses (each one with a conductance change g/N). Each one of the synaptic sites has about the same input impedance $\tilde{K}_{ii}$, the same transfer resistance to the soma $\tilde{K}_{is}$, and the same transfer resistance $\tilde{K}_{ij}$ between synaptic sites i and j. Taking account of the nonlinear interaction between the different synaptic inputs, it can be shown (Koch et al., 1982) that the combined change in somatic potential is

$$V_s = \frac{g\tilde{K}_{is}E}{1 + g\overline{K}_{ii}} ,$$

where $\overline{K}_{ii} = [\tilde{K}_{ii} + (N - 1)\tilde{K}_{ij}]/N$ (in other words, the more the synapses are de- coupled, that is, $\tilde{K}_{ij} \to 0$, the smaller $\overline{K}_{ii}$). Spreading the same conductance change among N at least partially decoupled sites enhances the maximal evoked somatic depolarization by a factor $\tilde{K}_{ii}/\overline{K}_{ii}$ (Koch et al., 1982). In the limit of N totally decoupled synapses, for instance on dendritic spines, this factor converges to one.

Nonlinear Interaction. Let us consider the nonlinear interaction in a passive dendritic tree between an excitatory synapse at location e with an associated conductance change $g_e(t)$ and reversal potential E, and an inhibitory synapse at i that increases the membrane conductance by $g_i(t)$ to an ionic species having an equilibrium potential close to the resting potential of the cell, $I = V_{rest} = 0$ (*silent or shunting inhibition;* Poggio and Torre, 1978; Torre and Poggio, 1978). Activating silent inhibition is similar to opening a hole in the membrane: Its effect is noticed only if excitatory input is present. The resulting somatic potential is given by a system of Volterra integral equations:

$$V_s(t) = \{g_e(t)(E - V_e(t))\} * K_{es}(t) - \{g_i(t)V_i(t)\} * K_{is}(t)$$

$$V_e(t) = \{g_e(t)(E - V_e(t))\} * K_{ee}(t) - \{g_i(t)V_i(t)\} * K_{ie}(t)$$

$$V_i(t) = \{g_e(t)(E - V_e(t))\} * K_{ei}(t) - \{g_i(t)V_i(t)\} * K_{ii}(t)$$

where $K_{ij}(t)$ is the Green function of the system, that is, the voltage response in time at location j if a δ pulse of current is injected at i. V_s, V_e, and V_i are the values of the membrane potential at the soma and at the excitatory and the inhibitory synapses, respectively. A simple measure of the effectiveness of silent inhibition is the ratio (F) between the maximum of somatic depolarization in the absence of inhibition and in the presence of inhibition. For steady-state conductance inputs, it is possible to prove rigorously that for passive and branched trees without loops, the most effective location for inhibition is always on the direct path between the location of the excitatory synapse and the soma (Koch, 1982; Koch et al., 1982). Rall observed earlier that in a single unbranched cable, silent inhibition effectively vetoes more distal excitation but not more proximal excitation (Rall, 1964).

Detailed biophysical simulations of highly branched neurons (under the assumption of passive membrane properties) show that this on-the-path condition is quite specific: If the amplitude of the inhibitory conductance change is above a critical value (50 nS or larger), F values can be quite high ($\approx$ 2–8) even when the excitatory inputs are much larger than the inhibitory ones, as long as the inhibition is between the excitatory synapse and the soma (Figure 6). Inhibition behind excitation or on a neighboring branch 10 μm or 20 μm off the direct path is ineffective in reducing excitation significantly. If the amplitude of the inhibitory conductance change is too small, the strength of the interaction depends mainly on the distance between the two sites, and F values are very low. When the inhibition is not of the silent type, that is, $I < V_{rest}$, inhibition at the soma is consistently more efficient (for more details, see Koch et al., 1982). This specificity carries over into the temporal domain. Silent inhibition must be activated shortly before or following the onset of excitation in order to veto excitation effectively (Figure 6; Koch et al., 1983; Segev and Parnas, 1983). In summary, the interaction between excitation and silent inhibition can be (1) strong, (2) specific with respect to the relative position of excitation and inhibition, and (3) tuned to their timing.

Our results hold also for the more unusual case of an input that decreases the membrane conductance for ions in equilibrium near the resting potential (see, for instance, Gerschenfeld and Paupardin-Trisch (1974), who provide evidence for a potassium-decreasing conductance in a molluscan neuron). In this case, the synaptic input facilitates the excitatory effect, thus implementing an analog approximation of a logical AND operation instead of the AND–NOT discussed previously (Koch et al., 1983).

Neuronal Operation. One operation implemented by synapses impinging upon the dendritic tree is a form of (nonlinear) addition. If the conductance change g is small in comparison with the input impedance $\tilde{K}_{ii}$ at that location ($g\tilde{K}_{ii} <$ 1), then the conductance change g can be approximated as current gE, and little interaction takes place between different synaptic inputs. This situation may easily occur if the synapse is located on the soma or a primary dendrite with their low input impedance $\tilde{K}_{ii}$. In these cases the addition will be linear. If the induced conductance change is large, synaptic saturation must be taken into account, and the resulting somatic potential is less than the sum of the individual contributions. The linear, nonsaturating operating range can be enhanced, however, by spreading the input among several at least partially decoupled sites, such as spines (see the section on dendritic spines below). Under these conditions, nonlinear saturation will be substantially reduced. Such linear addition most likely occurs in the morphological α- and β-cell classes of the cat retina, corresponding to Y- and X-cells, but not in the γ- and δ-cells (by exclusion identified with W-cells; Boycott and Wässle, 1974; Koch et al., 1982). It may also be used by bipolar cells to maintain a large dynamic range despite the high synaptic amplification at the photoreceptor synapse (Koch et al., 1986b).

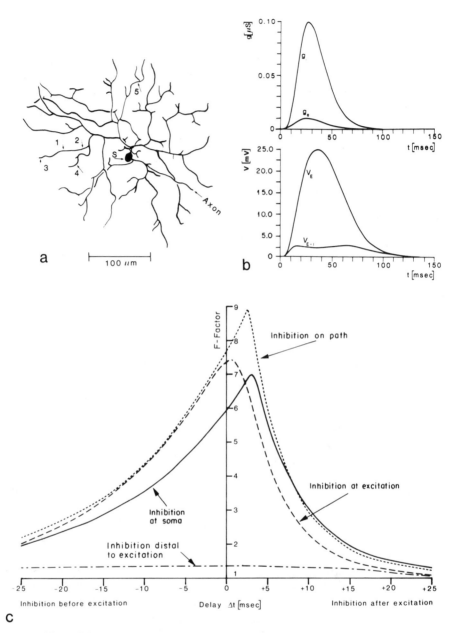

Figure 6. *Silent inhibition. a:* A cat retinal ganglion cell of the δ type (Boycott and Wässle, 1974). *b:* The depolarization in the soma of the δ cell for an excitatory conductance input g_e at location 1 and an inhibitory conductance input g_i at location 2. Both inputs have a rise time of 25 msec and decay to zero after about 90 msec. The location and the timing of inhibition are optimal (i.e., the inhibition is delayed by 2.5 msec). The excitatory battery is $E = 80$ mV and the inhibitory battery is $I = 0$ mV (relative to the resting potential). The corresponding somatic depolarization in the absence (V_E) and in the presence (V_{E+I}) of inhibition is also shown. Inhibition alone is "invisible" (because $I = 0$); its effect appears only when simultaneous excitation takes place, as expected from a multiplicationlike interaction. *c:* F factor (ratio of the maximum of the somatic depolarization without inhibition to the somatic depolarization with inhibition) for various locations of excitation and inhibition (as indicated in *a*) as a function of the relative timing. (From Koch et al., 1983.)

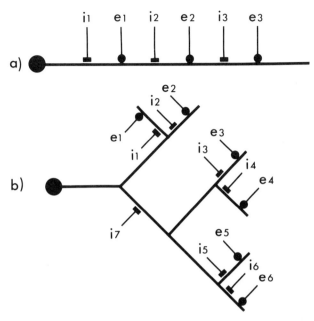

Figure 7. *Analog veto operation. a:* An idealized dendrite of a cat retinal ganglion cell of the γ type (Boycott and Wässle, 1974), receiving excitatory *(circles)* and inhibitory *(rectangles)* inputs of the silent or shunting type. Any inhibitory input can effectively veto only more distal excitation and does not affect other inputs more proximal to the soma. If the operation is described by an analog form of a digital AND–NOT gate, the operation "implemented" by the cell reads as [e_3 AND–NOT (i_1 OR i_2 OR i_3)] OR [e_2 AND–NOT (i_1 OR i_2) OR (e_1 AND–NOT i_1)]. *b:* An idealized dendrite of a δ cell (see also Figure 6a) with excitatory and inhibitory synapses of the silent type. Each inhibitory input (i_1–i_6) vetoes only the corresponding excitation (e_1–e_6) because it satisfies the on-the-oath condition. The operation implemented by this cell is (e_1 AND–NOT i_1) OR (e_2 AND–NOT i_2) OR {[(e_3 AND–NOT i_3) OR (e_4 AND–NOT i_4) OR (e_5 AND–NOT i_5) OR (e_6 AND–NOT i_6)] AND–NOT i_7}. (From Koch et al., 1982.)

The nonlinear interaction between an excitatory synapse and a silent inhibitory synapse implements an analog veto operation, functionally similar to a logical AND–NOT gate. (Note that AND–NOT is different from NAND.) Because of the strength and specificity of the veto operation, it may perform characteristic information processing operations in passive dendritic trees. Since inhibition vetoes more distal excitatory inputs only when it is near the excitatory synapse or on the direct path to the soma, a variety of local operations can be synthesized, exploiting the topology of the dendritic tree. Figure 7 shows a highly idealized picture of such "logical" operations implemented within a dendritic tree. Clearly, only certain types of logical operations can be carried out in a given dendritic topology. A cautionary note is in order here: This representation is primarily a convenient way of emphasizing some analogies between neuronal and logical information processing, while neglecting their substantial differences.

This behavior contrasts with the action obtained from a hyperpolarizing inhibitory synapse. In this case, the interaction between excitation and inhibition will be much more linear, that is, the inhibitory synapse will reduce the excitatory postsynaptic potential (EPSP) generated by the excitatory synapse by an amount roughly proportional to the inhibitory conductance change. Thus, hyperpolarizing inhibition is much less specific than silent inhibition, since neighboring excitatory synapses will be substantially inhibited even if the hyperpolarizing inhibitory synapse is not on the direct path between excitation and the soma (O'Donnell et al., 1985).

The predominant inhibitory neurotransmitter in the central nervous system appears to be γ-aminobutyric acid (GABA). GABAergic synapses are generally thought to operate via the classical, bicuculline-sensitive $GABA_A$ postsynaptic receptor by increasing chloride conductance (Curtis and Johnston, 1974; Ben-Ari et al., 1981; Dunlap, 1981; Segal and Barker, 1984). The resultant inhibitory postsynaptic potential does not markedly hyperpolarize the cell, since the equilibrium potential for chloride is generally close to the resting membrane potential of the cell (between −60 and −75 mV). Thus, activation of the $GABA_A$ receptor mediates silent inhibition. A different GABAergic effect has been described that acts via a distinctly different type of postsynaptic receptor, the $GABA_B$ receptor (Bowery et al., 1981; Simmonds, 1983; Newberry and Nicoll, 1984, 1985). This receptor binds the GABA agonist baclofen but is bicuculline-resistant. Newberry and Nicoll (1984, 1985) describe such a receptor on hippocampal cells, arguing that the receptors control potassium channels. Since the equilibrium potential for potassium (roughly −90 mV) is much more negative than the cell's resting potential, the activation of $GABA_B$ receptors results in significant hyperpolarization. Furthermore, little change in the cell's input resistance is seen during the GABAergic response. Thus, $GABA_A$ receptors will act in a local, highly nonlinear manner on the postsynaptic target cell, while $GABA_B$ receptors will subtract from the electrical activity throughout large portions of the postsynaptic cell (O'Donnell et al., 1985). In the more unusual case of the postsynaptic conductance decreasing in response to the neurotransmitter, this mechanism implements an analog form of a digital AND gate (see, for instance, Schulman and Weight, 1976).

Three Examples of Computations. *Computing the Direction of Motion in Retinal Cells.* Many neurons in both the retina and the visual cortex exhibit the property of direction selectivity; they respond maximally to stimuli moving in a particular (the preferred) direction and minimally to stimuli moving in the opposite (or null) direction (Figure 8A–C; Hassenstein and Reichardt, 1956; Hubel and Wiesel, 1959; Lettvin et al., 1959; Barlow and Levick, 1965; Oyster and Barlow, 1967; Cleland and Levick, 1974; Marchiafava, 1979; Jensen and DeVoe, 1983). Preferred and null directions are in general not predictable from the map of the receptive field nor can they be inferred from the global dendritic morphology of the direction selective cell (Amthor et al., 1984). Instead, direction selectivity has been postulated to be generated by asymmetries in the ganglion cell synaptic input (Torre and Poggio, 1978; Koch et al., 1982, 1986b).

The seminal work of Barlow and Levick (1965) implied that inhibition is crucial for direction selectivity: For motion in the null direction, excitatory inputs are vetoed by inhibitory inputs originating in adjacent regions of the dendritic tree. As shown by Barlow and Levick (Figure 8B; see also Wyatt and Daw, 1975), this veto operation must take place within small independent subunits contained within the receptive field that are extensively replicated. The neuronal substrate

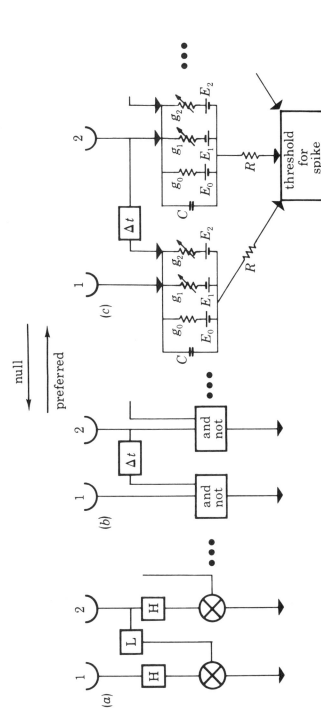

Figure 8. *Movement detection. a:* Part of the model of of Hassenstein and Reichardt (1956). The two inputs are multiplied after low-pass filtering with different time constants. If an average operation is made on the output, the overall operation is equivalent to cross-correlation of the two inputs. *b:* The scheme proposed by Barlow and Levick (1965) to account for direction selectivity of ganglion cells in the rabbit retina. A pure delay Δt is not really necessary: A low-pass filtering operation is sufficient (inhibition needs only to last longer than excitation). *c:* The equivalent electrical circuit of the synaptic interaction assumed to underlie direction selectivity, as proposed by Torre and Poggio (1978). The interaction implemented by the circuit is of the type $g_1 - \alpha g_1 g_2$. The ionic battery of the inhibitory input g_2 is assumed to be near the resting potential of the cell. (From Torre and Poggio, 1978.)

for this inhibition is likely to be GABA, since the application of picrotoxin, a GABA antagonist, abolishes direction selectivity: the ganglion cells respond equally well in both the preferred and the null directions (Caldwell et al., 1978; Ariel and Daw, 1982). Torre and Poggio (1978; see also Torre and Poggio, 1981) proposed that the nonlinear postsynaptic interaction between excitation and silent inhibition underlies this behavior. Direction selectivity is achieved by asymmetric delay (and/or low-pass properties) in the excitatory and inhibitory channels from the photoreceptors to the ganglion cell. Since the nonlinearity of interaction is an essential requirement of this scheme, Torre and Poggio suggested that the optimal location for excitation and inhibition is on distal fine dendrites, where the input impedance $\hat{K}_{ii}$ is expected to be high (Figure 8C).

If direction selectivity is based on a nonlinear interaction between excitation and inhibition, three alternative, but nonexclusive, retinal circuitries are compatible with current anatomical and electrophysiological evidence (Koch et al., 1986b). (1) Direction selectivity can be mediated by GABAergic amacrine cells inhibiting excitatory bipolar cells in an asymmetric manner; (2) excitatory bipolar (or amacrine) cells in conjunction with GABAergic amacrine cells can interact in a direction-selective manner at the level of the cholinergic amacrine cell; or (3) finally, GABAergic amacrine cells can interact nonlinearly with the cholinergic amacrine cell at the level of the ganglion cell. These three models can be roughly classified into two groups, according to whether the crucial nonlinear operation occurs before or at the level of the ganglion cell.

Postsynaptic Models.   Detailed biophysical simulations of cat retinal ganglion cells, with their highly branched dendritic trees, suggest that the AND–NOT mechanism is compatible with the available data about direction selectivity (Koch et al., 1982, 1983, 1986b; Mistler et al., 1985). In particular, intracellular recordings from turtle and frog direction-selective ganglion cells support activation of a silent inhibition in the null direction (Marchiafava, 1979; Watanabe and Murakami, 1984). This inhibition effectively and specifically shunts excitation as long as it is localized near excitation or between excitation and the soma. Since such a precise mapping (Figure 7) imposes a stringent requirement onto the specificity of the positioning of synapses during development, one particularly simple rule to follow is that a pair of excitatory and inhibitory inputs always contact the ganglion cell close to each other. Computer simulations show that if excitation and inhibition are located very close to each other (i.e., within a few micrometers), inhibition will effectively veto excitation (for g_e and $g_i \rightarrow \infty$, $F \rightarrow g_i/g_e + 1$; Koch et al., 1982). The direction of stimulus motion may thus be computed at many sites in the dendritic tree, independent of the threshold mechanism in the soma. On the basis of its nonlinear behavior and its highly branched dendritic architecture, Koch et al. (1982) conjectured that a δ-like cell morphology (in the cat; Boycott and Wässle, 1974) represents an ideal substratum for direction selectivity (Figure 6a).

Recently, Amthor and his colleagues stained physiologically identified on–off direction-selective cells in the rabbit retina with intracellular injections of horseradish peroxidase (HRP) (Amthor et al., 1983a, 1984). Their successfully stained cells always show a complex bistratified dendritic tree (Figure 9). These cells have extremely thin dendrites that carry spines or spinelike appendages;

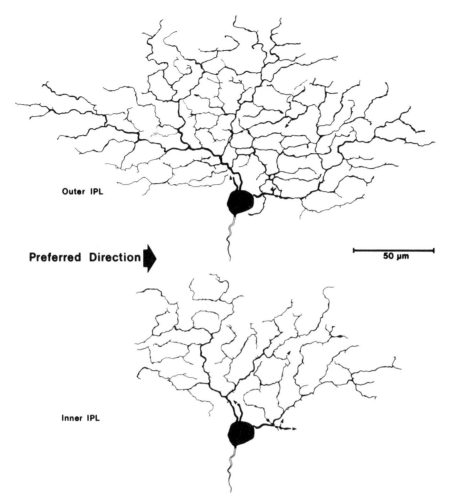

Figure 9. *Camera lucida drawing of an HRP-injected on–off direction-selective cell in the visual streak of the rabbit retina.* The dendritic fields have been drawn in two parts: "Outer" refers to the dendritic layer closest to the inner nuclear layer, while "inner" is the layer closest to the ganglion cell layer. (Modified from Amthor et al., 1984.)

a rather puzzling feature is the presence of apparent "loops" created by retroflexive branching within the dendritic fields. These loops seem to be a unique feature of direction-selective cells in the visual streak, for cells with such apparent loops have not been reported to occur in the less highly branched bistratified ganglion cells of the same type in the retinal periphery (Famiglietti, 1984). It is therefore doubtful that the loops are actually electrically closed structures. The cells studied by Amthor et al. (1984) appears to meet the requirement for numerous local nonlinear interaction sites, as postulated by Torre and Poggio (1978) and Koch et al. (1983). These distributed AND–NOT-like gates would compute direction selectivity throughout the dendritic tree, prior to somatic integration and impulse generation. Recent intracellular recordings in on–off direction-selective ganglion cells in the frog retina implicate such a postsynaptic interaction as being responsible for the direction-selective response (Watanabe and Murakami, 1984). The excitatory input in this model is likely to derive from motion-sensitive cholinergic "starburst" amacrine cells (see below), while inhibition could possibly be mediated by the γ-aminobutyric acid (GABA)-releasing population of transient on–off amacrine cells (Miller et al., 1977; Miller, 1979; Dowling, 1979; Vaughn et al., 1981).

Presynaptic Models.   An alternative to the postsynaptic models for direction se-lectivity in the rabbit is the hypothesis that the necessary computations occur prior to the ganglion cells. Although Werblin (1970) failed to record direction-selective responses in any neurons presynaptic to ganglion cells (see also Mar-chiafava, 1979), this possibility cannot be ruled out, especially if the large number of different amacrine cell classes is taken into consideration. Indeed, DeVoe and his collaborators (Criswell and DeVoe, 1984; DeVoe et al., 1985) have recorded from direction-selective amacrine and bipolar cells in the retina of the turtle. One candidate for the locus of the neuronal operation underlying direction selectivity is the so-called "starburst" amacrine cell, believed to provide the cholinergic input to direction-selective cells (Masland, 1980; Famiglietti, 1981, 1983b; Masland et al., 1984). Masland and his colleagues showed that these cells release acetylcholine (ACh) transiently at the on- or off-set of light. Starburst amacrine cells (Figure 10), thought to be nonspiking, have dendrites that are probably decoupled from each other and the soma (Miller and Bloomfield, 1983). Only the distalmost portion of the dendrites gives rise to conventional chemical synaptic output, while the bipolar and amacrine cell input is distributed throughout the cell (Famiglietti, 1983a). Since each dendrite may act essentially as an in-

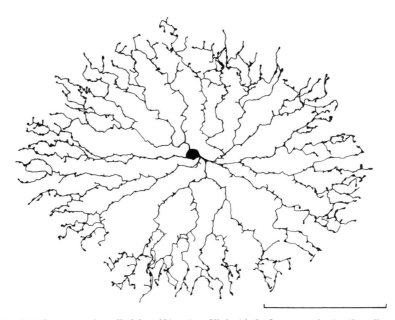

Figure 10.   *A starburst amacrine cell of the rabbit retina, filled with the fluorescent dye Lucifer yellow.* These cells release acetylcholine (ACh) transiently at the on- or off-set of the light stimulus. Calibration bar = 100 μm. (Modified from Tauchi and Masland, 1984.)

dependent subunit, it could be the morphological basis of Barlow's and Levick's subunits (1965).

Moreover, GABA appears to modulate the release of ACh (Massey and Neal, 1979), favoring the scheme whereby an excitatory (bipolar) input in conjunction with the GABAergic input implements an AND–NOT-like gate at the level of the starburst amacrine cell dendrites, whose output would then be direction selective itself. One would then predict that the application of an ACh potentiator should have little effect on the direction-selective response of the ganglion cell. Physostigmine, an acetylcholinesterase inhibitor, does, however, eliminate direction specificity, supporting the postsynaptic model (Ariel and Daw, 1982). A second class of presynaptic models postulates a hyperpolarizing inhibition vetoing excitation in the null direction. Because of the rectifying properties of the amacrine–ganglion cell synapse, this circuit is functionally equivalent to an AND–NOT gate. Although both presynaptic models are superficially rather similar, they correspond to different computations. Yet another possibility for the cellular site of direction selectivity is bipolar cells (DeVoe et al., 1985), though their dendritic trees may not be able to support complex information processing. Electron microscope immunocytochemical localization of glutamic acid decarboxylase (GAD)-positive synapses in rat retina indicates that there are GABAergic inputs to bipolar, amacrine, and ganglion cell processes in descending order of frequency (Vaughn et al., 1981), a result which is consistent with both the pre- and the postsynaptic models.

We emphasize that all models of direction selectivity that rely on the nonlinear interaction between excitation and inhibition to discriminate between different directions require a precise positioning of the different types of synapses (Swindale, 1983). The partial electron microscope reconstruction of a cat α-ganglion cell (Freed and Sterling, 1983), supports the notion that such precision is, at least for one type of excitatory input, biologically feasible. Although direction selectivity in the retina will probably represent the first critical test for the AND–NOT scheme, the proposed mechanism might play a role in other neurons of the central nervous system. In fact, the nonlinear synaptic interaction, perhaps augmented by membrane nonlinearities such as dendritic spikes evoked by EPSPs for a stimulus moving in the preferred direction, may also be responsible for computing the direction of motion in visual cortex neurons of the cat and primates, as well as underlying orientation selectivity in some cortical neurons (Emerson et al., 1984; Koch and Poggio, 1984). The idea that a vetolike operation may play an important role for computations in the central nervous system is not new, though its specific synaptic nature and properties are. Barlow has stressed before (e.g., Barlow, 1981) that a vetolike operation may be an important physiological mechanism for the retinal and cortical processes that underlie perception. Finally, it has recently been proposed that the synaptic veto mechanism underlies the direction-selective response of cells in the somatosensory cortex of the awake monkey when wheels with surface gratings are rolled over their skin (Warren et al., 1986).

Computing Relative Motion in the Fly.   It has been known for some time that the housefly can discriminate relative movement of an object and its background, even when the two have identical textures (Virsik and Reichardt, 1976). The ability to discriminate objects in front of a distant background in terms of the relative velocity induced by motion is probably of particular importance to fast-flying insects that cannot rely on binocular vision. Combining behavioral and electrophysiological experiments, Reichardt and his colleagues analyzed the optomotor response as a function of the spatial extent of motion and the velocity, contrast, and spatial structure of the image. They proposed the basic structure of a neuronal circuitry underlying the detection of motion discontinuities, relating it to known properties of cells in the third optic ganglion of flies (Reichardt and Poggio, 1979; Reichardt et al., 1983). A critical component of the model is the presynaptic action of silent inhibition on the output of the individual elementary movement detectors. This circuitry acts as gain control, making the optomotor response independent from the angular extent of the moving or oscillating figure, a well-established phenomenon (Reichardt et al., 1983).

Computing Disparity in Cortical Cells.   Studies in the alert monkey demonstrated that a large number of neurons in primary visual cortex (area V1) and an even higher proportion in prestriate cortex (area V2) are sensitive to horizontal binocular disparities (Barlow et al., 1967). Two main classes of stereoscopic neurons have been recognized (Poggio and Fischer, 1977; Poggio and Talbot, 1981): (1) cells that are selective for a very limited range of disparities, showing excitatory binocular facilitation (tuned excitatory neurons), or less frequently, inhibitory interaction (tuned inhibitory neurons); and (2) cells that are tuned either to disparities corresponding to objects in front of the fixation plane (NEAR neurons), or those corresponding to objects behind the plane of fixation (FAR neurons). These early studies used isolated line and bar stimuli in the visual field. Thus, there is no possibility of making an incorrect correspondence between elements in the left and the right image. Poggio (1980, 1984c) recently showed that roughly one fifth of all the cells whose depth sensitivity was examined responded to isolated lines as well as to random dot patterns, in which abundant ambiguous matches occur. Interestingly, all of these cells were of the complex type. Thus, these neurons "solve" the correspondence problem of stereopsis (Poggio and Poggio, 1984).

On the basis of the synaptic veto operation, we devised, together with Keith Nishihara, cellular models to account for the different types of disparity selectivity. Figure 11 shows two models for both excitatory and inhibitory neurons tuned to zero disparities, using edges as primitives. The synaptic input converging onto one dendritic branch and originating from the two eyes should have very similar receptive fields. Note that the synaptic inputs to this cell always originate in cells with monocular receptive fields. The excitatory, tuned, disparity-sensitive cell responds to an edge only if one eye signals ON activity and the other does not signal OFF activity for the same location, while the inhibitory cell always fires except if both eyes signal ON (or OFF) activity. The optimal disparity of these cells can be changed by varying the spatial offset between the receptive fields in the left and the right eyes. The processing occurs in many independent subunits throughout the dendritic field of these neurons, using the AND–NOT synaptic veto mechanism. This particular model seems consistent with Ferster's "multiplication" data concerning the synergistic interaction between the two eyes (Ferster, 1981). Because ON activity in one eye vetoes the EPSP evoked by

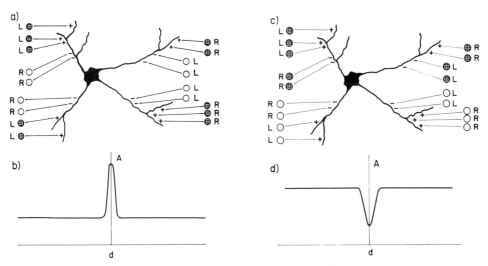

Figure 11. *Schematic drawings of two cortical cells excited (a) and inhibited (c) by a given disparity.* The excitatory, tuned, disparity-sensitive cell responds to an edge only if one eye signals ON activity (*clear circles*) while the other eye does not signal OFF activity (*hatched circles*) for the same location; the inhibitory tuned cell always fires except when both eyes signal ON (or OFF) activity. The disparity these cells optimally react to can be changed by varying the spatial offset between the monocular receptive fields in the left and right eyes. *b* and *d*: The expected response of the cell to different disparities is indicated.

OFF activity in the other eye, we predict that in an experiment using the pharmacological agent D,L-2-amino-4-phosphonobutyric acid (APB) to block the ON channel (Schiller, 1982), the excitatory tuned cell will lose its sensitivity to disparity. On the other hand, the inhibitory tuned disparity cell will continue to react to its tuned disparity in the presence of APB, although the signal-to-noise level will be decreased. Similar models, using AND–NOT and AND-like "synaptic logic," can be devised for NEAR and FAR disparity-sensitive neurons.

Finally, the synaptic veto operation can be used to compute locally some simple property in many subunits throughout the dendritic tree of a cortical cell, combining the result in a disjunctive manner at the soma. Thus, simple properties can be combined to yield a cell with a more complex receptive field.

DENDRITIC SPINES

Dendritic spines were originally discovered by Ramón y Cajal. Their existence was confirmed by Gray through electron microscopy (Gray, 1959). A spine usually consists of a thin and slender spine neck and a more bulbous spine head (Figure 12). Most important, every spine head has at least one synapse on its surface. These synapses are usually of the Gray type I and are therefore likely to be excitatory. Most neurons in the central nervous system can be classified as either spinous or aspinous. In the former case, the majority of excitatory inputs can be seen to be localized on spines. Examples of this cell type are pyramidal and stellate cells in the cerebral cortex and Purkinje cells in the cerebellum (Shepherd, 1979b).

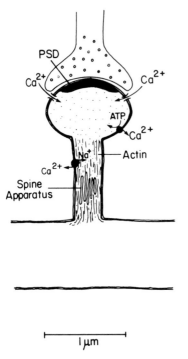

Figure 12. *A schematic drawing of a typcial dendritic spine in the mammalian cortex with some of its constituent elements.* The postsynaptic density (PSD) directly below the presynaptic terminal is a clump of electron-dense material made up of neurofilaments, actin, fodrin, tubulin, calmodulin, a microtubule-associated protein, and other proteins. The spine apparatus consists of two or three membrane-bound sacs alternating with thin laminae of dense material. Also shown are the proposed voltage-dependent calcium channels, the sodium-calcium exchange pump, and the ATP-driven calcium pump. The scale is only approximate. (From Robinson and Koch, 1984a.)

Biophysical Mechanism. *Dependence of the Synaptic Weight of a Spine on Its Geometry.* Since the synaptically injected current must pass through the relatively thin spine neck in order to reach the soma (Chang, 1952), the synaptic "weight" of the synapse is expected to depend strongly on the geometry of the spine. To study this effect, Koch and Poggio (1983a,b) modeled dendritic spines using one-dimensional cable theory. The spines are described by a thin cylinder of length l and diameter d and a thick, short spine head. The main assumption in this analysis is that the membrane is passive. Following the earlier studies of Rall (1974, 1978) it can be shown that the input resistance of a spine $\tilde{K}_{11}$ as seen by an imaginary electrode in the spine head is the sum of the input resistance in the dendrite just below the spine plus the resistance of the spine neck R_N: $\tilde{K}_{11} = \tilde{K}_{22} + R_N$.

R_N is simply the resistance of a cylinder, that is, $4R_i l/(\pi d^2)$. Thus, the spine input impedance depends strongly on the geometry of the spine neck. Since $\tilde{K}_{11}$ can be much higher than $\tilde{K}_{22}$ for small spine dimensions, current injected into the spine will produce a much larger local depolarization than if injected into the dendritic shaft. It turns out, however, that it is irrelevant from the point of view of somatic depolarization whether the current input is in the spine head or directly onto the dendritic stem next to the spine base. This is easy to understand. Since the membrane surface of the spine is minute ($\approx 1 \ \mu m^2$), essentially no current flows through the spine membrane (Koch and Poggio, 1983b). Thus, all the current injected into the spine head reaches the dendritic stem, or $\tilde{K}_{1s} = \tilde{K}_{2s}$, where $\tilde{K}_{1s}$ is the transfer impedance between the spine head and the soma, and $\tilde{K}_{2s}$ is the transfer impedance between the spine and the soma.

Because of their expected high input impedance, spines can show large saturation effects (Figure 13). Saturation occurs not only for stationary or slow, but also for very fast conductance changes (Koch and Poggio, 1983a; Perkel, 1983). Figure 14 shows the dependence of the somatic potential on the geometry of the spine neck. If the amplitude of the synaptic input is small with respect to the inverse of the spine neck impedance (i.e., if $R_N g < 1$), synaptic input can be considered as current and little of interest occurs. If, however, the synaptic input is large (i.e., $R_N g > 1$), significant saturation occurs, limiting the inflow of current into the spine. In this case, somatic depolarization induced by the synapse on the spine will depend strongly on spine morphology. The critical parameter determining the function of spines (for passive cable models) is thus the product of the spine neck resistance with the synaptic input rather than the spine input impedance (since both $\tilde{K}_{11}$ and $\tilde{K}_{22}$ can be quite large but R_N small; Turner, 1984). Unfortunately, little experimental data is available to bracket the size of these parameters. Kawato et al. (1984) estimated a peak conductance change of 43 nS and a time to peak of 0.3 msec for somatically recorded EPSPs in spiny rubrospinal neurons. Under these conditions, plausible changes in neck length could alter the "weight" of the synapse by a factor of two or three (Koch and Poggio, 1983b).

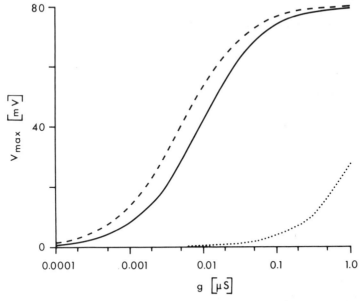

Figure 13. *The maximum of the depolarization in the distal apical tree of a cortical pyramidal cell, for a fast transient conductance input of peak amplitude g (with a time to peak of 0.25 msec and a total duration of 0.9 msec) of variable amplitude.* The *solid line* indicates the potential at a synapse located within a dendritic spine, while the *dotted line* indicates the depolarization for a synapse located just below the spine, directly on the dendritic shaft. The *dashed line* indictes that a steady-state conductance change yields essentially the same depolarization in the spine as the transient input. The membrane time constant is 8 msec. The spine membrane is assumed to be passive. (From Koch and Poggio, 1983a.)

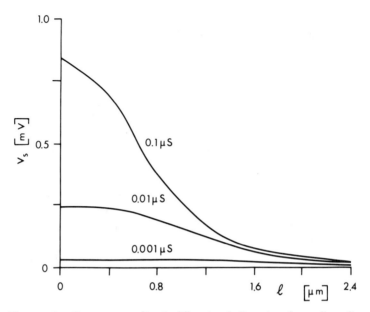

Figure 14. *The somatic voltage corresponding to different neck dimensions for small, medium, and large steady-state conductance inputs for a synapse located on a spine in the distal apical tree of a cortical pyramidal cell.* Fast transient inputs yield very similar curves for peak conductance values, except that the peak somatic depolarization is scaled down by about a factor of 10. The spine neck dimensions were changed in such a way as to leave the total neck surface constant and equal to $dl = 0.1$ μm^2. Plausible changes in neck length (for instance from 1.0 to 1.7 μm) could alter the "weight" of the synapse by a factor of two. (From Koch and Poggio, 1983a.)

Until now we have only considered the case of a passive spine membrane. However, if the number of active voltage-dependent channels in the spine head membrane is sufficient to trigger all-or-none impulses, the situation changes somewhat. Computer simulations show (Miller et al., 1985; Perkel and Perkel, 1985; Rall and Segev, this volume) that active, action potential-generating membrane nonlinearities in the spine head can produce amplification rather than attenuation of the postsynaptic potential. The presence and amount of amplification depend on the density of active channels and on the spine neck resistance. For a given spine head, there is an optimal range of spine neck resistances R_N that will lead to large EPSPs at the base of the spine. Outside of this range, the spine acts as a voltage attenuator.

Interaction Between Excitation and Inhibition. A significant exception to the rule that spines carry only excitatory synapses is spines that show both symmetrical and asymmetrical synaptic profiles, that is, excitation and inhibition, simultaneously. This situation occurs at about 5–15% of all cortical spines (Scheibel and Scheibel, 1968; Jones and Powell, 1969b; Peters and Kaiserman-Abramof, 1969, 1970; Sloper and Powell, 1979; Somogyi et al., 1983). Moreover, the retinal input to relay cells in the dorsal lateral geniculate nucleus (dLGN) of the cat of the physiological X-type terminates predominantly on dendritic appendages that always show a second, inhibitory, GABAergic synaptic terminal (Famiglietti and Peters, 1972; Hamori et al., 1974; Friedlander et al., 1981; Hamos et al., 1983)

The nonlinear interaction between an inhibitory conductance change, with a reversal potential close to V_{rest}, and an excitatory conductance change can be quite substantial and very specific, being essentially limited in its effect to the spine (Koch and Poggio, 1983a,b; Koch, 1985). Thus, if the amplitude of the inhibitory input is large enough ($g_i > 0.05 \cdot 10^{-6}$S and $g_i > g_e$), the depolarization evoked by the excitatory input is severely curtailed, dropping by a factor of five or more. Moreover, the potential at locations outside the spine is little affected by the inhibition. This is in accordance with the on-the-path principle (Koch et al., 1982). When transient inputs are considered, their relative timing is an important determinant for the degree of interaction. Figure 15 shows the "tuning curve" of the F factor (see the legend for Figure 6). As input functions we used fast transients with a time to peak of 0.25 msec and a total duration of about 1 msec. What is remarkable is that the vetoing effect of inhibition depends very sharply on relative timing between the two inputs. Whereas inhibition on the dendritic shaft can effectively veto excitation within a temporal window of the order of ±0.3 msec, inhibition on the spine is stronger and more selective, being effective only in a window of ±0.12 msec around the onset of excitation.

Activity-Dependent Change in Spine Shape.   It is well established that the form and shape of dendritic spines can vary following changes in environment and sensory input (see Purpura, 1974, for a study of mentally retarded children; Coss and Globus, 1978, for a study in goldfish; Bradley and Horn, 1979, for a study in

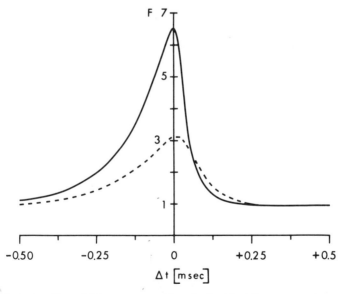

Figure 15. F factor (see Figure 6c) for synapses on the spine head (continuous curve) or on the dendritic shaft just below the spine (dashed line) in the distal apical tree of a cortical pyramidal cell. Both input functions have a time to peak of 0.25 msec and decay after 0.9 msec. Inhibition is 10 times stronger than excitation (see Figure 6b); that is $g_{i\ max} = 2 \times 10^{-7}$ S and $g_{e\ max} = 10^{-8}$ S. Inhibition on a spine is more powerful and specific than inhibition located on the dendritic shaft. (From Koch and Poggio, 1983.)

chicken; Boycott, 1982, for a study in hibernating ground squirrels; Brandon and Coss, 1982, for a study in bees). Stimulating briefly the afferents to hippocampal cells results in hypertrophy of the dendritic spines (Van Harreveld and Fifková, 1975; Fifková and Anderson, 1981; Fifková et al., 1982). The hippocampus is of particular interest, since it displays a prominent modification of synaptic efficiency termed long-term potentiation (LTP).

Free intracellular calcium is currently regarded as one of the key factors underlying certain forms of synaptic plasticity (e.g., in *Aplysia*, see Kandel, 1981; in mammalian hippocampus, see Baimbridge and Miller, 1981; Turner et al., 1982; Eccles, 1983). Preventing a rise in intracellular calcium concentration by injecting a calcium-chelating agent such as EGTA (Lynch et al., 1983) blocks the establishment of LTP. It is of interest that the spine apparatus, a unique organelle localized in the spine neck and consisting of two or more flattened sacs or cisternae, as well as the smooth endoplasmic reticulum inside the spine, has been shown to sequester calcium at high concentrations (Fifková et al., 1983). Once the concentration of intracellular calcium rises to substantial levels, the calcium can trigger a variety of mechanisms leading to a change in synaptic efficacy.

One such mechanism, possibly implementing a transient change in synaptic efficacy, has been proposed by Crick (1982). If contractile proteins, such as myosin and actin, were to be localized in the spine neck, they could lead to a rapid contraction of the neck, possibly within a fraction of a second. Functionally, this is equivalent to a rapid enhancement of the synaptic weight. Subsequently, different groups of researchers visualized actin in single neurons. While actin is present at all postsynaptic densities (PSDs), it concentrates in dendritic spines, where it is either organized in long filaments oriented parallel to the axis of the spine neck or extends throughout the spine head in a latticelike form (Fifková and Delay, 1982; Katsumaru et al., 1982; Matus et al., 1983; Fifková et al., 1984; for a review of actin in the nervous system, see Fifková, 1985).

A second mechanism, possibly underlying long-term synaptic modification, is based on the calcium-activated enzymes present in neuronal membranes, calpain I and II (for a summary see Eccles, 1983; Lynch and Baudry, 1984). In the presence of free calcium, this protease breaks up a localized portion of the subcellular fodrin network, irreversibly uncovering glutamate receptors (Siman et al., 1983). Since glutamate, or a closely related amino acid, most likely serves as transmitter in several hippocampal pathways, this uncovering will increase the postsynaptic conductance change $g(t)$ and thus the weight of the synapse. We would like to note, however, that for the unmasking of the receptors to increase the synaptic efficacy, two conditions must be met. First, the factor limiting the size of the postsynaptic conductance change must be the limiting number of postsynaptic receptors and not the amount of transmitter released by the presynaptic terminal. Second, the conductance change prior to the unmasking must be small in relation to the input impedance of the spine. If significant synaptic saturation occurs, increasing $g(t)$ will do little to increase the corresponding EPSP.

On the basis of computer simulations, Robinson and Koch (1984a,b; see also Gamble and Koch, 1987) modeled the dynamics of free calcium in dendritic spines. They assumed that presynaptic electrical activity induces, through the opening of aspartate or glutamate channels, a large depolarization in the spine head. The EPSP in turn activates voltage-dependent calcium channels, resulting in an influx of calcium into the spine. Such calcium channels are believed to exist in the dendritic arbors of *in vitro* Purkinje cells (Llinás and Hess, 1976; Llinás and Sugimori, 1980), olivary neurons (Llinás and Yarom, 1981), and *in vitro* thalamic neurons (Jahnsen and Llinás, 1984). The in-flowing calcium will be rapidly bound by high-affinity calcium buffers such as calmodulin and calcineurin, both of which have been localized in substantial amounts in the spine cytoplasm and PSD (Grab et al., 1980; Klee and Haiech, 1980; Wood et al., 1980). These buffers, together with the sodium–calcium exchange pump, the ATP-driven calcium pump, and the diffusion of calcium into the dendrites, keep intracellular calcium concentration low in response to moderate presynaptic activity. If, however, the presynaptic activity exceeds a critical amount, the calcium buffers will saturate. Since the volume of a dendritic spine is small, very few presynaptic spikes will be sufficient to drive the level of the calcium concentration from its resting value around 0.05 μM to values between 1.0 μM and 5.0 μM. As Robinson and Koch specifically point out, the optimal strategy to saturate the buffers are very closely timed spikes, that is, a burst of postsynaptic activity. As few as seven spikes in 20 msec can lead to micromolar levels of free intracellular calcium (Gamble and Koch, 1987).

The free intracellular calcium can now activate calpain I or II, leading to the irreversible uncovering of the glutamate receptors. Another possibility is the binding of calcium to calmodulin. Once calmodulin is fully activated, for which all four calcium sites must be occupied, it induces actin–myosin contractions (Klee and Haiech, 1980; Cheung, 1982). The time course of these contractions—and thus of synaptic enhancement—is governed by the rate at which calcium becomes unbound from the calmodulin, which in turn depends on intracellular calcium concentration. A hypothetical time course of calcium concentration and activated calmodulin for prolonged synaptic inputs is shown in Figure 16. Calmodulin will also interact strongly with another major cytoskeleton protein, fodrin or brain spectrin (Kakiuchi and Sobue, 1983), which is responsible for giving the neuronal membrane its rigidity. The strong binding of calmodulin directly to fodrin might cause a change in the fodrin–actin network such that loosening of the spine cytoskeleton occurs. Note that because of the fourth power relationship between the concentration of calcium and the concentration of the fully bound calcium/calmodulin complex, small increases in the former can lead to dramatic increases in the latter.

In brief, if calcium channels were to be found at the spine membrane, dendritic spines, because of their special geometry which limits the effects of diffusion and enhances local EPSPs, may implement a calcium-dependent modification in synaptic efficacy spanning different time scales. This mechanism itself is prone to modification, for instance, through voltage, giving rise to possible Hebb-like interactions between nearby spines. Cooperativity among afferents to CA1 cells in inducing and maintaining LTP has been reported (Lee, 1983).

Neuronal Operation.   Dendritic spines could be the morphological substrate for at least two different neuronal operations. First, they could serve as a locus for modifying the functional connectivity between individual neurons, changing synaptic weights within a fraction of a second (via actin–myosin contractions) to several days or even weeks (via structural changes in the cytoskeleton). It is likely that this synaptic modification is triggered by an activity-dependent calcium

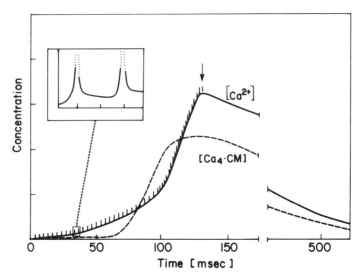

Figure 16. *Hypothetical time course of free intracellular calcium and of activated calmodulin in a dendritic*
spine during prolonged presynaptic activity (in this case at 300 Hz for 120 msec). The stimulus-induced
influx of calcium is buffered within a fraction of a millisecond. Each spike will, however, lead
to a small increase in intracellular calcium concentration and thus increase the fraction of calcium
bound to calmodulin (see *inset*). Once the presynaptic input ceases, both intracellular calcium
concentration and the activated calmodulin decay slowly, their time course being limited by
the low off-rate constants of the buffers (Klee and Haiech, 1980). A sudden increase in intracellular
calcium during and following repetitive presynaptic stimulation in hippocampal neurons has
been reported (Morris et al., 1983). Computer simulations, describing the time course of calcium
and the various calcium buffers in a three-compartment model as a function of presynaptic
activity, confirm such a behavior (Gamble and Koch, 1987; diagram from Robinson and Koch, 1984b).

influx. These mechanisms are crucially dependent on the potential buffering
abilities of the spine cytoplasm. The calcium buffers essentially act to delay the
onset of the synaptic enhancement and protect the system from noise induced
by spontaneous presynaptic activity. The change in functional connectivity is
primarily controlled by the amount and timing of the presynaptic input and
secondarily by postsynaptic electrical activity. In particular, if the proposed
calcium influx is mediated by voltage-dependent calcium channels, hyperpolarizing
the spine prevents these channels from opening, thus implementing a kind of
Hebbian rule (Hebb, 1948; Palm, 1982).

Second, the synthesis of a circuit consisting of an excitatory and an inhibitory
synapse localized onto the same spine may implement a localized AND–NOT
gate. Inhibition vetos excitation very efficiently as long as inhibition is activated
in a narrow temporal domain around the onset of excitation. Owing to the
particular geometry of the spine, inhibition will do little to influence the electrical
activity in the dendritic tree outside the spine. In other words, even though the
actual veto operation occurs at a postsynaptic site, it is functionally equivalent
to presynaptic inhibition.

Two Examples of Computations

Information Storage.   One obvious function of modifiable spines is information
storage over short and long time ranges (Rall, 1974, 1978; Jack et al., 1975; Koch

and Poggio, 1983a,b; Perkel, 1983; see especially Crick, 1982; Eccles, 1983; Lynch and Baudry, 1984). Differing from current digital computers, in which the memory resides in specialized hardware—usually kept separate from the logical processor—biological memory would be distributed throughout the information processing machinery, coded in the form of the strength of connectivity between the different computational machines. One instance of an experimentally well-known paradigm in which information could well be "stored" in dendritic spines is LTP in the mammalian hippocampus (for overviews, see Chung, 1977; Swanson et al., 1982). It is at the moment still unclear, however, how the actual storage and retrieval of information could take place.

Disabling Visual Input in the Lateral Geniculate Nucleus.   Recently, electron microscope studies of relay cells in the dLGN of the cat have shown that the retinal input to X-cells is associated with a particular synaptic circuitry, termed the spine triad complex (Famiglietti and Peters, 1972; Hamos et al., 1983, 1984; see also Wilson et al., 1984). The retinal afferent makes an asymmetrical synapse with both a dendritic appendage of the X-cell and a geniculate interneuron. The interneuron contacts in turn the same dendritic appendage with a symmetrical synaptic profile. Recent evidence shows that these geniculate interneurons stain for GAD, the synthesizing enzyme for GABA (Sterling and Davis, 1980; Fitzpatrick et al., 1984). The retinal input to geniculate Y-cells is predominantly found on dendritic shafts with no triadic arrangement.

On the basis of computer simulations of an anatomically reconstructed X-relay cell with a known somatic input resistance and time constant, Koch (1985) studied the effect of both types of GABAergic inhibition (i.e., $GABA_A$ and $GABA_B$) on the somatic potential of the neuron. Assuming that the geniculate interneuron mediates a silent inhibition, the retinal input to these cells can be vetoed very effectively within the dendritic appendage without depressing electrical activity in the rest of the cell. Evidence in favor of silent inhibition comes from the local application of bicuculline to cells in the cat's dLGN, resulting in a loss of inhibitory mechanisms in geniculate neurons (Sillito and Kemp, 1983; Berardi and Morrone, 1984). Moreover, inhibitory postsynaptic potentials (IPSPs) mediated by geniculate interneurons can easily be reversed by an injection of chloride into the cell (McIlwain and Creutzfeldt, 1967; Lindstrom, 1982). Since Y-cells lack the spine triad structure, inhibition in these cells will act globally, reducing and damping the general electrical activity of the cell.

Anatomical and electrophysiological evidence indicates that the geniculate interneurons receive an excitatory projection from the visual cortex (Jones and Powell, 1969a; Ahlsen et al., 1982) and inhibition from both the midbrain (Foote et al., 1977; Singer, 1977; Ahlsen et al., 1984) and the thalamic reticular nucleus (Guillery, 1969; Hamos et al., 1984; Wilson et al., 1984). Thus, Koch (1985) proposes that geniculate interneurons selectively gate the flow of visual information within the X-system, enhancing the center–surround antagonism of geniculate X-cells and possibly mediating reciprocal lateral inhibition and eye movement-related suppression in the movement-sensitive geniculate Y-cells (Noda, 1975). (Electrophysiological evidence in favor of a differential action of inhibition on geniculate X- and Y-cells can be found in Singer and Bedworth, 1973; Noda, 1975; Fukuda and Stone, 1976; Tsumoto and Suzuki, 1976; Foote et al., 1977; Bullier and Norton, 1979; Derrington and Fuchs, 1979; Berardi and Morrone, 1984.)

MEMBRANE NONLINEARITIES

Ever since Hodgkin and Huxley identified fast sodium and delayed rectifying potassium currents as the two major currents underlying the generation of action potentials, the total number of currents with widely different dependencies on voltage, time, and calcium has multiplied tremendously. What is the function of these currents in information processing? In the following, we focus on those currents that do not generate all-or-none impulses but modify the electrical behavior of the cell in different ways.

Quasi-Active Membranes

Biophysical Mechanism.   Usually, neuronal membranes are classified as either passive, that is, the voltage decays exponentially to zero, or as active, such as when the axonal membrane gives rise to action potentials. Between these two extremes, there is a range of membrane behavior we term quasi-active. Such a membrane still behaves linearly, that is, for instance, doubling the applied current doubles the voltage response, but it already shows oscillations. We define a membrane to be quasi-active if it shows band-passlike behavior, that is, if the membrane impedance has a prominent maximum at some nonzero frequency called the resonant frequency, f_{max} (see Figure 17). Such a membrane can always be modeled by an electrical circuit containing an inductance.

What are the biophysical mechanisms leading to such a behavior? An electrical component can be described on a phenomenological level by an inductance if its voltage is proportional to the current change. As Detwiler et al. (1980) pointed out, this situation arises for a time- and voltage-dependent potassium conductance activated by depolarization and inactivated by hyperpolarization. Examples are the currents mediated by potassium channels in the squid axon (Hodgkin and Huxley, 1952; Mauro et al., 1970), or by the calcium-dependent potassium current in sympathetic neurons and hair cells of the bullfrog (Adams et al., 1982; Lewis and Hudspeth, 1983). Alternatively, an inductance can mimic the small signal behavior of the sodium (or calcium) conductance inactivated by depolarization and activated by hyperpolarization, for instance the low-threshold calcium-mediated current in mammalian central nervous system neurons (Llinás and Yarom, 1981; Jahnsen and Llinás, 1984). For a small enough excursion of the voltage around a fixed potential $\overline{V}$, these channels can be described by a circuit similar to the one shown in Figure 19A.

The presence of an inductance can lead to resonant behavior, that is, the membrane impedance shows a maximum at f_{max}. A sinusoidal current of that frequency will therefore decay less than current with lower or higher frequency components, that is, the impedance will show band-passlike character (Figure 17). Thus, excitable membranes are capable of producing subthreshold oscillatory responses near 100 Hz when potassium and sodium carry the current (Hodgkin and Huxley, 1952; Mauro et al., 1970). The resonant frequency can be modulated

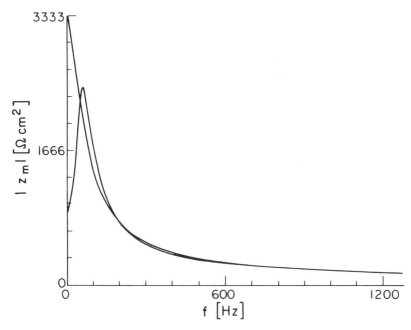

Figure 17. *The membrane impedance z_m for two types of membranes as a function of frequency.* Calculating the small signal impedance of a patch of squid axon membrane described by the Hodgkin–Huxley equations gives rise to the band-pass function, which peaks at 67 Hz. Reducing the channel density η to zero, leaving only the passive components, yields the monotonic decaying curve. Note that beyond 200 Hz the curves coincide. (From Koch, 1984.)

by the density η of active channels (Sabah and Leibovic, 1972; Koch, 1984a) and, perhaps less likely, by intracellular calcium concentration. It can be as low as 1 Hz, as in heart cell membrane (Clapham and DeFelice, 1982), or as high as several hundred hertz, as in the frog node of Ranvier (Clapham and DeFelice, 1976). Increasing η increases the degree of membrane excitability and the resonant frequency while decreasing the range of validity of the linear circuit approximation.

Neuronal Operation. Membranes showing quasi-active behavior within a given voltage range can implement at least two different operations. First, such membranes may act as an electrical resonant filter, preferentially responding to inputs within a certain frequency range. The value of the resonant frequency can be varied by modulating some of the parameters underlying excitability, such as the density of active channels or the level of free intracellular calcium (Ashmore, 1983; Koch, 1984). Second, quasi-active membranes may act as analog, temporal differentiators (Koch, 1984). Intuitively, this can be understood by noticing that differentiation is nothing but a high-pass filtering removing low frequencies. The differentiation of a function $f(t)$ corresponds to the multiplication of the Fourier transformed function with frequency, that is,

$$\frac{df(t)}{dt} \rightarrow iw\tilde{f}(w) \ .$$

If the frequency components above the resonant frequency are disregarded, the high-pass component of the membrane impedance can be approximated by $z_m(w) = a + bw$, with a and b positive constants and $b > a$. Injecting a current $I(t)$ containing little or no frequency components above f_{max} into a cable with a quasi-active membrane leads therefore to a change in potential

$$V(t) = aI(t) + b\frac{dI(t)}{dt}.$$

Figure 18 demonstrates such a case. The current $I(t)$ (Figure 18A) is injected into an infinite cylinder with a linearized Hodgkin–Huxley membrane (Hodgkin and Huxley, 1952). Figure 18B shows the analytical deriviate of $I(t)$, while in Figures 18C and D the "recorded" voltage change at two different locations in the cable is plotted. Such a situation may occur, for instance, in the photoreceptor of the fly. Its output process onto a lamina monopolar neuron does not generate spikes under physiological conditions. The visual evoked response in the post-synaptic neuron to a flash or to a step increase of light can be well approximated by the scaled derivative of the response of the photoreceptor as recorded in its soma (Hengstenberg, 1982). A third operation possibly implemented by quasi-active membranes is spatiotemporal filtering in visual neurons (Detwiler et al., 1978, 1980; Koch, 1984).

One Example of a Computation.   Individual sensory neurons, converting sound pressure or electrical fields into action potentials, have an optimal operating range in terms of the frequency of the input to which they are most sensitive. Such differential receptor tuning has been observed in hair cells of the cochlea in lower vertebrates (Crawford and Fettiplace, 1980, 1981a,b; Ashmore, 1983; Lewis and Hudspeth, 1983) or in fish electroreceptors thought to derive from hair cells (Hopkins, 1976; Meyer and Zakon, 1982). Hair cells, tonotopically organized along the basilar membrane in the cochlea according to their characteristic frequencies (the frequency of the sound stimuli the cell optimally responds to), reveal their electrical tuning by damped oscillations of the membrane potential induced by current injections. The frequency of the induced oscillations coincides with the characteristic frequency. In mammals, the basis of frequency discrimination is believed to be the mechanical traveling wave set up in the inner ear by the sound wave first described by von Békésy (1960). In some lower vertebrates, such as the turtle or the bullfrog, the tuning effect is believed to be an electrical resonance mechanism located in each hair cell (Crawford and Fettiplace, 1981a) and described by a circuit of the type shown in Figure 19A (Crawford and Fettiplace, 1981b).

The question of the ionic nature of the underlying mechanism has been investigated recently by Lewis and Hudspeth (1983) using the patch clamp whole-cell technique. They report the presence of three different voltage-dependent channels (calcium, potassium, and calcium-dependent potassium conductances), one or more of which is responsible for the tuning effect. In order to explain (1) the large range (70–700 Hz) of the characteristic frequency shown by hair cells and (2) the systematic variation of this frequency along the basilar membrane, it has been proposed that the nature of the individual channels remains invariant

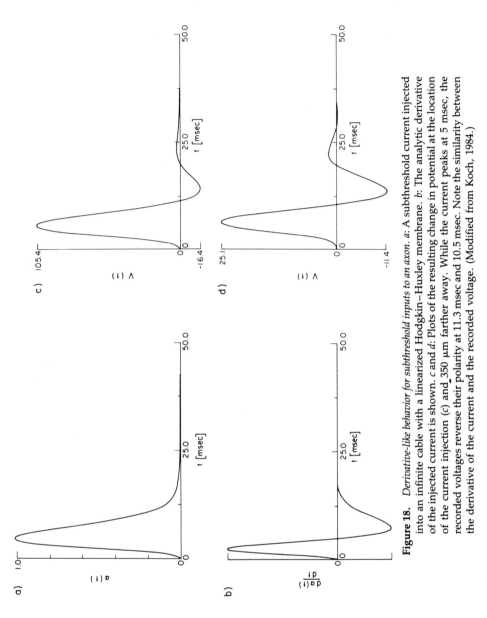

Figure 18. *Derivative-like behavior for subthreshold inputs to an axon.* a: A subthreshold current injected into an infinite cable with a linearized Hodgkin–Huxley membrane. b: The analytic derivative of the injected current is shown. c and d: Plots of the resulting change in potential at the location of the current injection (c) and 350 μm farther away. While the current peaks at 5 msec, the recorded voltages reverse their polarity at 11.3 msec and 10.5 msec. Note the similarity between the derivative of the current and the recorded voltage. (Modified from Koch, 1984.)

675

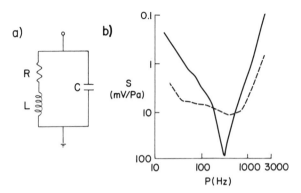

Figure 19. *Turtle hair cells. a*: Equivalent RLC circuit used to model the electrical resonance. *b*: The sensitivity of a hair cell (voltage response normalized to the sound pressure of the tone used) as a function of the frequency of the test tone (P). The cell operates in its linear range. The frequency selectivity derives from a broad band-pass filter common to all hair cells (most likely originating in the middle ear; indicated by the *dashed line*) and an electrical circuit like the one shown in *a*, which is unique to every cell. (Modified from Crawford and Fettiplace, 1981b.)

for all cells while the density of channels varies from cell to cell (Crawford and Fettiplace, 1981a; Koch, 1984). Because of this varying channel density and the concomitant varying degree of electrical excitability, Koch (1984) predicted a correlation between the characteristic frequency of individual hair cells and their degree of nonlinearity. While this mechanism leads to a fixed, stationary distribution of characteristic frequencies, transient effects might be achieved by a shift in the concentration of some ions like calcium (see Ashmore, 1983), neurotransmitters, or even hormones, as demonstrated in electric fish (Meyer and Zakon, 1982). Hair cells seem like ideal candidates for computer simulations, since their role in information processing relies in part on nonspiking membrane mechanisms that can be modeled using a Hodgkin–Huxley-like formalism (for a recent attempt, see Lewis, 1984).

Transmitter Regulation of Voltage-Dependent Channels

In the last few years, the habit of classifying conductances into those that depend only on voltage and those that depend only on the presence of a neurotransmitter (Grundfest, 1957) has gradually been eroded. There are now several examples in which a transmitter does not open ionic channels but modifies a voltage-dependent channel. Examples of such mechanisms include the control of cardiac calcium current by β-adrenergic agents (Reuter et al., 1982), the action of opiates on neurons of the myenteric plexus and locus coeruleus (North and Williams, 1983), the synaptic inhibition of voltage-sensitive currents in *Aplysia* (Klein and Kandel, 1980), and the muscarinic control of potassium conductances in bullfrog sympathetic neurons (Adams and Brown, 1982; Adams et al., 1982a,b; Kuffler and Sejnowski, 1983; Jones, 1985) and in the mammalian hippocampus (Halliwell and Adams, 1982; for a general survey, see Siegelbaum and Tsien, 1983). To illustrate this new development and its implications for neuronal computations, we describe the inhibition of two potassium currents by muscarinic and peptidergic agents.

Biophysical Mechanism.   Stimulation of cholinergic preganglionic fibers produces two different excitatory responses in amphibian (B-type) sympathetic neurons: a very fast EPSP with a superimposed spike and a subsequent slow EPSP of small amplitude (Figure 20A). The latter begins after a latency of some 200–300 msec, peaks at about 2 sec, and lasts some 10–20 sec (Adams and Brown, 1982; Brown, 1983; Kuffler and Sejnowski, 1983; for a review, see Adams et al., 1986). Both potentials result from the release of ACh from the same preganglionic fibers. The initial fast EPSP, analogous to the "classical" muscle end-plate potential, results from the action of ACh on curare-sensitive nicotinic receptors, while the slow response is a result of ACh acting on a muscarinic receptor. Adams and his collaborators showed that the mechanism underlying the slow EPSP is a selective inhibition of two potassium currents, called M (I_M)- and AHP (I_{AHP})-currents (Adams et al., 1982a,b, 1986; Jones, 1985; Koch and Adams, 1985). I_M shows no detectable inactivation, turns on rather slowly, starting at around −60 mV, and is maximally activated near −20 mV (Brown and Adams, 1980). Because it shows no inactivation, it strongly influences the steady-state $I–V$ relation near

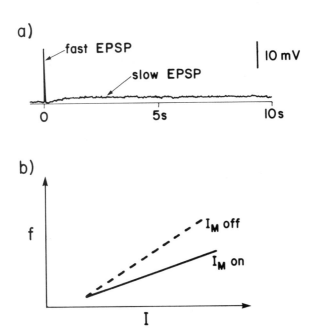

Figure 20.   *Bullfrog sympathetic neuron. a*: The intracellular potential following a single preganglionic stimulus. The fast excitatory postsynaptic potential (EPSP) and the thereby induced action potential are mediated by a nicotinic ACh receptor, while the slow EPSP results from the action of ACh on a muscarinic receptor, inhibiting M-current. (Modified from Adams and Brown, 1982.) *b*: One possible effect of M-current inhibition on the steady-state firing frequency of a neuron. Note that the current threshold remains unaffected, but that the total response of the cell to synaptic input increases.

the resting potential. I_{AHP} depends only on free intracellular calcium and not explicitly on potential and turns on rather slowly. It is responsible for the long afterhyperpolarization seen in a great variety of cells following action potentials.

Under normal conditions, the slow EPSP generated by a single preganglionic stimulus closes some 5–10% of the open M-channels; with repeated trains of stimuli up to 70% of the M-channels and about 30% of the AHP-channels can be closed. Muscarinic excitation usually produces a striking increase in the excitability of the neuron. This usually takes the form of long trains of spikes after the injection of a long depolarizing current pulse. Note that the essential action of I_M and I_{AHP} inhibition is not the slow EPSP but rather the facilitation of the neurons' response to some other excitation. Both conductances also seem to be sensitive to a neuropeptide similar to teleost luteinizing hormone-releasing hormone (LHRH; Adams et al., 1982b; Jan and Jan, 1983; see below).

A similar phenomenon is observed in the rodent hippocampus. When a prolonged depolarizing current pulse is injected into a hippocampal pyramidal cell, the cell responds with an initial burst of spikes, after which time it remains silent for the duration of the pulse. This spike frequency adaptation or accommodation is markedly attenuated by local application of norepinephrine or ACh, which causes the cell to fire throughout the depolarizing current pulse (Madison and Nicoll, 1982, 1984; Lancaster and Adams, 1985). The basis of this striking modification of spike frequency adaptation involves the blockage of I_{AHP} via a cAMP-dependent mechanism subsequent to calcium's entry into the cell.

Neuronal Operation. The inhibition of two sustained potassium-dependent currents, I_M and I_{AHP}, gives rise to an increase in cellular excitability, while the slow, low-amplitude EPSP may be more of an epiphenomenon. In particular, it leads to a blockage of the accommodation seen in a variety of neurons in response to a maintained excitatory input. While under normal conditions the cell will respond to such an input with a few action potentials at the start of the excitatory input, abolishing accommodation leads to a maintained output of action potentials throughout the duration of the input.

The operation implemented by this inhibition has thus the character of gain control, that is, modulating the input–output properties of the cell on a long-lasting time basis. By inhibiting the two potassium conductances, the neuron has lowered its threshold to synaptic input. Figure 20B graphically demonstrates the possible effect of I_M- and I_{AHP}- current inhibition on the $f-I$ curves of the cell. While the absolute current threshold changes little, the slope of the linear relation between f and I increases.

One Example of a Computation. In the mammalian visual system, the LGN is commonly thought to act as a mere relay for the transmission of visual information from the retina to the visual cortex, a relay without significant elaboration in receptive field properties or signal strength. However, morphological and electrophysiological observations are at odds with this view (see Sherman and Koch, 1986). For instance, the LGN receives input from the brain stem (McBride and Sutin, 1975; Singer, 1977; Hughes and Mullikin, 1984). In particular, norepinephrine-containing fibers that originate in the locus coeruleus provide a dense, uniform innervation of the dLGN (Kromer and Moore, 1980). In rats, electrical stimulation of the locus coeruleus, local application to cell bodies in the locus coeruleus of the excitatory amino acid glutamate, and direct iontophoretic application of norepinephrine to geniculate cells all lead to a delayed but dramatic increase in the firing rate of most spontaneously active geniculate neurons (Rogawski and Aghajanian, 1980; Kayama et al., 1982). This facilitation usually occurs 0.2 sec to a few seconds after the onset of the electrical stimulation and subsides gradually within several seconds after cessation of the stimulation (Kayama, 1985). If the optic nerve is sectioned to prevent visually mediated synaptic input, neither direct application of norepinephrine nor electrical stimulation of the locus coeruleus activates geniculate neurons, although the same cells can easily be excited by iontophoresis of glutamate (Rogawski and Aghajanian, 1980). In other words, the action of the pathway from the locus coeruleus onto geniculate relay cells is contingent upon prior or simultaneous excitation of the relay cells. Sherman and Koch (1986) propose that this blockage of the spike frequency adaptation in dLGN relay cells is mediated by the reduction of a sustained calcium-dependent potassium current, known to be present in thalamic neurons (Deschênes et al., 1984; Jahnsen and Llinás, 1984) via noradrenergic and/or cholinergic fibers originating in the brain stem reticular formation.

This biophysical mechanism may be responsible for the overall changes in geniculate cell responsiveness during sleep and arousal (Singer, 1977). Livingstone and Hubel (1981) report increased spontaneous firing rates and enhanced responses to optimal stimuli upon arousal (see also McCarley et al., 1983). Furthermore, neurons in the dorsal raphe nucleus and the locus coeruleus fire more rapidly during periods of increased alertness, such as paradoxical sleep and arousal (Chu and Bloom, 1973; Foote et al., 1980). These brain-stem afferents may thus modify retinogeniculate transmission during arousal by increasing the excitability of geniculate relay cells (Sherman and Koch, 1986).

Action of "Neurotransmitters" over Long Distances

Biophysical Mechanism. There is good experimental evidence that certain "neuroactive" substances, in particular neuropeptides, are capable of influencing the electrical behavior of neurons "at a distance," that is, over distances that are large compared to the metric employed for measuring the dimensions between the conventional presynaptic and postsynaptic elements. [Schmitt (1984) proposes the generic term informational substances to name these and similar chemical mediators.] Examples are the action of an LHRH-like peptide in bullfrog autonomic ganglion (Kuffler and Sejnowski, 1983; Jan and Jan, 1983; Jones et al., 1984), FMRFamide-like and proctolinlike peptides in the stomatogastric ganglion of crustaceans (Hooper and Marder, 1984; Marder and Hooper, 1985), substance P in cultured globus pallidus neurons (Stanfield et al., 1985), egg-laying hormone in *Aplysia* (Branton et al., 1978), and the proposed nonsynaptic release of norepinephrine and serotonin from the diffusely branching axons originating in the locus coeruleus and the raphe nucleus (Moore and Bloom, 1978; Dismukes, 1979). In order to understand some of the issues involved, we briefly examine the action of an LHRH-like peptide in the bullfrog.

Stimulation of cholinergic preganglionic fibers in the frog sympathetic ganglion gives rise to three different postsynaptic responses: the fast, nicotinic-mediated

EPSP and the slow, muscarinic-mediated EPSP (as discussed in the previous section). A third synaptic potential, termed the late slow potential, lasts for several minutes and is not mediated by ACh (Jan and Jan, 1983; Kuffler and Sejnowski, 1983). Its main action is to increase the excitability of the neuron, similar to I_M and I_{AHP} inhibition. In fact, blockage of these conductances is probably instrumental in generating the late slow EPSP (Adams et al., 1982a,b, 1986; Jones, 1985). It is believed that the late slow EPSP is mediated by a peptide structurally very similar to teleost LHRH (Jones et al., 1984). This peptide is contained in and released from the same preganglionic fiber as ACh. Stimulating a fiber presynaptic to a C-neuron gives rise to both the ACh-mediated synaptic event and to the late, slow EPSP. B-cells, thought not to be in any direct synaptic contact with the fibers presynaptic to C-cells, also show the late, slow EPSP upon stimulation of the preganglionic C-fibers. Thus, the LHRH-like peptide must diffuse for tens of microns from its release site before reaching the surface of B-cells. The longevity of the late slow EPSP is not limited by the diffusion time but is a consequence of the long lifetime of the peptide.

Three points are particularly noteworthy in this example and can be generalized to similar cases in other systems. (1) The influence of the peptide on the target cell is of long duration, typically much longer than the millisecond range of action potentials. (2) The action of the peptide on a nerve cell is contingent upon previous excitation in the target neuron. This attribute is crucial to the possible modulatory function of peptides (see the contribution by L. L. Iversen in Dismukes, 1979). Thus, M-current inhibition increases the excitability of the neuron without, or only with little, concomitant rise in voltage. Similarly, substance P acts on Renshaw cells in the spinal cord to antagonize the nicotinic actions of ACh, while having no effect when administered alone (Belcher and Ryall, 1977). (3) Lastly, the sphere of influence of these modulatory substances is not confined to the synaptic cleft, but may extend well beyond the 10 μm range. Their speed of action is usually limited, in the absence of any active transport process, by diffusion, that is, distance is proportional to the square (or cubic) root of the elapsed time. It is important then, that these substances are not degraded by enzymes during their diffusion from the release site to the receptor.

Increasing evidence from immunohistochemical studies reveals that neurons may contain one or more neuropeptides in addition to a monoamine neurotransmitter such as norepinephrine or ACh (Hökfelt et al., 1980; for an overview, see Lundberg and Hökfelt, 1983). Concomitantly, iontophoretic experiments demonstrate the presence of more than a single population of receptors on a particular postsynaptic neuron. Cells in the frog sympathetic ganglion respond to ACh, substance P, and LHRH (Jan and Jan, 1982), while locus coeruleus neurons bear both opiate and α-adrenoreceptors (Starke, 1981). Since all neuropeptides are made up of amino acids, the total number of possible peptides could be astronomically large, depending on the peptide chain length. Lastly, neuropeptides differ fundamentally from ACh, biogenic amines, and amino acids since they are not recycled or taken up. Peptidergic neurons rely entirely on the synthesis of the peptide in the cell body and on its axonal transport to the synaptic terminal. This might well have functional consequences under conditions of tonic firing.

Neuronal Operation.   We propose that the main action of neuropeptides and similar substances is a long-term modulation of cellular excitability without evoking direct, independent changes in the postsynaptic membrane potential (see Figure 20B). Applying the neuropeptide in the absence of any synaptic input will have little effect on the behavior of the neuron. The underlying biophysical mechanisms can be likened to a gain control. The major differences from the "conventional" mode of fast and focal chemical interaction are that neuropeptides can activate large areas in the central nervous system by diffusing throughout the extracellular matrix and that their time course is typically two to three orders of magnitude larger than the time course of postsynaptic conductance changes or of impulse initiation. This restricts the use of neuropeptides and similar substances to circumstances in which the global properties of a given hardwired circuit need to be modified to reflect a different situation requiring a different kind of information processing (see, for instance, Marder, 1984). Owing to their time course, it seems unlikely that neuropeptides underlie the fast computations required for visual perception and motor control.

An Example of a Computation.   Recent efforts to plan and build massive parallel computers have led to the growing realization that one major challenge facing the computer architecture designer is the problem of routing information efficiently among the individual processors, that is, using the least amount of time and connections (Hillis, 1984). The cortex, a computational structure comprising roughly 10^{11}–10^{12} individual processors operating in parallel, probably faces a similar problem. How is information routed among neurons without quickly exceeding space by connecting every neuron with every other neuron? One possible mechanism might involve neuropeptides. The basis of the mechanism is illustrated in Figure 21. Let us assume that a particular sensory neuron is presynaptic to a large number of neurons, that is, establishes conventional synapses with them. In the absence of any modulatory input, electrical activity in the sensory neuron evokes some activity in the corresponding postsynaptic elements. In the presence of a particular neuropeptide A, for which only a subset M_A of all neurons has a receptor, the excitability of all neurons in M_A is enhanced. The neuropeptide is released from a local, diffusely branching interneuron. Activity in the sensory neuron will now evoke a much stronger response in the affected neurons than before and the information about the occurrence of a specific stimulus has been routed to a certain subset of neurons. If another population of neurons has receptors to a different peptide, the information is routed to a different target.

In order for such an addressing scheme to work efficiently, a large number of different peptides are required in order to "program" different paths. The number and location of neurons that could be addressed in this way depends critically on the transport mechanism of the neuropeptide, that is, on diffusion in the extracellular space. Thus, addressing works by selectively and temporarily increasing the gain of the active membrane properties of the class of neurons to be addressed, without actually exciting them. This solution to the addressing problem is similar to the traditional telephone system, in which connections are made and broken as required for exchanging information. It is conceivable that

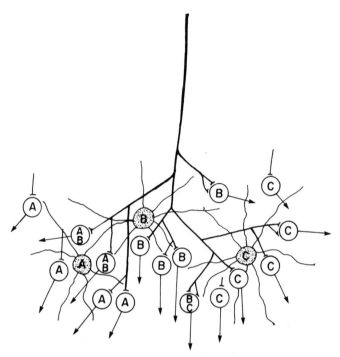

Figure 21.   *A highly speculative addressing scheme in a closely packed neuronal ganglion.* The axon *(heavy line)* is presynaptic to a variety of cells that project outside the ganglion. Each one of these cells has receptors for one or two different neuromodulators, such as neuropeptides (A, B, and C). They are released by local interneurons projecting diffusely throughout parts of the ganglion. Once a specific neuromodulator has been released, it diffuses to its receptor sites, enabling the postsynaptic cell to fire much more vigorously in response to a presynaptic input than before. Thus, information from the axon has been routed to a subset of all its postsynaptic neurons. This mechanism requires a large number of neuropeptides or similar substances, which may diffuse for many microns before binding to a receptor. Moreover, neurons are assumed to have receptors for a few of these substances.

neuropeptides or other modulators may route information within the branched axonal tree of a single neuron by controlling in a differential way the active membrane properties of the axonal branches.

BIOPHYSICS OF COMPUTATION

From the point of view of information processing, an important difference among the biophysical mechanisms we have reviewed above is likely to become increasingly clear. Action potential generation and propagation, synaptic transmission, and the interaction between synaptic inputs usually occur on a time scale of milliseconds, what we term the primary logical time scale. The lower limit on this time scale is given by the speed of propagation of the electrical potential in axons and other excitable tissues and by the chemical kinetics of the binding of receptors and transmitters. The primary time scale can be likened to the basic cycle time of a digital computer. However, some of the newly discovered currents, such as the slow, muscarinic-mediated, cholinergic excitation (Brown, 1983) or the effects of neuropeptides on the firing behavior of neurons, take many hundreds of milliseconds to be noticeable, and may last many seconds and even minutes. Their use in information processing would be one of modulating the existing hardwired circuitry, adapting the circuit to different stimuli or to different modes of operation (e.g., Marder, 1984). They act in what we call the secondary modulatory time scale. Biophysical mechanisms operating in the primary time range most likely underlie visual perception and the computation required for motor output. Mechanisms acting on the modulatory time scale, on the other hand, may increase the excitability of a neuronal population following some stimuli alerting the animal to a potential danger, or may mediate sensory aftereffects or habituation. While the biophysical mechanisms in the primary time scale correspond to the physical mechanisms underlying the operation of transistors and gates, there are at present no counterparts to the biophysical mechanisms operating in the modulatory time range.

We still know too little about the computational style used by nervous systems. As a consequence, there is a large gap between computational theories of vision and motor control and their possible implementation in neural hardware. The model of computation provided by the digital computer is clearly unsatisfactory for the neurobiologist, given the increasing evidence that neurons are complex devices, very different from the simple digital switches suggested by the McCulloch and Pitts (1943) model. It is especially difficult to imagine how networks of neurons may solve the equations involved in vision algorithms in a way similar to digital computers.

Recently, Poggio and Koch (1985) have suggested a powerful analog model of computation in electrical or chemical networks for a large class of vision problems that maps more easily into biologically plausible mechanisms of the type we discussed in this chapter. Their suggestion is based on a new theoretical framework for early vision—regularization theory—introduced by Poggio and Torre (1984; for a review, see Poggio et al., 1985). Regularization methods solve early vision problems in terms of variational principles of a specific type. Poggio and Koch begin by recognizing that analog electrical networks are a natural hardware for computing the class of variational principles suggested by regularization analysis. Because of the well-known isomorphism between electrical and chemical networks (see, for instance, Busse and Hess, 1973; Eigen, 1974) that derives from the common underlying mathematical structure (i.e., Kirchoff's laws), appropriate sets of chemical reactions can be devised, at least in principle, to "simulate" exactly the electrical circuits (Figure 22).

Electrical and chemical systems of this type therefore offer a computational model for early vision that is quite different from the digital computer. Equations are "solved" in an implicit way, exploiting the physical constraints provided by Kirchoff's laws. It is not difficult to imagine how this model of computation could be extended to mixed electrochemical systems by the use of transducers such as chemical synapses that can decouple two parts of a system, similar to operational amplifiers (Koch et al., 1986a).

Could neural hardware exploit this model of computation? Several researchers, most notably Jerry Lettvin and John Hopfield (Hopfield, 1984; Hopfield and Tank, 1985), have in the past proposed analog models of computation for the

a)

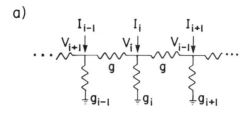

b)

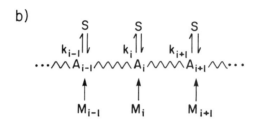

c)

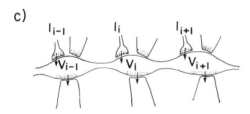

Figure 22. *Analog electrical networks. a:* A resistive network solving a particular visual task—computing the smoothest velocity field of a moving contour (Hildreth, 1984). The input data, injected current of amplitude I_i, correspond to the measured perpendicular velocity component $v_i^\perp$. The solution of the network, the voltages V_i, corresponds to the unknown normal velocity components $v_i^\top$. Sampling the output, that is, the voltage, between nodes corresponds to linear interpolation between the node values. Notice that the value of the conductance g_i varies from location to location. *b:* A chemical network that is formally equivalent to the electrical circuit shown in *a*. A substance *A*, the concentration of which corresponds to the desired $v^\top$, diffuses along a cable while reacting with an extracellular substance *S* (first-order kinetics). The corresponding ON rate k_i varies from location to location. This could be achieved, for instance, by a differential concentration of an enzyme. The inputs $v_i^\perp$ are given by the influxes of substance *A*. *c:* This scheme illustrates a hypothetical neuronal implementation of the electrical and chemical circuit shown above. A dendrite, acting as both a pre- and postsynaptic element, has a membrane resistance that can be locally controlled by suitable synaptic input, preferentially from channels with a reversal potential close to the resting potential of the dendrite. The output, the voltage V_i, is sampled by dendrodendritic synapses. (Modified from Poggio and Koch, 1985.)

nervous system. The evidence reviewed here shows that for implementing electrical networks in equivalent neuronal hardware, one can draw upon a large number of elementary circuit elements. Patches of neuronal membrane or cytoplasm can be treated as resistances and capacitances. Voltage sources may be mimicked by synapses on dendritic spines or thin dendrites, whereas synapses on large dendrites may act as current sources. Chemical synapses could effectively serve to decouple different parts of a network (see Poggio and Koch, 1985). Chemical processes such as the reactions associated with postsynaptic effects or with neuropeptides could also be thought of as part of a complex electrochemical network. Obviously, the analogy cannot be taken too literally. We are convinced, however, that the style of computation represented by analog circuits represents a very useful model for neural computations (in particular, see Koch et al., 1986a).

In the brief history of computer technology, several different physical effects have been exploited to perform elementary operations, mostly digital. Within a single, very specific technology, however, a small number of physical mechanisms and corresponding operations are typically used, such as the inverter and NAND gating in MOS technology. Most of the more complex operations are synthesized beginning from these two basic ones. It would be very surprising if evolution were to choose a very small number of basic mechanisms in the nervous system. This is certainly the "old" view, in which the only operation was a thresholding operation, implemented through the mechanism of spike initiation. The evidence accumulated over the last several years by research on membranes and synapses has made it abundantly clear, however, that several different mechanisms are likely to be exploited by the brain for information processing (Schmitt, 1979; Bullock, 1979). It seems unlikely, on the other hand, that the number of basic mechanisms is much larger than, say, a dozen or so. This general class of mechanisms includes voltage-dependent channels, neurotransmitter-dependent channels, modifications of subcellular components, and spatiotemporal integration in neuronal structures.

Our approach—to identify and characterize some of the basic mechanisms for information processing—may provide powerful constraints for interpreting morphological and physiological data and for connecting them with computational theories. Clearly, this plan can only be successful if the number of basic biophysical mechanisms in information processing is small. The final answer to these questions can only be obtained with experimental methods. A case in point is provided by our conjecture about silent inhibition being a basic mechanism for implementing operations of the analog AND–NOT type. We have isolated a few computations, such as the computation of directional motion, in which silent inhibition may have a critical role. We have shown with theoretical methods and computer simulations based on anatomical data that the properties of the biophysical mechanisms are consistent with our conjecture in the case of retinal ganglion cells. We have also made specific experimental predictions. Several of them are supported by recent data. If our conjecture turns out to be correct in the case of directional selectivity of retinal ganglion cells, the next task will be to demonstrate that the same mechanism is, or is not, used in other parts of the nervous system for other computations.

REFERENCES

Adams, P. R., and D. A. Brown (1982) Synaptic inhibition of the M-current: Slow excitatory post-synaptic mechanism in bullfrog sympathetic neurones. *J. Physiol. (Lond.)* **332**:263–272.

Adams, P. R., D. A. Brown, and A. Constanti (1982a) M-currents and other potassium-currents in bullfrog sympathetic neurones. *J. Physiol. (Lond.)* **330**:537–572.

Adams, P. R., D. A. Brown, and A. Constanti (1982b) Pharmacological inhibition of the M-current. *J. Physiol. (Lond.)* **332**:223–262.

Adams, P. R., A. Constanti, D. A. Brown, and R. B. Clark (1982c) Intracellular Ca^{2+} activates a fast voltage-sensitive K^+ current in vertebrate sympathetic neurones. *Nature* **296**:746–749.

Adams, P. R., S. W. Jones, P. Pennefather, D. A. Brown, C. Koch, and B. Lancaster (1986) Slow synaptic transmission in frog sympathetic ganglia. *J. Exp. Biol.* **124**:259–285.

Ahlsen, G., K. Grant, and S. Lindstrom (1982) Monosynaptic excitation of principal cells in the lateral geniculate nucleus by corticofugal fibers. *Brain Res.* **234**:454–458.

Ahlsen, G., S. Lindstrom, and F.-S. Lo (1984) Inhibition from the brain stem of inhibitory interneurones of the cat's dorsal lateral geniculate nucleus. *J. Physiol. (Lond.)* **347**:593–609.

Amthor, F. R., C. W. Oyster, and E. S. Takahashi (1983a) Do major physiological retinal ganglion cell classes have distinct morphologies? *Neurosci. Abstr.* **9**:896.

Amthor, F. R., C. W. Oyster, and E. S. Takahashi (1983b) Quantitative morphology of rabbit ganglion cells. *Proc. R. Soc. Lond. (Biol.)* **217**:341–355.

Amthor, F. R., C. W. Oyster, and E. S. Takahashi (1984) Morphology of on–off direction-selective ganglion cells in the rabbit retina. *Brain Res.* **298**:187–190.

Ariel, M., and N. W. Daw (1982) Pharmacological analysis of directionally sensitive rabbit retinal ganglion cells. *J. Physiol. (Lond.)* **324**:161–185.

Ashmore, J. F. (1983) Listening with one cell. *Nature* **304**:489–490.

Ashmore, J. F., and G. Falk (1976) Absolute sensitivity of rod bipolar cells in a dark-adapted retina. *Nature* **263**:248–249.

Ashmore, J. F., and G. Falk (1979) Transmission of visual signals to bipolar cells near absolute threshold. *Vision Res.* **19**:419–423.

Attwell, D., and M. Wilson (1980) Behavior of the rod network in the tiger salamander retina mediated by membrane properties of individual rods. *J. Physiol. (Lond.)* **309**:287–315.

Baimbridge, K. G., and J. J. Miller (1981) Calcium uptake and retention during long-term potentiation of neuronal activity in the rat hippocampal slice preparation. *Brain Res.* **221**:299–305.

Barlow, H. B. (1981) Critical limiting factors in the design of the eye and visual cortex. *Proc. R. Soc. Lond. (Biol.)* **212**:1–35.

Barlow, H. B., and R. W. Levick (1965) The mechanism of directional selectivity in the rabbit's retina. *J. Physiol. (Lond.)* **173**:477–504.

Barlow, H., C. Blakemore, and J. D. Pettigrew (1967) The neural mechanism of binocular depth discrimination. *J. Physiol. (Lond.)* **193**:327–342.

Belcher, G., and R. W. Ryall (1977) Substance P selectively blocks nicotinic receptors on Renshaw cells: A new concept of inhibitory synaptic interaction. *J. Physiol. (Lond.)* **272**:105–119.

Ben-Ari, Y., K. Krnjević, R. J. Reiffenstein, and W. Reinhardt (1981) Inhibitory conductance changes and action of γ-aminobutyrate in rat hippocampus. *Neuroscience* **6**:2445–2463.

Bennett, M. V. L. (1977) Electrical transmission: A functional analysis and comparison to chemical transmission. *Handb. Physiol., Cellular Biology of Neurons* **1**:357–416.

Berardi, N., and M. C. Morrone (1984) The role of γ-aminobutyric acid-mediated inhibition in the response properties of cat lateral geniculate nucleus neurones. *J. Physiol. (Lond.)* **357**:505–524.

Bittner, G. D. (1968) Differentiation of nerve terminals in the crayfish opener muscle and its functional significance. *J. Gen. Physiol.* **51**:731–758.

Blodgett, A. J., and D. R. Barbour (1982) Thermal conduction module: A high-performance multilayer ceramic package. *IBM J. Res. Dev.* **26**:30–36.

Bowery, N. G., A. Doble, D. R. Hill, A. L. Hudson, J. S. Shaw, M. J. Turnbull, and R. Warrington (1981) Bicuculline-insensitive GABA receptors on peripheral autonomic nerve terminals. *Eur. J. Pharmacol.* **71**:53–70.

Boycott, B. B. (1982) Experiments on dendritic spines. *Trends Neurosci.* **5**:328–329.

Boycott, B. B., and H. Wässle (1974) The morphological types of ganglion cells of the domestic cat's retina. *J. Physiol. (Lond.)* **240**:397–419.

Bradley, P., and G. Horn (1979) Neuronal plasticity in the chicken brain: Morphological effects of visual experience on neurons in hyperstriatum accessorium. *Brain Res.* **162**:148–153.

Brandon, J. G., and R. G. Coss (1982) Rapid dendritic spine stem shortening during one-trial learning: The honeybee's first orientation flight. *Brain Res.* **252**:51–61.

Branton, W. D., E. Mayeti, P. Brownell, and S. B. Simon (1978) Evidence for local hormonal communication between neurones in *Aplysia*. *Nature* **274**:70–72.

Brayton, R. K., and J. K. Moser (1964) A theory of nonlinear networks—Part I. *Quart. Appl. Math.* **22**:1–33.

Brown, D. A. (1983) Slow cholinergic excitation—A mechanism for increasing neuronal excitability. *Trends Neurosci.* **6**:302–307.

Brown, D. A., and P. Adams (1980) Muscarinic suppression of a novel voltage-sensitive K^+-current in a vertebrate neurone. *Nature* **283**:673–676.

Bullier, J., and T. T. Norton (1979) Comparison of receptive-field properties of X and Y ganglion cells with X and Y lateral geniculate cells in the cat. *J. Neurophysiol.* **42**:274–291.

Bullock, T. H. (1979) Evolving concepts of local integrative operations in neurons. In *The Neurosciences: Fourth Study Program*, F. O. Schmitt and F. G. Worden, eds., pp. 43–49, MIT Press, Cambridge, Massachusetts.

Busse, H., and B. Hess (1973) Information transmission in a diffusion-coupled oscillatory chemical system. *Nature* **244**:203–205.

Caldwell, J. H., N. W. Daw, and H. J. Wyatt (1978) Effects of picrotoxin and strychnine on rabbit retinal ganglion cells: Lateral interactions for cells with more complex receptive fields. *J. Physiol. (Lond.)* **276**:277–298.

Chang, H. T. (1952) Cortical neurons with particular reference to the apical dendrites. *Cold Spring Harbor Symp. Quant. Biol.* **17**:189–202.

Cheung, W. Y. (1982) Calmodulin. *Sci. Am.* **246**:48–56.

Chiu, S. Y., and J. M. Ritchie (1982) Evidence for the presence of potassium channels in the internode of frog myelinated nerve fibres. *J. Physiol. (Lond.)* **322**:485–501.

Chiu, S. Y., and J. M. Ritchie (1984) On the physiological role of internodal potassium channels and the security of conduction in myelinated fibres. *Proc. R. Soc. Lond. (Biol.)* **220**:415–422.

Chiu, S. Y., J. M. Ritchie, R. B. Rogart, and D. Stagg (1979) A quantitative description of membrane currents in rabbit myelinated nerve. *J. Physiol. (Lond.)* **292**:149–166.

Chu, N.-S., and F. E. Bloom (1973) Norepinephrine-containing neurons: Changes in spontaneous discharge patterns during sleeping and waking. *Science* **179**:908–910.

Chung, S.-H. (1977) Synaptic memory in the hippocampus. *Nature* **266**:677–678.

Chung, S.-H., S. A. Raymond, and J. Y. Lettvin (1970) Multiple meaning in single visual units. *Brain Behav. Evol.* **3**:70–101.

Clapham, D. E., and L. J. DeFelice (1976) The theoretical small signal impedance of the frog node, *Rana pipiens. Eur. J. Physiol.* **366**:273–276.

Clapham, D. E., and L. J. DeFelice (1982) Small signal impedance of heart cell membranes. *J. Membr. Biol.* **67**:63–71.

Cleland, B. G., and W. R. Levick (1974) Properties of rarely encountered types of ganglion cells in the cat's retina. *J. Physiol. (Lond.)* **240**:457–492.

Copenhagen, D. R., and W. G. Owen (1976) Functional characteristics of lateral interaction between rods in the retina of the snapping turtle. *J. Physiol. (Lond.)* **259**:251–282.

Coss, R. G., and A. Globus (1978) Spine stems on tectal interneurons in jewel fish are shortened by social stimulation. *Science* **200**:787–789.

Crawford, A. C., and R. Fettiplace (1980) The frequency selectivity of auditory nerve fibres and hair cells in the cochlea of the turtle. *J. Physiol. (Lond.)* **306**:79–125.

Crawford, A. C., and R. Fettiplace (1981a) An electrical tuning mechanism in turtle cochlear hair cells. *J. Physiol. (Lond.)* **312**:377–412.

Crawford, A. C., and R. Fettiplace (1981b) Non-linearities in the responses of turtle hair cells. *J. Physiol. (Lond.)* **315**:317–338.

Crick, F. (1982) Do dendritic spines twitch? *Trends Neurosci.* **5**:44–46.

Crill, W. E., and P. C. Schwindt (1983) Active currents in mammalian central neurons. *Trends Neurosci.* **6**:236–240.

Criswell, M. H., and R. D. DeVoe (1984) Responses of turtle retinal bipolar cells to moving stimuli. *Invest. Ophthalmol. Vis. Sci. (Suppl.)* **25**:119.

Curtis, D. R., and G. A. R. Johnston (1974) Amino acid transmitters in the mammalian central nervous system. *Ergeb. Physiol. Biol. Chem. Exp. Pharmakol.* **69**:97–188.

Derrington, A. M., and A. F. Fuchs (1979) Spatial and temporal properties of X and Y cells in the cat lateral geniculate nucleus. *J. Physiol. (Lond.)* **293**:347–364.

Deschênes, M., M. Paradis, J. P. Roy, and M. Steriade (1984) Electrophysiology of neurons of lateral thalamic nuclei in cat: Resting properties and burst discharges. *J. Neurophysiol.* **51**:1196–1219.

Detwiler, P. B., and A. L. Hodgkin (1979) Electrical coupling between cones in the turtle retina. *J. Physiol. (Lond.)* **291**:75–100.

Detwiler, P. B., A. L. Hodgkin, and P. A. McNaughton (1978) A surprising property of electrical spread in the network of rods in the turtle's retina. *Nature* **274**:562–565.

Detwiler, P. B., A. L. Hodgkin, and P. A. McNaughton (1980) Temporal and spatial characteristics of the voltage response of rods in the retina of the snapping turtle. *J. Physiol. (Lond.)* **300**:213–250.

DeVoe, R. D., R. G. Guy, and M. H. Criswell (1985) Directionally selective cells of the inner nuclear layer in the turtle retina. *Invest. Ophthalmol. Vis. Sci. (Suppl.)* **26**:311.

Dismukes, R. K. (1979) New concepts of molecular communication among neurons. *Behav. Brain Sci.* **2**:409–448.

Dowling, J. E. (1979) Information processing by local circuits: The vertebrate retina as a model system. In *The Neurosciences: Fourth Study Program*, F. O. Schmitt and F. G. Worden, eds., pp. 163–181, MIT Press, Cambridge, Massachusetts.

Dowling, J. E., and B. B. Boycott (1966) Organization of the primate retina: Electron microscopy. *Proc. R. Soc. Lond. (Biol.)* **166**:80–111.

Eccles J. C. (1983) Calcium in long-term potentiation as a model for memory. *Neuroscience* **10**:1071–1081.

Eigen, M. (1974) Molecules, information and memory: From molecules to neural networks. In *The Neurosciences: Third Study Program*, F. O. Schmitt and F. G. Worden, eds., pp. xix–xxvii, MIT Press, Cambridge, Massachusetts.

Ellias, S. A., and J. K. Stevens (1972) The dendritic varicosity: A mechanism for electrically isolating the dendrites of cat retinal amacrine cells? *Brain Res.* **196**:365–372.

Emerson, R. C., M. C. Citron, D. J. Felleman, and J. H. Kaas (1985) A proposed mechanism and site for cortical directional selectivity. In *Models of the Visual Cortex*, D. Rose and V. G. Dobson, eds., pp. 420–442, Wiley, Chichester.

Famiglietti, E. V. (1981) Starburst amacrines: 2 mirror-symmetric retinal networks. *Invest. Ophthalmol. Vis. Sci. (Suppl.)* **20**:204.

Famiglietti, E. V. (1983a) On and off pathways through amacrine cells in mammalian retina: The synaptic connections of "starburst" amacrine cells. *Vision Res.* **23**:1265–1279.

Famiglietti, E. V. (1983b) "Starburst" amacrine cells and cholinergic neurons: Mirror-symmetric on and off amacrine cells of rabbit retina. *Brain Res.* **261**:138–144.

Famiglietti, E. V. (1984) Postnatal development of ganglion cells in rabbit retina. *Neurosci. Abstr.* **10**:10–13.

Famiglietti, E. V., and A. Peters (1972) The synaptic glomerulus and the intrinsic neuron in the dorsal lateral geniculate nucleus of the cat. *J. Comp. Neurol.* **144**:285–334.

Ferster, D. (1981) A comparison of binocular depth mechanisms in areas 17 and 18 of the cat visual cortex. *J. Physiol. (Lond.)* **311**:623–655.

Fifková, E. (1985) Actin in the nervous system. *Brain Res. Rev.* **9**:187–215.

Fifková, E., and C. L. Anderson (1981) Stimulation-induced changes in dimensions of stalks of dendritic spines in the dentate molecular layer. *Exp. Neurol.* **74**:621–627.

Fifková, E., and R. Delay (1982) Cytoplasmic actin in dendritic spines as a possible mediator of synaptic plasticity. *J. Cell Biol.* **95**:345–350.

Fifková, E., C. L. Anderson, S. J. Young, and A. Van Harreveld (1982) Effect of anisomycin on stimulation-induced changes in dendritic spines of the dentate granule cells. *J. Neurocytol.* **11**:183–210.

Fifková, E., J. A. Markham, and R. Delay (1983) Calcium in the spine apparatus of dendritic spines in the dentate molecular layer. *Brain Res.* **266**:163–168.

Fifková, E., J. A. Markham, and K. Cullen-Dockstader (1984) Association of the actin lattice with cytoplasmic organelles and the plasma membrane in dendrites and dendritic spines. *Neurosci. Abstr.* **10**:127.2.

Fitzpatrick, D., G. R. Penny, and D. E. Schmechel (1984) Glutamic acid decarboxylase-immunoreactive neurons and terminals in the lateral geniculate nucleus of the cat. *J. Neurosci.* **4**:1809–1819.

Foote, S. L., G. Aston-Jones, and F. E. Bloom (1980) Impulse activity of locus coeruleus neurons in awake rats and monkeys is a function of sensory stimulation and arousal. *Proc. Natl. Acad. Sci. USA* **77**:3033–3037.

Foote, W. E., J. P. Mordes, C. L. Colby, and T. A. Harrison (1977) Differential effect of midbrain stimulation on X-sustained and Y-transient neurons in the lateral geniculate nucleus of the cat. *Brain Res.* **127**:153–158.

Fox, A. P. (1981) Voltage-dependent inactivation of a calcium channel. *Proc. Natl. Acad. Sci. USA* **78**:953–956.

Freed, M., and P. Sterling (1983) Spatial distribution of input from depolarizing cone bipolars to dendritic tree of On-center alpha ganglion cell. *Neurosci. Abstr.* **9**:234.

Friedlander, M. J., C.-S. Lin, L. R. Stanford, and S. M. Sherman (1981) Morphology of functionally identified neurons in lateral geniculate nucleus of the cat. *J. Neurophysiol.* **46**:80–129.

Fukuda, Y., and J. Stone (1976) Evidence of differential inhibitory influences on X- and Y-type relay cells in the cat's lateral geniculate nucleus. *Brain Res.* **113**:188–196.

Funch, P. G., and D. S. Faber (1984) Measurement of myelin sheath resistances: Implications for axonal conduction and pathophysiology. *Science* **225**:538–540.

Furshpan, E. J., and D. D. Potter (1959) Transmission at the giant motor synapses of crayfish. *J. Physiol. (Lond.)* **145**:289–325.

Gamble, E., and C. Koch (1987) The dynamics of free calcium in dendritic spines in response to repetitive synaptic input. *Science* (in press).

Gerschenfeld, H. M., and D. Paupardin-Tritsch (1974) Ionic mechanisms and receptor properties underlying the responses of molluscan neurons to 5-hydroxytryptamine. *J. Physiol. (Lond.)* **243**: 427–456.

Gilbert, C. D., and T. N. Wiesel (1983) Clustered intrinsic connections in cat visual cortex. *Neuroscience* **3**:1116–1133.

Goldstein, S. S., and W. Rall (1974) Changes of action potential shape and velocity for changing core conductor geometry. *Biophys. J.* **14**:731–757.

Grab, D. J., R. K. Carlin, and P. Siekevitz (1980) The presence and functions of calmodulin in the postsynaptic density. *Ann. N.Y. Acad. Sci.* **1980**:55–72.

Graubard, K. (1978) Synaptic transmission without action potentials: Input–output properties of a nonspiking presynaptic neuron. *J. Neurophysiol.* **41**:1014–1025.

Graubard, K., J. A. Raper, and D. K. Hartline (1980) Graded synaptic transmission between spiking neurons. *Proc. Natl. Acad. Sci. USA* **77**:3733–3735.

Graubard, K., J. A. Raper, and D. K. Hartline (1983) Graded synaptic transmission between identified spiking neurons. *J. Neurophysiol.* **50**:508–521.

Gray, E. G. (1959) Axo-somatic and axo-dendritic synapses of the cerebral cortex: An electron microscope study. *J. Anat.* **93**:420–433.

Grossman, Y., I. Parnas, and M. E. Spira (1979a) Differential conduction block in branches of a bifurcating axon. *J. Physiol. (Lond.)* **295**:283–305.

Grossman, Y., I. Parnas, and M. E. Spira (1979b) Ionic mechanisms involved in differential conduction of action potentials at high frequency in a branching axon. *J. Physiol. (Lond.)* **295**:307–322.

Grundfest, H. (1957) Electrical inexcitability of synapses and some consequences in the central nervous system. *Physiol. Rev.* **37**:337–361.

Guillery, R. W. (1969) The organization of synaptic interconnections in the laminae of the dorsal lateral geniculate nucleus of the cat. *Z. Zellforsch. Mikrosk. Anat.* **96**:1–38.

Hagiwara, S. (1983) *Membrane Potential-Dependent Ion Channels in Cell Membrane*, Raven, New York.

Halliwell, J. V., and P. R. Adams (1982) Voltage-clamp analysis of muscarinic excitation in hippocampal neurons. *Brain Res.* **250**:71–92.

Hamori, J., T. Pasik, P. Pasik, and J. Szentagothai (1974) Triadic synaptic arrangements and their possible significance in the lateral geniculate nucleus of the monkey. *Brain Res.* **80**:379–393.

Hamos, J. E., D. Raczkowski, S. C. van Horn, and S. M. Sherman (1983) The ultrastructural substrates for synaptic circuitry of an X retinogeniculate axon. *Neurosci. Abstr.* **9**:814.

Hamos, J. E., S. C. van Horn, D. Raczkowski, D. J. Uhlrich, and S. M. Sherman (1984) Input and output organization of a local circuit neuron in the cat's lateral geniculate nucleus. *Neurosci. Abstr.* **10**:622.

Harris A. L., D. C. Spray, and M. V. L. Bennett (1983) Control of intercellular communication by voltage dependence of gap junctional conductance. *J. Neurosci.* **3**:79–100.

Hassenstein, B., and W. Reichardt (1956) Systemtheoretische Analyse der Zeit-, Reihenfolgen- und Vorzeichenauswertung bei der Bewegungs-perzeption der Russelkafers, *Chlorophanus. Z. Naturforsch.* **11b**:513–524.

Hebb, D. O. (1948) *The Organization of Behavior*, Wiley, New York.

Hengstenberg, R. (1982) Common visual response properties of giant vertical cells in the lobula plate of the blowfly *Calliphora. J. Comp. Physiol.* **149**:179–193.

Hildreth, E. C. (1984) *The Measurement of Visual Motion*, MIT Press, Cambridge, Massachusetts.

Hillis, W. D. (1984) The connection machine: A computer architecture based on cellular automata. *Physica* **10D**:213–228.

Hodgkin, A. L. (1964) *The Conduction of the Nervous Impulse*, Charles C Thomas, Springfield, Illinois.

Hodgkin, A. L., and A. F. Huxley (1952) A quantitative description of membrane current and its application to conduction and excitation in nerve. *J. Physiol. (Lond.)* **117**:500–544.

Hökfelt, T., O. Johansson, A. Ljungdahl, J. M. Lundberg, and M. Schultzberg (1980) Peptidergic neurones. *Nature* **284**:515–521.

Hopfield, J. J. (1984) Neurons with graded response have collective computational properties like those of two-state neurons. *Proc. Natl. Acad. Sci. USA* **81**:3088–3092.

Hopfield, J. J., and D. W. Tank (1985) "Neural" computation of decisions in optimization problems. *Biol. Cybern.* **52**:141–152.

Hopkins, C. D. (1976) Stimulus filtering and electroreception: Tuberous electroreceptors in three species of gymnotoid fish. *J. Comp. Physiol.* **111**:171–207.

Hooper, S. L., and E. Marder (1984) Modulation of a central pattern generator by two neuropeptides, proctolin and FMRFamide. *Brain Res.* **305**:186–191.

Hubel, D. H., and T. N. Wiesel (1959) Receptive fields of single neurons in the cat's striate cortex. *J. Physiol. (Lond.)* **148**:574–591.

Hughes, H. C., and W. H. Mullikin (1984) Brainstem afferents to the lateral geniculate nucleus of the cat. *Exp. Brain Res.* **54**:253–258.

Jack, J. J., D. Noble, and R. W. Tsien (1975) *Electric Current Flow in Excitable Cells*, Clarendon, Oxford.

Jahnsen, H., and R. Llinás (1984) Ionic basis for the electroresponsiveness and oscillatory properties of guinea-pig thalamic neurones *in vitro. J. Physiol. (Lond.)* **349**:227–247.

Jan, Y. N., and L. Y. Jan (1983) A LHRH-like peptidergic neurotransmitter capable of "action at a distance" in autonomic ganglia. *Trends Neurosci.* **6**:320–325.

Jensen, R. J., and R. D. DeVoe (1983) Comparisons of directionally selective with other ganglion cells of the turtle retina: Intracellular recording and staining. *J. Comp. Neurol.* **217**:271–287.

Jones, E. G., and T. P. S. Powell (1969a) An electron microscopic study of the mode of termination of cortico-thalamic fibres within the sensory relay nuclei of the thalamus. *Proc. R. Soc. Lond. (Biol.)* **172**:173–185.

Jones, E. G., and T. P. S. Powell (1969b) Morphological variations in the dendritic spines of the neocortex. *J. Cell Sci.* **5**:509–529.

Jones, S. W. (1985) Muscarinic and peptidergic excitation of bullfrog sympathetic neurons. *J. Physiol. (Lond.)* **366**:63–87.

Jones, S. W., P. R. Adams, M. J. Brownstein, and J. E. Rivier (1984) Teleost luteinizing hormone-releasing hormone: Action on bullfrog sympathetic ganglia is consistent with role as neurotransmitter. *J. Neurosci.* **4**:420–429.

Kakiuchi, S., and K. Sobue (1983) Control of the cytoskeleton by calmodulin and calmodulin-binding proteins. *Trends Biochem. Sci.* **9**:59–62.

Kandel, E. R. (1981) Calcium and the control of synaptic strength by learning. *Nature* **293**:697–700.

Kaneko, A. (1976) Electrical connections between horizontal cells in the dogfish retina. *J. Physiol. (Lond.)* **213**:95–105.

Katsumaru, H., F. Murakami, and N. Tsukahara (1982) Actin filaments in dendritic spines of red nucleus neurons demonstrated by immunoferritin localization and heavy meromysin. *Biomed. Res.* **3**:337–340.

Katz, B. (1966) *Nerve, Muscle and Synapse*, McGraw-Hill, New York.

Katz, B., and R. Miledi (1967) A study of synaptic transmission in the absence of nerve impulses. *J. Physiol. (Lond.)* **192**:407–436.

Kawato, M., T. Hamaguchi, F. Murakami, and N. Tsukahara (1984) Quantitative analysis of electrical properties of dendritic spines. *Biol. Cybern.* **50**:1–8.

Kayama, Y. (1985) Ascending, descending and local control of neuronal activity in the rat lateral geniculate nucleus. *Vision Res.* **25**:339–347.

Kayama, Y., T. Negi, M. Sugitani, and K. Iwama (1982) Effects of locus coeruleus stimulation on neuronal activities of dorsal lateral geniculate nucleus and perigeniculate reticular nucleus of the rat. *Neuroscience* **7**:655–666.

Kernell, D. (1970) Cell properties of importance for the transfer of signals in nervous pathways. In *Excitatory Synaptic Mechanisms*, P. O. Andersen and J. Jansen, eds., pp. 269–273, Universitetsforlag, Oslo.

Klee, C. B., and J. Haiech (1980) Concerted role of calmodulin and calcineurin in calcium regulation. *Ann. N.Y. Acad. Sci.* **1980**:43–53.

Kleene, S. C. (1956) Representation of events in nerve nets and finite automata. In *Automata Studies*, C. E. Shannon and J. McCarthy, eds., pp. 3–41, Princeton Univ. Press, Princeton.

Klein, M., and E. R. Kandel (1980) Mechanism of calcium current modulation underlying presynaptic facilitation and behavioral sensitization in Aplysia. *Proc. Natl. Acad. Sci. USA* **77**:6912–6916.

Kleinhaus, A. L., and J. W. Prichard (1975) Calcium-dependent action potentials produced in leech Retzius cells by tetraethylammonium chloride. *J. Physiol. (Lond.)* **246**:351–361.

Koch, C. (1982) Nonlinear information processing in dendritic trees of arbitrary geometry. PhD Thesis, University of Tübingen, Federal Republic of Germany.

Koch, C. (1984) Cable theory in neurons with active, linearized membranes. *Biol. Cybern.* **50**:15–33.

Koch, C. (1985) Understanding the intrinsic circuitry of the cat's dLGN: Electrical properties of the spine-triad arrangement. *Proc. R. Soc. Lond. (Biol.)* **225**:365.

Koch, C., and P. R. Adams (1985) Computer simulation of bullfrog sympathetic ganglion cell excitability. *Neurosci. Abstr.* **11**:642.

Koch, C., and T. Poggio (1983a) Electrical properties of dendritic spines. *Trends Neurosci.* **6**:80–83.

Koch, C., and T. Poggio (1983b) A theoretical analysis of electrical properties of spines. *Proc. R. Soc. Lond. (Biol.)* **218**:455–477.

Koch, C., and T. Poggio (1985) The synaptic veto mechanism: Does it underlie direction and orientation selectivity in the visual cortex? In *Models of the Visual Cortex*, D. Rose and V. G. Dobson, eds., pp. 408–419, Wiley, Chichester.

Koch, C., T. Poggio, and V. Torre (1982) Retinal ganglion cells: A functional interpretation of dendritic morphology. *Philos. Trans. R. Soc. Lond. (Biol.)* **298**:227–264.

Koch, C., T. Poggio, and V. Torre (1983) Nonlinear interaction in a dendritic tree: Localization, timing and role in information processing. *Proc. Natl. Acad. Sci. USA* **80**:2799–2802.

Koch, C., J. Marroquin, and A. Yuille (1986a) Analog "neuronal" networks in early vision. *Proc. Natl. Acad. Sci. USA* **83**:4263–4267.

Koch, C., T. Poggio, and V. Torre (1986b) Computations in the vertebrate retina: Motion discrimination, gain enhancement and differentiation. *Trends Neurosci.* **9**:204–211.

Kocsis, J. D., and S. G. Waxman (1980) Absence of potassium conductance in central myelinated axons. *Nature* **287**:348–349.

Korn, H., and D. S. Faber (1979) Electrical interactions between vertebrate neurons: Field effects and electrotonic coupling. In *The Neurosciences: Fourth Study Program*, F. O. Schmitt and F. G. Worden, eds., pp. 333–358, MIT Press, Cambridge, Massachusetts.

Kromer, L. F., and R. Y. Moore (1980) A study of the organization of the locus coeruleus projections to the lateral geniculate nuclei in the albino rat. *Neuroscience* 5:255–271.

Krnjević, K., and R. Miledi (1959) Presynaptic failure of neuromuscular propagation in rats. *J. Physiol. (Lond.)* 149:1–22.

Kuffler, S. W., and T. J. Sejnowski (1983) Peptidergic and muscarinic excitation at amphibian sympathetic synapses. *J. Physiol. (Lond.)* 341:257–278.

Lancaster, B., and P. R. Adams (1985) Components of a Ca-activated K-current in rat hippocampal neurons in vitro. *J. Neurophysiol. (Lond.)* 362:23.

Laughlin, S. B. (1973) Neural integration in the first optic neuropil of dragonflies. I. Signal amplification in dark-adapted second order neurons. *J. Comp. Physiol.* 84:335–355.

Lee, K. S. (1983) Cooperativity among afferents for the induction of long-term potentiation in the CA1 region of the hippocampus. *J. Neurosci.* 3:1369–1372.

Lettvin, J. Y., R. R. Maturana, W. S. McCulloch, and W. H. Pitts (1959) What the frog's eye tells the frog's brain. *Proc. Inst. Radio Eng.* 47:1940–1951.

Lewis, R. S. (1984) A biophysical model for electrical resonance in hair cells of the bullfrog sacculus. *Neurosci. Abstr.* 10:7.3.

Lewis, R. S., and A. J. Hudspeth (1983) Voltage- and ion-dependent conductances in solitary vertebrate hair cells. *Nature* 304:538–541.

Lindstrom, S. (1982) Synaptic organization of inhibitory pathways to principal cells in the lateral geniculate nucleus of the cat. *Brain Res.* 234:447–453.

Livingstone, M. S., and D. H. Hubel (1981) Effects of sleep and arousal on the processing of visual information in the cat. *Nature* 291:554–561.

Llinás, R. (1979) The role of calcium in neuronal function. In *The Neurosciences: Fourth Study Program*, F. O. Schmitt and F. G. Worden, eds., pp. 555–572, MIT Press, Cambridge, Massachusetts.

Llinás, R., and R. Hess (1976) Tetrodotoxin-resistant dendritic spikes in avian Purkinje cells. *Proc. Natl. Acad. Sci. USA* 73:2520–2523.

Llinás, R., and M. Sugimori (1980) Electrophysiological properties of *in vitro* Purkinje cell dendrites in mammalian cerebellar slices. *J. Physiol. (Lond.)* 305:197–213.

Llinás, R., and Y. Yarom (1981) Properties and distribution of ionic conductances generating electroresponsiveness of mammalian inferior olivary neurons *in vitro*. *J. Physiol. (Lond.)* 315:569–584.

Lundberg, J. M., and T. Hökfelt (1983) Coexistence of peptides and classical neurotransmitters. *Trends Neurosci.* 6:325–333.

Lynch, G., and M. Baudry (1984) The biochemistry of memory: A new and specific hypothesis. *Science* 224:1057–1063.

Lynch, G., J. Larson, S. Kelso, G. Barrionuevo, and F. Schottler (1983) Intracellular injections of EGTA block induction of hippocampal long-term potentiation. *Nature* 305:719–721.

Madison, D. V., and R. A. Nicoll (1982) Noradrenalin blocks accommodation of pyramidal cell discharge in the hippocampus. *Nature* 299:636–638.

Madison, D. V., and R. A. Nicoll (1984) Control of the repetitive discharge of rat CA1 pyramidal neurones *in vitro*. *J. Physiol. (Lond.)* 354:319–334.

Marchiafava, P. L. (1979) The responses of retinal ganglion cells to stationary and moving visual stimuli. *Vision Res.* 19:1203–1211.

Marder, E. (1984) Mechanisms underlying neurotransmitter modulation of a neuronal circuit. *Trends Neurosci.* 7:48–53.

Marder, E., and S. L. Hooper (1985) Neurotransmitter modulation of the stomatogastric ganglion of decapod crustaceans. In *Model Neural Networks and Behavior*, pp. 319–337, A. I. Selverston, ed., Plenum, New York.

Marr, D. (1982) *Vision*, Freeman, San Francisco.

Marr, D., and T. Poggio (1977) From understanding computation to understanding neural circuitry. *Neurosci. Res. Program Bull.* 15:470–488.

Martin, A. R., and G. L. Ringham (1975) Synaptic transfer at a vertebrate central nervous system synapse. *J. Physiol. (Lond.)* **251**:409–426.

Masland, R. H. (1980) Acetylcholine in the retina. In *Neurochemistry of the Retina*, N. Bazan and R. N. Lolley, eds., pp. 501–518, Pergamon, New York.

Masland, R. H., W. Mills, and C. Cassidy (1984) The functions of acetylcholine in the rabbit retina. *Proc. R. Soc. Lond. (Biol.)* **223**:121–139.

Massey, S. C., and M. J. Neal (1979) The light evoked release of ACh from the rabbit retina *in vivo* and its inhibition by GABA. *J. Neurochem.* **32**:1327–1329.

Matus, A., M. Ackermann, G. Pehling, H. R. Byers, and K. Fujiwara (1983) High actin concentrations in brain dendritic spines and postsynaptic densities. *Proc. Natl. Acad. Sci. USA* **79**:7590–7594.

Mauro, A., F. Conti, F. Dodge, and R. Schor (1970) Subthreshold behavior and phenomenological impedance of the squid giant axon. *J. Gen. Physiol.* **55**:497–523.

McBride, R. L., and J. Sutin (1976) Projections of the locus coeruleus and adjacent pontine tegmentum in the cat. *J. Comp. Neurol.* **165**:265–284.

McCarley, R. W., O. Benoit, and G. Barrionuevo (1983) Lateral geniculate nucleus unitary discharge in sleep and waking: State- and rate-specific aspects. *J. Neurophysiol.* **50**:798–817.

McCulloch, W. S., and W. Pitts (1943) A logical calculus of ideas immanent in neural nets. *Bull. Math. Biophys.* **5**:115–137.

McIlwain, J. T., and O. D. Creutzfeldt (1967) Microelectrode study of synaptic excitation and inhibition in the lateral geniculate nucleus of the cat. *J. Neurophysiol.* **30**:1–21.

Mead, C., and L. Conway (1980) *Introduction to VLSI Systems*, Addison-Wesley, Reading, Massachusetts.

Meyer, J. H., and H. H. Zakon (1982) Androgens alter the tuning of electroreceptors. *Science* **217**: 634–637.

Miller, R. F. (1979) The neuronal basis of ganglion-cell receptive field organization and the physiology of amacrine cells. In *The Neurosciences: Fourth Study Program*, F. O. Schmitt and F. G. Worden, eds., pp. 227–245, MIT Press, Cambridge, Massachusetts.

Miller, R. F., and S. A. Bloomfield (1983) Electroanatomy of a unique amacrine cell in the rabbit retina. *Proc. Natl. Acad. Sci. USA* **80**:3069–3073.

Miller, R. F., R. F. Dacheux, and T. Frumkes (1977) Amacrine cells in *Necturus* retina: Evidence for independent GABA and glycine releasing neurons. *Science* **198**:748–749.

Miller, J. P., W. Rall, and J. Rinzel (1985) Synaptic amplification by active membrane in dendritic spines. *Brain Res.* **325**:325–330.

Mistler, L. A., F. R. Amthor, and C. Koch (1985) Modeling HRP-injected, physiologically-characterized direction-selective ganglion cells in rabbit retina. *Invest. Ophthalmol. Vis. Sci. (Suppl.)* **26**:165.

Moore, R. Y., and F. E. Bloom (1978) Central catecholamine neuron systems: Anatomy and physiology. *Annu. Rev. Neurosci.* **1**:129–170.

Morris, M. E., K. Krnjević, and N. Ropert (1983) Changes in free Ca recorded inside hippocampal pyramidal neurons in response to fimbrial stimulation. *Neurosci. Abstr.* **9**:118.5.

Newberry, N. R., and R. A. Nicoll (1984) A bicuculline-resistant inhibitory post-synaptic potential in rat hippocampal pyramidal cells *in vitro*. *J. Physiol. (Lond.)* **348**:239–254.

Newberry, N. R., and R. A. Nicoll (1985) Comparison of the action of baclofen with γ-aminobutyric acid on rat hippocampal pyramidal cells *in vitro*. *J. Physiol. (Lond.)* **360**:161–185.

Noda, H. (1975) Depression in the excitability of relay cells of lateral geniculate nucleus following saccadic eye movements in the cat. *J. Physiol. (Lond.)* **249**:87–102.

North, R. A., and J. T. Williams (1983) How do opiates inhibit neurotransmitter release? *Trends Neurosci.* **6**:337–339.

O'Donnell, P., C. Koch, and T. Poggio (1985) Demonstrating the nonlinear interaction between excitation and inhibition in dendritic trees using computer-generated color graphics: A film. *Neurosci. Abstr.* **11**:465.

Oster, G. F., A. Perelson, and A. Katchalsky (1971) Network thermodynamics. *Nature* **234**:393–399.

Oyster, C. W., and H. B. Barlow (1967) Direction-selective units in rabbit retina: Distribution of preferred directions. *Science* **155**:841–842.

Palm, G. (1982) *Neural Assemblies*, Springer, Berlin.

Parnas, I., and I. Segev (1979) A mathematical model for conduction of action potentials along bifurcating axons. *J. Physiol. (Lond.)* **295**:323–343.

Perkel, D. H. (1983) Functional role of dendritic spines. *J. Physiol. (Paris)* **78**:695–699.

Perkel, D. H., and D. J. Perkel (1985) Dendritic spines: Role of active membrane in modulating synaptic efficacy. *Brain Res.* **325**:331–335.

Peters, A., and I. R. Kaiserman-Abramof (1969) The small pyramidal neuron of the cerebral cortex. *Z. Zellforsch. Mikrosk. Anat.* **100**:498–506.

Peters, A., and I. R. Kaiserman-Abramof (1970) The small pyramidal neuron of the rat cerebral cortex. The perikaryon, dendrites and spines. *Am. J. Anat.* **127**:321–356.

Pickard, W. F. (1969) Estimating the velocity of propagation along myelinated and unmyelinated fibers. *Math. Biosci.* **5**:305–319.

Poggio, G. F. (1980) Neurons sensitive to dynamic random-dot stereograms in areas 17 and 18 of the rhesus monkey cortex. *Neurosci. Abstr.* **6**:672.

Poggio, G. F. (1984) Processing of stereoscopic information in primate visual cortex. In *Dynamic Aspects of Neocortical Function*, G. Edelman, W. E. Gall, and W. M. Cowan, eds., pp. 613–635, Wiley, New York.

Poggio, G. F., and B. Fisher (1977) Binocular interaction and depth sensitivity of striate and prestriate cortical neurons of the behaving rhesus monkey. *J. Neurophysiol.* **40**:1392–1405.

Poggio, G. F. and T. Poggio (1984) The analysis of stereopsis. *Annu. Rev. Neurosci.* **7**:379–412.

Poggio, G. F., and W. H. Talbot (1981) Mechanisms of static and dynamic stereopsis in focal cortex of the rhesus monkey. *J. Physiol. (Lond.)* **315**:469–492.

Poggio, T. (1984) Vision by man and machine. *Sci. Am.* **250**:106–116.

Poggio, T., and C. Koch (1985) Ill-posed problems in early vision: From computational theory to analog networks. *Proc. R. Soc. Lond. (Biol.)* **226**:303–323.

Poggio, T., and V. Torre (1978) A new approach to synaptic interaction. In *Theoretical Approaches to Complex Systems*, Vol. 21, R. Heim and G. Palm, eds., pp. 28–38, Springer, Berlin.

Poggio, T., and V. Torre (1984) Ill-posed problems and regularization analysis in early vision. *Artificial Intelligence Lab. Memo*, **No. 773**, MIT.

Poggio, T., H. K. Nishihara, and K. R. K. Nielsen (1982) Zero-crossings and spatiotemporal interpolation in vision: Aliasing and electrical coupling between sensors. *Artificial Intelligence Lab. Memo*, **No. 675**, MIT.

Poggio, T., V. Torre, and C. Koch (1985) Computational vision and regularization theory. *Nature* **317**:314–319.

Purpura, D. (1974) Dendritic spine "dysgenesis" and mental retardation. *Science* **186**:1126–1128.

Rall, W. (1964) Theoretical significance of dendritic trees for neuronal input–output relations. In *Neuronal Theory and Modeling*, R. F. Reiss, ed., pp. 73–97, Stanford Univ. Press, Palo Alto.

Rall, W. (1967) Distinguishing theoretical synaptic potentials computed for different soma-dendritic distributions of synaptic input. *J. Neurophysiol.* **30**:1138–68.

Rall, W. (1974) Dendritic spines, synaptic potency and neuronal plasticity. *Brain Info. Service Res. Report* **3**:13–21.

Rall, W. (1978) Dendritic spines and synaptic potency. In *Studies in Neurophysiology*, R. Porter, ed., Cambridge Univ. Press, Cambridge, England.

Raymond, S. A. (1979) Effects of nerve impulses on threshold of frog sciatic nerve fibres. *J. Physiol. (Lond.)* **290**:273–303.

Reichardt, W., and T. Poggio (1979) Figure–ground discrimination by relative movement in the visual system of the fly. Part I. Experimental results. *Biol. Cybern.* **35**:81–100.

Reichardt, W., T. Poggio, and K. Hausen (1983) Figure–ground discrimination by relative movement in the visual system of the fly. Part II. Towards the neural circuitry. *Biol. Cybern.* **46S**:1–30.

Reuter, H., C. F. Stevens, R. W. Tsien, and G. Yellen (1982) Properties of single calcium channels in cardiac cell culture. *Nature* **297**:501–504.

Ritchie, J. M. (1982) On the relation between fibre diameter and conduction velocity in myelinated nerve fibers. *Proc. R. Soc. Lond. (Biol.)* **217**:29–35.

Robinson, H., and C. Koch (1984a) An information storage mechanism: Calcium and spines. *Artificial Intelligence Lab. Memo*, **No. 779**, MIT.

Robinson, H. P. C., and C. Koch (1984b) Free calcium in dendritic spines: A biophysical mechanism for rapid memory. *Neurosci. Abstr.* **10**:53.

Rogawski, M. A., and G. K. Aghajanian (1980) Modulation of lateral geniculate neurone excitability by noradrenalin microiontophoresis or locus coeruleus stimulation. *Nature* **287**:731–734.

Rushton, W. A. H. (1951) A theory of the effects of fibre size in medullated nerve. *J. Physiol. (Lond.)* **115**:101–122.

Sabah, N. H., and K. N. Leibovic (1972) The effect of membrane parameters on the properties of the nerve impulse. *Biophys. J.* **12**:1132–1144.

Schiller, P. H. (1982) Central connections of the retinal ON and OFF pathways. *Nature* **297**:580–583.

Scheibel, M. E., and A. B. Scheibel (1968) On the nature of dendritic spines. Report of a workshop. *Commun. Behav. Biol. (Series A)* **1**:231–265.

Schmitt, F. O. (1979) The role of structural, electrical, and chemical circuitry in brain function. In *The Neurosciences: Fourth Study Program*, F. O. Schmitt and F. G. Worden, eds., pp. 5–20, MIT Press, Cambridge, Massachusetts.

Schmitt, F. O. (1984) Molecular regulators of brain function: A new view. *Neuroscience* **13**:991–1002.

Schmitt, F. O., and F. G. Worden, eds. (1979) *The Neurosciences: Fourth Study Program*, MIT Press, Cambridge, Massachusetts.

Schulman, J. A., and F. F. Weight (1976) Synaptic transmission: Long-lasting potentiation by a postsynaptic mechanism. *Science* **194**:1437–1439.

Schwartzkroin, P. A., and M. Slawsky (1977) Probable calcium spikes in hippocampal neurons. *Brain Res.* **135**:157–161.

Schwindt, P. C., and W. E. Crill (1982) Factors influencing motoneuron rhythmic firing: Results from a voltage-clamp study. *J. Neurophysiol.* **48**:875–890.

Segal, M., and J. L. Barker (1984) Rat hippocampal neurons in culture: Properties of GABA-activated Cl^- ion conductance. *J. Neurophysiol.* **51**:500–515.

Segev, I., and I. Parnas (1983) Synaptic integration mechanisms. *Biophys. J.* **41**:41–50.

Shannon, C. E., and W. Weaver (1949) *The Mathematical Theory of Communication*, Univ. Illinois Press, Urbana.

Shaw, S. R. (1981) Anatomy and physiology of identified non-spiking cells in the photoreceptor–lamina complex of the compound eye of insects, especially *Diptera*. In *Neurones without Impulses*, A. Roberts and B. M. H. Bush, eds., pp. 61–116, Cambridge Univ. Press, Cambridge, England.

Shepherd, G. M. (1979a) Synaptic and impulse loci in olfactory bulb dendritic circuits. In *Neurones without Impulses*, A. Roberts and B. M. H. Bush, eds., pp. 255–267, Cambridge Univ. Press, Cambridge, England.

Shepherd, G. M. (1979b) *The Synaptic Organization of the Brain*, Oxford Univ. Press, New York.

Sherman, S. M., and C. Koch (1986) The control of retinogeniculate transmission in the mammalian lateral geniculate nucleus. *Exp. Brain Res.* **63**:1–20.

Siegelbaum, S. A., and R. W. Tsien (1983) Modulation of gated ion channels as a mode of transmitter action. *Trends Neurosci.* **6**:307–313.

Sillito, A. M., and J. A. Kemp (1983) The influence of GABAergic inhibitory processes on the receptive field structure of X and Y cells in the cat dorsal lateral geniculate nucleus (dLGN). *Brain Res.* **277**:63–77.

Siman, R., M. Baudry, and G. Lynch (1983) Purification from synaptosomal plasma membranes of calpain I, a thiol protease activated by micromolar calcium concentrations. *J. Neurochem.* **41**:950–956.

Simmonds, M. A. (1983) Multiple GABA receptors and associated regulatory sites. *Trends Neurosci.* **6**:279–281.

Singer, W. (1977) Control of thalamic transmission by corticofugal and ascending reticular pathways in the visual system. *Physiol. Rev.* **57**:386–420.

Singer, W., and N. Bedworth (1973) Inhibitory interaction between X and Y units in the cat lateral geniculate nucleus. *Brain Res.* **49**:291–307.

Sloper, J. J., and T. P. S. Powell (1979) An experimental electron microscopic study of afferent connections to the primate motor and somatic sensory cortices. *Philos. Trans. R. Soc. Lond. (Biol.)* **285**:199–226.

Spira, M. E., and M. V. L. Bennett (1972) Synaptic control of electrotonic coupling between neurons. *Brain Res.* **37**:294–300.

Spray, D. C., A. L. Harris, and M. V. L. Bennett (1981) Gap junctional conductance is a simple and sensitive function of intracellular pH. *Science* **211**:712–714.

Somogyi, P., Z. F. Kisvaraday, K. A. Martin, and D. Whitteridge (1983) Synaptic connections of morphologically identified and physiologically characterized large basket cells in the striate cortex of cat. *Neuroscience* **10**:261–294.

Stanfield, P. R., Y. Nakajima, and K. Yamaguchi (1985) Substance P raises neuronal membrane excitability by reducing inward rectification. *Nature* **315**:498–501.

Sterling, P., and T. L. Davis (1980) Neurons in the cat lateral geniculate nucleus that concentrate exogenous [^{3}H]γ-aminobutyric acid (GABA). *J. Comp. Neurol.* **192**:737–749.

Swanson, L. W., T. J. Teyler, and R. F. Thompson (1982) Hippocampal long-term potentiation: Mechanisms and implications for memory. *Neurosci. Res. Program Bull.* **20**:613–769.

Swindale, N. V. (1983) Anatomical logic of retinal nerve cells. *Nature* **303**:570–571.

Tauc, L., and G. M. Hughes (1963) Modes of initiation and propagation of spikes in the branching axons of molluscan central neurons. *J. Gen. Physiol.* **46**:533–549.

Tauchi, M., and R. H. Masland (1984) The shape and arrangement of the cholinergic neurons in the rabbit retina. *Proc. R. Soc. Lond. (Biol.)* **223**:101–119.

Torre, V. (1976) A theory of synchronization of heart pace-maker cells. *J. Theor. Biol.* **61**:55–71.

Torre, V., and T. Poggio (1978) A synaptic mechanism possibly underlying directional selectivity to motion. *Proc. R. Soc. Lond. (Biol.)* **202**:409–416.

Torre, V., and T. Poggio (1981) A new approach to synaptic interaction. In *Theoretical Approaches in Neurobiology*, W. Reichardt and T. Poggio, eds., pp. 39–46, MIT Press, Cambridge, Massachusetts.

Torre, V., and W. G. Owen (1983) High-pass filtering of small signals by the network of rods in the retina of the toad, *Bufo marinus*. *Biophys. J.* **41**:305–324.

Torre, V., W. G. Owen, and G. Sandini (1983) The dynamics of electrically interacting cells. *IEEE Trans. Systems, Man & Cybern.* **SMC-13**:757–765.

Tsumoto, T., and D. A. Suzuki (1976) Effects of frontal eye field stimulation upon activities of the lateral geniculate body of the cat. *Exp. Brain Res.* **25**:291–306.

Turner, D. A. (1984) Conductance transients onto dendritic spines in a segmental cable model of hippocampal neurons. *Biophys. J.* **46**:85–96.

Turner, R. W., K. G. Baimbridge, and J. J. Miller (1982) Calcium-induced long-term potentiation in the hippocampus. *Neuroscience* **7**:1411–1416.

Virsik, R., and W. Reichardt (1976) Detection and tracking of moving objects by the fly *Musca domestica*. *Biol. Cybern.* **23**:83–98.

Van Harreveld, A., and E. Fifková (1975) Swelling of dendritic spines in the fascia dentata after stimulation of the perforant fibers as a mechanism of post-tetanic potentiation. *Exp. Neurol.* **49**:736–749.

Vaughn, J. E., E. V. Famiglietti, R. P. Barber, K. Saito, E. Roberts, and C. E. Ribak (1981) GABAergic amacrine cells in rat retina: Immunocytochemical identification and synaptic connectivity. *J. Comp. Neurol.* **197**:113–127.

von Békésy, G. (1960) *Experiments in Hearing*, McGraw-Hill, London.

Warren, S., H. A. Hamalainen, and E. P. Gardner (1986) Coding of the spatial period of gratings rolled across the receptive fields of somatosensory cortical neurons in awake monkeys. *J. Neurophysiol.* **56**:623–639.

Watanabe, S.-I., and M. Murakami (1984) Synaptic mechanisms of directional selectivity in ganglion cells of frog retina as revealed by intracellular recordings. *Jpn. J. Physiol.* **34**:497–511.

Waxman, S. G., and M. V. L. Bennett (1972) Relative conduction velocities of small myelinated and non-myelinated fibres in the central nervous system. *Nature New Biol.* **238**:217–219.

Werblin, F. S. (1970) Responses of retinal cells to a moving spot: Intracellular recording in *Necturus maculosus. J. Neurophysiol.* **33**:342–350.

Wilson, J. R., M. J. Friedlander, and S. M. Sherman (1984) Fine structural morphology of identified X- and Y-cells in the cat's lateral geniculate nucleus. *Proc. R. Soc. Lond. (Biol.)* **221**:411–436.

Wong, R. K. S., P. A. Prince, and A. I. Basbaum (1979) Intradendritic recordings from hippocampal neurons. *Proc. Natl. Acad. Sci. USA* **76**:986–990.

Wood, J. G., W. Wallace, J. N. Whitaker, and W. Y. Cheung (1980) Immunocytochemical localization of calmodulin and a heat-labile calmodulin-binding protein (CaM–BP$_{80}$) in basal ganglia of mouse brain. *J. Cell Biol.* **84**:66–76.

Wyatt, H. J., and N. W. Daw (1975) Directionally sensitive ganglion cells in the rabbit retina: Specificity for stimulus direction, size and speed. *J. Neurophysiol.* **38**:613–626.

Chapter 24

Specific Consequences of General Brain Properties

CHARLES F. STEVENS

ABSTRACT

This work explores some consequences of general brain properties. Neighbor inhibitory interactions, structural homogeneity, and symmetry lead, in the simplest theory, to a difference of Gaussian-type receptive field structure; this same form of spatial information processing can be anticipated to occur also in cortical structures. Accuracy of brain function is limited by various noise sources, two important ones of which are the imprecision with which neuronal connections are made and synaptic noise. Both of these noise sources limit the spatial accuracy with which neuronal circuits can function, but their effects tend to be in opposite directions. These general brain properties are formalized, using the methods of functional calculus, and a brief summary of the mathematical techniques is included.

The complexity of the brain is certainly one of its dominant characteristics. The numbers of neurons, their intricate and variable shape, the number and richness of the interconnections, and the variety of structures from one region to another all tend to discourage the search for global principles of brain organization. Nevertheless, certain regular features stand out: recurrent inhibitory loops are present through which neurons commonly influence their neighbors; the circuitry in a region tends to consist of the same modules repeated over and over; circuit connections are symmetric in that—in cortex, for example—mirror reversal would seem not to change the pattern of connections; connections are orderly but not completely precise, and functional studies have revealed randomness in the behavior of individual neurons. The purpose of this discussion is to explore some of the simplest implications of these typical aspects of brain structure and function. Although the differences that exist between one brain structure and another are certainly most interesting and important for function, common features are responsible for some general brain properties; one must investigate the usual as well as the unique. An indication of how some global properties of synaptic organization can arise from regularities is presented here. The discussion will, for convenience, consider structures like retina and cortex that can be viewed as surfaces.

The goal here is to explore some consequences of several general brain properties: recurrent inhibition, symmetry, local homogeneity, and imprecision in neuronal connections and function. These general properties lead in a natural way to the center–surround receptive field structure described by a difference of Gaussian functions. Physiological and anatomical noise sources predict spatial fluctuations in excitation across a cortex subjected to a constant input, and the general properties provide the basis for a quantitative description of the spatial correlations. Although the focus is on some of the simplest possible consequences, the approaches used should be applicable for exploring more complex situations.

THREE GENERAL CIRCUIT PROPERTIES

Neighbor Interactions

A neuron influences neighboring neurons through excitation and inhibition (see Jones, 1984; Peters, this volume). To study these interactions, certain simplifications are convenient but not essential. The cortex will be taken as one-dimensional so that position is specified by the single variable x. Furthermore, we focus on the behavior of only a single class of neurons, although the interactions themselves would in general be mediated through interneurons. Cell state will be given by a single variable $f(x)$, which denotes a Fourier component of the cell's discharge frequency; that is, firing rate as a function of time is decomposed into sinusoidal components, and the amplitude of a component is taken to represent excitation at a particular location (with the frequency variable suppressed). This representation is used because the concern here is with spatial and not temporal effects. We also assume that cells in our one-dimensional neuronal sheet can be stimulated with an input function $S(x)$. This function for the retina, for example, would be the intensity of light at position x.

These restrictions are made primarily for notational convenience. Thus, a more general treatment would assume a two- or three-dimensional structure (x would be a vector) and multiple populations of cells would be included (e.g., Jones, 1984); the field variable f would also be a vector, with possibly a large number of dimensions. Also, more than one variable might be required to specify the state of a cell or the stimulus function.

The existence of neighbor interactions, then, can be expressed by the relation

$$f(x) = M[f,S] ,\tag{1}$$

where $M[\cdot]$ is a functional (see the Appendix for a description of functionals); the quantity of excitation $f(x)$ at one point x thus depends on the behavior of the excitation over the cortex as well as the entire input function S. This notation therefore expresses the fact that the behavior of the neurons at x depends on the excitation in neighboring neurons and on the overall stimulation pattern, not just the stimulus at a single location. For simplicity, we consider here only dominant inhibitory interactions, although lateral excitation could also be included without materially altering the method of argument.

Homogeneity

As far as one can tell, circuits are the same across the extent of the cortex (or retina) (Jones, 1984; Peters, this volume; see also Rockel et al., 1980). The overall organization, then, reflects the continuous spatial repeat of a single pattern of synaptic connections. This property is implicitly assumed, for example, when one draws a representation of cortical circuitry that uses only a few neurons from one location. In some instances, as in the retina, neuronal density varies systematically with position so that strict homogeneity does not hold. We assume that our distance scale has been appropriately transformed to take account of such effects as decreased cell densities or sizes. Because of the homogeneity property, when a stimulus pattern is displaced on the cortex the response pattern is shifted to the same extent; cortical excitation does not depend on absolute position but only on relative distance from sites of stimulation.

Symmetry

Generally, cortical circuits seem to have the property that one cannot distinguish a circuit viewed directly from one seen as a reflection in a mirror. That is, x may be replaced by $-x$ without altering the sense of the synaptic connections.

A SIMPLE CONSEQUENCE

We assume that $M[\cdot]$ in Equation 1 is a continuous functional, an assumption that supposes that all neurons have a resting impulse discharge, and that our stimulus conditions do not drive any cortical regions below the discharge threshold. This assumption is made for simplicity and is not a necessary one: For example, synaptically generated current flow into the spike-generating region could be used as a measure of excitation to avoid the problem.

Use the neighbor interactions *property 1* and expand (see the Appendix) the right side of Equation 1 as a functional power series, retaining only the linear terms, to obtain

$$f(x) = \int_{-\infty}^{\infty} K(x,\xi)f(\xi)d\xi + \int_{-\infty}^{\infty} A(x,\xi)S(\xi)d\xi , \qquad (2)$$

where the zero order term has been taken as zero (excitation is absent without external stimulus S). $K(\cdot)$ and $A(\cdot)$ are functions that are specified by the properties of $M[\cdot]$; K defines inhibitory influences and A describes the spread of the stimulus $S(x)$. Of course, higher order terms must in general be retained, but the simplest case is one for which the stimulus function $S(x)$ can be considered not to drive the system appreciably out of its linear range.

Use the homogeneity *property 2*. Homogeneity implies that only relative distances are involved in $K(\cdot)$ and $A(\cdot)$, so that Equation 2 may be written as a convolution

$$f(x) = \int_{-\infty}^{\infty} K(x - \xi)f(\xi)d\xi + \int_{-\infty}^{\infty} A(x - \xi)S(\xi)d\xi . \qquad (3)$$

A further approximation is necessary to obtain an expression for the simplest form for K and A. These functions can be expected to vary too rapidly for a power series expansion to be useful in obtaining approximations, but they can be transformed logarithmically into slowly varying functions. The arguments will be carried out only for K. Define

$$W(x) = -\ln K(x) \qquad (4)$$

so that

$$K(x) = \exp(-W(x)) . \qquad (5)$$

Because of the logarithmic function, $W(x)$ should now be slowly varying, and one can expect it to be well approximated by the early terms in a power series expansion. Because of the symmetry *property 3*, $W(x)$ is an even function with only even terms in the power series. To the lowest order then,

$$W(x) = ax^2 , \qquad (6)$$

where a is a constant and the zero order constant term in the expansion has been included in a scale factor for the integral. Symmetry implies, then, that the simplest form for the functions K and A is the Gaussian. With the appropriate scale factors α and β, Equation 3 is approximately

$$f(x) = -\alpha \int_{-\infty}^{\infty} e^{-a(x-\xi)^2}f(\xi)d\xi + \beta \int_{-\infty}^{\infty} e^{-b(x-\xi)^2}S(\xi)d\xi . \qquad (7)$$

The first term describes lateral inhibitory interactions, and the second term specifies the distribution of the stimulus.

Equation 7 has been used previously to describe the response of *Limulus* eye and vertebrate retina to light ($S(x)$); Ratliff (1965) has summarized the history of this equation in the visual system and has explored the functional implications. More recently, Marr and Hildreth (1980) have investigated the role of such differences of Gaussians in edge detection in the visual system. Lateral inhibition appears to be a quite common cortical property, and Equation 7 is in at least semiquantitative agreement with experimentally determined inhibitory spread. In the present context, it is seen to be the result of the three basic properties, together with lowest order approximations in power series expansions.

BRAIN STRUCTURE AND FUNCTION IS UNCERTAIN

The precision of brain function is limited by the presence of noise arising through various mechanisms. Noise sources are conveniently divided into two classes, functional and structural. These two classes are considered in turn.

Functional Noise Sources

Functional noise sources produce time-varying fluctuations (see Calvin and Stevens, 1968). At least five independent mechanisms contribute to the uncertainty of neuronal function, with different mechanisms dominating in one circumstance or another: (1) All stimulus sources have inherent variability, and this can be of appreciable importance for brain function. For example, at low light levels, photon noise can be limiting for signal detection in vision, and at low sound pressure levels, thermal agitations of air molecules and of hair cells can produce an unfavorable signal-to-noise ratio. (2) Channels behave probabilistically (Anderson and Stevens, 1973), and the fluctuations in current flows produced can be limiting in those situations where small numbers of channels are responsible for function. This has been reported to occur in small cells (Fenwick et al., 1982) and can be anticipated in any small structure such as a dendritic spine. (3) In small processes, thermal noise in membrane impedances can, as Fatt and Katz (1950) first noted, become significant. (4) Neurotransmitter release is probabilistic, and the central nervous system quantal contents are sufficiently small to make this a relatively important noise source (see Korn and Faber, this volume). (5) In at least some circumstances, however, the predominant source of variability is synaptic noise. This noise arises through the noncoherent activation of many synapses: It is an inevitable result of a neuronal computation scheme that uses a pulse code and must integrate information from a large number of sources. Calvin and Stevens (1968) demonstrated that all of the variability in spinal motoneuron discharge is attributable to this source, and their findings suggest that synaptic noise is probably the fundamental time domain limitation on the precision of information processing (see Green and Swets, 1966).

The present concern is not with time-varying noise, but rather with the spatial aspects of information processing. The temporal noise sources just enumerated are, however, distributed through the lateral inhibitory network and thereby give rise to spatial correlations in the firing of neurons. Here, as before, we deal with the temporal Fourier components of neuronal activity and thus focus on the spatial patterns of activity without the necessity of considering the structure of temporal properties; the frequency variable is suppressed in our expressions, but all parameters depend upon it.

Noise sources are best considered in a hypothetical "resting" situation in which all of the input neurons to a one-dimensional cortex are firing at a constant rate. Let $f(x)$ indicate the deviation from the average in the discharge rate of the neurons at position x. This state of excitation reflects two factors: (1) the constant stimulus arriving over all inputs, and (2) synaptic noise and other sources of variability (such as randomness in the behavior of a neuron's channels). The noise sources considered here arise independently in each neuron and therefore have no inherent spatial correlations. The excitation $f(x)$ of a neuron at x thus is described by a modified version of Equation 7,

$$f(x) = \varphi(x) - \alpha \int_{-\infty}^{\infty} e^{-a(x-\xi)^2} f(\xi) d\xi ,\qquad (8)$$

in which the lateral inhibitory term is present but the term corresponding to the spatial spread of excitation is replaced by a function that represents the inherent noise arising independently in each neuron; this spatial distribution of noise should thus be white. The spatial spectrum of excitation is found by Fourier transforming and squaring the expression in Equation 8 to give

$$S(\omega) = \frac{1}{\left(1 + \alpha\sqrt{\dfrac{N}{a}}e^{-\omega^2/4a}\right)^2} .$$

(9)

Here $S(\omega)$ is the spectrum of excitation with spatial frequency ω, and N is the amplitude of the white noise $\varphi(x)$ arising independently in each cell; note that N varies with the temporal frequency of synaptic noise, but that this dependence has not been explicitly expressed. Synaptic noise arising independently in each cell thus is processed through the lateral inhibitory network to give rise to spatial correlations in excitation. The effect is to suppress the low spatial frequency components below the inherent white noise level given by N.

Structural Noise Sources

The source of the spatial noise just discussed is dynamic, rather than static, in that it changes from moment to moment. In addition to the dynamic physiological sources just discussed, however, are spatial noises that arise from the imprecision of synaptic connections (see Cowan et al., 1984). This imprecision causes a variation of innervation density across the cortex, and the variation in turn produces, in a situation where all incoming axons have a steady "resting" discharge, a static spatial noise (static because it is different from place to place, but is time-invariant at one location). Spatial fluctuations in excitation arising from spatial variations in innervation density can be estimated as follows.

Let $n(x)$ be the variation from the average value in the density of input axon terminals at location x in our one-dimensional cortex. During development and subsequent periods of readjustment in connections, each cortex would establish its own $n(x)$ with a probability determined by the underlying mechanisms of the development process. A resting constant input would then appear to cause variations in excitation along the cortex because of the spatial fluctuations in innervation density specified by $n(x)$. Our goal is to calculate the spectrum of these spatial fluctuations.

The generating functional for these paths $n(x)$ is given by the path integral (see the Appendix)

$$\mathcal{L} = \int \mathcal{P}[n(x)]\mathcal{D}[n(x)] ,$$

(10)

where $\mathcal{P}$ assigns a probability density to each path. By arguments like those that led to Equation 6, the generating functional may be approximated to the first order by

$$\mathcal{L} = \int e^{-\int_0^L [\alpha^2 n^2(x) + \beta^2 \dot{n}^2(x)]dx} \mathcal{D}[n(x)] ,$$

(11)

where α and β are constants and the cortex is supposed to stretch from O to L; $\dot{n}(x) = dn(x)/dx$. Squared terms represent the lowest order approximation because of symmetry. This generating functional is useful because it permits calculation of the mean path, the covariance of the path, and other such quantities by taking functional derivatives (see the Appendix) of the accessory generating function $Q(y)$:

$$Q(y) = \int e^{-\int_O^L(\alpha^2 n^2 + \beta^2 \dot{n}^2)dx + \int_O^L y(x)n(x)dx} \mathcal{D}[n(x)] , \qquad (12)$$

where $y(x)$ is an arbitrary function. For example, the mean path is given by

$$\frac{1}{\mathcal{Z}} \frac{\delta Q(y)}{\delta y(x)} \bigg|_{y=0} , \qquad (13)$$

and the covariance (for a zero mean path) is

$$\frac{1}{\mathcal{Z}} \frac{\delta^2 Q(y)}{\delta y(O)\delta y(x)} \bigg|_{y=0} . \qquad (14)$$

Equation 11 is, for many purposes, easier to deal with if the function $n(x)$ is replaced by its Fourier representation. For convenience, we suppose that $n(x)$ vanishes at the boundaries O and L so that only the sine terms need be considered:

$$n(x) = \sum_{j=1}^{\infty} b_j \sin \frac{\pi j x}{L} . \qquad (15)$$

In this representation, the spatial integral of n^2 and of the squared derivative are given by

$$\int_O^L n^2(x)dx = \sum_{j=1}^{\infty} b_j^2 \qquad (16)$$

and

$$\int_O^L \dot{n}^2(x)dx = \left(\frac{\pi}{L}\right)^2 \sum_{j=1}^{\infty} j^2 b_j^2 . \qquad (17)$$

The probability generating functional becomes, with the changed variables,

$$\mathcal{Z} = J \int_{-\infty}^{\infty} \left(\prod_{j=1}^{\infty} \frac{db_j}{B}\right) e^{-\sum_{j=1}^{\infty}[\alpha^2 + \beta^2(\pi/L)^2 j^2]b_j^2} . \qquad (18)$$

Here J is the Jacobian associated with the change for Fourier representation, and B is a normalizer. Associate the functional $Q(g)$ defined by

$$Q(g) = J \int_{-\infty}^{\infty} \left(\prod_{j=1}^{\infty} \frac{db_j}{B} \right) e^{-\Sigma_{j=1}^{\infty}[\alpha^2 + \beta^2(\pi/L)^2 j^2] b_j^2 + \Sigma_{j=1}^{\infty} g_j b_j} , \qquad (19)$$

where the g_j are arbitrary. The spectrum of spatial fluctuations $S(k)$ in excitation is given by

$$S(k) = \frac{1}{\mathcal{L}} \frac{\partial^2 Q(g)}{\partial g_k^2} \bigg|_{g=0} = \frac{\int_{-\infty}^{\infty} db_k e^{-[\alpha^2 + \beta^2(\pi/L)^2 k^2] b_k^2} b_k^2}{\int_{-\infty}^{\infty} db_k e^{-[\alpha^2 + \beta^2(\pi/L)^2 k^2] b_k^2}} . \qquad (20)$$

This expression gives the mean of the squared amplitude of each spatial frequency component. These Gaussian integrals yield

$$S(\omega) = \frac{1}{2(\alpha^2 + \beta^2 \omega^2)} , \quad \omega = \frac{\pi k}{L} , \qquad (21)$$

where ω is the spatial frequency in cm^{-1}. Thus, the spatial correlations resulting from variation in innervation density decay, in this simplest theory, exponentially. The value of the spectrum is greatest for the low frequencies and decreases for the higher frequencies; it behaves roughly opposite to the spatial fluctuations caused by synaptic noise.

In summary, then, both physiological and anatomical factors produce spatial fluctuations in excitation for a constant, noise-free input. The effects are in opposite directions, at least at the level of the approximations treated here. Insofar as the characteristic lengths involved in the two effects are similar—a plausible situation—they would tend to cancel to produce a white spectrum. In any event, these factors should be taken into account as placing a limitation on the accuracy of neuronal computations that involve spatially distributed functions.

SUMMARY

The point made here is that very general properties of brain structure and function can be formalized with simple theories to yield predictions about such features as receptive field structure and the spatial correlations of excitation for nonvarying inputs. A unifying theme has been the use of functional calculus, a tool that seems particularly well suited for approaching questions at this level of generality. Further studies can perhaps begin to delineate those general aspects common to neuronal processing machinery as a basis for discovering the interesting specializations responsible for actual computations.

APPENDIX

Because functional techniques have not been widely used in biological sciences, I provide here a brief informal summary of some definitions and methods. Just as the value of a function of N variables $f(u_1, u_2, \ldots, u_N)$ depends on all of the u_j, so does the functional $F[g(x)]$ depend on all values of the function $g(x)$; its argument is not, then, a single value for g for a particular x, but the entire path specified by $g(x)$ for some range of x (Volterra, 1959). For example,

$$F[g(x)] = \int_0^\infty g^2(x)dx \ .$$

Here the value of the integral depends upon the entire path $g(x)$ from zero to infinity. A continuous functional is one whose value changes by an arbitrarily small amount when the argument function is altered slightly.

Functional Derivatives

A variation of a functional is written as

$$\delta F[g(x)] = F[g(x) + \eta(x)] - F[g(x)]$$

for arbitrarily small η. One formulation of the functional derivative is given by

$$\frac{\delta F[g(x)]}{\delta g(\xi)} = \lim_{\epsilon \to 0} \frac{1}{\epsilon} (F[g(x) + \epsilon \delta(\xi - x)] - F[g(x)]) \ .$$

For example, if

$$F[g(x)] = \int_0^\infty K(x)g(x) \ dx$$

then

$$\frac{\delta F}{\delta g(\xi)} = \lim_{\epsilon \to 0} \frac{1}{\epsilon} \left(\int_0^\infty K(x)[g(x) + \epsilon \delta(\xi - x)]dx - \int_0^\infty K(x)g(x)dx \right)$$

$$= K(\xi) \ .$$

Another example comes from Equation 13:

$$\bar{n}(x) = \text{mean} = \frac{1}{\mathcal{Z}} \frac{\delta Q(y)}{\delta y(x)} \bigg|_{y=0}$$

$$= \lim_{\epsilon \to 0} \frac{1}{\mathcal{Z}} \frac{1}{\epsilon} \left(\int e^{-S[n] + \int \delta n[y + \epsilon \delta(x - \xi)]d\xi} \mathcal{D}[n] - Q(y) \right)$$

$$= \lim_{\epsilon \to 0} \frac{1}{\mathcal{Z}} \int \mathcal{D}[n]e^{-S[n]}(e^{\epsilon n(x)} - 1) = \frac{1}{\mathcal{Z}} \int \mathcal{D}[n]n(x)e^{-S[n]} \ ,$$

where

$$S[n] = \int_O^L [\alpha^2 n^2(\xi) + \beta^2 \dot{n}^2(\xi)]d\xi .$$

Note that the functional derivative depends on the "index" x just as the partial derivative of the function $f(u_1, u_2, \ldots, u_N)$ of N variables $\delta f / \delta u_k$ depends on the index k.

Functional Power Series

A continuous functional $F[g]$ for a spatially homogeneous sytem (one where only relative distances matter) may be represented (Volterra, 1959) as

$$F_x[g] = K_0(x) + \int_{-\infty}^{\infty} K_1(x - x_1)g(x_1)dx_1$$

$$+ \frac{1}{2} \iint_{-\infty}^{\infty} K_2(x - x_1, x - x_2)g(x_1)g(x_2)dx_1 dx_2 + \cdots$$

The subscript x here indicates that the functional depends on the value of x in the kernels K. This may be written to look more like a power series as

$$F_x[g] = \sum_k \frac{1}{k!} K_k * g^k ,$$

where * indicates convolution and the superscript k denotes a k-fold convolution. From the definition of the functional derivatives given earlier, it may be seen that K_k in the expression above are the kth order functional derivatives of $F[\ ]$ with respect to the argument function. Thus, for example,

$$\frac{\delta F_x}{\delta g(\xi)} = K(x, \xi) .$$

Functional Integration

In the ordinary integral

$$\int_0^{\infty} f(x)dx ,$$

each value $f(x)$ is weighted by a small length dx, and all of the weighted values are added up. In a functional integral

$$\int F[g(x)] \mathcal{D}[g(x)] ,$$

each value of the functional $F[g]$ is weighted by a small length in function space. $\mathcal{D}[g(x)]$, and these weighted values are added up. A clear explanation of how one can assign these weights in function space is given by Kac (1951), who makes use of the *Weiner measure*. If $d_w x$ represents the Weiner measure, then the path integral, as given in the Feynman and Hibbs' $\mathcal{D}$ (1965) notation, is

$$\int F[g(x)]d_w x = \int F[g(x)]e^{-1/2\int\dot{g}^2 dx}\mathcal{D}[g(x)] .$$

An early and still useful review of path integrals is Gel'fand and Yaglom (1960). Feynman and Hibbs (1965) is especially readable, and Schulman (1981) includes many recent applications and references to the literature. The conversion of path integrals to the Fourier representation is discussed by Feynman and Hibbs (1965) and, most recently, by Royer (1984), who briefly reviews the intervening literature.

REFERENCES

Anderson, C. R., and C. F. Stevens (1973) Voltage clamp analysis of acetylcholine-produced end-plate current fluctuations at frog neuromuscular junction. *J. Physiol. (Lond.)* **235**:655–691.

Calvin, W. H., and C. F. Stevens (1968) Synaptic noise and other sources of randomness in motoneuron interspike intervals. *J. Neurophysiol.* **31**:574–587.

Cowan, W. M., J. W. Fawcett, D. D. M. O'Leary, and B. B. Stanfield (1984) Regressive events in neurogenesis. *Science* **225**:1258–1265.

Fatt, P., and B. Katz (1950) Some observations on biological noise. *Nature* **166**:597–598.

Fenwick, E. M., A. Marty, and E. Neher (1982) A patch-clamp study of bovine chromaffin cells and of their sensitivity to acetylcholine. *J. Physiol. (Lond.)* **331**:577–597.

Feynman, R. P., and A. R. Hibbs (1965) *Quantum Mechanics and Path Integrals*, McGraw-Hill, New York.

Gel'fand, I. M., and A. M. Yaglom (1960) Integration in functional spaces and its applications in quantum physics. *J. Math. Phys.* **1**:48–69.

Green, D. M., and J. A. Swets (1966) *Signal Detection Theory and Psychophysics*, Wiley, New York.

Jones, E. G. (1984) Identification and classification of intrinsic circuit elements in the neocortex. In *Dynamic Aspects of Neocortical Function*, G. M. Edelman, W. E. Gall, and W. M. Cowan, eds., pp. 7–40, Wiley, New York.

Kac, M. (1951) On some connections between probability theory and differential and integral equations. *Proc. Berkeley Symp. Math. Stat. Probab.* **2**:189–215.

Marr, D., and E. Hildreth (1980) Theory of edge detection. *Proc. R. Soc. Lond. (Biol.)* **207**:187–217.

Ratliff, F. (1965) *Mach Bands: Quantitative Studies on Neural Networks in the Retina*, Holden-Day, Oakland, California.

Rockel, A. J., R. W. Hiorns, and T. P. S. Powell (1980) The basic uniformity in structure of the neocortex. *Brain* **103**:221–244.

Royer, A. (1984) On the Fourier series representations of path integrals. *J. Math. Phys.* **25**:2873–2884.

Schulman, L. S. (1981) *Techniques and Applications of Path Integration*, Wiley, New York.

Volterra, V. (1959) *Theory of Functionals and of Integral and Integro-Differential Equations*, Dover, New York.

Chapter 25

Population Rules for Synapses in Networks

LEIF H. FINKEL
GERALD M. EDELMAN

ABSTRACT

In this chapter, we consider how different presynaptic and postsynaptic modifications interact when allowed to operate at the same time in a neural network. Presynaptic and postsynaptic efficacies are both considered to be modifiable, but according to separate and independent rules. Population properties of such rules embedded in networks of neurons result in significant interactions between short-term and long-term changes. We review possible mechanisms for synaptic modifications and formulate two separate modification rules. The postsynaptic rule regulates predominantly short-term changes at specific, individual postsynaptic processes. These changes are influenced by the firing patterns of many of the other synaptic inputs to the postsynaptic neuron and are carried out by a family of biochemical mechanisms that selectively modify ion channels or transmitter receptors that are in particular conformational states. The presynaptic rule deals with stable, long-term changes in the amount of neurotransmitter released by a neuron. This change affects most or all of the presynaptic terminals of a neuron, and occurs in response to significant firing of that neuron over a period of time. This long-term presynaptic change affects numerous synapses, distributed widely throughout the network by the ramifications of the axon.

The main finding of this analysis is that the properties of the interactions between synaptic rules depend critically upon the anatomy and pharmacology of the network. Organization of the network into neuronal groups is found to give rise to a useful relationship between short- and long-term changes. In particular, the presence of neuronal groups guarantees that long-term changes differentially enhance related short-term modifications while also generating increased variability in unrelated short-term modifications. This links short- and long-term synaptic modifications, allows them both to occur within the same population of neurons without overwhelming interference, and provides interesting properties for a system of memory.

Shortly after the first anatomical descriptions of the synapse nearly a century ago, the idea arose that the modification of synaptic function might provide the basis for memory (Ramón y Cajal, 1937). Numerous models have subsequently been proposed in which various cognitive activities are represented by the firing patterns of individual neurons and in which learning or memory is due to activity-dependent changes at individual synapses. These models rely on the principle that the synaptic modifications that result from a particular pattern of neural activity act preferentially to enhance subsequent occurrences of that activity pattern. However, with the exception of some extraordinary synapses such as those onto Mauthner cells or those made by climbing fibers in the cerebellum, the complexity of real nervous systems prohibits any simple relationship between changes at an individual synapse and changes in the behavior of the network. The complex relationship between synapse and network, and the fact that multiple synaptic modifications are likely to occur together at various sites in the network, motivates a consideration of the population properties of synaptic modifications.

In this chapter, we propose a model of synaptic modifications within populations of neurons, and in the course of developing the model we review the experimental results on the variables influencing presynaptic and postsynaptic change. The model assumes that both presynaptic and postsynaptic modifications occur, but that the two are governed by separate and independent rules. We propose rules that are based on biochemical and biophysical mechanisms and that give rise to experimentally testable predictions. The detailed mechanisms of the rules are of some interest, but they only represent particular choices from a large family of possible mechanisms. Our main objective is to consider the interactions between multiple rules synchronously operating in parallel within a structurally defined network and to examine how such interactions are constrained by the structure of the network.

Our motivation in studying these interactions comes from the theory of neuronal group selection (Edelman, 1978, 1981; Edelman and Reeke, 1982; Edelman and Finkel, 1984; Finkel and Edelman, 1985). This theory is based on the idea that the nervous system operates as a selective system, akin to natural selection in evolution, but operating during somatic time on groups of neurons. Particular groups of neurons are "selected" over other potential groups based on their responses to stimuli. Neuronal groups are determined by the strengths of their synaptic connections: Neurons within a group are more tightly coupled than neurons in different groups and tend to share functional properties such as receptive fields. The modification of synaptic function serves as the principal mechanism for the selection of groups and for their competitive interactions. Just as there are multiple genetic mechanisms for altering gene frequencies in animal populations, we must consider the joint effects of multiple synaptic mechanisms operating within the same neuronal population.

There is experimental evidence for the occurrence of both presynaptic modifications (see Magleby, this volume) and postsynaptic modifications (see Changeux and Heidmann, this volume). If both types of changes occur at the same synapse, they could occur in either a dependent or an independent fashion. In an independent synaptic rule, presynaptic and postsynaptic modifications can occur independently, a reasonable property given the individuality of the two neurons involved. Nonetheless, since the work of Hebb (1949) and von Hayek (1952), most theoretical models have opted for some form of dependent synaptic rule. In a dependent rule, the locus of the change in synaptic efficacy can be presynaptic and/or postsynaptic (and usually is not specified), but the change is contingent upon events at both loci. For example, the Hebb rule (1949) states that "when an axon on cell A is near enough to excite a cell B and repeatedly or persistently takes part in firing it, some growth process or metabolic change takes place in one or both cells such that A's efficiency, as one of the cells firing B, is increased."

There are both experimental and theoretical difficulties with dependent modification rules. Such rules make the firing of both cells necessary and sufficient for modification. Yet, evidence from *Aplysia* (Carew et al., 1984) and from rat hippocampus (Wigstrom et al., 1982) indicates that firing of both cells is neither necessary nor sufficient. Andersen (this volume) has argued that synaptic modifications require that the postsynaptic process be depolarized to a certain "threshold" value, but that the postsynaptic cell need not fire an action potential. In the visual cortex, Singer (Singer and Rauschecker, 1982) has discussed the notion of central "gating" inputs that are necessary but not sufficient for the modification of synaptic efficacies. Such gating effects have also recently been reported in the hippocampus (Hopkins and Johnston, 1984). In contrast, there is no experimental support of the Hebb synapse at the *synaptic* level; most experiments that are cited in support of the Hebb synapse (e.g., Rauschecker and Singer, 1981) only support the notion that intense, correlated firing of the cells in a region leads to synaptic modifications.

From a theoretical point of view, dependent rules are unable to explain many of the heterosynaptic effects that have been reported. We use the term "heterosynaptic" modifications for changes in the efficacy of synapses as a result of stimulation to other synapses on the same neuron. "Homosynaptic" modifications are those in which only the synapse that has received direct, intense stimulation is modified (Kandel, 1976). Dependent rules make synaptic modification contingent upon the firing of both the presynaptic and the postsynaptic cells; implying, at least statistically, that when a threshold number of presynaptic inputs fire together, all of the active synapses are strengthened and all of the unaffected synapses are weakened. But we know that an individual presynaptic input can be strengthened (for example, by facilitation) without firing the postsynaptic cell and without inducing postsynaptic changes. Moreover, heterosynaptic facilitations (presumably of postsynaptic origin) have been reported in which the various presynaptic inputs did not fire together (Swanson et al., 1982).

These considerations lead us to propose that presynaptic and postsynaptic modifications both occur but are controlled by independent mechanisms. The two proposed rules governing the separate modifications operate concurrently in parallel at each synapse and jointly contribute to the net modification of the individual synapse. An important consequence of this idea is that at the level of the individual synapse, presynaptic and postsynaptic modifications will be functionally indistinguishable. However, the two rules differ markedly with regard to how the modifications are anatomically distributed within a network, and the two types of modifications may be distinguished by considering the distribution of these changes over the population of synapses. For this reason, the anatomical and pharmacological details of a given network assume major importance in determining the interactions among synapses.

We first discuss the postsynaptic rule, which proposes that coactivated heterosynaptic inputs to a neuron alter the states of ion channels at a given synapse, thereby changing the susceptibility of these channels to local biochemical alterations. The resultant change in the population distribution of local channel states affects the postsynaptic potential produced at that synapse by subsequent inputs. This postsynaptic rule applies, in general, to short-term changes at specific individual synapses. In contrast, the presynaptic rule, which we discuss next, applies to long-term changes in the whole neuron resulting in an altered probability of transmitter release. Because of neuroanatomical constraints, the presynaptic rule affects large numbers of synapses defined by the connectivity of that neuron and distributed nonspecifically over the population.

The central aim of this chapter is an analysis, based both on an analytical mathematical model and on computer simulations, of the properties of the two modification rules acting within a network with group structure. The analysis specifically addresses the fundamental problem of how short-term and long-term modifications evoked by the same history of activation can both occur in the same network without interference and loss of information. Indeed, we show that not only can the two processes operate concurrently over the same population of synapses, but that in doing so significant emergent properties can be gained. We suggest that independent presynaptic and postsynaptic mechanisms acting together over the same period can account for: (1) the existence of heterosynaptic as well as homosynaptic modifications; (2) the occurrence of stable network changes over several different time scales while producing a continual source of variance in the synaptic couplings of neurons; (3) the coexistence of long- and short-term changes distributed within the same network based upon modifications of the same population of synapses; and (4) the property that these long- and short-term modifications are functionally related to each other despite independent biochemical mechanisms of pre- and postsynaptic change.

THE POSTSYNAPTIC RULE

The postsynaptic rule describes a family of local biochemical modifications of postsynaptic structures and the effect of other synaptic inputs upon these local modifications. These modifications can change the local postsynaptic potential resulting from the release of a given amount of neurotransmitter by altering either the effective number or the functional properties of receptors, channels, or various other regulatory or ultrastructural proteins. In its most general form, the postsynaptic rule says that the change in the postsynaptic efficacy of a given synapse is governed by the positional pattern and timing of heterosynaptic inputs with respect to the homosynaptic inputs to that synapse. As a result of diffusional constraints, the substances responsible for the modifications (cAMP, calcium, etc.) must be produced either locally at the synapse being modified, or at nearby synapses. However, the influences of heterosynaptic inputs to both nearby and distant synapses can be communicated through a variety of mechanisms including: paracrine diffusion of transmitter, intracellular diffusion of modifying substances or messengers, cell surface modulation, and active or electrotonic conduction. Any one or more of these mechanisms are compatible with our combined model of interactions of different rules within a network. We discuss the evidence for some of these mechanisms later. Here we discuss only the electrotonic mechanism in detail because it is exemplary; its plausibility depends most critically on temporal and morphological constraints, and many of these same constraints apply to the other mechanisms.

In this specific example, homosynaptic inputs give rise to a substance that modifies local voltage-sensitive channels assumed to be present in postsynaptic processes, but the susceptibility of these channels to modification can be altered by heterosynaptic inputs (Figure 1). We suggest that a possible result of the biochemical modification is a change in the voltage-dependent probability of the channel switching between functional states, for example, open, closed, and inactivated. However, other possible mechanisms could involve a change in the effective lifetime of the membrane channel, the maximum open channel conductance, the spectrum of kinetic states the channel exhibits, or the actual kinetics of these states. In any case, the modification alters both the postsynaptic potential evoked by subsequent homosynaptic inputs and the sensitivity to subsequent heterosynaptic inputs.

The main assumption of the proposed mechanism is that the local biochemical modifications are *state-dependent*: The probability of modifying a channel depends upon its functional state. Because of the steric properties of different channel conformations, one particular conformational state, for example the "inactivated" conformation, could be more susceptible to phosphorylation by a particular protein kinase. Conducted voltages from other synapses will transiently alter the channel population distribution (i.e., the ratio of voltage-sensitive channels

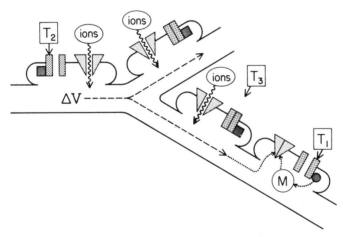

Figure 1. *Operation of the postsynaptic mechanism.* Schematic of four synapses on a branching dendritic tree. *Shaded triangles* represent voltage-sensitive channels and *shaded rectangles* represent receptor-operated channels. Transmitter (T_1) has bound to the synapse at the *lower right*, leading to the opening of the receptor-operated channels and also to the production of a modifying substance M through the activation of a membrane-associated protein (*small shaded circles*). M modifies voltage-sensitive channels that are in the modifiable state. More recently, a potentially different transmitter, T_2, has bound to the *leftmost* synapse, opening local receptor-operated and voltage-sensitive channels. The resulting change in membrane potential (ΔV) is propagated through the dendritic tree (*dashed line*), changing the states of voltage-sensitive channels as they are reached. If the potential reaches the synapse at the *bottom right* (*dotted line*) at a time when the concentration of M is still high, the fraction of voltage-sensitive channels in the modifiable state at the synapse will be altered, and consequently, so will the number of channels modified by M. Synapses that have not yet bound transmitter (e.g., T_3), and synapses not yet reached by the potential, will not be affected.

in the different possible functional states) and thereby alter the number of channels susceptible to modification. Thus, appropriately timed heterosynaptic inputs can modulate the degree of local synaptic modification. Depending upon whether the heterosynaptic inputs are depolarizing or hyperpolarizing, the fraction of channels in the modifiable state may be increased or decreased. However, the modifications are always specific in terms of target and action regardless of whether they strengthen or weaken a particular synapse.

Without a state-dependent assumption, heterosynaptic effects would be obligately nonspecific. Conducted voltages would give rise to modifications at all or most postsynaptic sites (within several space constants) regardless of the state of activity of those synapses. To some degree, postsynaptic state dependence serves as a record of local presynaptic activity, but modulated by heterosynaptic activity. Making the state-dependent assumption at the molecular level assures proper context dependence at the neuronal and network levels. Note that the Hebb rule achieves context dependence at the neuronal level by definition: Postsynaptic sites are strengthened only if they are being activated by presynaptic inputs. The state-dependent assumption provides an explicit mechanism for this Hebbian property.

In this model, the degree of postsynaptic modification therefore depends upon (1) the timing of the different synaptic inputs to a neuron; (2) the number and intensity of the heterosynaptic inputs occurring during the modification period; (3) the spatial distribution of synapses on the postsynaptic cell (conduction delays); and (4) the types of transmitters, receptors, and ion channels present.

Formal Model of the Postsynaptic Mechanism

The plausibility of this particular instantiation of the postsynaptic mechanism based on electrotonically mediated heterosynaptic effects rests upon its capacity to produce a physiologically significant change in the magnitude of the postsynaptic potential (PSP). In order to demonstrate this property, we will consider the number of channels that are modified, the magnitude of that modification as a function of heterosynaptically conducted voltages, and the temporal constraints upon the inputs necessary to effect a modification.

The synaptic current is the sum of three terms: the current flowing through receptor-operated ionophores (ROC), the current flowing through voltage-sensitive ionophores (VSC), and the capacitative current.

$$I_l(t) = I_{ROC}(t) + \sum_i N_i \cdot g_i(V) \cdot (V(t) - E_i) + C \cdot \frac{dV}{dt}, \qquad (1)$$

where N_i is the number of voltage-gated channels for ionic species i of conductance g_i, with reversal potential E_i. Let us consider the case in which a single species of voltage-sensitive channel, species k, undergoes biochemical modification, and suppose that N_k^* of the N_k total species k channels are modified. Then, assuming that the change in the capacitative currents can be neglected, the change in local current resulting from the modification is

$$\Delta I_l = N_k^* \cdot (g_k^*(V) - g_k(V)) \cdot (V - E_k) , \qquad (2)$$

where g_k^* is the modified voltage-dependent conductance.

Modifying the conductance will alter both the local input impedance K_{ll} and the transfer impedances. We will neglect the change in these impedances inasmuch as only a small fraction of the channels will be modified, and because the resistance of the nonsynaptic region is unchanged. Thus, to a first approximation, channel modification leads to a PSP change of

$$\Delta V_l = K_{ll} \cdot N_k^* \cdot \Delta g_k \cdot (V - E_k) , \qquad (3)$$

or to a relative change of

$$\frac{\Delta V}{V} = (N_k^*/N_k) \cdot (\Delta g_k/g_k) . \qquad (4)$$

In other words, the relative change in the PSP resulting from modification depends upon the fraction of channels modified and the fractional change in conductance because of the modification. We now consider these two fractional changes.

As mentioned above, we assume that the conductance change results from a shift in the voltage-dependent probability of the modified channels switching functional states. Figure 2 illustrates a typical sigmoidal curve for the state transitions obtained by using the Hodgkin–Huxley equations (1952) to calculate the inactivation of regenerative sodium channels as a function of voltage. Also shown

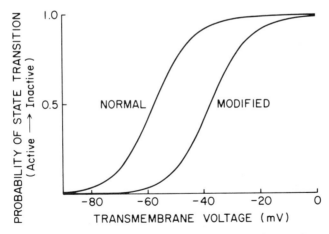

Figure 2. *Effect of postsynaptic modification.* Plot of the probability of channel inactivation versus membrane potential for a regenerative sodium channel (*curve* labeled "normal") using the Hodgkin–Huxley equations (1952). *Curve* labeled "modified" shows the effect of modifying the voltage-dependent inactivation parameter (β) by 20 mV in the depolarizing direction. At the same membrane potential, the modified channel has a smaller probability of inactivating. Thus, fewer modified channels will be inactivated, leading to a larger depolarization of the modified synapse.

is the effect of changing the voltage dependence of the closing parameter (β) by 20 mV in the depolarizing direction.

It is difficult to estimate a realistic range of values for the shift in conductance because of biochemical modifications, although some examples are available. Shifts of tens of millivolts in the current–voltage plots of various channels have been reported as a result of channel phosphorylation (de Peyer et al., 1982; Siegelbaum et al., 1982). The toxin allethrin shifts the sodium inactivation curve 16 mV in the hyperpolarizing direction in crayfish axons and tetramethrin results in a 17–20-mV shift in squid axons (Murayama et al., 1972; Lund and Narahashi, 1981). Scorpion toxins (Catterall, 1979) or batrachotoxin (Huang et al., 1982) can shift conductance curves to even greater extents. Although we might not expect normal cellular modifications such as those resulting from second messenger mechanisms to be as dramatic as modifications resulting from specific toxins, these examples provide an indication of the approximate range of effects.

To determine the size of the change in the PSP, we still need to know the fraction N_k^*/N_k of channels that are modified. In all likelihood, the several conformational states of a channel will be differentially modifiable; for simplicity, let us assume that only a single state is modifiable. Suppose the modifiable state is I, the inactivated state. We will not treat all the complexities of the microkinetics of state transitions; instead we consider only a two-state model consisting of a lumped active state, A, and a lumped inactivated state, I.

Such a two-state model is shown in Figure 3, in which M is the concentration of modifying substance. The starred quantities in the lower tier represent the modified channels; $a(v)$ and $b(v)$ are voltage-dependent parameters—one or both of which are modified by the biochemical mechanism. Decay of the modification may be state-specific, but we assume here that it is not; thus, $K_b = K_{b2}$.

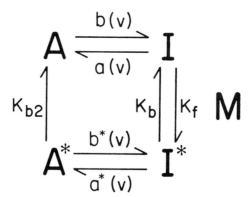

Figure 3. *Kinetics of state-dependent modification; a two-state model of channel modification. A* represents lumped activated states, and *I* represents lumped inactivated states, which we take to be the modifiable states. Channels in state *I* can be modified, in the presence of modifying substance *M,* to state *I**. The forward and backward rate constants for modification are K_f and K_b. The effect of modification is to change the voltage-dependent state transition probabilities (see Figure 2) governed by parameters *a(v)* and *b(v)* to modified parameters *a*(v)* and *b*(v)*. Modification is short-term and decays from *I** according to K_b and according to the potentially different constant K_{b2} from the activated state.

It also seems reasonable to assume that the time constants for state transitions, $(a + b)^{-1}$ and $(a^* + b^*)^{-1}$, are small with respect to the time constant for modification, $(K_f + K_b)^{-1}$. Thus,

$$\frac{dN^*(t)}{dt} = K_f \cdot I(t) \cdot M(t) - K_b \cdot (I^*(t) + A^*(t)) . \qquad (5)$$

In general, the reaction could be higher order, that is,

$$\frac{dN^*}{dt} = K_f \cdot I \cdot M^n - K_b \cdot N^* , \qquad (6)$$

but we take the reaction to be first order (i.e., $n = 1$), without cooperative effects at the molecular level.

To find the steady-state amount of modified channels, we assume that the channels have reached their equilibrium distribution for the ambient voltage

$$\frac{dN^*(t)}{dt} = K_f \cdot (N - N^*) \cdot \frac{b(v)}{a(v) + b(v)} \cdot M(t) - K_b \cdot N^* . \qquad (7)$$

Setting $dN^*(t)/dt = 0$, we find

$$\frac{N^*}{N} = \frac{M \cdot b/(a + b)}{M \cdot b/(a + b) + K_b/K_f} , \qquad (8)$$

which is a Michaelis–Menten-like equation. This represents the number of channels that would be modified if the membrane potential were voltage clamped. Depending upon the topology of the kinetic scheme (which state transitions are allowed and which are forbidden), channels may have to pass through an intermediate state to reach one another. For example, channels may have to open before they can inactivate. In that case, if the modifiable state is an intermediate state, its equilibrium distribution may be a small fraction of the number of channels that pass through it transiently. The number of channels that would actually be modified would then also depend on how long the channels remain in the state, and how long it takes to modify them. The K_D for phosphorylation has been estimated to be approximately 10 μM, hence, $K_b/K_f = K_D \cong 10^{-7}$ (Nestler and Greengard, 1984).

Values for M are more difficult to estimate since there is some question as to what the "modifying substance" actually represents. For example, if the modification is a phosphorylation, should we take $M(t)$ to be the concentration of bound transmitter, adenylate cyclase, cAMP, cAMP-dependent protein kinase, and so forth? Even if we assume $M(t)$ to be the concentration of activated protein kinase, the value of $M(t)$ must still be guessed from values of the K_m (the concentration at which an enzyme is half-maximally activated). These values typically range from 0.01 to 0.10 μM (Nestler and Greengard, 1984). If we assume that $M(t)$ never exceeds a factor of 10 times the K_m, then

$$0 \leq \frac{N^*}{N} = \frac{b/(a + b)}{b/(a + b) + 10} \leq \frac{1}{11} . \qquad (9)$$

Typical values for $b/(a + b)$ are shown in Table 1 for the regenerative sodium channel and the voltage-dependent potassium channel, as calculated from the Hodgkin–Huxley (1952) equations for the squid giant axon.

The table also indicates the change in the number of channels in each functional state resulting from a depolarization of 20 mV. Using values from Table 1 for the inactivated sodium channels in Equation 9, we find that a 20-mV depolarization more than doubles the number of modifiable channels and increases the value of N^*/N by 0.0357. If, as discussed above, we assume that the modification changes the conductance by roughly an order of magnitude, then, using Equation 4, the relative change in the PSP would be around 35%.

We should also note that the values in Table 1 represent the equilibrium values of the channel state population; under transient voltages, these values are never attained. Furthermore, a large fraction of the channels may transiently pass through intermediate kinetic states (e.g., as mentioned above, some channels may have to open before they can inactivate). Channels may be modified while they are in these intermediate states (albeit briefly), yet this process is not reflected in the equilibrium values given in the table.

The final consideration in this analysis concerns the time window within which the homosynaptic and heterosynaptic inputs must occur in order to produce a modification. Suppose, as shown in Figure 4, that homosynaptic inputs lead to the production of some modifying substance which persists for a time t_M after a lag time of t_L, and that conducted heterosynaptic inputs produce a local change in membrane potential which persists for a time t_V after a conduction delay of t_D. Then the time window for synaptic modification requires that the heterosynaptic inputs occur no earlier than a time $(t_V + t_D - t_L)$ before the occurrence of the homosynaptic inputs, and no later than a time $(t_M + t_L - t_D)$ after them. It is possible that one or both of these quantities will be negative for a given synapse. In that case, the presentation of the inputs in that particular order will not lead to a modification. Multisynaptic circuits with dense reentrant connections would be ideal to synchronize inputs to a cell such that heterosynaptic inputs arrive during the peak of the local production of modifying substance. Viewed in

Table 1. The Fraction of Channels in Each Functional State

	Ambient Voltage	
	−60 mV	−40 mV
Regenerative sodium		
Open	0.0001	0.004
Closed	0.6	0.1
Inactive	0.4	0.9
Voltage-dependent potassium		
Open	0.01	0.15
Closed	0.99	0.85

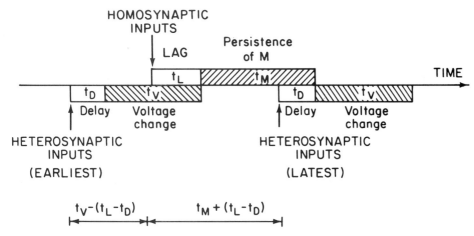

Figure 4. *Timing constraints for postsynaptic modification.* A time axis showing the window before and after a homosynaptic input during which the occurrence of heterosynaptic inputs can lead to modification. After a barrage of homosynaptic inputs, a biochemical cascade of duration t_L leads to the production of modifying substance M, which persists for a time t_M. Heterosynaptic inputs lead to a depolarization (or hyperpolarization) at the local synapse that begins after a conduction delay, t_D, and then persists for t_V. *Arrows* indicate the earliest and the latest times that the heterosynaptic inputs can occur with respect to the homosynaptic inputs so that the effect of the conducted voltage temporally overlaps with the prevalance of M. Depending on the values of the time constants t_V, t_M, and so forth (see text), heterosynaptic inputs may be constrained to either exclusively follow or precede the homosynaptic inputs in order to achieve modification.

another way, those circuits whose time delays and patterns of activation are such that the reentrant input returns at the appropriate time will be the circuits that are differentially selected.

Postsynaptic Rule Computer Results

The postsynaptic rule, as modeled in Equations 1–8, was simulated with a FORTRAN program run on an IBM 4331. The postsynaptic strengths of all the synapses onto a single cell were computed as a function of stimulation over time.

The local synaptic voltage at synapse i is given by

$$V_i(t) \ = \ \sum_j A_{ij}\xi_j\eta_{ij}S_j(t) \, f_{open} \ + \ \delta V_i(t - 1) , \tag{10}$$

where A_{ij} is the voltage attenuation between synapses i and j, ξ_j is the presynaptic efficacy of cell j, $S_j(t)$ is the activity of cell j at time t (and $\xi_j \cdot S_j$ is the amount of transmitter released from j), η_{ij} is the postsynaptic efficacy of the connection from cell j to cell i, f_{open} is a sigmoidal function of voltage that gives the fraction of channels in the open state, and δ is the decay constant of the voltage. The postsynaptic rule involves a number of kinetic processes governing channel transitions and modifying substance production, the fraction of open channels being one specific example. These fractions should be calculated using a kinetic scheme similar to that shown in Figure 3. However, to increase computational speed, we assume that the state transitions occur instantaneously (compared to the duration of an iteration step), and f_{open} is determined by the function

$$f_{open} = \frac{1}{1 + \exp(-(V - U_{1/2})/U_{KT})} ,$$

where $U_{1/2}$ and U_{KT} are input parameters (in the simulations presented here $U_{1/2} = 10$ mV and $U_{KT} = 5$ mV).

The local voltage at each synapse is used to calculate the fraction of channels at that synapse which are in the modifiable state (assumed to be the inactivated state). This fraction is calculated in the same manner as the fraction of open channels is calculated, namely,

$$f_{inact} = \frac{1}{1 + \exp(-(V - V_{1/2})/V_{KT})} .$$

A second sigmoidal curve, generated with the same V_{KT} but with $V_{1/2}$ shifted to the right, is used to calculate the fraction of modified channels in the inactivated state, f^*_{inact}.

We make the assumption that the production of modifying substance increases in a sigmoidal fashion with the amount of transmitter released by the local presynaptic input:

$$M_p(\xi S) = \frac{1}{1 + \exp(-(\xi S - M_{1/2})/M_{KT})} .$$

The concentration of modifying substance is determined by the following equation:

$$M(t + 1) = m_1 M_p S - m_2 M(t) . \tag{11}$$

This equation represents a simple accumulation of modifying substance at a rate proportional to M_p whenever the local afferent input fires, together with an exponential decay of the substance with rate constant m_2 (see the discussion of Equation 13 below).

The fraction of channels modified, N^*, is determined from Equation 5, where K_f and K_b are input parameters. The postsynaptic efficacy η is given by

$$\eta = \eta^0[(1 - N^*)(1 - f_{inact})g + N^*(1 - f^*_{inact})g^*] , \tag{12}$$

where η^0 is the baseline postsynaptic efficacy, and g and g^* are the conductances of the unmodified and the modified channels, respectively.

Figure 5 shows the basic operation of the postsynaptic rule. We consider the case of afferents from group A and group B synapsing onto cell C. The mean postsynaptic efficacy η_{CA} of the inputs from group A is plotted versus time (cycle number). The run began with no channels in the modified state and with $\eta^0 = 0.25$. An initial burst of five spikes (cycles 3–7) gives rise to a modest increase in η. This follows from the local production of modifying substance concurrently with inactivation of channels. The modification of postsynaptic efficacy is short-term and thus η starts to decay back to its baseline value η^0 with a decay constant determined by K_b and K_{b2}. A large stimulus burst from the group B (heterosynaptic) inputs (cycles 17–26) produced no detectable change in η. Despite the inactivation of channels resulting from the conducted voltage, no modifying substance is being locally produced at the CA synapse, and that which was present has

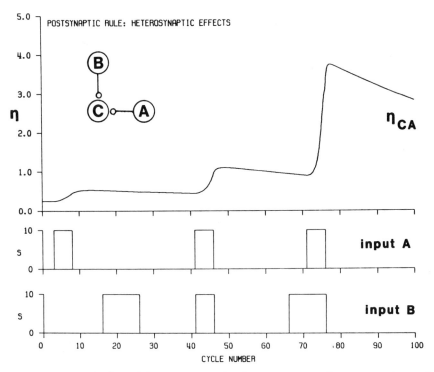

Figure 5. *Heterosynaptic effects of the postsynaptic rule.* The postsynaptic efficacy, η_{CA}, of input from cell A to cell C as a function of stimuli from cell A and from heterosynaptic input (cell B) is shown. A stimulus burst to cell A increases η_{CA}, a lone heterosynaptic burst has no effect, and paired homosynaptic and heterosynaptic bursts produce a larger increase in η_{CA}. However, a large heterosynaptic burst with an appropriately timed homosynaptic burst (final pair) produces a much larger increase. This demonstrates that heterosynaptic inputs can modulate local post-synaptic modifications. The parameters used in the simulation were: intragroup voltage attenuation = 0.5; intergroup voltage attenuation = 0.25; $\delta = 0.9$; $U_{\frac{1}{2}} = 10.0$; $U_{KT} = 5.0$; $V_{\frac{1}{2}} = 40.0$; $V_{KT} = 10.0$; $V^*_{\frac{1}{2}} = 100.0$; $V^*_{KT} = 10.0$; $M_{\frac{1}{2}} = 1.0$; $M_{KT} = 0.5$; $m_1 = 5.0$; $m_2 = 0.5$; $K_f = 0.1$; $K_b = K_{b2} = 0.986$; $\eta^0 = 0.25$; $g = 1.0$; $g^* = 9.0$. No channels are initially modified, and the presynaptic parameters are as given in Figure 9.

already decayed away. In contrast, simultaneous bursts from both the group A and group B inputs (cycles 42–46) lead to a larger change in η. In this case, production of M and inactivation were concurrent. However, if the group B inputs are given a large burst and the group A inputs are stimulated at the appropriate time, the increase in η is dramatically greater (cycles 67–76). This result demonstrates the basic property of the postsynaptic rule, namely, that appropriately timed heterosynaptic inputs can dramatically modulate local postsynaptic modifications.

Figure 6 shows the same scheme as Figure 5 except that in the final burst pair the heterosynaptic input burst is now shorter in duration than the homosynaptic input burst. This figure shows that a large homosynaptic burst is equally effective in increasing postsynaptic efficacy. The locally generated voltage is able to inactivate channels at least as well as can be done by the attenuated voltage from heterosynaptic inputs.

Figure 7 addresses the question of the time window (see Figure 4) within which the homosynaptic and heterosynaptic inputs must occur. The middle stimulus sequence shown is delivered by the heterosynaptic (group B in Figure 5) inputs. The two superposed plots of postsynaptic efficacy correspond to the upper and lower stimulus sequences applied to the homosynaptic (group A in

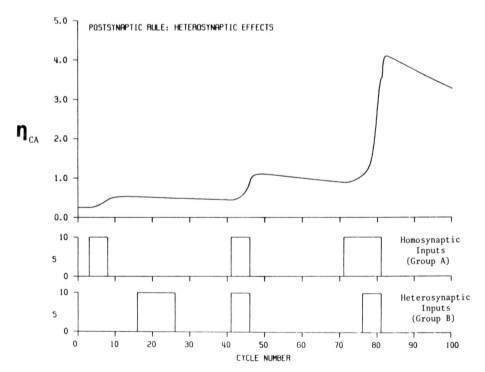

Figure 6. *Further heterosynaptic effects of the postsynaptic rule.* Same as in Figure 5, except the final pair of bursts has been switched. The figure illustrates that a large homosynaptic burst coupled with a shorter heterosynaptic burst is equally effective in producing postsynaptic modification (in fact the change is slightly larger than in Figure 5).

Figure 5) inputs. Note that if the homosynaptic inputs precede the onset of the heterosynaptic inputs (bottom curve) the increase in η is far less dramatic than if the heterosynaptic inputs precede the homosynaptic inputs (top curve). This is because, given the time constants of M and inactivation chosen here, if the homosynaptic inputs occur too early the modifying substance all decays away before enough channels inactivate to produce significant modification. As shown in Figure 4, by adjusting these time constants we could obtain various timing relationships between the classes of inputs required to produce large modifications. What is important in this case is that, given the appropriate timing relationship, a dramatic increase in postsynaptic efficacy can be achieved.

Properties of the Postsynaptic Rule

The postsynaptic mechanism can account for heterosynaptic changes and for the differential strengthening or weakening of certain subsets of synapses. While the geometry and pharmacology of the synapses on a given neuron are fixed, depending upon the play of inputs over the cell, different combinations of synapses will be modified. Certain cohorts of synapses may be in privileged anatomical positions to influence or to be influenced by others. The degree of voltage attenuation between two synaptic sites reflects the neuronal geometry. As noted by Rall and Rinzel (1973) and by Poggio and his coworkers (Koch et al., 1982) the voltage attenuation in the retrograde direction (i.e., going from more proximal to more distal sites) is, in general, far less than that in the orthograde direction. In cat retinal ganglion cells, the retrograde attenuation is on the average *10 times smaller* (Koch et al., 1982).

Dendritic spines constitute an extreme example of this principle. Their high input impedances make the voltage attenuation from spine to shaft much greater than from shaft to spine; they thus act as voltage rectifiers. It has been suggested that the function of spines is to electrically isolate inputs (Chang, 1952; Rall, 1974; Koch and Poggio, 1983). But any voltage changes in the dendritic shaft should be acutely felt within the spine. Therefore, any hypothesis regarding the role of spines in controlling synaptic efficacy should consider conducted voltage effects within the cell in addition to those produced by afferents to the spine. Indeed, within the framework of the proposed model, spines are ideally suited to "listen into" long-distance voltage communications.

All of this analysis suggests that instead of dividing inputs into only two classes—excitatory and inhibitory—and considering neuronal operations in Boolean terms, it may be more valuable to consider a kind of *transmitter logic* in which each transmitter (in association with its postsynaptic partners) can lead to characteristic modifications of synapses receiving only certain other transmitters and located on only certain other parts of the dendritic tree. Such a system would generate a great diversity of classes of synaptic modifications, all specific, but varying with respect to magnitude, time course, origin, and target.

Postsynaptic modification based on such an electrotonic model depends on (1) the number and intensity of heterosynaptic inputs occurring during the modification period; (2) the timing of the heterosynaptic inputs relative to the homosynaptic inputs; (3) the spatial distribution of synapses on the postsynaptic cell (attenuations and conduction delays); and (4) the types of transmitters,

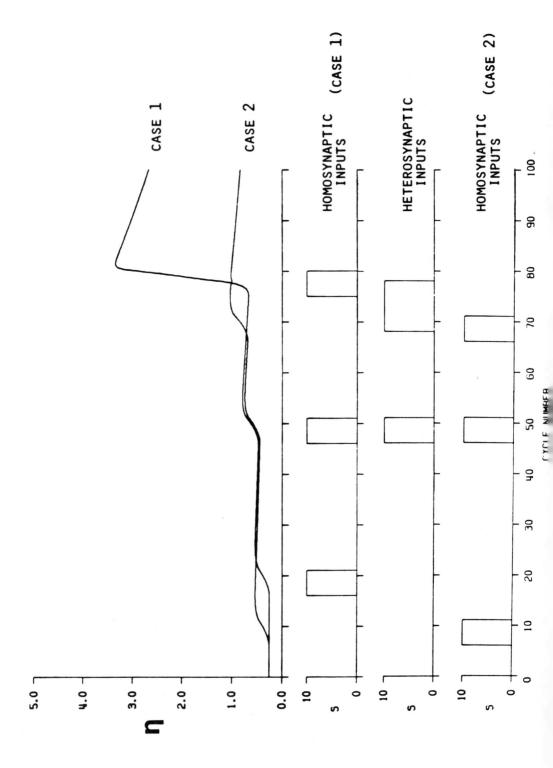

Figure 7. *Timing relationships of heterosynaptic effects.* Same anatomical setup as in Figures 5 and 6. *Middle* stimulus sequence is applied to the heterosynaptic inputs. Plotted is the local postsynaptic modification resulting from either the *top* stimulus sequence (*upper plot*) or the *bottom* stimulus sequence (*lower plot*) applied as the homosynaptic inputs. This shows that if homosynaptic inputs precede heterosynaptic inputs, the induced change is much smaller than if homosynaptic inputs follow heterosynaptic inputs. This is due to the particular choice of parameters (see Figure 4). With this particular set of parameters, if the homosynaptic burst precedes the heterosynaptic burst, the modifying substance will have mostly decayed away before most channels inactivate. This favors the situation in which the homosynaptic burst follows the heterosynaptic burst. By adjusting the input parameters, we could favor various different temporal relations between the synaptic inputs.

receptors, and ion channels present. These factors apply not only to the particular voltage-dependent mechanisms detailed here, but also to the other mechanisms (diffusion of modifier, cell surface modulation) through which the postsynaptic rule might operate.

Biochemical Basis of the Modification Mechanism

Before considering the possible biochemical mechanisms that could mediate the proposed postsynaptic rule, we should perhaps briefly review several related mechanisms. Changeux (1981; Heidmann and Changeux, 1982) has proposed a model of allosteric changes in transmitter receptors resulting from a substance produced by transmitter binding to nearby receptors. He argues that such a mechanism can account for conditioning effects. This mechanism has some experimental support from data on the effects of intracellular calcium upon acetylcholine and glutamate receptors (see Changeux and Heidmann, this volume). Lynch and his colleagues (Lynch and Baudry, 1984; Siman et al., this volume) have proposed a mechanism in which calcium entering the postsynaptic process acts through a calcium-dependent protease to uncover reserve glutamate receptors. Andersen (this volume) and Ito (Ito et al., 1982, and this volume) have interpreted their experiments as consistent with the notion that intracellular calcium modifies the efficacy of postsynaptic receptors. These proposals all share the idea that postsynaptic receptors are modified by calcium produced through the activation of either the receptor itself or other nearby receptors.

This class of mechanism can account for homosynaptic modifications and for effects of a synaptic input on other nearby synaptic inputs (with the distance over which inputs can interact determined by the diffusion of calcium or a calcium-dependent molecule). However, this mechanism cannot explain long-distance heterosynaptic effects by any direct means. The same holds true for the mechanism reported by Kandel's group (Hawkins et al., 1983; Kandel et al., this volume) in collaboration with Greengard and his colleagues. In this mechanism, firing of a serotonergic (or serotoninlike) input leads to a cAMP-dependent phosphorylation of potassium channels in presynaptic terminals of sensory neurons in *Aplysia*. The modified potassium channels lengthen the depolarization of the terminal, allowing more calcium influx and more transmitter release. We should note, however, that in this case the presynaptic terminal is actually serving as a postsynaptic structure for the presumed serotonergic input.

These mechanisms, which act locally at the postsynaptic site, may be seen as one component of a more general postsynaptic modification mechanism; our formal example may also be viewed as a particular example of this general mechanism. In general, the target of the modification can be either voltage-sensitive channels or receptor-operated channels. Nestler and Greengard (1984) have reviewed the evidence for modification by phosphorylation of a variety of ion channels and transmitter receptors in the nervous system. At present, the main candidates for modifying substances are calcium and the seven known protein kinases (which include cAMP-dependent and calcium/calmodulin-dependent kinases). The modifying substances can be produced either by the binding of specific transmitters or by conducted voltages in the case of calcium-dependent processes. A number of different mechanisms (see Table 2) given by

Table 2.   Family of Postsynaptic Modifications

Local modifier
   Receptor-associated second messenger
   Calcium
   Voltage
   pH
   Direct structural interaction (see text)
Heterosynaptic mediator
   External paracrine diffusion of transmitter
   Internal second messenger diffusion
   Calcium diffusion
   Voltage (electronic or active conduction)
   Global cell surface modulation
Target
   Receptors
   Ionophores
   Other ultrastructural or regulatory proteins
Effect
   Change in effective number of channels or receptors
   Change in maximal conductance of channels or binding of receptors
   Change in kinetics of state transitions for channels or receptors

the various possible combinations of modifying substances and targets of modification may come into play. It may be useful to summarize some examples of these combinations, as observed by experiment.

There are numerous examples of interactions between transmitters which could be due to cross modifications of receptor-operated channels either directly or through second messengers. In the superior cervical ganglion, cGMP disrupts the enhanced response to acetylcholine (ACh) normally produced by application of dopamine (Libet et al., 1975). In dog myocardium, muscarinic agonists have been shown to increase β-adrenergic binding threefold in the presence of GTP (Watanabe et al., 1978). Interactions have also been documented between ACh and α-1 agonists, ACh and dopaminergic agonists, ACh and vasoactive intestinal polypeptide (VIP), enkephalins and glutamate, and between γ-aminobutyric acid (GABA) and the benzodiazepines (for a review, see Birdsall, 1982).

Transmitter binding can lead to modification of voltage-sensitive channels (Kupfermann, 1979). The best example of this, as discussed above, is the cAMP-dependent action of serotonin to phosphorylate channels in *Aplysia* (Hawkins et al., 1983). There is also evidence that both the β-adrenergics and histamine (through H-2 receptors) act in this manner (Haas and Konnerth, 1983).

Any voltage dependency in a receptor-operated channel [such as is found for ACh receptors (Magleby and Stevens, 1972)] will allow the receptor to be modulated by ionophores. Calcium produced by activation of calcium channels affects the binding of several transmitters, including ACh and glutamate (Changeux and Heidmann, this volume). Finally, calcium can modify the conductances of other voltage-sensitive channels, notably the calcium-dependent potassium channel, and the calcium channel itself (Reuter, 1983).

In addition to second messenger-mediated modifications, the types of post-synaptic changes necessary for our proposed mechanism could be carried out by direct structural interactions between different channels. There are several conceivable ways in which this could occur: (1) channels may be close enough to interact directly; (2) parts of the molecules, such as regulatory subunits, may be exchanged; (3) initially mobile channels may finally couple irreversibly to other channels; or (4) channels may cluster within the synaptic membrane so that they experience different electric fields (Fraser and Poo, 1982).

The postsynaptic mechanism that we have proposed centers upon the assumption that modification takes place in a state-dependent fashion. Most likely, the various conformational states of a channel are differentially modifiable— and we may imagine that there are a spectrum of intermediate possibilities whose extremes are represented by the cases in which (1) only one channel state is modifiable, or (2) all states are equally modifiable. While there is, at present, no direct experimental support for state-dependent modifications, Catterall (1979) has shown that the mechanisms by which scorpion toxins block the inactivation of sodium channels is voltage dependent. He argues that the toxin binds with different specificities to sodium channels in different conformational states (active, inactive, etc.). While this result concerns a foreign toxin, as opposed to an internal second messenger, it nonetheless supports the possibility of the proposed state-dependent modifications.

It is interesting to note that the assumptions of the postsynaptic mechanism are also compatible with observations in the lobster stomatogastric ganglion (Selverston et al., 1976; Eisen and Marder, 1982; Marder et al., this volume) in which different transmitters interact to couple neural subnetworks and thereby give rise to qualitatively different behaviors. We should further note that the electrical synapses characteristic of this invertebrate ganglion exhibit voltage-dependent rectifying properties (Margiotta and Walcott, 1983) that would be very sensitive to the kinds of long-distance voltage effects that we have been discussing.

The postsynaptic mechanism proposed above involves modifications of the functional properties of channels occurring over a time scale on the order of 100 msec and persisting for minutes, hours, or at most for perhaps days. The pre-synaptic mechanism we discuss in the next section gives rise to long-term modification that could potentially last for years. It should be noted, however, that such long-term changes could also occur postsynaptically through changes in the *number* of channels or receptors. Perhaps the best-studied example of such a long-term change is the phenomenon of "down-regulation" of receptor synthesis by cells that have been intensely stimulated. This has been documented for the ACh receptor on muscle cells (Fambrough, 1979), and for α-bungarotoxin receptors in retina (Betz, 1983). It may be that down-regulation of synthesis is a general way to select only those modifications that exceed a viable threshold. For example, if the total number of receptors is reduced, the number in any conformational state will likewise be reduced, and the shifts in the population distribution induced by conducted voltages might then only affect a minuscule number of channels. Thus, down-regulation may terminate the ability of synapses to modify each other.

Finally, it should be mentioned that long-term changes would likely be reflected in ultrastructural alterations in the synapse. Such changes have been reported in several systems after various stimulation protocols (Fifková and van Harreveld, 1977; Desmond and Levy, 1981; Vrensen and Nunes-Cardoza, 1981; Brandon and Coos, 1982; Bailey and Chen, 1983; Carlin and Siekevitz, 1983).

THE PRESYNAPTIC RULE

The presynaptic rule describes the amount of neurotransmitter released by a presynaptic terminal in response to a given depolarization. There is a substantial experimental literature documenting short-term (milliseconds to seconds) facilitations and depressions of transmitter release as a result of the recent history of activation of the synapse (see Magleby, this volume). There are fewer examples of intermediate-term modifications lasting hours to days (Hawkins et al., 1983; Andersen, this volume; Ito, this volume), and at present there are no examples of truly long-term changes in transmitter release persisting for more than several weeks. Understandably, it would be difficult to track such long-term changes experimentally; nevertheless, the biochemical mechanisms that have been proposed for short-term and intermediate-term modifications cannot produce changes capable of persisting for long periods of time. However, such long-term changes are presumably necessary to account for the persistence of memories over several decades. The basic premise of our proposed presynaptic rule is that such long-term changes do indeed occur, that they occur at the cellular and populational levels rather than just at the synaptic level, and that they reflect a change in the homeostatic set level of transmitter release by a cell in response to appropriate or "significant" fluctuations in release over shorter time scales.

The release of transmitter is a complex cellular process, and it could be regulated at any of a number of steps: invasion of the terminal by action potentials (safety factor), depolarization of the terminal, activation of voltage-sensitive calcium channels in the membrane, diffusion and buffering of calcium within the terminal, active pumping of calcium out of the cell or into internal spaces, interactions of vesicles with the ultrastructural specializations of the release sites, modulation of release by autoreceptors or other transmitters, or transmitter availability because of synthesis, transport, storage, degradation, or re-uptake.

The macroscopically measured facilitations and depressions must be explicable in terms of biophysical and biochemical alterations. Our earlier model of presynaptic modification (Edelman and Finkel, 1984) is framed at the molecular level and involves changes in calcium and transmitter concentrations, and it can be shown to be consistent with the model of facilitation and depression that is developed here. However, there are several cogent reasons for describing the present model at the macroscopic rather than the microscopic level: (1) insufficient data exist about the component processes listed above; (2) the same macroscopic behavior of facilitation and depression could be equivalently produced by several different but equally plausible microscopic models; (3) a model pitched at the level of macroscopic effects is easier to test experimentally; and (4) with regard to the *interactions* between neurons, it is the amount of transmitter released, as described macroscopically, that is the main variable.

Our model of long-term changes in transmitter release will depend upon the ongoing short-term changes in release, and for this reason we first consider these transient changes. Evidence from a variety of preparations, including avian ciliary ganglion (Martin and Pilar, 1964), frog neuromuscular junction (Mallart and Martin, 1968; Magleby and Zengel, 1982), *Aplysia* ganglia (Hawkins et al., 1983), crayfish neuromuscular junction (Parnas et al., 1984), squid giant synapse (Smith et al., 1984), and Mauthner cells (Korn et al., 1984), demonstrate that the level of transmitter release from a presynaptic terminal can be transiently increased or decreased after various stimulation sequences. In general, there appear to be several components of increased release (Mallart and Martin, 1968; Magleby, this volume), as well as of decreased release (Bryan and Atwood, 1981; Magleby, this volume), each with characteristic time constants. These separable components may be thought of as different regulatory steps in the kinetic pathways governing release. In perhaps the most elegantly analyzed system, the frog neuromuscular junction, Magleby and Zengel (see Magleby, this volume) have described four separate components of increased transmitter release, each decaying with a different time course: facilitation I ($T = 60$ msec), facilitation II ($T = 400$ msec), augmentation ($T \cong 7$ sec), and potentiation ($T = 10\text{--}1000$ sec). The frequency and duration of stimulation necessary to maximally evoke each of these processes differ.

The mechanism most commonly offered to explain increased release is the accumulation of calcium in the presynaptic terminal (Katz and Miledi, 1968; Dodge and Rahamimoff, 1967). In general, this is due to a shift in the balance between calcium influx and calcium sequestration or efflux. A change in the amount of influx could result from an increase in the number of active calcium channels, from an increase in the conductance of the calcium channels present, or from an increase in the time during which the calcium channels are open [one mechanism for this is to prolong the deplorization of the terminal (Hawkins et al., 1983)]. Most models of facilitation have been based on the residual calcium hypothesis (Katz and Miledi, 1968), in which frequent action potentials result in a transient accumulation of calcium before sequestration and pumps can equilibrate the ionic load. Action potentials invading the terminal during this time will release supranormal amounts of transmitter. There are several technical problems with the simple residual calcium hypothesis (Bittner and Schatz, 1981; Stockbridge and Moore, 1984); for example, the hypothesis cannot account for four separate components of increased release. An additional difficulty arises in reconciling changes in amplitude and frequency of miniature end-plate potentials (MEPPs) with the amplitude of evoked release. Two recent developments may resolve some of these problems. The first is the demonstration by Smith et al. (1984) that in squid giant synapse, postsynaptic potentials (which are assumed to reflect transmitter release) vary as the third power of the presynaptic calcium current. A small change in the calcium current then results in a large change in transmitter release. The second development is the appreciation of the role of calcium diffusion in release (Stockbridge and Moore, 1984; Llinás, this volume). Only the ions very near the ultrastructural release sites (perhaps within 100 nm) actually contribute to release. Diffusion of calcium ions away from the release sites will limit the time during which release can occur.

Synaptic depression is less well understood. Various mechanisms have been proposed, including depletion of a finite store of releasable transmitter, or transient inactivation of release sites involved in vesicular exocytosis. Korn and Faber (Korn et al., 1984) have presented evidence, using a binomial model of release on data from Mauthner cell inhibitory synapses, that the number of available release sites does not change, but that the probability of release from these sites does change. At the macroscopic level of the model proposed below, the alternatives are formally similar.

These observations can be formalized in a model. In order to keep the model simple, we will pick only a single component of increased release, a generic "facilitation," and only one component of "depression." Facilitation can be described by an equation similar to that used by Magleby and Zengel (1982) and others,

$$\frac{dF_i}{dt} = \epsilon S_i(t) - \lambda F_i(t) , \tag{13}$$

where $F_i(t)$ is the degree of facilitation in the presynaptic terminal of neuron i; λ is the decay time constant; $S_i(t)$ is the firing rate of the neuron at time t; and ϵ is the amount of increase in facilitation per spike. We assume, for simplicity, that the increase in facilitation ϵ is a constant corresponding to a constant bolus of calcium entering with every spike. It is more likely that ϵ is a nonlinear function of voltage and calcium concentration. Equation 13 represents the simplest formal description of a facilitatory process—it increases in constant increments each time a spike occurs, and decays exponentially with a single time constant. We must bear these extreme simplifications in mind when we apply the model to real experimental data.

Synaptic depression can be described by a similar equation,

$$\frac{dD_i(t)}{dt} = \kappa \xi_i(t) S_i(t) - \beta D_i(t) , \tag{14}$$

where $D_i(t)$ is the degree of depression in the presynaptic terminal, β is the time decay constant, and κ is the constant of proportionality between release and depression. The first term describes the increase in depression because of the release of transmitter. The $S(t)$ in the first term indicates that substantial (i.e., nonspontaneous) levels of release only occur when significant depolarization has occurred due to the rapid diffusion of calcium away from the release site. The first term as a whole indicates that depression increases linearly with the amount of release. In a more detailed model, it would perhaps be more realistic to assume a nonlinear dependence, with significant levels of depression only arising after a substantial amount of release has already occurred. The second term represents the decay of depression due to, as discussed above, replenishment of depleted transmitter, return of previously inactivated release sites, or return to equilibrium of whatever molecular process is actually involved.

A final equation relates the amount of release to the degree of facilitation and depression,

$$\xi_i(t) = \xi_i^0 \cdot (1 + F_i(t))^3 \cdot (1 - D_i(t)) , \tag{15}$$

where ξ^0 is the baseline amount of release that would occur in response to an isolated action potential in the absence of facilitation or depression. F is defined to range between zero and some maximum value, while D ranges from 0 to 1. Equation 15 resembles those studied by Magleby and Zengel (1982) and could be generalized to include products of all the components of facilitation and depression. Magleby and Zengel found that raising the facilitatory term to the third power resulted in a better fit to their data. We adopt this nonlinearity, which also agrees with the results of Smith and colleagues (1984) on the dependence of PSP magnitude on calcium current.

Note that these facilitatory and depressive changes are intrinsically stable because of the decay terms. Whereas most synaptic models demand stability as a system property, we have built local stability directly into the mechanism as a reflection of the biological tendency toward homeostasis.

The pattern of activity will determine the relative changes in facilitation and depression. The specific changes depend upon the values of the kinetic constants; however, for the case when the time decay constant of depression β is slightly smaller than that for facilitation λ, the behavior in general is as follows. Short high-frequency bursts favor facilitation; longer low-frequency bursts may favor depression, and lack of activity or low levels of activity will leave transmitter release unchanged. This property has been observed in many experimental preparations. For instance, stimulation of the right pleural connective in *Aplysia* at 5 Hz for 30 sec leads to several minutes of posttetanic potentiation, but stimulation at 0.1 Hz leads only to homosynaptic depression (Kandel, 1976).

Thus far we have considered short-term changes in transmitter release from individual terminals in response to cell activity. These changes are unable to serve as long-term modifications since, by definition, the time constants for their decay are on the order of milliseconds to a few seconds. In the absence of any direct experimental evidence, we assume that the long-term change in transmitter release occurs through a shift in the baseline amount of transmitter release, ξ_i^0, rather than from a change in the properties of the facilitation or depression. It is, however, conceivable that other parameters (ϵ, λ, κ, or β) could change. Our assumption is based on the idea that the long-term modification in ξ^0 results from a total cell response to time-averaged fluctuations, both facilitatory and depressive, in presynaptic strength ξ.

The basic idea is shown in Figure 8. The presynaptic efficacy of a neuron, ξ, depends upon three factors, as given by Equation 15: the degree of facilitation, the degree of depression, and the baseline presynaptic efficacy ξ^0. Firing of the neuron leads to both facilitation and depression in a manner dependent on the temporal pattern of activity, as described by Equations 13–15. The *presynaptic rule* says that if the long-term average (perhaps on the order of a second) of the instantaneous value of the presynaptic efficacy exceeds a threshold, then the baseline presynaptic efficacy, ξ^0, is reset to a new value.

We further assume that the direction in which ξ^0 is reset corresponds to the direction of the deviation in ξ. Namely, sufficiently large facilitatory fluctuations give rise to an *increase* in ξ^0, while large depressive fluctuations result in a *decrease* in ξ^0. Although there is no time decay of this shift in ξ^0, at a later time, given the required stimulation sequence, a cell may be induced to reverse the direction of the shift.

The shift in ξ^0 will alter the dynamic properties of the neuron with respect to the amount of transmitter released for a given temporal pattern of stimulation.

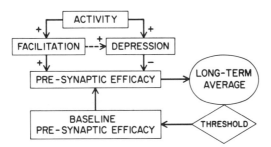

Figure 8. *Flowchart of the presynaptic rule.* Activity increases the degree of both facilitation and
depression, which are also coupled, as greater facilitation increases depression (see Equations
14, 15). Facilitation increases and depression decreases presynaptic efficacy ξ, which also depends
on the baseline presynaptic efficacy, ξ^0. The presynaptic rule states that a long-term average is
kept of ξ as it fluctuates because of the temporal pattern of activity. If this average reaches a
threshold, the baseline value of presynaptic efficacy is reset to a new value. This changes the
response of the cell to future inputs.

It is important to observe that even though the baseline presynaptic efficacy has
been increased, the actual efficacy ξ can still be driven to zero by transient
depressions or further increased by transient facilitations.

The assumption regarding the direction of the shift in ξ^0 gives the system a
useful stability property: Stronger synapses will be harder to strengthen and
easier to weaken. For as ξ^0 increases, the degree of facilitation is unchanged,
but the amount of transmitter released increases, leading to a greater degree of
depression for a similar sequence of stimulation. It will then be more difficult
to evoke short-term facilitations necessary to further increase ξ^0. This property
will tend to maintain stronger synapses, which in some sense may be considered
functionally more important, while weaker synapses are more adaptable to change.
Note that we have not assumed any negative feedback for long-term changes;
indeed, there is positive feedback in that facilitatory fluctuations lead to long-
term strengthening and depressive fluctuations to long-term weakening.

There are two reasons for postulating that the long-term modification occurs
on a total cell basis rather than independently at individual synapses. The first
reason is that we have assumed all presynaptic modifications are dependent
upon the firing of the cell. It is known that transmitter release can occur in the
absence of action potentials (Miledi, 1973), particularly at presynaptic dendrites.
However, axonic presynaptic terminals will release transmitter primarily in response to action potentials. The essential point is that most of the terminals
given off by a given axon will experience a similar history of activation. The
series of facilitatory and depressive fluctuations will thus be similar at the various
terminals of an axon. We do not wish, however, to diminish the possibility that
variation occurs among axonal terminals—indeed, the raison d'être of a selective
theory is to emphasize such variability and to utilize it for selective amplifications.
The sources for such variation are abundant: Axonal branch conduction block
(safety factor) has been observed in several species (Parnas, 1972; Henneman,
1984), autoreceptors or receptors to other transmitters (Chesselet, 1984) influence
presynaptic transmitter release, and the initial distribution of presynaptic strengths
must itself have a finite variance. In addition, influences of local circuits will

give each axonal terminal an essentially unique environment. But as we discuss in detail later, such variability will only serve to increase the combinatorial richness of the behavior of the system—one cell may have several quasi-independent functional domains both for input (as proposed by Koch et al., 1982, 1983) and for output. The main point remains that all (or at least large parts) of the cell will experience nearly identical long-term changes.

The second reason for assuming that presynaptic modification must occur across the entire cell rather than at individual synapses concerns the physical limitations of any synaptic mechanism. We are implicitly supposing that these long-term modifications involve a change in gene expression, potentially in response to second messengers produced at synapses and retrogradely transported (Greengard and Kuo, 1970; Nestler and Greengard, 1984). In this case, the net effect would reflect an average of the individual synaptic short-term fluctuations. Given the inherent time lags in the production and transport of newly synthesized gene products, there is no currently known way to selectively route the new material to those individual synapses that originally experienced the short-term changes. In any case, a long-term modification will reflect a fairly long temporal average (otherwise the synaptic state would thrash about unstably) and such an average will necessarily involve a loss of specificity of the contributions of individual synapses.

We have previously argued (Edelman and Finkel, 1984) that such a presynaptic mechanism can give rise to a Hebb-like property at the group level without using a Hebb synapse. The essential requirement is that there be a group structure with stronger and/or more numerous intragroup connections than intergroup connections. In this case, correlated activity among the neurons in a group will give rise to higher firing rates, facilitatory short-term changes, and long-term increases in synaptic strength. Conversely, uncorrelated activity will give rise to short-term depression and long-term decreases in synaptic strength. The present presynaptic mechanism differs from the Hebb synapse since it depends upon the temporal pattern of activity of the cell itself and not upon the correlation of firing across synapses. It is based on empirical observations of short-term changes and the physiological constraints incumbent upon the as yet unknown detailed mechanism for long-term presynaptic modification.

Presynaptic Rule Computer Results

The presynaptic rule was simulated using an IBM 4331 computer. One presynaptic terminal of a single cell was simulated. The firing level of the cell as a function of time, $S_i(t)$, was given as input to the program. The program simulated Equations 13, 14, and 15 with the four parameters ϵ, λ, κ, and β specified as input parameters.

Long-term changes in ξ were effected whenever the running average of a parameter L surpassed a threshold, θ_S. L was determined by the equation

$$L(t + 1) = \alpha L(t) + \gamma \frac{(\xi(t) - \xi^0)}{\xi^0} \tag{16}$$

Thus L represents a running average of the deviation of ξ from its steady-state value, with α the averaging time constant and γ a constant of proportionality.

Figure 9 shows the results of two runs that demonstrate the operation of the presynaptic rule. First a run was done with two bursts of stimulation separated by five cycles of rest (the first two bursts in Figure 9). The threshold θ_S was chosen to be 4.0, and L never reached this threshold. During the next 65 cycles, no stimuli were applied, so that ξ and L both returned toward resting values. A test burst at cycle 85 yielded a change in ξ similar to that observed with the initial burst. The next run (plotted as the upper curve in Figure 9) involved three initial bursts of stimuli (the extra "third" burst is distinguished by an asterisk). This was sufficient to allow L to surpass θ_S, and a long-term change resulted. The long-term change is seen as the sharp rise in ξ at cycle 32. As discussed above, such long-term changes are proposed to result from changes in gene expression and would require minutes to hours to be fully manifested. For simplicity, we opted to make the change take place instantaneously. Such discontinuities could potentially introduce spurious oscillations into the network, but in our simulations we never observed such effects. The change in ξ^0 was 0.6, and ξ underwent a proportionate increase. During the 55 rest cycles, ξ decreased with the same decay constant as before the long-term change, since λ and β were unchanged. The test pulse at cycle 85 reveals a much larger response than was initially produced—this is the result of the long-term change. The increase in ξ would give rise to greater stimulation of any follower cells. It might be objected that the increase in ξ seen at cycle 85 is due to the shorter recovery time from the preceding bursts. This is not the case; the same result is obtained with identical resting times between the last stimulus and the test burst.

The cause of the increase in ξ is shown in Figure 10. Here the same set of stimuli were applied to neurons with $\xi^0 = 0.5$, 1.0, and 2.0. This corresponds to long-term changes in ξ^0 evoked when L exceeds θ_S. It is apparent that as ξ^0 increases, there is an increase in the fluctuations in the values of ξ with bursts of stimulation. Less apparent is the gentle wave of increase in the mean value of ξ, and the fact that the peak of this wave occurs earlier for larger ξ^0. This effect is due to the fact that the magnitude of ξ affects the amount of depression (see Equation 14), and larger values of ξ^0 lead to an earlier onset of significant depression, which depresses the ξ curve.

Figure 10 also illustrates the plasticity property of the presynaptic rule: Stronger synapses are harder to strengthen. Note that as ξ^0 increases (the upper curves) the ratio of ξ/ξ^0 decreases. For instance, when $\xi^0 = 0.5$ (bottom curve) ξ reaches a value of 1.4 ($\xi/\xi^0 = 2.8$). However, when $\xi^0 = 2.0$ (upper curve), ξ never exceeds 3.8 ($\xi/\xi^0 = 1.9$). Furthermore, the general depressive trend of the upper curve discussed in the last paragraph keeps the running average of ξ/ξ^0 lower as ξ^0 increases. It can be seen from the equation for L above that lowering ξ/ξ^0 will lower L and thus make further long-term changes more difficult to achieve.

INTERACTION OF PRESYNAPTIC AND POSTSYNAPTIC MODIFICATIONS

The assumption of independence of the mechanisms regulating presynaptic and postsynaptic modifications prompts the question of how the two types of changes interact to produce functional alterations in network behavior. In considering

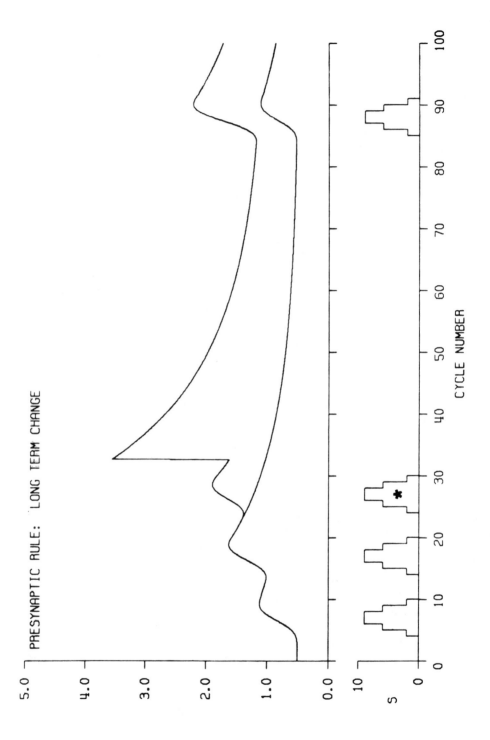

PRESYNAPTIC RULE: LONG TERM CHANGE

CYCLE NUMBER

738

Figure 9. *Long-term presynaptic change.* Two superposed plots of presynaptic efficacy ξ versus the number of cycles; the *bottom panel* shows the applied stimulation. Two stimulus bursts produce the *lower curve,* which does not achieve a long-term change, and which shows a response to test burst at cycle 85 that is virtually identical to the initial response. Three stimulus bursts (including the burst marked with an *asterisk*) give rise to a long-term change (*upper curve*) manifested as increased baseline presynaptic strength. A test burst at cycle 85 produced an enhanced response. In this simulation, each iteration was broken into 10 substeps, and the values of the parameters used were: $\lambda = 0.04$; $\beta = 0.01$; $\epsilon = 0.10$; $\kappa = 0.02$; $\xi^0 = 0.5$; $\alpha = 0.90$; $\gamma = 0.20$.

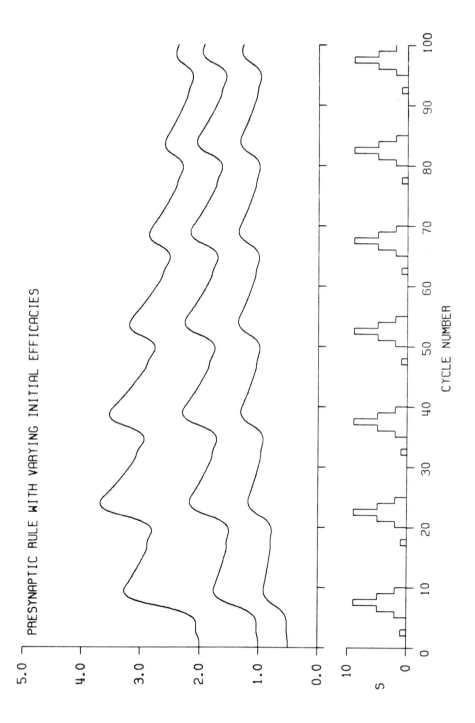

PRESYNAPTIC RULE WITH VARYING INITIAL EFFICACIES

CYCLE NUMBER

Figure 10. *Effect of changing baseline presynaptic efficacy.* Plots of ξ versus cycle number for $\xi^0 = 2.0$ (*top curve*), $\xi^0 = 1.0$ (*middle curve*), and $\xi^0 = 0.5$ (*bottom curve*). Note that as the baseline value increases, the absolute magnitude of the fluctuations increases, but the relative value of the peak efficacy to the baseline value decreases. This results in the plasticity property that stronger synapses (higher baseline values) are more difficult to strengthen. Parameter values are the same as in Figure 9.

this question, we consider synaptic modifications occurring on only two time scales, short-term postsynaptic modifications and long-term presynaptic modifications. We realize that modifications occurring over several different time scales probably take place at both sites (pre- and postsynaptic). For example, we have discussed short-term presynaptic facilitations and depressions in addition to the long-term presynaptic change; and we have mentioned long-term changes in the number of postsynaptic receptors in addition to our model of short-term postsynaptic modifications. The main point is that long-term modifications cannot be localized to particular individual synapses, and changes that can be so localized are obligately short term in nature. Inasmuch as any synaptic modification alters the patterns of network activity in response to input stimulation, long-term modifications will alter the probability and distribution of subsequent short-term changes, and vice versa. The central question we address here is what is gained and what is lost when short-term and long-term modifications both operate on the same population of synapses in a particular network.

Some degree of specificity must be lost in going from short-term postsynaptic changes to long-term presynaptic changes. The mechanism for inducing presynaptic changes involves a temporal integration of transient fluctuations in presynaptic strength. Thus the long-term change will not be specifically tied to the activity during any single shorter interval. The long-term presynaptic modification will affect large numbers of synapses distributed across a wide area by the ramifications of the axon. Thus, in addition to the loss of temporal specificity involved in the induction of a long-term change, the effect of the long-term change is rather nonspecifically distributed over many synapses.

Repeated presentations of a pattern of stimuli lead to both short- and long-term modifications. Ostensibly, there should be a "link" between these two sets of modifications such that each fortifies the occurrence of the other when the stimulus is again presented. However, each type of modification may be sensitive to different characteristics of the stimulus. For instance, short-term postsynaptic modifications reflect the occurrence of particular context-dependent patterns of inputs. Long-term modifications are context-free and represent a type of stable "generalization" of the short-term changes—with a loss of some specificity, yet maintaining a link between the particular long-term modification and the precipitating short-term changes.

The point to emphasize is that the actual translation between long- and short-term modifications depends upon minute cytoarchitectonic details of connectivity and will be effected in an idiosyncratic fashion by each particular network. Indeed, we show that in a randomly connected network there is no statistical link between short-term and long-term modifications; in other words, everything gets lost in the translation. But in a network with neuronal group structure, in which groups of neurons interact with each other to a greater degree than with other groups, there is a well-defined relationship between short-term and long-term changes.

This relationship has four main characteristics: (1) Short-term changes in a group lead to long-term changes primarily within that same group. (2) The presence of group structure is sufficient to ensure that long-term changes arising from short-term changes in a particular group differentially affect future short-term changes in that particular group. (3) Long-term presynaptic changes increase the variance of the distribution of subsequent short-term postsynaptic strengths. (4) Although short-term changes are differentially affected in the group originating the long-term change, the group still retains a significant capacity to respond to novel input with novel short-term modifications. In other words, the repertoire of possible short-term modifications does not become entrained, stereotyped, or overgeneralized.

These points arise from considering the constraints placed by anatomy on any synaptic modification rule. Axons spread over several groups (Edelman and Finkel, 1984), and presynaptic changes of a neuron in one group will therefore affect neighboring groups. A neuron receives afferents from cells in its own group as well as from cells in other groups, and the postsynaptic mechanism will lead to strengthening of some subset of these synapses. We show that synaptic modifications originating in a particular group have very different effects on that group as compared to those on neighboring groups. In general, the group originating the changes will become more cohesive and more tightly connected, while neighboring groups will be weakened. Because synaptic changes are occurring in all groups in parallel, there will be an ongoing competition between groups to maintain a set of synaptic states.

These arguments are pursued first in a simplified analytical treatment of the interaction of the pre- and postsynaptic mechanisms, and then with results from computer simulations of a network of neurons that uses the pre- and postsynaptic mechanisms to modify synaptic strengths. We shall assume that short-term modifications have given rise to long-term modifications and will examine the change in future short-term modifications. For simplicity, in this analysis we neglect the presence of different cell types in the population, the individual patterns of connections, the particular electrotonic properties of individual neurons, and the differential effects of the variety of transmitters, receptors, and channels present at synapses. Instead, we consider networks consisting of groups of a single type of neuron. We assume that the attenuation of voltages between all pairs of synapses on a neuron is identical. We weaken the dependence of postsynaptic modification upon the precise relationship between the timing and voltage attenuation of heterosynaptically conducted voltages and the local production of modifying substance, and we require only a statistical relationship between the inputs. This will destroy the tremendous diversity and selectivity of the actual postsynaptic mechanism. Yet even this weakest version of the mechanism is sufficient to yield the four properties that we have asserted to be characteristic of the relationship between short- and long-term changes.

Consider a formal version of the postsynaptic rule,

$$\Delta\eta_{ij} = c_1 \langle \eta_{ij} \xi_j \overline{S_j}(t) \cdot \sum_k \eta_{ik} \xi_k S_k(t) \rangle - c_2(\eta_{ij} - \eta_{ij}^0), \qquad (17)$$

where $\Delta\eta_{ij}$ is the modification of η_{ij}, the strength of the postsynaptic connection from neuron j to neuron i, ξ_j is the presynaptic strength from neuron j, $S_j(t)$ is the activity of neuron j at time t, $\overline{S_j}(t)$ is this activity averaged over some time period, and $\langle \cdot \rangle$ represents an average over time. The terms in the brackets can be appreciated by reference to Figure 11. The first term in the product represents the amount of modifying substance present at time t. The averaging of activity

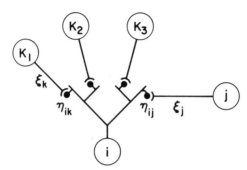

Figure 11. *Schematic of inputs received by a neuron.* Circles represent neurons. Neuron i receives inputs on its dendritic tree. Presynaptic efficacy ξ is the amount of transmitter released by cell j for a given depolarization. Postsynaptic efficacy η_{ij} is the local depolarization produced at the post-synaptic process for a given amount of released transmitter. Changes in η_{ij} depend on the statistical relationship between the firing of cell j and the firing of the heterosynaptic inputs K_1, K_2, K_3, and so forth, as given by Equation 17 in the text.

$\overline{S}_j(t)$ reflects the relatively slower time course of production and decay of the modifying substance compared to activity. The summation term in the product represents the magnitude of conducted voltages at time t from all other synapses on the cell to the jth synapse. We have taken the net synaptic strength to be simply the product of postsynaptic and presynaptic strengths $\eta \cdot \xi$. This represents a first-order kinetic scheme between the amount of transmitter released and the number of postsynaptic receptors.

We assume that the synaptic strengths η and ξ change slowly with regard to the change in activity S; some manipulation then shows

$$\Delta\eta_{ij} = c_1\eta_{ij}\xi_j \sum_k \eta_{ik}\xi_k\langle\overline{S}_j(t) \cdot S_k(t)\rangle - c_2(\eta_{ij} - \eta_{ij}^0) . \tag{18}$$

Figure 11 points out how the postsynaptic rule, even in this weakened version, differs from the Hebb rule. Changes in the postsynaptic strengths of neuron i do not depend upon the firing of neuron i, but upon the coactivity of the inputs to i. In this way, we retain the population effects of synaptic alterations.

Now assume that the neurons are segregated into groups. Let I, J, and K denote the groups, rather than individual neurons, and as shown in Figure 12, let N_{IJ} be the number of connections from group J to group I, and N_{II} be the number of intragroup connections in group I. Furthermore, assume that all connections between the two groups are identical in strength (or equivalently, only consider the mean of the individual synaptic strengths). We are interested in changes in the synaptic strengths between the groups.

$$\Delta\eta_{IJ} = c_1'\eta_{IJ}\xi_J \sum_K N_{IK}\eta_{IK}\xi_K R_{JK} - c_2'(\eta_{IJ} - \eta_{IJ}^0) , \tag{19}$$

where $R_{JK} = \langle\overline{S}_J(t) \cdot S_K(t)\rangle$ averaged over all connections from group K to group J.

Now suppose that because of short-term fluctuations, a long-term presynaptic modification has occurred in group I: $\xi_I \to \xi_I + \delta_I$. We can do a simple perturbation analysis to see how this affects future short-term changes in various groups (see Figure 12). Neglecting the effect of the modification in I on the statistical relationship between firing of neurons R_{IJ} and so forth,

$$\Delta \eta'_{IJ} = c'_1 \eta_{IJ} \xi_J [\sum_{K \neq I} N_{IK} \eta_{IK} \xi_K R_{JK} + N_{II} \eta_{II} (\xi_I + \delta_I) R_{JI}] - c'_2 (\eta_{IJ} - \eta^0_{IJ})$$

(20)

$$= \Delta \eta_{IJ} + \delta_I c'_1 N_{II} \eta_{II} \eta_{IJ} \xi_J R_{JI}.$$

By similar calculations, we can find the changes in all other classes of connections between groups as shown in Figure 12. These changes in the short-term modifications, $\Delta^2 \eta_{IJ} = \Delta \eta'_{IJ} - \Delta \eta_{IJ}$, are listed below.

$$\Delta^2 \eta_{II} = \delta_I c'_1 \left[N_{II} \eta^2_{II} \xi_I R_{II} + \eta_{II} \sum_K N_{IK} \eta_{IK} \xi_K R_{IK} \right]$$

(21)

$$\Delta^2 \eta_{JI} = \delta_I c'_1 \left[N_{JI} \eta^2_{JI} \xi_I R_{II} + \eta_{JI} \sum_K N_{JK} \eta_{JK} \xi_K R_{IK} \right]$$

(22)

$$\Delta^2 \eta_{IJ} = \delta_I c'_1 [N_{II} \eta_{II} \eta_{IJ} \xi_J R_{JI}]$$

(23)

$$\Delta^2 \eta_{JJ} = \delta_I c'_1 [N_{JI} \eta_{JI} \eta_{JJ} \xi_J R_{JI}]$$

(24)

$$\Delta^2 \eta_{JK} = \delta_I c'_1 [N_{JI} \eta_{JI} \eta_{JK} \xi_K R_{KI}] .$$

(25)

What conditions are sufficient to guarantee that $\Delta^2 \eta_{II}$ is the biggest change, or namely that short-term changes in the set experiencing the long-term modification are differentially affected? There are three sufficient conditions:

$$N_{II} \eta_{II} > N_{JI} \eta_{JI} ;$$

(26a)

$$R_{II} > R_{JI} ;$$

(26b)

$$\sum_K N_{IK} \eta_{IK} \xi_K R_{IK} \approx 0 .$$

(26c)

These conditions state that (1) connectivity within a group is stronger than between groups (Equation 26a); (2) neurons in the same group fire together more often than neurons in different groups (Equation 26b); and (3) on the average, input from different groups is uncorrelated (Equation 26c).

The key point of this analysis is that within the context of this simple model, these three sufficient conditions define a neuronal group (Edelman, 1978; Edelman and Finkel, 1984): A group is a set of strongly connected cells which predominantly fire together and constitute the smallest neural functional unit for selection. The

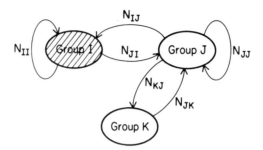

Figure 12. *Classes of group connections. Ellipses* represent groups, and *arrows* represent all connections
between the groups. There are N_{IJ} connections from group J to group I, N_{JI} connections from
group I to group J, and N_{II} from group I to itself, and so forth. The analysis (see text) assumes
a long-term change has occurred in group I (*cross-hatching*) and examines the effect on subsequent
short-term changes in the various connections between the groups.

present analysis thus indicates that the organization of a network into neuronal
groups provides a *sufficient* condition for long-term modifications to differentially
affect those short-term modifications that gave rise to them.

Given the group condition, we can rank the classes of connections according
to the magnitude of the change in short-term modifications. The changes within
group I ($\Delta^2\eta_{II}$) are always the greatest, those between unaffected groups ($\Delta^2\eta_{JK}$)
are always the least; but the three remaining classes may have different relative
positions depending upon the relative values of N_{II}/N_{JI}, $\eta_{II}/\eta_{JI}/\eta_{JJ}$, and R_{II}/R_{JI}.
We would usually expect $\Delta^2\eta_{JJ}$ to be the smallest of the three, for $\Delta^2\eta_{IJ}$ to be
the largest for a few select groups J that are highly correlated with group I, but
for $\Delta^2\eta_{JI}$ to be the largest for most other groups J. In other words, a long-term
change in group I gives rise to increased subsequent short-term changes in the
internal connections of group I, in the connections from group I to other groups,
in the connections from related groups to group I, and to smaller internal changes
in other groups themselves, and yet smaller changes between other unrelated
groups.

Results of Computer Simulations

We now turn to computer simulations of the dual pre- and postsynaptic rules
operating within a network. We present results from two separate programs;
the first is based on the simplified analytical model just presented, and the
second uses the more detailed individual formulations of the rules presented
earlier. The network used for the first program, a typical example of which is
shown in Figure 13, consists of a chosen number of groups (typically eight) with
a chosen number of cells in each group (usually eight per group in all groups).
Neurons within each group are interconnected randomly with a fixed average
density of connections, and each connection is randomly assigned an initial
presynaptic and postsynaptic strength from a normal distribution. Each cell is
also randomly connected to neurons in a fixed number of other groups. Within
each of these groups, a fixed average number of intergroup connections are
made and randomly assigned initial pre- and postsynaptic strengths. This is
supposed to reflect the property that if an axon reaches a certain group, it is
likely to contact several cells in that group, whereas other groups might be

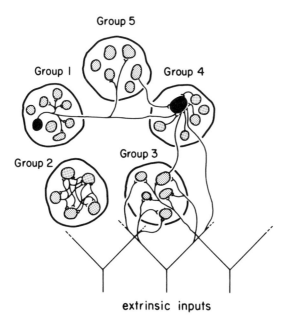

Figure 13. *Schematic network connectivity used in computer simulations.* Five groups are shown with some of their cells indicated. Each group illustrates one aspect of the connectivity. Group 1 shows that each cell contacts cells in its own group and in other groups. Group 2 shows the dense internal connectivity of groups. Group 3 shows that each group also receives inputs from a set of overlapped extrinsic inputs that can be selectively stimulated. Group 4 shows that each cell thus receives inputs from cells in its own group, from cells in other groups, and from extrinsic sources. The computer simulation allows the observation of changes in the presynaptic and postsynaptic efficacies of the various connections after different stimulation paradigms.

entirely bypassed. The baseline presynaptic strengths ξ^0 of all terminals of each neuron are set equal, and the mean baseline postsynaptic strength of intragroup connections exceeds that of intergroup connections.

Note that this network does not contain any inhibitory neurons. It is well known that an intrinsically excitatory network, aside from being unrealistic, is also intrinsically unstable—but in practice we stimulate the network at very low levels to avoid large-scale excitations. We felt that the drawbacks of not including inhibition were acceptable at this stage, since the exact location of inhibitory connections would have profound effects on the postsynaptic rule, and would require more extensive consideration of the details of electrotonic delays and attenuations.

Each cell in the network also receives extrinsic fibers with fixed synaptic strengths. These connections were not generated randomly, but consisted of an orderly topographic mapping onto the network. We included adjustable parameters for the magnification factor and degree of overlap of the incoming fibers. These inputs were stimulated in patterns designed to elicit activity in various regions of the network, in a fashion not unlike placing a stimulating electrode in a real neural tissue.

The input fibers are stimulated, and the voltage V_i of each neuron i is determined by summing all its intrinsic, S_j, and extrinsic, X_i, inputs.

$$V_i(t) = \delta \cdot V_i(t - 1) + \sum_j \eta_{ij}\xi_j S_j(t - 1) + X_i , \qquad (27)$$

where δ is the decay constant for voltage. If V_i surpasses a threshold, cell i fires at a rate proportional to the voltage; otherwise it does not fire at all.

Each iteration represents roughly 5–10 msec of real time, approximately the membrane time constant of many cells. After a set number of iterations (usually 10), the change in postsynaptic strengths is computed from Equation 18 and the change in presynaptic strength from Equations 13 to 15. If the running average of $(\xi - \xi^0)$ exceeds a set upper threshold, ξ^0 is incremented; and if it decreases below a set lower threshold, ξ^0 is decremented. Statistics are kept of these changes, as well as of the distribution of synaptic strengths and of the firing patterns.

Figure 14 shows the results of one computer simulation. Two groups, called I and J for convenience, were arbitrarily chosen; and the first group, I, was stimulated via its extrinsic inputs to induce short-term postsynaptic changes in its intrinsic connections. The actual stimulation used was a burst of five cycles of stimulation to half the cells in the group, followed by a five-cycle rest, followed by five cycles of the same stimulation. After allowing time (50 cycles) for the activity in the system to return to its resting state, the same stimulation protocol was applied to the other group, J. The magnitude of the short-term changes, averaged over all group connections, is shown as the solid lines in Figure 14. Note that the second barrage of stimulation induced a larger synaptic change than the first barrage. If the barrages are repeated, eventually the threshold for a presynaptic modification is surpassed. We thus repeated the stimulus barrages to group I 10 times, without rest, to produce a change in ξ^0 for several of the cells in group I. After 50 cycles of rest, the initial stimulation protocol (two barrages of five cycles of stimulation separated by five cycles of rest) was repeated, first to group I; then, after a rest, to group J. The dashed curve in Figure 14 shows the resultant short-term postsynaptic changes in both group I and group J subsequent to the long-term change induced in group I.

It is clear from Figure 14 that there is no significant change in subsequent short-term modifications of the group that did not receive the long-term presynaptic modification (solid and dashed curves are practically superposed). However, in the group with the long-term change, repetition of the stimuli that induced the long-term change gives rise to an amplified pattern of short-term changes.

We also examined the change in the variability of short-term modifications as a result of a long-term modification. The definition of variability is elusive and model-dependent, however, and we have not yet been able to satisfactorily study changes in variability in a true population biology sense. We are currently investigating models of changes in the number of partitions of short-term modifications. In the present study, we did examine the effect of modifications upon the variance of the postsynaptic strengths, η, and also upon the variance of the changes of these strengths, $\Delta\eta$. Values of the former are shown in Figure 14. The variance of postsynaptic strengths in a group increases after a long-term change in that group (here by 30%); but significantly, it also increases in groups which did not experience the long-term change (here by 10%). Thus, groups that do not directly experience a long-term change themselves, but which receive

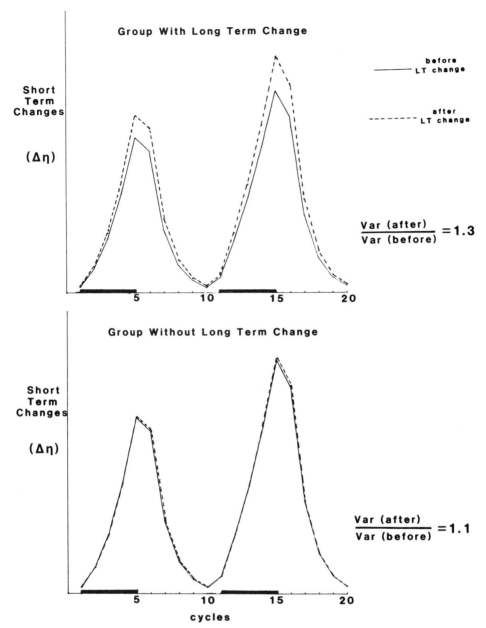

Figure 14. *Results of a simulation of the formal model.* Plots of the magnitude of change in postsynaptic efficacy η versus time (iteration of the simulation). Two groups were chosen at random and were stimulated (*dark bars* on *abscissa*) for five cycles, allowed to rest for five cycles, and then stimulated again for five cycles. The *solid line* shows the resulting short-term changes. One group (plotted at *top*) was then repeatedly stimulated for 50 cycles to produce a long-term presynaptic change in some of the cells in the group. After allowing 50 cycles of rest, the initial stimulation sequence (five cycles stimulation/five cycles rest/five cycles stimulation) was given again. The short-term changes after this stimulation are shown by the *dashed line*. Only the group that received the long-term change shows an alteration in subsequent short-term changes. Also shown is the ratio of the variance in η of the group (measured at cycle 15) before and after the long-term change. The variance increases in both groups.

inputs from a group that did, are still affected by an increased variance in their subsequent short-term modifications. Since each group contacts many other groups, the variability-generating property of long-term presynaptic changes will have wide effects upon the network.

Given the results of the simulations of the presynaptic and postsynaptic rules, and that of the simplified version of the interaction between these rules in a network (Figure 14), we finally attempted to use the actual formulations of the presynaptic and postsynaptic rules in the same neural network. Thus the programs for simulating the presynaptic and postsynaptic rules were merged into a single network program, and the test applied in Figure 14 was repeated. This represents a stringent test of the total synaptic modification model developed here.

The network used was similar to that used above and consisted of two groups of 10 cells each. Five cycles of stimuli were applied to the first five cells of group 1, and then after 10 cycles of rest the stimulus burst was repeated. The resulting postsynaptic changes are plotted in Figure 15. After allowing the network to return to rest, a burst of 13 cycles of stimulation was applied to the same five cells, and this gave rise to a long-term change in the presynaptic efficacy of all five of these cells (and none of the others), as described by the presynaptic rule. After allowing the system to return to rest (500 cycles), the initial testing sequence was repeated, with the results plotted in Figure 15A.

Note that the pattern of short-term changes has been enhanced. Unlike the result in Figure 14, the stimulus bursts now lead to an initial decrease in η, followed by an increase. This is because in the previous case, any coactivation of the stimuli led to an increase in η, whereas in the present case, the initial increase in voltage inactivates channels leading to an initial decrease in η via Equation 12, and only after the concentration of modifying substance begins to rise does the postsynaptic efficacy increase. The present result is more appropriate, since during the first few impulses it is unclear whether the inputs are going to be significantly coactivated. Also note that after the long-term change, the rise time of the curve has been shortened. This allows the group to respond more rapidly to the same set of inputs.

Figure 15B represents the control case in which the long-term change was produced in group 2. Note that, in contrast to Figure 15A, the long-term change

---

Figure 15. *Simulation of the combined model.* Effect of a long-term change in one group on subsequent short-term changes in various groups. Simulation employed the same parameters used in the presynaptic and postsynaptic simulations previously discussed (except that $\lambda = 0.06$). The network was composed of two groups with 10 cells each; each cell had eight intragroup and four intergroup connections. $\eta^0 = 1.0$ and $\xi^0 = 1.0$ for all connections, and ξ^0 was incremented by 1.0 when a long-term change occurred. Stimulation and testing protocol is identical to that given in Figure 14. Two bursts of five spikes separated by 10 cycles of rest are delivered to five cells in a group. *A: Lower curve* is a plot of the mean of the short-term changes $\Delta\eta$ in the five stimulated cells. *Upper curve* is a plot of short-term changes in response to the repetition of the same stimuli to the same cells after a long-term change has occurred in the presynaptic strengths of these five cells (resulting from 13 cycles of stimulation to these cells). Note that the pattern has been amplified, and that the time rise is faster after long-term change. *B:* Control plot (see Figure 14) of short-term changes in response to the same stimuli as in *A*, except now the long-term change has been induced in five cells of the other group; the plot of the postsynaptic modifications after the long-term change is virtually identical to the initial plot.

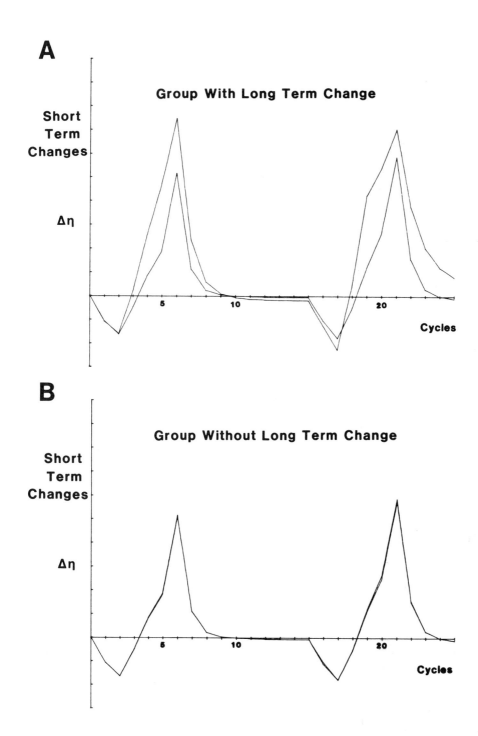

751

in group 2 has virtually no effect on the magnitude of subsequent short-term changes in group 1. In fact, the magnitude of the changes decreased to a small extent. This demonstrates that the equations for the presynaptic and postsynaptic rules developed earlier give rise to a differential enhancement of short-term changes in a group as a result of long-term changes in that group.

The fact that we have found similar results in Figures 14 and 15, despite the very different formulations of the synaptic rules in each case, argues for the robustness of the model. In addition, corroboration of our analytically derived results by the detailed versions of the presynaptic and postsynaptic rules provides support for the formulation of the rules as given.

CONCLUSIONS AND PREDICTIONS

There are several conclusions we can draw from the interaction between the pre- and postsynaptic rules. Synaptic efficacy depends upon both pre- and postsynaptic mechanisms and upon the short- and long-term state of the synapse. At the level of individual synapses, short- and long-term modifications are functionally indistinguishable, but they differ with regard to their distribution across the population. This helps to refine the notion of a distributed memory. The distribution of modifications reflects the anatomical, physiological, and pharmacological properties of a region. The interaction of short- and long-term modifications in a random network would not lead to useful properties. But in a network with group structure, there is a functional link between different components of modification arising within the same group. Short-term modifications in a group increase the likelihood of generating a long-term change in the cells in that group. Once generated, the long-term change has two effects: It differentially increases the ability of the group to generate short-term changes to inputs similar to those precipitating the modification, and it also increases the variability of short-term modifications both in the group itself and in surrounding groups. Without this introduction of new variability, a selective system would eventually lose its ability to respond to novel inputs. Indeed, every selective system operates to reduce variability, and each utilizes different mechanisms to generate new variability (Edelman, 1978).

There will be a competition between groups to retain the integrity of their short-term modification repertoires—each group acts to increase the likelihood of its own set of short-term responses while acting to decrease the likelihood of those of surrounding groups. Clearly this requires a delicate balance to maintain a state intermediate between completely rigid stereotyped response and amnesic *de novo* trial and error. This balance may shift with input history and experience.

Differential interference with the postsynaptic mechanism through loss of spines, decreased channel synthesis, or changes in electrotonic properties will lead to the differential loss of short-term modifications, particularly in the face of a continued increase in the variance of firing. Long-term modifications are harder to lose since they are intrinsically more stable, and they are distributed over a larger population of neurons.

It would be naive to jump from synaptic modification on short and long time scales to cognitive processes occurring over different time scales—no such link can be made at present, and in any case, such higher level processes most likely reflect the combined influences of many brain regions operating in parallel. Nevertheless, this model of short- and long-term modifications interacting over synaptic populations does have useful memorial properties. The independence of short- and long-term modifications allows specific responses on a short time scale in a context-dependent fashion without altering the long-term properties of the group. Long-term modifications reflect generalization of short-term changes and act to bias future responses toward the precipitating changes. The more distributed nature of the long-term changes allows associations to be made more easily—but in a relatively context-independent fashion. Most important, the existence of synaptic modifications as a population property of networks of degenerate groups implies that a very long-term memory can be constructed with cells having fewer long-term changes but overlapping lifetimes.

Although both modification rules discussed here can act synchronously (but independently), one or the other may predominate in different regions of the brain, depending upon anatomical or pharmacological differences. Moreover, a more general treatment than the one presented here would allow changes at several overlapping time scales in both pre- and postsynaptic populations.

The critical predictions of the present model are:

1. Pre- and postsynaptic modifications occur independently through separate mechanisms and in no case will be found to be contingent only upon correlated firing across individual synapses.

2. Each class of biochemical modifications will primarily affect those channels or receptors that are in a particular conformational state. Such modifications will lead to measurable changes in the magnitude and time course of the PSP, shifts in the current–voltage curve, and possibly to measurable changes in the time constants for state transitions. This prediction could be tested by controlling the voltage across a patch clamped postsynaptic membrane and studying the relationship between the voltage level and the degree of channel modification (conductance changes, transition probability changes, or phosphorylations, etc.) as a function of ionto-phoresed transmitter.

3. Heterosynaptic interactions are dependent on the relative timing of inputs, the relative position of synapses on the postsynaptic neuron, and the types of transmitters, receptors, and channels present. The details of the constraints on the timing of inputs depend upon the distance between the synapses and the duration of the depolarization and the persistence of the modifying substance, as shown in Figure 4. The longer the de-polarization or the persistence of the modifying substance, the greater the distance over which heterosynaptic effects can take place.

4. Transmitter release will exhibit homeostasis—small perturbations in the amount of release resulting from a given pattern of activity (because of previous activity or biochemical fluctuations) will be rapidly brought back to steady state.

5. The same transient change in the efficacy of transmitter release may be observed after many different sequences of stimulation. Any permanent

change reflects only the magnitude of the transient change, not the specific stimulus sequence from which the transient change arose.

6. The change in efficacy of transmitter release will be similar at all presynaptic terminals given off by a particular axon.

7. Long-term presynaptic modifications occur on a cell-wide basis.

8. For long-term presynaptic modifications, stronger synapses are more difficult to strengthen and easier to weaken. For short-term postsynaptic modifications, stronger synapses are, in general, easier to strengthen.

9. Short-term and long-term modifications are differentially distributed over the same neuronal population.

10. The presence of neuronal groups guarantees that long-term modifications differentially enhance the short-term changes that led to those modifications.

11. Cooling of intrinsic afferents, and thus slowing of axonal conduction, should change the pattern of heterosynaptic couplings.

12. Drastic changes in the retention of abnormal connections, or the shedding of normal connections, can be induced by directing fibers with the appropriate transmitters onto developing neurons.

13. Long-term memories will largely reflect presynaptic alterations; short-term memories will largely reflect postsynaptic alterations. Some amnesic syndromes featuring abnormalities of long-term and short-term memory will be associated with corresponding loci of *neuronal* pathology.

The accuracy with which the proposed presynaptic and postsynaptic rules describe synaptic modifications in the nervous system remains to be experimentally demonstrated. In any case, a system that operated according to rules similar to these, and that had several different types of modifications occurring in parallel, as well as a network anatomy which constrained the interactions between the modification rules, would possess interesting properties with regard to memory and categorization.

REFERENCES

Bailey, C. H., and M. Chen (1983) Morphological basis of long-term habituation and sensitization in *Aplysia*. *Science* **220**:81–93.

Betz, H. (1983) Regulation of alpha-bungarotoxin receptor accumulation in chick retina cultures—Effects of membrane depolarization, cyclic-nucleotide derivatives, and Ca^{++}. *J. Neurosci.* **3**: 1333–1341.

Birdsall, N. J. M. (1982) Can different receptors interact directly with each other? *Trends Neurosci.* **5**:137–138.

Bittner, G. D., and R. A. Schatz (1981) An examination of the residual calcium theory for facilitation of transmitter release. *Brain Res.* **210**:431–436.

Brandon, J. G., and R. G. Coos (1982) Rapid dendritic spine stem shortening during one-trial learning: The honeybee's first orientation flight. *Brain Res.* **353**:51–61.

Bryan, J. S., and H. L. Atwood (1981) Two types of synaptic depression at synapses of a single crustacean motor axon. *Mar. Behav. Physiol.* **8**:99–121.

Carew, T. J., R. D. Hawkins, T. W. Abrams, and E. R. Kandel (1984) A test of the Hebb postulate at identified synapses which mediate classical conditioning in *Aplysia*. *J. Neurosci.* **4**:1217–1224.

Carlin, R. K., and P. Siekevitz (1983) Plasticity in the central nervous system—Do synapses divide? *Proc. Natl. Acad. Sci. USA* **80**:3517–3521.

Catteral, W. A. (1979) Binding of scorpion toxin to receptor sites associated with sodium channels in frog muscle—Correlation of voltage-dependent binding with activation. *J. Gen. Physiol.* **74**:375–391.

Chang, H. T. (1952) Cortical neurons with particular reference to the apical dendrites. *Cold Spring Harbor Symp. Quant. Biol.* **17**:189–202.

Changeux, J.-P. (1981) The acetylcholine receptor: An "allosteric" membrane protein. *Harvey Lect.* **75**:85–254.

Chesselet, M.-F. (1984) Presynaptic regulation of neurotransmitter release in the brain—Facts and hypothesis. *Neuroscience* **12**:347–375.

de Peyer, J. E., A. B. Cachelin, I. B. Levitan, and H. Reuter (1982) Ca^{++}-activated K^+ conductance in internally perfused snail neurons is enhanced by protein phosphorylation. *Proc. Natl. Acad. Sci. USA* **79**:4207–4211.

Desmond, N. L., and W. B. Levy (1981) Ultrastructural and numerical alteration in dendritic spines as a consequence of long-term potentiation. *Anat. Rec.* **199**:68A–69A.

Dodge, F. A., and R. Rahamimoff (1967) Co-operative action of calcium ions in transmitter release at the neuromuscular junction. *J. Physiol. (Lond.)* **193**:419–432.

Edelman, G. M. (1978) Group selection and phasic reentrant signaling: A theory of higher brain function. In *The Mindful Brain: Cortical Organization and the Group-Selective Theory of Higher Brain Function*, by G. M. Edelman and V. B. Mountcastle, pp. 55–100, MIT Press, Cambridge, Massachusetts.

Edelman, G. M. (1981) Group selection as the basis for higher brain function. In *Organization of the Cerebral Cortex*, F. O. Schmitt, F. G. Worden, G. Adelman, and S. G. Dennis, eds., pp. 51–100, MIT Press, Cambridge, Massachusetts.

Edelman, G. M., and L. H. Finkel (1984) Neuronal group selection in the cerebral cortex. In *Dynamic Aspects of Neocortical Function*, G. M. Edelman, W. E. Gall, and W. M. Cowan, eds., pp. 653–695, Wiley, New York.

Edelman, G. M., and G. N. Reeke, Jr. (1982) Selective networks capable of representative transformations, limited generalizations, and associative memory. *Proc. Natl. Acad. Sci. USA* **79**:2091–2095.

Eisen, J. S., and E. Marder (1982) Mechanisms underlying pattern generation in lobster stomatogastric ganglion as determined by selective inactivation of identified neurons. III. Synaptic connections of electrically coupled pyloric neurons. *J. Neurophysiol.* **48**:1329–1415.

Fambrough, D. M. (1979) Control of acetylcholine receptors in skeletal muscle. *Physiol. Rev.* **59**:165–227.

Fifková, E., and A. van Harreveld (1977) Long-lasting morphological changes in dendritic spines of dentate granular cells following stimulation of the entorhinal area. *J. Neurocytol.* **6**:211–230.

Finkel, L. H., and G. M. Edelman (1985) Interaction of synaptic modification rules within populations of neurons. *Proc. Natl. Acad. Sci. USA* **82**:1291–1295.

Fraser, S. E., and M. M. Poo (1982) Development, maintenance, and modulation of patterned membrane topography—Models based on the acetylcholine receptor. *Curr. Top. Dev. Biol.* **17**:77–100.

Greengard, P., and J. F. Kuo (1970) On the mechanism of action of cyclic AMP. *Adv. Biochem. Psychopharmacol.* **3**:287–306.

Haas, H. L., and A. Konnerth (1983) Histamine and noradrenaline decrease calcium-activated potassium conductance in hippocampal pyramidal cells. *Nature* **302**:432–434.

Hawkins, R. D., T. W. Abrams, T. J. Carew, and E. R. Kandel (1983) A cellular mechanism of classical conditioning in *Aplysia*—Activity-dependent amplification of pre-synaptic facilitation. *Science* **219**:400–405.

Hebb, D. O. (1949) *The Organization of Behavior*, Wiley, New York.

Heidmann, T., and J.-P. Changeux (1982) Un modèle moléculaire de régulation d'efficacité au niveau postsynaptique d'une synapse chimique. *C. R. Seances Acad. Sci. (Paris)* **295**:665–670.

Henneman, E., H. R. Luscher, and J. Mathis (1984) Simultaneously active and inactive synapses of single Ia fibers on cat spinal motoneurones. *J. Physiol. (Lond.)* **352**:147–161.

Hodgkin, A. L., and A. F. Huxley (1952) A quantitative description of membrane current and its application to conduction and excitation in nerve. *J. Physiol. (Lond.)* **117**:500–544.

Hopkins, W. F., and D. Johnston (1984) Frequency-dependent noradrenergic modulation of long-term potentiation in the hippocampus. *Science* **226**:350–352.

Huang, L.-Y. M., N. Moran, and G. Ehrenstein (1982) Batrachotoxin modifies the gating kinetics of sodium channels in internally prefused neuroblastoma cells. *Proc. Natl. Acad. Sci. USA* **79**: 2082–2085.

Ito, M., M. Sakurai, and P. Tongroach (1982) Climbing fiber-induced depression of both mossy fiber responsiveness and glutamate sensitivity of cerebellar Purkinje cells. *J. Physiol. (Lond.)* **324**: 113–134.

Kandel, E. R. (1976) *The Cellular Basis of Behavior*, Freeman, San Francisco.

Katz, B., and R. Miledi (1968) The role of calcium in neuromuscular facilitation. *J. Physiol. (Lond.)* **199**:729–741.

Koch, C., and T. Poggio (1983) Electrical properties of dendritic spines. *Trends Neurosci.* **6**:80–83.

Koch, C., T. Poggio, and V. Torre (1982) Retinal ganglion cells: A functional interpretation of dendritic morphology. *Philos. Trans. R. Soc. Lond. (Biol.)* **298**:227–264.

Koch, C., T. Poggio, and V. Torre (1983) Nonlinear interactions in a dendritic tree: Localization, timing, and role in information processing. *Proc. Natl. Acad. Sci. USA* **80**:2799–2802.

Korn, H., D. S. Faber, Y. Burnod, and A. Triller (1984) Regulation of efficacy at central synapses. *J. Neurosci.* **4**:125–130.

Kupfermann, I. (1979) Modulatory actions of neurotransmitters. *Annu. Rev. Neurosci.* **2**:447–465.

Libet, B., H. Kobayashi, and T. Tanaka (1975) Synaptic coupling into the production and storage of a memory trace. *Nature* **258**:155–157.

Lund, A. E., and T. Narahashi (1981) Modification of sodium-channel kinetics by the insecticide tetramethrin in crayfish giant-axons. *Neurotoxicology (Little Rock)* **2**:213–229.

Lynch, G., and M. Baudry (1984) The biochemistry of memory: A new and specific hypothesis. *Science* **224**:1057–1063.

Magleby, K. L., and C. F. Stevens (1972) The effect of voltage on the time course of end-plate currents. *J. Physiol. (Lond.)* **223**:151–171.

Magleby, K. L., and J. E. Zengel (1982) Quantitative description of stimulation-induced changes in transmitter release at the frog neuromuscular junction. *J. Gen. Physiol.* **80**:613–638.

Mallart, A., and A. R. Martin (1968) An analysis of facilitation of transmitter release at the neuromuscular junction of the frog. *J. Physiol. (Lond.)* **193**:679–694.

Margiotta, J. F., and B. Walcott (1983) Conductance and dye permeability of a rectifying electrical synapse. *Nature* **305**:52–55.

Martin, A. R., and G. Pilar (1964) Presynaptic and postsynaptic events during post-tetanic potentiation and facilitation in the avian ciliary ganglion. *J. Physiol. (Lond.)* **175**:17–30.

Miledi, R. (1973) Transmitter release induced by injection of calcium ions into nerve terminals. *Proc. R. Soc. Lond. (Biol.)* **183**:421–425.

Murayama, K., N. J. Abbott, T. Narahashi, and B. I. Shapiro (1972) Effects of allethrin and *Condylactis* toxin on the kinetics of sodium channel conductance of crayfish membranes. *Comp. Gen. Pharmacol.* **3**:391–400.

Nestler, E. J., and P. Greengard (1984) *Protein Phosphorylation in the Nervous System*, Wiley, New York.

Parnas, I. (1972) Differential block at high frequency of branches of a single axon innervating two muscles. *J. Neurophysiol.* **35**:903–914.

Parnas, I., J. Dudel, and H. Parnas (1984) Depolarization dependence of the kinetics of phasic transmitter release at the crayfish neuromuscular junction. *Neurosci. Lett.* **50**:157–162.

Rall, W. (1974) Dendritic spines, synaptic potency, and neuronal plasticity. *Brain Info. Service Res. Report* **3**:13–21.

Rall, W., and J. Rinzel (1973) Branch input resistance and steady state attenuation for input to one branch of a dendritic model. *Biophys. J.* **13**:648–688.

Ramón y Cajal, S. (1937) *Recollections of My Life*, MIT Press, Cambridge, Massachusetts.

Rauschecker, J. P., and W. Singer (1981) The effects of early visual experience on the cat's visual cortex and their possible explanation by Hebb synapses. *J. Physiol. (Lond.)* **310**:215–239.

Reuter, H. (1983) Calcium channel modulation by neurotransmitters, enzymes and drugs. *Nature* **301**:569–574.

Selverston, A. I., D. G. King, D. F. Russell, and J. P. Miller (1976) The stomatogastric nervous system: Structure and function of a small neural network. *Prog. Neurobiol.* **7**:215–290.

Siegelbaum, S. A., J. S. Camardo, and E. R. Kandel (1982) Serotonin and cyclic AMP close single K$^+$ channels in *Aplysia* sensory neurones. *Nature* **299**:413–417.

Singer, W., and J. P. Rauschecker (1982) Central core control of developmental plasticity in the kitten visual cortex. II. Electrical activation on mesencephalic and diencephalic projections. *Exp. Brain Res.* **47**:223–233.

Smith, S. J., G. J. Augustine, and M. P. Charlton (1984) Transmission at voltage-clamped giant synapse of the squid—Evidence for cooperativity of presynaptic calcium action. *Proc. Natl. Acad. Sci. USA* **82**:622.

Stockbridge, N., and J. W. Moore (1984) Dynamics of intracellular calcium and its possible relationship to phasic transmitter release and facilitation at the frog neuromuscular junction. *J. Neurosci.* **4**:803–811.

Swanson, L. W., T. J. Teyler, and R. F. Thompson, eds. (1982) *Hippocampal Long-Term Potentiation: Mechanisms and Implications for Memory*, Neurosci. Res. Program Bull. 20, MIT Press, Cambridge, Massachusetts.

von Hayek, F. A. (1952) *The Sensory Order: An Inquiry into the Foundations of Theoretical Psychology*, Univ. Chicago Press, Chicago.

Vrensen, G., and J. Nunes-Cardozo (1981) Changes in size and shape of synaptic connections after visual training: An ultrastructural approach of synaptic plasticity. *Brain Res.* **218**:79–97.

Watanabe, A. M., M. M. McConnaughey, R. A. Strawbridge, J. W. Fleming, L. R. Jones, and H. R. Besch (1978) Muscarinic cholinergic receptor modulation of beta-adrenergic receptor affinity for catecholamines. *J. Biol. Chem.* **253**:4833–4836.

Wigstrom, H., B. L. McNaughton, and C. A. Barnes (1982) Long-term synaptic enhancement in hippocampus is not regulated by post-synaptic membrane potential. *Brain Res.* **233**:195–199.

Contributors and Participants

Thomas W. Abrams
Department of Biology
Leidy Laboratories
University of Pennsylvania
Philadelphia, Pennsylvania 19104

Paul R. Adams
Department of Neurobiology
State University of New York
Graduate Biology Building 576
Stony Brook, New York 11794

Per O. Andersen
Institute of Neurophysiology
University of Oslo
Karl Johans Gt. 47
Oslo
Norway

Elena Battenberg
Division of Preclinical Neuroscience &
    Endocrinology
Research Institute of Scripps Clinic
10666 North Torrey Pines Road
La Jolla, California 92037

Michel Baudry
Center for the Neurobiology of Learning
    & Memory
University of California/Irvine
Irvine, California 92717

Michael V. L. Bennett
Department of Neuroscience
Albert Einstein College of Medicine
1300 Morris Park Avenue
Bronx, New York 10461

Floyd E. Bloom
Division of Preclinical Neuroscience &
    Endocrinology
Research Institute of Scripps Clinic
10666 North Torrey Pines Road
La Jolla, California 92037

Vincent F. Castellucci
College of Physicians & Surgeons
Columbia University
722 West 168th Street
New York, New York 10032

William A. Catterall
Department of Pharmacology
University of Washington
Seattle, Washington 98195

Jean-Pierre Changeux
Department of Molecular Neurobiology
Institut Pasteur
28 rue du Dr. Roux
75015 Paris
France

Marie-Francoise Chesselet
Laboratory of Cell Biology
National Institute of Mental Health
Bethesda, Maryland 20205

W. Maxwell Cowan
Office of the Provost
Washington University
1 Brookings Drive
St. Louis, Missouri 63130

Benson M. Curtis
Department of Pharmacology
University of Washington
Seattle, Washington 98195

James Douglass
Institute for Advanced Biomedical
    Research
The Oregon Health Sciences University
3181 SW Sam Jackson Park Road
Portland, Oregon 97201

Gerald M. Edelman
The Rockefeller University
1230 York Avenue
New York, New York 10021

759

Judith S. Eisen
Neurosciences Institute
University of Oregon
Eugene, Oregon 97403

Donald S. Faber
Division of Neurobiology
SUNY School of Medicine
Buffalo, New York 14214

Daniel J. Feller
Department of Pharmacology
University of Washington
Seattle, Washington 98195

Andre Ferron
Division of Preclinical Neuroscience &
    Endocrinology
Research Institute of Scripps Clinic
10666 North Torrey Pines Road
La Jolla, California 92037

Leif H. Finkel
The Rockefeller University
1230 York Avenue
New York, New York 10021

Gerald D. Fischbach
Department of Anatomy &
    Neurobiology
Washington University School of
    Medicine
St. Louis, Missouri 63110

W. Einar Gall
The Rockefeller University
1230 York Avenue
New York, New York 10021

David L. Glanzman
College of Physicians & Surgeons
Columbia University
722 West 168th Street
New York, New York 10032

Paul Greengard
The Rockefeller University
1230 York Avenue
New York, New York 10021

Susan Hassler
The Neurosciences Institute
1230 York Avenue
New York, New York 10021

Robert D. Hawkins
College of Physicians & Surgeons
Columbia University
722 West 168th Street
New York, New York 10032

Thierry Heidmann
Department of Molecular Neurobiology
Institut Pasteur
28 rue du Dr. Roux
75015 Paris
France

Hugh C. Hemmings, Jr.
The Rockefeller University
1230 York Avenue
New York, New York 10021

Edward Herbert
Institute for Advanced Biomedical
    Research
The Oregon Health Sciences University
3181 SW Sam Jackson Park Road
Portland, Oregon 97201

Bertil Hille
Department of Physiology & Biophysics
SJ-40, Health Sciences Building
University of Washington
Seattle, Washington 98195

Binyamin Hochner
Department of Neurobiology
Life Sciences Institute
Hebrew University
Jerusalem, Israel

Tomas Hökfelt
Department of Histology
Karolinska Institute
S-10401 Stockholm
Sweden

Scott L. Hooper
Neurobiology Comparée
CNRS
Université de Bordeaux
Arcachon, France 33120

Anya Hurlbert
Department of Psychology
Massachusetts Institute of Technology
Cambridge, Massachusetts 02139

Masao Ito
Department of Physiology
Faculty of Medicine
University of Tokyo
Tokyo
Japan 113

Eric R. Kandel
College of Physicians & Surgeons
Columbia University
722 West 168th Street
New York, New York 10032

Harvey J. Karten
Department of Psychiatry & Behavioral
    Science
SUNY School of Medicine
Stony Brook, New York 11794

Mark Klein
College of Physicians & Surgeons
Columbia University
722 West 168th Street
New York, New York 10032

Christof Koch
Divisions of Biology & Engineering,
    216-76
California Institute of Technology
Pasadena, California 91125

Henri Korn
Laboratory of Cellular Neurobiology
Institut Pasteur
25 rue du Dr. Roux
75724 Paris Cedex 15
France

Christopher J. Lingle
Department of Biological Sciences
Biology Unit 1
Florida State University
Tallahassee, Florida 32306

Rodolfo R. Llinás
Department of Physiology & Biophysics
New York University Medical Center
550 First Avenue
New York, New York 10016

Gary S. Lynch
Department of Psychobiology
University of California/Irvine
Irvine, California 92717

Karl L. Magleby
Department of Physiology & Biophysics
University of Miami School of Medicine
P.O. Box 016430
Miami, Florida 33101

Jorge Mancillas
Division of Preclinical Neuroscience &
    Endocrinology
Research Institute of Scripps Clinic
10666 North Torrey Pines Road
La Jolla, California 92037

Eve E. Marder
Department of Biology
Brandeis University
Waltham, Massachusetts 02254

Robert J. Milner
Division of Preclinical Neuroscience &
    Endocrinology
Research Institute of Scripps Clinic
10666 North Torrey Pines Road
La Jolla, California 92037

Vernon B. Mountcastle
Department of Neuroscience
The Johns Hopkins University School of
    Medicine
725 North Wolfe Street
Baltimore, Maryland 21205

Eric J. Nestler
Department of Psychiatry
Yale University
25 Park Street
New Haven, Connecticut 06519

Richard W. Olsen
Department of Pharmacology
UCLA School of Medicine
Los Angeles, California 90024

Charles C. Ouimet
The Rockefeller University
1230 York Avenue
New York, New York 10021

Alan Peters
Department of Anatomy
Boston University School of Medicine
80 East Concord Street
Boston, Massachusetts 02118

Tomaso Poggio
Artificial Intelligence Laboratory
Massachusetts Institute of Technology
545 Technology Square
Cambridge, Massachusetts 02142

Wilfrid Rall
Mathematical Research Branch
National Institute of Arthritis &
  Metabolic Diseases
Bethesda, Maryland 20014

Idan Segev
Mathematical Research Branch
National Institute of Arthritis &
  Metabolic Diseases
Bethesda, Maryland 20014

Michael Shuster
Departments of Biochemistry &
  Biophysics
University of California School of
  Medicine
San Francisco, California 94143

Steven A. Siegelbaum
College of Physicians & Surgeons
Columbia University
722 West 168th Street
New York, New York 10032

George R. Siggins
Division of Preclinical Neuroscience &
  Endocrinology
Research Institute of Scripps Clinic
10666 North Torrey Pines Road
La Jolla, California 92037

Adam M. Sillito
Department of Physiology
University College
Cardiff CF1 1XL, Wales
United Kingdom

Robert Siman
Experimental Station
Central Research & Development
  Department
DuPont at Wilmington
Wilmington, Delaware 19898

Solomon H. Snyder
Department of Neuroscience
The Johns Hopkins University School of
  Medicine
725 North Wolfe Street
Baltimore, Maryland 21205

David C. Spray
Department of Neuroscience
Albert Einstein College of Medicine
1300 Morris Park Avenue
Bronx, New York 10461

Charles F. Stevens
Section on Molecular Neurobiology
Yale University School of Medicine
333 Cedar Street
New Haven, Connecticut 06510

J. Gregor Sutcliffe
Department of Molecular Biology
Research Institute of Scripps Clinic
10666 North Torrey Pines Road
La Jolla, California 92037

Nakaakira Tsukahara*
Faculty of Engineering Science
Osaka University
Osaka
Japan

S. Ivar Walaas
The Rockefeller University
1230 York Avenue
New York, New York 10021

Neale Ward
The Neurosciences Institute
1230 York Avenue
New York, New York 10021

*Died August 12, 1985.

Index

AB neurons
  action potentials, 309–310
  bursting pacemakers, 311–315
  coupled to PD neurons, 309–311
  DA, 5-HT, and pilocarpine effects, 317, 319
  evoked IPSPs, 310–312
  inferior ventricular nerve stimulation response, 317, 319
  neurotransmitter release, 310, 313–315
ACE
  action, 250
  binding to captopril, 251–252
  brain, 251
  role in blood pressure regulation, 251
  striatonigral substrate, 252–253
  and substance K, 251
  and substance P, 251
Acetylcholine. *See* ACh
Acetylcholinesterase. *See* AChE
ACh
  actions in dLGN, 337–339
  α-toxin binding sites, 558
  coexistence with VIP, 183, 336–337
  distribution, 183
  ion channel model, 559–560
  muscarinic and nicotinic synaptic actions, 472, 510–511
  regulation of neuromuscular junction ion channels, 259–260
  SSt actions, 291–292, 355–356
  VIP actions, 357
  visual cortex actions, 357–361
AChE
  bipolar cell binding, 391
  composition, 579–580
  localization, 579–580
ACh receptors
  AChE localization, 579–580
  adult muscle fiber distribution, 573
  amino acid sequences, 557–558
  binding sites, 558–560
  biosynthesis and turnover, 578–579
  embryonic muscle fiber distribution, 573
  extrinsic modifications, 575–578

intrinsic modifications, 573–575
  ion channel interactions, 559–560
  long-term changes, 572–580
  neuromuscular half-life, 581
  postsynaptic densities, 577–578
  reconstitution into lipid vesicles, 575–576
  subunits, 557–558
ACTH, distribution, 273
Actin
  dendritic spines, 668
  fodrin binding, 529
Action potentials
  AB neurons, 309–310
  all-or-none events, 641
  Aldrovanda, 169
  axonal sodium and dendritic calcium, 642
  conduction failure, 646–647
  conduction velocity and fiber diameter, 645
  effect of calcium/phosphatidylserine-dependent protein kinases, 217, 219
  hippocampal afferent fibers, 406–414
  information coding, 643–644
  initiation and propagation, 641–647
  PY neurons, 307–308
  S-channel effect, 491
  sodium and potassium currents, 672
  spike
    frequency, 643–644
    threshold, 641–642
Active zone, 8–10
Adaptive filter model, cerebellum, 442
Adenylate cyclase
  activation and inhibition by dopamine receptors, 224
  allosteric properties, 508
  Aplysia classical conditioning, 508
  calmodulin inhibition, 505–508
  cerebellum, 230
  complex, amplification of neurotransmitter response, 500–509
  5-HT activation, 500–508
Adrenocorticotropic hormone. *See* ACTH
Adult muscle fiber, ACh receptor distribution, 573